£32.50
12/97

D1145537

WITHDRAWN
FROM STOCK
QMUL LIBRARY

WITHDRAWN
FROM STOCK
DCU LIBRARY

Hematology

A Combined Theoretical and Technical Approach

Second Edition

Arthur Simmons, F.I.B.M.S.

Associate Vice President, Laboratory Corporation of America,
Burlington, North Carolina

With a Foreword by

Bernard E. Statland, M.D., Ph.D.

Clinical Professor, Department of Pathology,
Vanderbilt University School of Medicine, Nashville, Tennessee

Butterworth–Heinemann

Boston • Oxford • Johannesburg • Melbourne • New Delhi • Singapore

Copyright © 1997 by Butterworth–Heinemann

 A member of the Reed Elsevier group

All rights reserved.

No part of this publication may be reproduced, stored in a retrieval system, or transmitted in any form or by any means, electronic, mechanical, photocopying, recording, or otherwise, without the prior written permission of the publisher.

Every effort has been made to ensure that the drug dosage schedules within this text are accurate and conform to standards accepted at time of publication. However, as treatment recommendations vary in the light of continuing research and clinical experience, the reader is advised to verify drug dosage schedules herein with information found on product information sheets. This is especially true in cases of new or infrequently used drugs.

The opinions represented in this text are solely those of the author and do not necessarily represent those of the Laboratory Corporation of America Holdings.

∞ Recognizing the importance of preserving what has been written, Butterworth–Heinemann prints its books on acid-free paper whenever possible.

Library of Congress Cataloging-in-Publication Data

Simmons, Arthur.
Hematology : a combined theoretical and practical approach /
Arthur Simmons; foreword by Bernard E. Statland. -- 2nd ed.
p. cm.
Includes bibliographical references and index.
ISBN 0-7506-9848-9
1. Hematology. 2. Blood--Diseases--Diagnosis. I. Title.
[DNLM: 1. Hematologic Diseases. 2. Hematologic Tests--laboratory
manuals. WH 100 S592h 1996]
RB145.S525 1996
616.1'5--dc21
DNLM/DLC   96-47476
for Library of Congress   CIP

British Library Cataloguing-in-Publication Data

A catalogue record for this book is available from the British Library.

The publisher offers special discounts on bulk orders of this book.
For information, please contact:
Manager of Special Sales
Butterworth–Heinemann
313 Washington Street
Newton, MA 02158-1626
Tel: 617-928-2500
Fax: 617-928-2620

For information on all Butterworth–Heinemann medical publications available, contact our
World Wide Web home page at: http://www.bh.com/med

10 9 8 7 6 5 4 3 2 1

Printed in the United States of America

SBRLSMD		
CLASS MARK	WH100 SIM	
CIRC TYPE		
SUPPLIER	WESTONS £24.00	3/98 ✓
BINDING		

Contents

Foreword

Observers of medicine often make a distinction between the content of the discipline and the context in which it is practiced. The content over the years has generally been consistent and unchanging (i.e., the same diseases that plagued humans in the past continue to cause anguish, morbidity, and death today). However, the context continues to undergo dramatic change and upheaval. I am referring here to changes in the manner that medicine is practiced, evaluated, and reimbursed. The buzz words for this generation of practitioners are *cost/benefit analysis, decentralization of diagnosis and treatment, merging of services,* and *outcomes management.* Moreover, we have witnessed a new group of emerging diseases: iatrogenic diseases, virus-induced diseases, and diseases associated with patients surviving into their 80s and 90s.

The practice of hematology and, in particular, laboratory hematology should be viewed increasingly in terms of its changing context. The laboratory hematologist may be a clinician, a pathologist, or a medical technologist; he or she may be a technician in a physician's office laboratory or a physician's assistant. There is a great need to gain the necessary knowledge base in hematology, the skills appropriate to practice high-quality work, and the appreciation for maximizing efficiency and effectiveness in this world of changing demands. This text will serve you well in meeting those requirements.

Art Simmons is an experienced academician in hematology, as well as a hands-on supervisor and director, who has practiced hematology in various clinical settings, including large university hospital laboratories and various commercial laboratories. I can attest to his ability to combine the theoretical aspects of hematology with the practical aspects of quality assurance and cost containment.

A quick perusal of the table of contents of this book highlights the spectrum of issues covered in the text. It begins with the theoretical bases of the discipline of hematology, continues with the choice of tests that have diagnostic utility, and concludes with practical concerns in the choice of instrumentation.

Some laboratory medicine books are meant to be placed on the shelf for future reference. Others are meant to be kept near the phone when clinicians call or on the bench when doing an assay. This text is unique in that it can serve both needs. I trust that you will use this book as a guide as you practice laboratory hematology over the coming years. It will assist you in quickly giving the information you need to serve the ultimate customer—the patient—and his or her physician.

Bernard E. Statland

Preface

The second edition of this text is, in effect, the fifth edition of the original work entitled *Technical Hematology*. Over 25 years have passed since the original publication, and much has changed both in laboratory medicine and in health care in general.

Changes in laboratory medicine are reflected in the shift from hospital-based operations and reference laboratories to "point-of-care" testing, physician office laboratories, and hospital consortiums. Managed care systems and health maintenance organizations are becoming commonplace in an attempt to control overall health costs; one can only speculate as to the future of the clinical laboratory as we know it today. Along with these dramatic changes have arisen changes in technologist training and licensing by individual states, the consolidation and renaming of medical technologist professional societies, and the slow erosion of the numbers of well-trained technologists and schools of medical technology.

This text is intended for the student, graduate medical technologist, medical technician, and nursing staff, as well as other ancillary individuals who may have occasion to become involved in laboratory hematology both in the conventional manner and in physician offices and point-of-care practices.

This edition has been totally revised, with the emphasis on updating chapters on anemias, neoplasms, and blood coagulation. Of note is the rewriting and expansion of the thalassemia and hemoglobinopathy chapters, as well as the updating of hematologic neoplasms and cell surface markers. Blood coagulation discussions have also been revised to include recent advances in the area of hypercoagulation and the influences of protein C, protein S, and lupus anticoagulants.

Testing procedures have been expanded to cover these changes. Specifically, methods for the assay of protein C and protein S, venous occlusion tests, and additional methods for the detection of lupus anticoagulants and E rosettes have been added. The chapter on automated equipment has been curtailed due to the plethora of available equipment. The ever-changing availability of various cell counters, coagulometers, and aggregometers make discussions obsolete before the publication of the text; no useful purpose is served in describing equipment when the manufacturers' manuals are readily available. The sole exception, however, is the description of a universal principle, such as the common volume displacement technique used by Coulter and other manufacturers.

This edition presents an affordable, more complete text attuned to recent advances in the field of laboratory hematology and an accessible reference for students, technicians, technologists, nurses, paramedics, medical students, and physicians' office staff. The text will allow the reader to quickly reference a problem associated with laboratory hematology without delving into the many excellent tomes on the subject.

My thanks are extended to the staff of Butterworth–Heinemann, particularly to Susan Pioli, Director of Medical Publishing, and to Jana Friedman, Assistant Editor, for much support, encouragement, and help in the preparation of the manuscript. In addition, the diligence and patience of Jenn Nagaj, Production Editor at Silverchair Science + Communications, is much appreciated. My thanks are also extended to the staff of Laboratory Corporation of America who provided the inspiration and encouragement to undertake this revision.

A.S.

Hematology

A Combined Theoretical and Technical Approach

Chapter 1

Hematopoiesis

Embryonic Hematopoiesis

Blood is a complex liquid tissue composed of three main cellular elements: red cells (erythrocytes), white cells (leukocytes), and platelets (thrombocytes). These cells are suspended in an aqueous fluid, the plasma, that contains a wide variety of minerals and proteins.

In the embryo, blood production, or *hematopoiesis* (Figure 1.1), begins in the yolk sac, which probably is derived from embryonic connective tissue mesenchymal cells, which are morphologically identical to adult connective tissue cells. Cells capable of replicating under appropriate conditions are found here as well as in the fetal liver. This suggests the presence in these organs of both cells that can give rise to cells of all orders (totipotential) and, possibly, cells that possess the ability to develop or act in several ways (pluripotential).

During the third week of embryonic life, mesenchymal cells produce blood islands composed of cell clusters, the outer layers of which ultimately grow to form a continuous tubular pathway. This is the primitive vascular system. The remainder of the blood island cells begin to produce primitive erythroidlike cells, termed *hematocytoblasts,* which are characterized by a large nucleus containing spongy chromatin, several nucleolar condensations, and a deeply basophilic cytoplasm. This primitive mesoblastic erythropoietic activity is recognizable as early as the fourteenth day of development and lasts for approximately 10 weeks.

By the third month of embryonic development, this mesoblastic stage fades, and the liver becomes the main focus of blood production. This liver activity (hepatic phase) begins between the sixth and ninth weeks of embryonic life and represents the chief site of red-cell and granulocyte production. It is aided secondarily by the spleen, thymus, and lymph nodes. The spleen is first active in red-cell production (erythropoiesis), granulocyte production (myelopoiesis), and lymphocyte production (lymphopoiesis) but, by the fifth month, granulocyte production disappears. Splenic activity continues until the end of gestation, whereas lymphopoiesis continues throughout life.

The liver remains active until just after birth but, by the fourth month of embryonic life, the bone marrow starts to play an increased role in the production of both granulocytes and erythroid cells. At birth, this organ is the principal source of both these cells as well as of thrombocytes. Such bone marrow–derived, or medullary, hematopoiesis occurs in most bones, particularly in the flat bones of the sternum, ribs, skull, vertebrae, and pelvis. As the marrow cavities enlarge, the long bone shafts filled with active tissue gradually are replaced with fatty marrow, leaving the principal source of blood-cell production to the sternum and other flat bones.

Regulation of Hematopoiesis

The structure of the hematopoietic stem-cell compartment has been discerned from in vitro assays

1

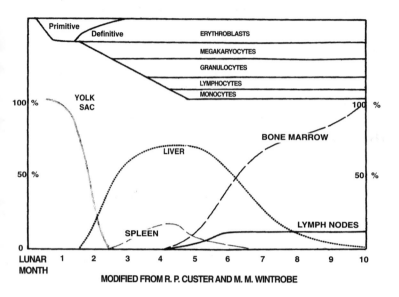

Figure 1.1. Hematopoiesis during antenatal life. Hematopoiesis takes place principally in the liver until the fifth to sixth month of gestation. Thereafter, the bone marrow becomes the principal site of hematopoietic activity. (Reprinted from BH Hyun, JK Ashton, K Dolan. Practical Hematology. Philadelphia: Saunders, 1975.)

and functional studies in the mouse. Originally, a totipotential stem cell was postulated. This is supported by splenic, bone marrow, and diffusion chamber cultures as well as by changes seen during disease. Present-day theories postulate a multicell compartment, as shown in Figure 1.2. In such a scheme, primitive mesenchymal cells of the embryo differentiate to produce hemocytoblasts. Such cells are believed to be precursors of all blood cells and are thought to be the totipotential hematopoietic stem cell (THSC). The slightly more mature, but still primitive, pluripotential (myeloid) stem cell (PMSC or colony-forming unit–spleen [CFU_S]) is postulated to give rise to at least four cell variations: CFU_D (myeloid-monocytic), CFU_{EOS} (eosinophil), burst-forming unit–erythroid (BFU_E), and the megakaryocyte (CFU_{MEG}). In addition, two other CFUs producing basophils and mast cells have been reported (Denburg and Temesuari, 1983).

Granulopoiesis

Most specific CFUs give rise to progenitor cells capable of replication, enabling them to produce mature elements within each cell lineage. The one known exception is in the neutrophil-monocyte cell line. Here, three distinct cells are interposed between the pluripotential cell and the first recogniz-

able granulocyte and monocyte. These three types of cells (CFU_D cells [growing in diffusion chambers], CFU_{NM} [primitive neutrophil-monocytic] cells producing colonies in semisolid media, and cluster-forming cells in semisolid media) are believed to play an important role in DNA synthesis. This is in contrast to the restricted synthesis provided by the CFU_S cell. Consequently, the CFU_D and some CFU_{NM} elements possess the ability to synthesize DNA in greater amounts than their own precursor cell (CFU_S) and thus are able to provide an emergency reserve of DNA for cell synthesis when required.

The theory that the THSC produces the PMSC and other elements, including lymphocytes, has resulted from mouse studies and from data obtained from patients with pluripotential stem-cell disorders, such as aplastic anemia, paroxysmal hemoglobinuria, and cyclic hematopoiesis (Abrahamson et al., 1977). CFU_D are composed mainly of neutrophils and monocytes (CFU_{NM}). The CFU_D cell differs from its progeny mainly in that DNA synthesis is not as abundant. At this time, it is unknown whether the pluripotential cell differs at all or in some minor way from the CFU_D cell. Eosinophils derived from CFU_{EOS} and platelets derived from CFU_{MEG} also are believed to be produced directly from the PMSC as the result of the action of a specific poietin, such as thrombopoietin.

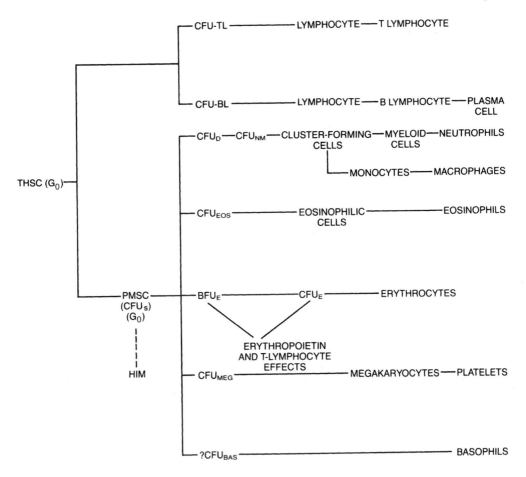

Figure 1.2. Stem-cell compartments (theorized). (THSC = totipotential hematopoietic stem cell; G_0 = resting stage, no growth; PMSC = pluripotential myeloid stem cell; CFU_S = colony-forming unit–spleen; HIM = hematopoietic inductive microenvironment; CFU-TL = colony-forming unit–T lymphocyte; CFU-BL = colony-forming unit–B lymphocyte; CFU_D = colony-forming unit–diffusion [chamber]; CFU_{NM} = colony-forming unit–neutrophil-monocyte; CFU_{EOS} = colony-forming unit–eosinophil; BFU_E = burst-forming unit–erythroid; CFU_E = colony-forming unit–erythroid; CFU_{MEG} = colony-forming unit–megakaryocyte; CFU_{BAS} = colony-forming unit–basophil.)

Erythropoiesis

Colonies of erythroid cells can be produced in vitro if erythropoietin is added to CFU_E cell cultures. If a sufficiently large amount of erythropoietin is added to these cells, large clusters are produced, resulting in a BFU_E. This, in turn, requires erythropoietin to produce hemoglobin-forming red cells. Significantly, the ability of BFU_E to proliferate and differentiate in culture depends also on a helper effect of added T lymphocytes, which may promote hematopoiesis by increasing the PMSC proliferation rate (Beck,

1982a). Lymphoid cells are believed to arise from separate CFUs (T lymphocyte [CFU_{TL}] and B lymphocyte [CFU_{BL}]), which are themselves the result of the THSC activity. These CFU_{TL} and CFU_{BL} cells, under the stimulus of a specific poietin, give rise to T and B lymphocytes, the B cell being the precursor of the plasma cell.

Megakaryocytopoiesis

Megakaryocytes are derived from the PMSC by an unknown stimulus that produces committed

Table 1.1. Life Cycle of Hematopoietic Cells

Phase	Time	Principal Activity
Postmitotic (G_1)	~10 hrs	RNA and protein synthesis
DNA synthesis (S)	~9 hrs	DNA synthesis
Premitotic (G_2)	~4 hrs	Accelerated metabolic activity
Mitotic (M)	~0.5–1.0 hr	Cell division

progenitor cells. However, two classes of human marrow megakaryocyte progenitor cells have been described: CFU_{MEG}-derived colonies and BFU_{MEG}-derived colonies (Briddell et al., 1989). The earliest detectable progeny of PMSC is CFU_{MEG}. This cell is thought to be heterogeneous in several respects. First, one type consists of colonies composed exclusively of small lymphoid-appearing cells that carry platelet glycoproteins. These cells are believed to be immature mega-karyocytes (Gerwitz, 1986). Another type of colony is composed of both large, recognizable megakaryocytes and small cells. A third type is made up of cells of mixed lineages (Gerwitz and Hoffman, 1984).

The small, transitional megakaryocytes pass through four stages of maturation, which are distinguishable by differences in the nuclear-to-cytoplasmic ratio, the nuclear configuration, and size. Stage 1 megakaryocytes (megakaryoblasts) have lobulated nuclei and basophilic cytoplasm containing granules and dense bodies. Stage 2 megakaryocytes possess an indented, horseshoe-shaped nucleus and more abundant and less basophilic cytoplasm. There are also increased platelet organelles. Stage 3 megakaryocytes are large cells with abundant granular eosinophilic cytoplasm. Stage 4 cells show a more compact and denser nucleus with a more intensely and evenly stained eosinophilic cytoplasm. The number of platelets produced by a given megakaryocyte is related more to its ploidy level and the state of cytoplasmic maturation than to its stage of development. The process of platelet release is uncertain, but three mechanisms have been suggested. First, megakaryocytes extend pseudopodia through the walls of the marrow sinusoids, which fracture releasing platelets (Penington, 1981). Second, megakaryocytes pass through the marrow sinusoids intact; they then travel to the lung, fracture in the capillary beds, and release

platelets (Kaufman et al., 1965). Last, it has been proposed that megakaryocytes fracture in the bone marrow environment itself and release platelets (Zucker-Franklin and Peturrson, 1984).

Cell Formation and Division

Hematopoiesis in health is maintained in a steady state that is the result of equal production and destruction of cells. When physiologic alterations in health are produced, increased cell production often is required. Such control of cellular replication is poorly understood, although it is believed that a feedback mechanism is involved. If the entire CFU compartment is reduced chemically or by radiation, the PMSCs (CFU_S) or THSCs normally in a resting stage (G_0) will become activated and enter a growth phase (G) to produce CFU cells of the specific and required lineage.

Cell culture techniques have shown that the life cycle of a cell has four phases (Ellis, 1961): the G_1 phase, which is the postmitotic phase, lasting approximately 10 hours; the S phase of DNA synthesis and chromosomal replication, which lasts approximately 9 hours; the G_2, or premitotic, phase, lasting approximately 4 hours; and the mitotic phase (M), lasting approximately 0.5–1.0 hour (Table 1.1).

In the generative cell cycle, the first, or G_1, phase is involved with both RNA and protein synthesis. During this activity, the S phase becomes triggered by an unknown mechanism to cause the cell to synthesize DNA. The shorter G_2 phase is characterized by decreased protein synthesis and apparent cellular preparation to enter mitotic division. Characteristics of this phase are accelerated metabolic reactions, including synthesis of cytoplasmic lipids, membrane phospholipids, proteins, and RNA. The G_2 phase is followed by the mitotic phase, normally resulting in the formation of two daughter cells possessing normal chromosomal components (Figure 1.3).

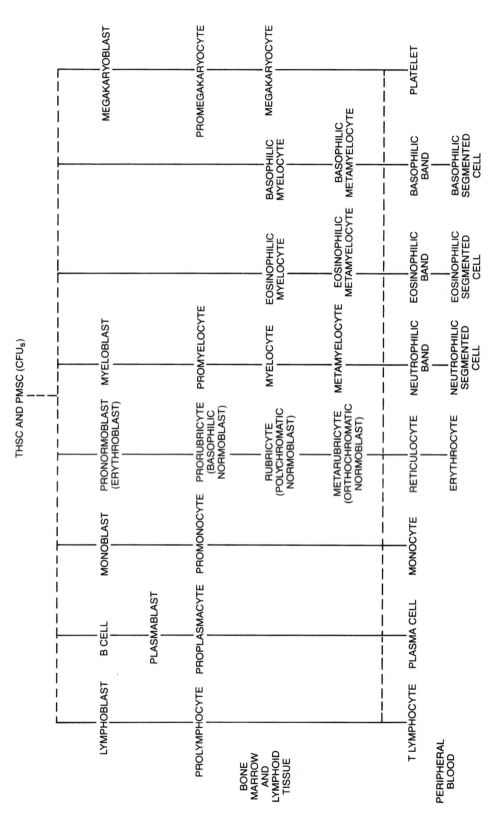

Figure 1.3. Expanded cell compartment. (THSC = totipotential hematopoietic stem cell; PMSC = pluripotential myeloid stem cell; CFU$_S$ = colony-forming unit–spleen.)

Chapter 2

Erythropoiesis

Erythropoietin

Under physiologic conditions, the red-cell mass is maintained in equilibrium by appropriate adjustments of red-cell production. This erythropoiesis results from the action of erythropoietin on colony-forming unit–erythroid (CFU_E) cell cultures. Erythropoietin is a heat-stable glycoprotein that is present in small amounts in the serum and in higher concentration in the urine. The protein is produced by the action of renal erythropoietic factor (REF), which is derived from the kidneys under the secondary influence of hypoxic conditions. REF acts on a plasma substrate produced in the liver to form erythropoietin. Consequently, tissue hypoxia resulting from anemia leads to an increase in REF, which, in turn, controls the increase of erythropoietin production. In situations in which oxygen affinity is reduced, such as in hypertransfused individuals, erythropoietin activity is decreased proportionally. Decreases in erythropoietin can be found in renal disease, chronic disease, and polycythemia. In renal disease, the degree of erythropoietin production impairment is roughly proportional to the degree of renal excretory loss. In chronic diseases such as chronic infections, inflammation, and neoplastic states, decreased production of erythropoietin also is noted. In polycythemia, erythrocytic production occurs independent of erythropoiesis stimulation; erythropoietin production is suppressed by a negative feedback mechanism.

Increases in erythropoietin are found in neoplasms that may produce the hormone (renal cell or hepatocellular carcinomas) and in secondary polycythemia.

Besides being the major stimulus in differentiating primitive erythropoietin-sensitive cells to produce immature erythroid elements, erythropoietin aids in the acceleration of primitive red cells to produce more mature forms and promotes reticulocyte release from the bone marrow. Erythropoietin also influences DNA and RNA synthesis, the rate of hemosynthesis, the glycolysis rate of the pentose-phosphate shunt, and the transfer of iron from transferrin to the early red cells (Graber and Krantz, 1978; Beck, 1982b).

The average life of a red cell approximates 120 days, and fewer than 2% of the circulating cells are newly produced and released from the bone marrow as reticulocytes. When fixed and stained, the mature cells are approximately 7.2–7.6 μ in diameter but, if measured in wet preparation, they have an average diameter of 8.3–8.5 μ.

Red-Cell Shape

In vivo, the mature erythrocyte is a biconcave disc with a surface-to-volume ratio that enables optimal gaseous interchange. The cell also is deformed easily and, consequently, can pass through small vessels and capillaries without rupturing. Cell shape is believed to be maintained by a variety of conditions, including elastic forces within the membrane surface, osmotic pressure, steric interference, and the presence of polymeric

Table 2.1. Factors Affecting Red-Cell Shape

Mechanism	Cause
Echinocyte transformation (crenated)	Intracellular adenosine triphosphate decrease and calcium increase
	Exposure to stored plasma and to increased environmental pH
Stomatocyte transformation (cup-shaped)	Exposure to reduction in environmental pH and to cationic detergents
Osmotic swelling	Exposure to hypotonic solutions

proteins. The maintenance of cell shape depends as well on external forces, such as the osmotic and pH environment. Factors affecting red-cell shape are described in Table 2.1.

Alterations in normal red-cell shape to produce spiculated cells (echinocytes) take place in several stages. First, the cell becomes irregularly outlined (*echinocyte I*) and proceeds to form a crenated red cell, termed an *echinocyte II*. The next stage is the formation of an ovoid or spheric cell with approximately 30 evenly spaced spicules. This cell, termed an *echinocyte III,* slowly becomes more spheric, and smaller spicules are formed to produce a *spheroechinocyte I*. At this point the cell is irreversible. It is in its final prelytic stage and is termed a *spheroechinocyte II*.

Stomatocytic, or cup-shaped cellular, transformation can be seen in vitro as well as in certain hereditary and acquired hemolytic diseases. If the pH is decreased, the red cell assumes a profound cup shape that, when viewed on a slide by light microscopy, appears to possess a large central elongated region of pallor.

Characteristics of the Red-Cell Membrane

The red-cell membrane is composed of a matrix formed from a double layer of phospholipids. Phosphoric acid moieties are found on the outer and inner surfaces, and hydrophobic fatty-acid chains are anchored by the outer layers of the membrane directing inward. Embedded in this lipid matrix are globular proteins, some of which penetrate the membrane completely, whereas others are exposed only at one surface. However, all these sialoglycoproteins are exposed on the outer membrane surface and carry red-cell antigens, predominantly ABH antigens (blood group A, B, and O antigens) and Lewis antigen. Membrane proteins

that lack carbohydrates are confined to the cytoplasmic membrane surface. They include enzymes (glyceraldehyde-3-phosphate dehydrogenase) and structural proteins (spectrin, actin, hemoglobin). The transmembrane proteins, glycophorins, may function as transportation systems for cations, whereas the cytoplasmic proteins, spectrin and actin, may constitute a type of cellular exoskeleton accounting for the ability of the membrane to maintain a cellular shape. The fluid mosaic model of the structure of cell membranes is shown in Figure 2.1.

The lipids of the cell membrane are composed of nonesterified cholesterol, phospholipids, and glycolipids. The cholesterol is in equilibrium with plasma cholesterol, but most of the membrane is composed of phospholipids (phosphatidylcholine, sphingomyelin, phosphatidylserine), which, when liberated into the circulation following brisk hemolysis, often can produce a severe coagulopathy or disseminated intravascular coagulopathy.

Maintenance of the normal shape of the red cell depends on the spectrin skeleton, on the lipid bilayer makeup, and on control of the ionic composition of the cell. The cellular anions, such as hemoglobin and glutathione, are not permeable and, consequently, do not cross the red-cell membrane. However, water and sodium ions do cross the membrane but, under normal conditions, this is regulated by active cation transport pumps. This system controlling the transportation of sodium and potassium ions is operated on energy derived from adenosine triphosphate (ATP), obtained from glycolysis.

Membrane Function

The main physiologic functions of the red-cell membrane are to maintain cell-shape deformability for osmotic balance between plasma and cell

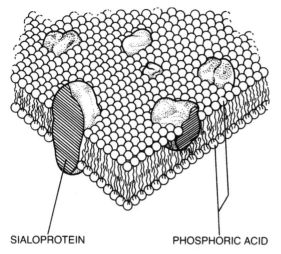

SIALOPROTEIN   PHOSPHORIC ACID

Figure 2.1. The structure of cell membranes. (Reprinted from SJ Singer, GL Nicolson. The fluid mosaic model of the structure of cell membranes. Science 175:720, 1972. Copyright 1972 by the AAAS.)

cytoplasm, to help in the transportation of essential cellular ions and gases, and to act as a supporting skeletal system for surface antigens. Red-cell stability in large part requires ATP as an energy source. Depletion of ATP ultimately leads to spectrin aggregation and loss of membrane material. The role of the membrane in the movement of gases and essential cellular substances is biphasic. Passive transportation occurs by simple diffusion through cell pores, but active movement of substance occurs against an electrochemical gradient. This requires energy obtained by ATP resulting from cellular glycolysis. An example of passive transfer is the transportation of gases and glucose, and an example of active transport is the passage of sodium and potassium ions.

The membrane acts as a partial barrier to the penetration of all solutes. Nonpolar substances diffuse through the membrane at a rate proportional to their solubility in organic solvents. Polar solutes cross the membrane at specialized sites. Glucose and other monosaccharides easily cross the membrane barrier, whereas the more lipid-soluble disaccharides do not, the speed of such a process depending on the molecular structure. Of the more common isomers, the D forms are transported to the exclusion of the L forms. Of the common D isomers, glucose, galactose, xylose, and arabinase are transported in that order. Glucose enters the red cell by diffusion that is mediated by a transmembrane protein known as a *glucose transporter*. This material constitutes approximately 5% of the red-cell membrane protein. Of the polar materials, water, chlorides, and bicarbonates diffuse most freely. In contrast, the red-cell membrane is only slightly permeable to the major monovalent cations, sodium and potassium. Within the red cell, potassium is the predominant and sodium the minor cation.

Cell Maturation

Maturation entails changes in the nucleus and the cytoplasm of cells. In all the very early stages of development, the nucleus of the cell is round. While maturing, it normally remains round and is not segmented in the red-cell series nor in lymphocytes or plasma cells. Only in the monocytes is the nucleus often indented or irregular in outline, even in the monoblast stage. It seldom is segmented in the mature stage. The nuclei of basophils, eosinophils, and neutrophils undergo not only indentation but also segmentation while maturing, the segments being linked by thin, short bridges of chromatin. Most nuclei in mature eosinophils have two typical segments, whereas the majority of nuclei of neutrophils have three segments. No such regularity is present in basophils, and the large nuclei of megakaryocytes often exhibit bizarre shapes.

As maturation progresses, the nuclei gradually become smaller, and their structure becomes denser and more coarse. The most immature of cells show the presence of nucleoli, the number and appearance of which can vary according to the cell species. Most lymphocytes have only one nucleolus, whereas all other cell species generally have two or more. Nucleoli are most clearly discernible and are largest and most numerous in the blasts. During maturation, they become smaller and less numerous. In the granulocytic and red-cell series, the nucleoli disappear and the basophilic cytoplasm becomes more mature and less blue. In the monocytic and lymphoid cells, the nucleoli fade less quickly and occasionally may be seen in more mature cells.

The maturation of erythrocytes follows the common pathway of all hematologic cells. In general, cell aging is reflected in the following summary:

1. Cell size is reduced.
2. Cytoplasmic RNA production decreases, producing less basophilia. (In the erythrocyte, hemoglobinization starts at the polychromatic normoblast stage and increases until the cell reaches maturity.)
3. Cytoplasmic granules in the granulocytic cells are developed and gradually become finer in texture.
4. The cytoplasm-to-nucleus ratio becomes greater (nucleus becomes smaller).
5. Nuclear chromatin becomes more aggregated.
6. Nucleoli disappear.

In identifying hematopoietic cells, it is important to decide whether the cell is a leukocyte, erythrocyte, or thrombocyte, or not of hematopoietic origin. An easy and convenient method of arriving at the correct morphologic answer is to carry out the following exercise:

1. Describe the cell size in relation to a normal red cell. Is the cell twice the size, one and one-half the size, or three times the size of a red cell? The advantage of using such a format is that a mature erythrocyte is nearly always present in the same microscopic field and can be used for comparison.
2. Describe the cell shape. Is it round, oval, or irregular? Does it appear to possess pseudopodia?
3. Describe the cytoplasm: First, determine its nucleus-to-cytoplasm ratio; then detail the staining qualities using a standard Romanowsky stain such as Wright's or Giemsa. Is the cytoplasm stained hyaline blue, is it basophilic, or does it possess a foamy or cloudy consistency? Are there cytoplasmic granules present? If so, describe their size, quantity, color, and position within the cell. Are there cytoplasmic vacuoles? If present, describe their approximate number, size, and position within the cell. Is there a perinuclear halo? If so, where is it positioned? Detail its size.
4. Describe the nucleus: Where is it positioned? Is it eccentrically or centrally placed, or is it partially extruded from the cell? Is the nuclear shape round, oval, lobulated, indented, or cleaved? How does the nuclear chromatin stain? Does it appear densely staining without visible chromatin present, or is it immature with an open reticular pattern showing free chromatin? Are there nucleoli? If so, approximate the number seen.

Normal Red-Cell Maturation

Pronormoblast (Rubriblast)

Cell size	Approximately twice that of a mature red cell (10–16 μ)
Cell shape	Irregular or round
Cytoplasm	Nucleus-to-cytoplasm ratio: 5:1
	Staining: basophilic
	Granules: none seen
	Vacuoles: none seen
	Perinuclear halo: possible pale halo
Nucleus	Position: centrally placed but can occasionally be positioned eccentrically
	Shape: oval or round
	Structure: stains irregularly showing fine, dense, and uniformly close-meshed, reddish purple chromatin network
	Nucleoli: normally 2–5 present; occasionally fading and difficult to identify; may be larger than those found in myeloblast and may stain with a blue hue
Main points of recognition	General size and shape of cell similar to other immature cells, but cell differs in its nuclear characteristics; nucleus smaller and staining properties more pronounced; cell usually easy to identify as it frequently is found amid mature normoblasts

Basophilic Normoblast (Prorubricyte)

Cell size	Slightly smaller than its precursor, the pronormoblast (8–18 μ)
Cell shape	Irregular or round; cytoplasmic protrusions common
Cytoplasm	Nucleus-to-cytoplasm ratio: 3:2
	Staining: less basophilic than that of the pronormoblast; still lacking reddish color

	Granules: none seen
	Vacuoles: none seen
	Perinuclear halo: none seen
Nucleus	Position: centrally placed
	Shape: oval or round
	Structure: coarse, trabecular, lumpy radial structure, often in a cartwheel arrangement; possible sharp contrast between chromatin and parachromatin
	Nucleoli: no longer visible
Main points of recognition	Coarse chromatin arrangement of the nucleus with abundant basophilic cytoplasm typical of this cell

Polychromatic Normoblast (Rubricyte)

Cell size	Up to twice the size of a mature red cell (8–12 μ)
Cell shape	Irregular
Cytoplasm	Nucleus-to-cytoplasm ratio: 3:2–1:1
	Staining: polychromatic; occasional hemoglobin-tinged cytoplasm, turning to a muddy gray-brown color
	Granules: none seen
	Vacuoles: none seen
	Perinuclear halo: none seen
Nucleus	Position: centrally placed
	Shape: round
	Structure: prominent; presence of deeply staining, condensed chromatin masses; chromatin clumped and coarse
	Nucleoli: none seen
Main points of recognition	Blue-gray to pink polychromatic cytoplasm and coarse, deeply staining nuclear chromatin, which differentiate this cell from the basophilic normoblast

Orthochromatic Normoblast (Metarubricyte)

Cell size	Slightly larger than the mature red cell (8–10 μ)
Cell shape	Round
Cytoplasm	Nucleus-to-cytoplasm ratio: 1:1–1:4
	Staining: more hemoglobinized than in the polychromatic normoblast;

	appearance of full hemoglobinization in some cells
	Granules: none seen
	Vacuoles: none seen
	Perinuclear halo: none seen
Nucleus	Position: centrally or eccentrically placed or, on occasion, partially extruded from the cell
	Shape: round
	Structure: pyknotic nucleus, appearing homogeneous without chromatin structure; may assume various bizarre forms, such as buds, rosettes, or clover leaves
	Nucleoli: none seen
Main points of recognition	Small cell possessing well-hemoglobinized cytoplasm and small, densely staining pyknotic nucleus, which may be eccentrically positioned

Reticulocyte

Cell size	Slightly larger than that of a mature red cell (7–9 μ)
Cell shape	Round
Cytoplasm	Fully hemoglobinized; nucleus extruded from cell, leaving a slightly polychromatic red cell when stained by Romanowsky dyes; differentiation possible only by staining the cytoplasmic organelles that are left (ribosomes, mitochondria, Golgi apparatus) with vital dyes such as new methylene blue or brilliant cresyl blue (see page 273)

Mature Erythrocyte

Cell size	6.7–7.7 μ
Cell shape	Round
Cytoplasm	Staining: pink, with slightly more intense color at the periphery and lighter color in the center
	Granules: none seen
	Vacuoles: none seen
Nucleus	Not present

Abnormal Red-Cell Maturation

Promegaloblast

Cell size	Up to four times that of an abnormal mature red cell (18–25 μ)
Cell shape	Irregular
Cytoplasm	Nucleus-to-cytoplasm ratio: 5:1–4:1
	Staining: deeply basophilic, varying to purple-blue
	Granules: none seen
	Vacuoles: none seen
	Perinuclear halo: possible pale halo
Nucleus	Position: centrally placed
	Shape: round or irregular
	Structure: fine, very close-meshed chromatin network with a pronounced radial disposition
	Nucleoli: possible presence of multiple nucleoli, often as many as eight
Main points of recognition	Cell size, typical close-meshed nunuclear chromatin, and multiple nucleoli

Basophilic Megaloblast

Cell size	Up to three times that of a normal mature red cell (16–20 μ)
Cell shape	Round
Cytoplasm	Nucleus-to-cytoplasm ratio: 4:1–3:1
	Staining: less basophilic than the promegaloblast, with unevenly stained areas of basophilia; may show very early hemoglobinization
	Granules: none seen
	Vacuoles: none seen
	Perinuclear halo: possible faint halo
Nucleus	Position: centrally or eccentrically placed
	Shape: round
	Structure: chromatin appears coarser than in the preceding stage, but still a persistent fine stippled appearance
	Nucleoli: none seen
Main points of recognition	Coarser nuclear chromatin and paler, more hemoglobinized cytoplasm, which primarily distinguish this cell from the basophilic normoblast

Polychromatic Megaloblast

Cell size	Approximately twice that of a mature normal red cell (12–16 μ)
Cell shape	Round or irregular
Cytoplasm	Nucleus-to-cytoplasm ratio: 3:1–2:1
	Staining: hemoglobinized, with only faint blue tinges; occasional uneven areas of light basophilia
	Granules: none seen
	Vacuoles: none seen
	Perinuclear halo: frequently found
Nucleus	Position: centrally placed
	Shape: round
	Structure: coarse chromatin network, radially laid out; persistent fine, stippled appearance
	Nucleoli: none seen
Main points of recognition	Coarse, open nuclear chromatin, which differentiates this cell from the polychromatic normoblast; hemoglobinization more advanced than in normal red-cell maturation

Orthochromatic Megaloblast

Cell size	Up to twice that of a mature normal red cell (10–15 μ)
Cell shape	Round or irregular
Cytoplasm	Nucleus-to-cytoplasm ratio: 1:1–1:2
	Staining: pink, fully hemoglobinized
	Granules: none seen; occasional Howell-Jolly bodies (DNA nuclear remnants) present
	Vacuoles: none seen
	Perinuclear halo: none seen
Nucleus	Position: centrally or eccentrically placed
	Shape: round but can be slightly irregular
	Structure: densely stained, often homogeneous in appearance; chromatin structures sometimes seen
	Nucleoli: none seen
Main points of recognition	Cell size and presence of occasional chromatin structures

Proliferation of Erythroid Cells

Within the red-cell compartment (i.e., circulating mature cells and their precursors, the erythron), proliferation and maturation take place simultaneously. All recognizable erythroid cells are incapable of undergoing mitotic division and replication after the polychromatic normoblastic stage, and consequently they all become mature erythrocytes. From this point, maintenance of the erythron depends principally on the ability of its stem-cell compartment to meet physiologic demands, because production must equal destruction. The time interval required by selective cells for development is uncertain. The pronormoblast stage lasts approximately 30 hours; the basophilic normoblast stage may last between 12.4 and 95 hours; the polychromatic normoblast stage may last between 8.8 and 37.5 hours; and the orthochromatic normoblast stage may last 19 hours. Thus, an immature red cell takes 70–180 hours to pass from the pronormoblast stage to the reticulocyte stage, and it takes an additional 2–3 days for the cell to be released from the bone marrow into the peripheral circulation. Three to five separate cell divisions take place after erythropoietin stimulation of the blast-forming unit–erythroid (BFU_E) cell. The pronormoblast produces two basophilic normoblasts, each of which divides, in turn, to form two polychromatic normoblasts. Thus, between eight and 32 mature red cells are derived from each pronormoblast. Orthochromatic cells cannot synthesize DNA, and so cell division of the polychromatic stage of maturation ceases.

Nutritional Requirements of the Red Cell

Vitamin B_{12}

Vitamin B_{12} is essential for normal nuclear maturation, playing an important role in DNA synthesis. A deficiency of vitamin B_{12} results in impairment of nuclear maturation and in megaloblastic red-cell changes. The principal effect is of retarded nuclear growth in the presence of normal cytoplasmic maturation.

Vitamin B_{12} is not synthesized by higher plants but is produced by many bacteria and fungi. It is found in large quantities in soil. Its bacterial synthesis in the alimentary tract is carried out distal to the intestinal segments, at which point absorption occurs. Consequently, dietary sources are the sole method of obtaining sufficient vitamin for normal hematopoiesis. Such sources are chiefly foods of animal origin, such as liver, muscle, eggs, cheese, and milk.

Normal absorption of vitamin B_{12}—approximately 70% of the dietary vitamin level—takes place when the vitamin is bound to a gastric juice protein, intrinsic factor. However, if the vitamin B_{12} remains unbound because of lack of intrinsic factor, only approximately 2% is used. Intrinsic factor is a pH-sensitive thermolabile glycoprotein that possesses the ability to bind vitamin B_{12} and its analogs with high affinity. It is absorbed principally from the lower level of the ileum, the intrinsic factor–vitamin B_{12} complex becoming attached to specific receptor sites on the mucosal cells. This process requires an acidic pH greater than 5.7 and the presence of calcium ions. The mode of entry of bound vitamin B_{12} into the plasma is unknown but, once in the blood, it is bound to specific proteins called *transcobalamins*. Three such proteins are recognized. The first is transcobalamin I (TC I) arising from granulocytes, which probably serves as a backup system for endogenous vitamin B_{12}. It is not required for the release of vitamin B_{12} from the mucosal cells, and it appears to be a passive reservoir that is in equilibrium with the body stores in the liver. Transcobalamin II (TC II) is the chief transport protein, acting as a vitamin receptor and main carrier to the liver, hematopoietic cells, and other dividing cells. This protein is probably produced by the liver, macrophages, and ileum. A third binding protein, transcobalamin III (TC III), is derived from granulocytes. It does not appear to bind large amounts of vitamin B_{12} and is believed to differ from TC I only in its carbohydrate proportions. Lack of TC II results in severe megaloblastic anemia despite a normal serum vitamin B_{12} level, but a similar reduction of TC I is not accompanied by anemia, despite a decrease in serum vitamin B_{12}.

TC I and TC III are believed to be related to other *R proteins* or cobalophilins. These proteins bind vitamin B_{12} and are found in gastric juice, saliva, plasma, tears, and milk, accounting for

Table 2.2. Properties of the Transcobalamins

Property	TC I	TC II	TC III
Electrophoretic mobility	α_1	$\alpha_2\beta$	α_1
Protein type	R	S	R
Half-life	9–12 days	1.0–1.5 hrs	<1 hr
Complex	Chronic myeloid leukemia, polycythemia vera	Pregnancy, acute leukemia, polycythemia vera	Chronic myeloid leukemia
Likely function	Storage	Transport	Storage

TC = transcobalamin.
Source: Data from RH Allen, PW Majerus. Isolation of vitamin B binding proteins using affinity chromatography III. Purification and properties of human plasma transcobalamin II. J Biol Chem 247:7709, 1972; RK Burger et al. Human plasma R-type vitamin B binding proteins: I. Isolation and characterization of transcobalamin I, transcobalamin III and normal granulocytic vitamin B binding protein. J Biol Chem 110:7700, 1975; and B Rachmilewitz, M Rachmilewitz. The synthesis of transcobalamin II, a vitamin B_{12} transport protein by stimulated mouse peritoneal macrophages. Biomedicine 27:213, 1977.

nearly 20% of the vitamin B_{12} binding capacity of gastric juice. Cobalophilins are glycoproteins that possess rapid electrophoretic mobility, which gives rise to the term *R protein*. In humans, total levels of cobalamins in the body are high (800–1,000 µg) relative to the daily requirements (Grasbeck and Salonen, 1976). Loss of cobalamins from the body occurs at a rate of 0.1%, equivalent to approximately 1–4 µg (Herbert, 1987). Table 2.2 illustrates some of the properties of the transcobalamins.

Folic Acid

Like vitamin B_{12}, folic acid is essential in the synthesis of nuclear proteins. The major clinical manifestations of human folate deficiency are produced by impairment of thymidylate synthesis, which impairs DNA synthesis, producing megaloblastic cell transformations.

Folates are synthesized by higher plants and are widely distributed in nature. Green leafy vegetables are particularly rich sources and include asparagus, broccoli, spinach, and lettuce. Folates also are found in liver, kidney, yeast, eggs, and mushrooms. They are absorbed after deconjugation in the small intestine, mainly in the jejunum, and are transported in the plasma bound to protein, mainly in the methyltetrahydrofolate form. This conversion takes place in the intestine or liver. Within these organs, part of the folate becomes polyglutaminated, and the remainder is excreted in the bile ducts. It is then reabsorbed from the intestines. Increased alcohol ingestion interferes with this process, resulting in

retention of folate by the liver and the production of a megaloblastic anemia.

Folate transfer to the tissues is rapid. Approximately one-third of the total body stores are found in the liver but, when folate intake is reduced, these stores become depleted within 3–4 months. This leads to impaired DNA synthesis in the erythroid cells and results in the megaloblastic dyserythropoiesis also seen in vitamin B_{12} deficiency. The precursor of DNA is thymidylate, which is derived from deoxyuridylate. Dihydrofolate is reduced to tetrahydrofolate by the enzyme dihydrofolate reductase. Tetrahydrofolate is the principal folate form found in red cells and the liver. This reduction of dihydrofolate to tetrahydrofolate is important in chemotherapy. Some drugs used in cancer treatment (such as methotrexate, aminopterin, and pyrimethamine) inhibit dihydrofolate reductase; consequently, DNA synthesis is impaired, leading to a megaloblastic blood picture.

Vitamin B_6

Vitamin B_6 is composed of a group of naturally occurring compounds of which pyridoxine is the most common. The vitamin is found widely in nature in plants and animals, especially in meats and grains. A deficiency of vitamin B_6 results in a microcytic hypochromic anemia, iron overload, and abnormal neurologic findings. The vitamin is absorbed rapidly from the intestine and participates in amino acid metabolism. Its principal role in erythropoiesis is as a cofactor in the formation of aminolevulinic acid, a necessary precursor for heme synthesis.

Naturally occurring dietary deficiency is rare because of the ubiquitous distribution of the vitamin. Certain drugs such as isoniazid and penicillamine inactivate vitamin B_6 and can cause a deficiency.

Trace Metals

Serum copper is found in the plasma in two forms: that bound to albumin (approximately 7% of the total) and that bound to an α_2-globulin, ceruloplasmin. The full role of copper in erythropoiesis is not well documented, but ceruloplasmin appears to be required for optimal flow of iron from the erythroid cells to the plasma. When severe reductions are present, iron is not released from macrophages at the normal rate, thus leading to hypoferremia in the presence of normal iron stores. Reductions in copper are believed to be responsible also for the inability of normoblasts to use iron fully for hemoglobin synthesis. This results in accumulation of cytoplasmic iron granules in the nucleated red cell and the formation of sideroblasts. The abnormality is probably due to defective mitochondrial iron uptake caused by a decrease in a copper enzyme, cytochrome oxidase.

Cobalt is a component of the vitamin B_{12} molecule and is an essential trace metal. It is present in many foods and required only in extremely small amounts. Cobalt deficiency does not appear to occur naturally, and its absorption is thought to be similar to that of iron.

Iron

Because of the ease with which it is oxidized and reduced, iron is a component of many metabolically active substances. The most important of these substances are cytochrome, myoglobin, and hemoglobin. Iron-containing heme moieties function as oxygen carriers.

Iron is the most abundant heavy metal in the body and is used mainly for hemoglobin synthesis. The daily requirement approximates 20–25 mg, most of which is obtained through hemoglobin recycling. The remainder (approximately 1 mg) is obtained from dietary sources in amounts sufficient to achieve a delicate balance with that lost by excretion in the feces and urine, in perspiration, and from desquamated skin.

To be absorbed, dietary iron must first be reduced from its ferric state to the ferrous form. Such reduction takes place with the aid of gastric acids. Chelation with low-molecular-weight compounds, such as fructose and amino acids, also solubilizes the iron prior to absorption in the upper and middle small intestine. The regulation of iron absorption is believed to be carried out by the intestinal epithelia. The mucosal cells appear to act as attractions to the iron molecule, reflecting within their own cytoplasm the state of the body iron stores. Mucosal uptake occurs rapidly at the brush borders of the cell, and the soluble iron passes across the cell membrane. High concentrations of cellular iron discourage further uptake, whereas iron-poor cells seem to encourage further absorption. Increased erythropoietic activity also appears to activate this process. The exact mechanism of iron passage from the mucosal cell to the plasma is unclear, but such transmucosal activity likely is aided by chelation to cellular amino acids. Once in the plasma, most of the ferrous iron becomes attached to a plasma β-globulin, *transferrin,* for transportation to storage sites.

The metabolic pathway of iron is shown in Figure 2.2. The absorption of iron, folate, and vitamin B_{12} is demonstrated in Figure 2.3.

Transferrin is usually measured and expressed as the amount of iron that it binds, an index known as the *total iron-binding capacity* (TIBC). Each transferrin molecule binds two molecules of ferric iron (Fe^{+++}). Under normal conditions, approximately one-third of the available binding sites are occupied. Free plasma iron exhibits a diurnal variation, with the highest values found in the morning and the lowest values in the evening. However, transferrin does not show such physiologic fluctuations.

Iron is incorporated mainly into newly synthesized hemoglobin molecules derived from recycled effete red cells. Such cells are phagocytosed by macrophages in the liver, spleen, and bone marrow. The hemoglobin within the cell is degraded, and the resulting salvaged iron is combined with apoferritin (an iron-free protein) to form highly iron-concentrated molecules of ferritin, each of which may contain up to 4,000 atoms of iron.

Ferritin molecules, in turn, are compressed into still larger aggregates of amorphous material known

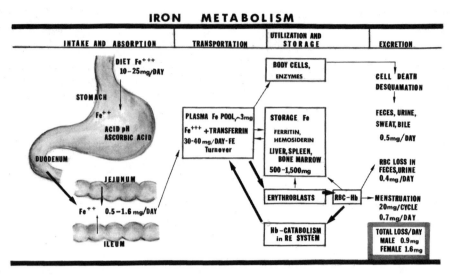

Figure 2.2. The metabolic pathway of iron. (RBC = red blood cell; Hb = hemoglobin; RE = reticuloendothelial.) (Reprinted from BH Hyun, JK Ashton, K Dolan. Practical Hematology. Philadelphia: Saunders, 1975. P 14.)

as *hemosiderin*. It is these ferritin-hemosiderin complexes that become the main source of iron reserves in the body. If apoferritin levels are insufficient to bind all the available iron, it becomes deposited in

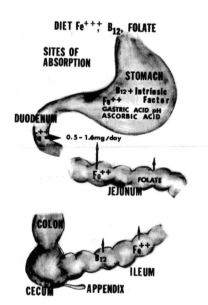

Figure 2.3. The absorption of iron, folate, and vitamin B_{12} in the alimentary tract. (Reprinted from BH Hyun, JK Ashton, K Dolan. Practical Hematology. Philadelphia: Saunders, 1975. P 15.)

the bone marrow, liver, and other tissues. Ferritin thus functions in a storage-site capacity, particularly within the red cell, and provides a pathway by which iron may be made available for hemoglobin synthesis under abnormal conditions. Ferritin deposits in the red cell can be stained by the Prussian blue reaction and are known as *siderocytes*.

The iron in the ferritin complex is stored in the trivalent state predominantly in hepatocytes and cells of the monocyte-macrophage systems. It is then reduced to the ferrous form for removal from apoferritin and is carried in the ferric state by transferrin. This protein delivers the iron at the surface of nucleated red cells. The transfer of the transferrin-bound iron from the protein molecule to the red cell is poorly understood, but it is postulated that the reaction occurs in four stages. In the first phase, transferrin iron becomes electrostatically bound to the cells, and the protein-iron complex enters the cell by micropinocytosis (Wheby, 1970). Once inside the cell, the iron is released from the transferrin, a process requiring an intact mitochondrial electron-transport chain.

Other Vitamins

Vitamin C depletion classically produces scurvy. This is characterized by mucous membrane bleed-

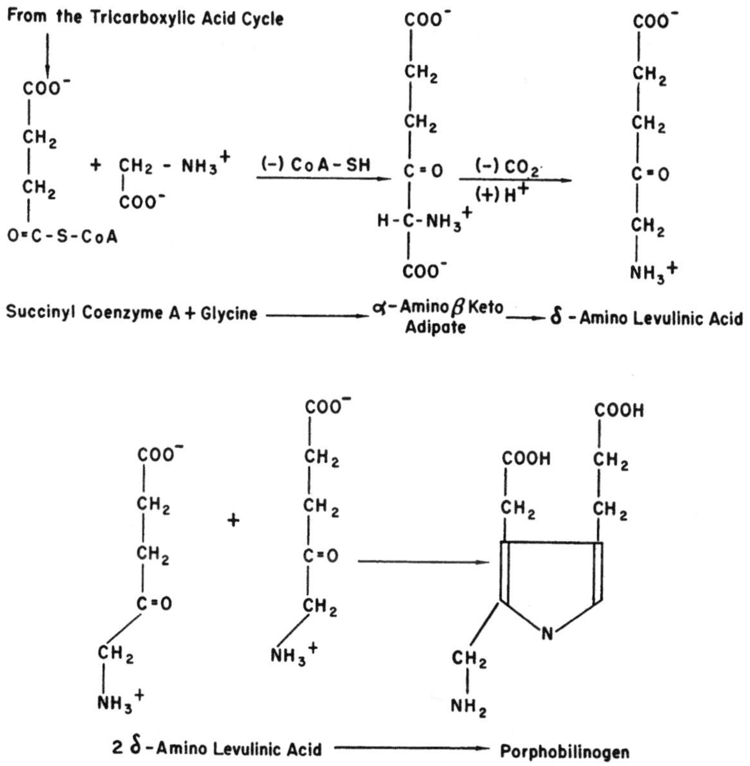

Figure 2.4. The formation of porphobilinogen from succinyl coenzyme A and glycine. (Reprinted from BS Leavell, O Thorup. Fundamentals of Clinical Hematology [4th ed]. Philadelphia: Saunders, 1976. P 38.)

ing, particularly in the gums, and skin hemorrhages on the legs and thighs. Most individuals with scurvy have a mild-to-moderate normocytic normochromic anemia, but the disease can also produce a macrocytic picture. Reticulocytes and hemoglobin catabolic products may be increased in the disease. The bone marrow picture is one of a normoblastic hyperplasia and, on occasion, a megaloblastic picture is present.

The role of vitamin A in erythropoiesis is not proven, although an experimental deficiency of the vitamin leads to anemia that responds to treatment with beta-carotene (Hodges, 1978).

Vitamin E is essential in erythropoiesis and in the maintenance of red-cell integrity. A deficiency of the vitamin in humans is rare, as it is distributed in many foods, particularly fats, oils, and grains; deficiency is associated with hemolytic anemias and red-cell sensitivity to peroxide hemolysis (Grutcher et al., 1984). Absorption of vitamin E depends on the ability to absorb fat. The deficiency has been suspected in some patients with malabsorption syndrome.

Hemoglobin Synthesis and Structure

Hemoglobin is a pigment composed of heme and the protein globin. The synthesis of heme begins with the formation of δ-aminolevulinic acid (ALA) in the erythrocytic mitochondria. This ALA is produced from glycine and succinylcoenzyme A to form an unstable intermediate product, α-amino β-ketoadipic acid, which, in turn, is converted to ALA in the presence of a cofactor, pyridoxal phosphate (vitamin B_6). Two molecules of ALA then condense to produce porphobilinogen in the presence of ALA-dehydrase. Four molecules of porphobilinogen react to form uroporphyrin III in the presence of uroporphyrinogen I synthetase and uroporphyrinogen III cosynthetase. The formation of porphobilinogen from succinyl coenzyme A and glycine is shown in Figure 2.4, and the formation of heme from porphobilinogen is shown in Figure 2.5.

Coproporphyrinogen is then converted to protoporphyrinogen IX, and the protoporphyrin is attached to iron in the presence of the enzyme heme synthetase to produce a heme moiety. This reaction

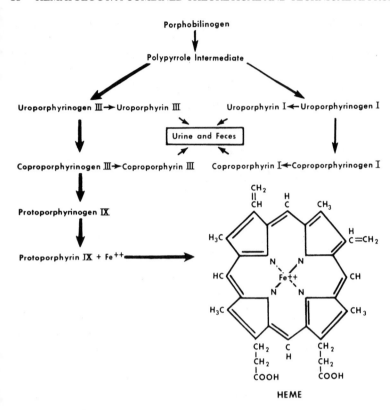

Figure 2.5. The formation of heme from porphobilinogen. (Reprinted from BS Leavell, O Thorup. Fundamentals of Clinical Hematology [4th ed]. Philadelphia: Saunders, 1976. P 39.)

takes place in the nucleated red-cell mitochondria. When uroporphyrinogen I synthetase is present, the type I isomers of uroporphyrinogen and coproporphyrins are formed, and their oxidized products are excreted in both feces and urine. Consequently, the heme molecule is not produced.

Globin synthesis takes place in the cytoplasm of the nucleated red cell and in cells as mature as reticulocytes. This synthesis takes place under the influence of RNA polymerases. The polypeptide globin chains are produced on the cellular ribosomes. Specific soluble RNA (sRNA) molecules determine the placement of each amino acid according to the messenger RNA (mRNA) code.

The synthesis of heme is coordinated with that of globin synthesis and requires control of protoporphyrin and globin synthesis as well as control of the entry of iron into the red cell. The major rate-limiting enzyme is ALA-synthetase (ALA-S), which possesses high activity in the early red cell and gradually diminishes as the cell matures. Heme depresses the formation of ALA-S and also inhibits its activity. A low concentration of iron activates ALA-S, whereas a high concentration is inhibitory.

The resulting hemoglobin molecule is composed of a four-membered, iron-containing heme structure that binds oxygen in a molecular ratio to the iron. The globin part of the molecule is a convoluted protein, within which are the specific binding sites for heme, so that one globin chain binds with one heme molecule. Although all the heme molecules are structurally identical, the globin chains differ in their amino acid sequence as well as in their composition (Figure 2.6).

Normally, four types of chains are synthesized: α, β, γ, and δ. Each hemoglobin molecule consists of two α chains and two other chains. Most adults possess hemoglobin A, made up of two α and two β chains ($\alpha_2\beta_2$), and this constitutes approximately 98% of the total hemoglobin, with the balance being hemoglobin A$_2$ ($\alpha_2\delta_2$) and hemoglobin F ($\alpha_2\gamma_2$). Hemoglobin F is found predominantly in the fetus and newborn but, by 6 months of age, the principal pigment is hemoglobin A. The relative proportion of polypeptide chains of hemoglobin present during fetal and neonatal life is shown in Figure 2.7.

The α chain of hemoglobin molecule contains 141 amino acids, and the non-α chains are com-

Table 2.3. Normal Embryonic and Adult Hemoglobins

Hemoglobin	Structure	Comments
A	$\alpha_2\beta_2$	—
A$_2$	$\alpha_2\delta_2$	Increased in β-thalassemia
F	$\alpha_2\gamma_2$	Present from the third month of gestation; increased in β-thalassemia
A$_{1c}$	$\alpha_2(\beta$-NH-glucose$)$	Increased in uncontrolled diabetes
H	β_4	Increased in α-thalassemia; unstable nonfunctional
Barts	γ_4	Present in homozygous α-thalassemia; nonfunctional
Gower 1	ε_4	Unknown function
Gower 2	$\alpha_2\varepsilon_2$	Unknown function

posed of 146 residues. Besides the different sequences of these amino acids, the different hemoglobin chains are structurally dissimilar in three main ways: (1) the organization of amino acids into stabilized helices, (2) the manner in which the polypeptide chains are folded to produce a three-dimensional spheric unit, and (3) the way in which several chains join to produce a simple molecule. Table 2.3 summarizes the "normal" hemoglobins produced from embryonic to postembryonic stages. In addition, there are three embryonic hemoglobins—Portland, Gower 1, and Gower 2—composed of one pair of α or α-like chains (ε), and one pair of non-α non-ε globin chains.

Hemoglobin Metabolism and Function

The developing red cell contains all the required components for replication, maturation, and differentiation. The cell also is able to synthesize proteins, carbohydrates, and lipids and becomes involved in the production of both heme and globin. To enable the erythrocyte to meet these functions, glucose is metabolized by two major routes: the Embden-Meyerhof pathway and the pentose-phosphate shunt, with approximately 90% of the glycolysis following the Embden-Meyerhof pathway (Figure 2.8).

However, the use of glucose is relatively inefficient. In the breakdown of a molecule of glucose to lactate, 2 mol ATP are consumed during the hexose portion of the pathway, but 3–4 mol are generated at the triose level. It is this net gain in ATP that provides high-energy phosphate for maintenance of membrane lipids and for energizing free metabolic pumps that control sodium and potassium flux. The essential role of ATP in the red cell is shown in two conditions: early cell death, which occurs when ATP is deficient because of inherited defects in glycolysis, and the loss of cell viability that is found accompanying ATP depletion of stored blood.

The absence of respiration, associated with the lack of mitochondria and cell enzymes of the tricarboxylic acid cycle, results in both less efficient energy production and the unavailability of the reduced form of nicotinamide adenine dinucleotide phosphate (NADPH). This coenzyme is required as a reducing

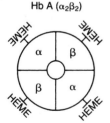

Hb A ($\alpha_2\beta_2$)

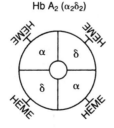

Hb A$_2$ ($\alpha_2\delta_2$)

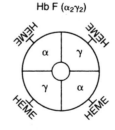

Hb F ($\alpha_2\gamma_2$)

α — α-polypeptide chain
β — β-polypeptide chain
γ — γ-polypeptide chain
δ — δ-polypeptide chain

Figure 2.6. Normal hemoglobin (Hb) molecules. (Adapted from BH Hyun, JK Ashton, K Dolan. Practical Hematology. Philadelphia: Saunders, 1975. P 11.)

Figure 2.7. The relative proportions of polypeptide chains of hemoglobin (Hb) present during fetal and neonatal life. (Reprinted from HF Bunn, BG Forget, HM Ranney. Human Hemoglobins. Philadelphia: Saunders, 1975. P 107. Modified from WS Beck [ed]. Hematology [2nd ed]. Boston: MIT Press, 1976.)

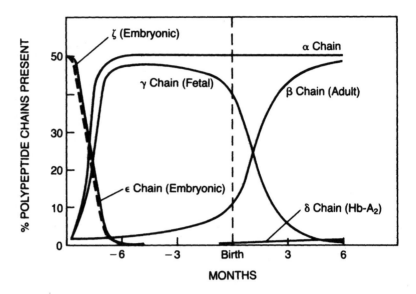

agent in the prevention of hemoglobin oxidation. It is generated in the red cell during glucose metabolism by the alternate pentose-phosphate shunt.

Most of the methemoglobin produced by the normal cell is reduced by nicotinamide adenine dinucleotide–linked methemoglobin reductase. In the pentose-phosphate shunt, NADPH is generated by glucose, which is converted to pentose through the action of glucose-6-phosphate dehydrogenase (G6PD) and 6-phosphogluconide dehydrogenase. For each molecule of glucose, one molecule of nicotinamide adenine dinucleotide phosphate (NAPD) is converted to its reduced form, NADPH. Lack of G6PD results in the lowering of the concentration of reduced glutathione (GSH) in the cell, which normally is present intracellularly in relatively high concentrations. GSH acts as a buffer, protecting the cell against injury by exogenous and endogenous oxidants produced by macrophages following infections and by a variety of drugs and chemicals. If these oxidants are allowed to accumulate intracellularly, injury to the cell proteins occurs, resulting in premature cell lysis. These events are prevented by GSH, which inactivates the oxidants. The enzyme glutathione-peroxidase enhances the reaction during which glutathione becomes converted to its oxidized form, GSSG. This process is balanced by GSH, which, in turn, catalyzes the NADPH-mediated reduction of GSSG back to GSH.

In primaquine-sensitive individuals, the erythrocytes possess a decreased level of G6PD. Primaquine then acts to oxidize GSH faster than it can be reduced by NADPH. Young cells with normal enzyme levels survive, but cells that have enzyme deficiencies ultimately fail to continue to provide ATP for cellular integrity, and they hemolyze. Other common drugs that act in a manner similar to primaquine include quinine, quinidine, aspirin, chloramphenicol, vitamin K, and some sulfonamides.

The principal function of hemoglobin is to bind blood gases. When fully saturated, each gram of hemoglobin binds 1.34 ml oxygen, the degree of saturation being related to the blood oxygen tension (Figure 2.9).

Delivery of adequate oxygen to the tissues involves the chest muscles, heart, lungs, red cells, blood vessels, and neurocontrol mechanisms. The process can be divided into four parts: (1) pulmonary perfusion and gas exchange, (2) transport capacity, (3) systemic and regional transport and gas exchange, and (4) use in the tissues.

The oxygen-carrying capacity of the blood is based on the physical and chemical characteristics of the hemoglobin molecule. The normal hemoglobin molecule possesses a cyclic affinity for oxygen bound to iron. When the first iron atom binds to oxygen, three remaining atoms of iron exhibit an increased affinity so that the oxygen affinity of the

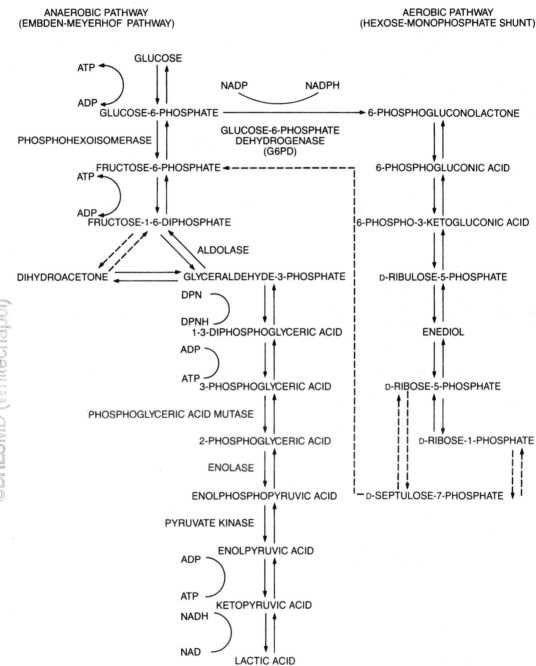

Figure 2.8. The anaerobic and aerobic pathways of glucose metabolism by red cells. (ATP = adenosine triphosphate; ADP = adenosine diphosphate; NADP = nicotinamide adenine dinucleotide phosphate; NADPH = reduced nicotinamide adenine dinucleotide phosphate; DPN = diphosphopyridine nucleotide; DPNH = reduced diphosphopyridine nucleotide; NAD = nicotinamide adenine dinucleotide; NADH = reduced nicotinamide adenine dinucleotide. (Reprinted from JB Henry. Clinical Diagnosis and Management by Laboratory Methods [17th ed]. Philadelphia: Saunders, 1984.)

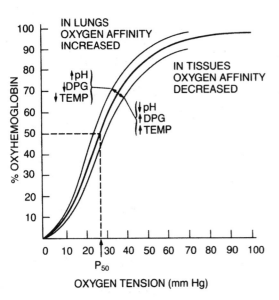

Figure 2.9. The normal oxygen-hemoglobin dissociation curve and the effects on oxygen affinity of changes in pH, temperature, and red-cell 2,3-diphosphoglycerate (DPG) level. (Adapted from WS Beck [ed]. Hematology [3rd ed]. Cambridge: MIT Press, 1981. P 135.)

hemoglobin molecule increases as more oxygen is bound. This phenomenon is known as the *heme-heme interaction*. The oxygen affinity of hemoglobin also is influenced directly by a pH greater than 6.0–8.5; this is termed the *Bohr effect*. It is a benefit to the tissues when the decrease in pH resulting from carbon dioxide uptake lowers the oxygen affinity and aids in oxygen release. In the lungs, carbon dioxide expulsion raises pH levels and thereby increases oxygen affinity and uptake. Oxygen affinity also depends on the concentration of red-cell 2,3-diphosphoglycerate (2,3-DPG). This phosphate-containing enzyme combines reversibly with deoxygenated hemoglobin, decreasing the affinity of hemoglobin for oxygen without disturbing the heme-heme interaction or the Bohr effect.

Each of the divalent iron atoms of the hemoglobin molecule can bind reversibly with oxygen to form oxyhemoglobin. This exchange alters the quaternary structure of the molecule, which in turn affects the molecule's buffering capacity for hydrogen ions. It also alters the oxygen affinity of the other iron atoms of the molecule, the net result being substantial oxygen-carrying capacity. Thus, the amount of oxygen delivered to the tissues is related to the total hemoglobin, the amount of hemoglobin carrying oxygen, and the cardiac output.

Whereas oxyhemoglobin and reduced hemoglobin (deoxygenated) can transport oxygen, the dyshemoglobins are hemoglobin derivatives that are incapable of reversing binding with oxygen and of carrying oxygen. Three dysfunctional hemoglobins are of interest: *Methemoglobin* incorporates an oxidized iron (trivalent) atom into the heme moiety. Elevated methemoglobin levels occur when there is excess production due to the presence of oxidants such as nitrites or if there is a decreased affinity of methemoglobin reductase.

Carboxyhemoglobin is the result of covalent binding of carbon monoxide to the divalent iron, which can occur at very low levels of carbon monoxide tensions. This is because hemoglobin possesses more than 200 times the affinity for carbon monoxide as for oxygen.

Sulfhemoglobin is a rare and poorly characterized dyshemoglobin that contains sulfur and trivalent iron. Hemoglobin-oxygen saturation is the amount of oxyhemoglobin in the blood expressed as a fraction of the total hemoglobin available to bind oxygen. In contrast to saturation, fractional oxyhemoglobin is the amount of oxyhemoglobin expressed as a fraction of the total hemoglobin.

Hemoglobin Catabolism

When red cells come to the end of their normal life span, they are removed extravascularly from the circulation by the reticuloendothelial (RE) system, principally by the spleen but, in pathologic states, also by the liver and bone marrow. Within the RE cell, hemoglobin is catabolized by the cleavage of the heme from the globin moiety. This is followed by the opening of the porphyrin ring at the α-methane bridge, producing biliverdin and carbon monoxide. The released globin is returned to the plasma protein pool, and the heme iron then is stored in the iron pool of the liver.

The biliverdin, under the influence of biliverdin reductase, is converted to bilirubin, is passed out of the RE cell, and is bound to plasma albumin. In this state, it is known as *unconjugated* or *indirect bilirubin* and is cleared rapidly from the blood by the liver parenchymal cells. Here it is conjugated with glucuronic acid with the aid of glucuronyl trans-

Figure 2.10. The catabolic pathways of hemoglobin. (R.E. = reticuloendothelial; Hb = hemoglobin; RBC = red blood cell.) (Reprinted from BH Hyun, JK Ashton, K Dolan. Practical Hematology. Philadelphia: Saunders, 1975. P 13.)

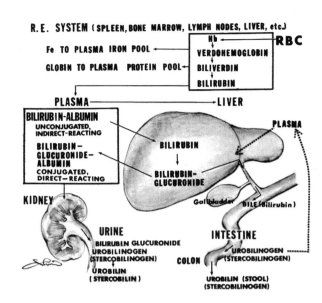

ferase. In this form, it is then passed into the bile ductules and common bile duct to the small intestine, at which point it is reduced by bacterial action to mesobilirubinogen. This product undergoes conversion to urobilinogen and urobilin, and the urobilinogen is partially reabsorbed from the colon to the blood. Some urobilinogen is excreted by the urine, but the majority is returned to the liver (a process known as *enterohepatic recirculation*), at which point it is excreted once more. Catabolic pathways of hemoglobin are shown in Figure 2.10.

The intravascular hemolytic pathway takes up approximately 10–20% of normal effete red cells, but it plays an important role in many forms of pathologic lysis. When red cells are hemolyzed in the plasma, the resulting free hemoglobin becomes bound to a liver-synthesized α_2-globulin known as *haptoglobin*, a specific hemoglobin-binding protein that can be divided into two groups by electrophoresis. The two allelic autosomal codominant genes Hp1 and Hp2 produce three phenotypes: Hp1-1, Hp2-2, and Hp2-1. The main difference between them is in the composition of their light chains. These phenotypes are of interest in paternity studies and in the study of genetic diseases.

If not complexed with hemoglobin, haptoglobin has a half-life in the plasma of approximately 5 days. If bound to hemoglobin, it has a half-life of less than 30 minutes. The complex is cleared by parenchymal liver cells, but the molecule is too large to filter across the glomerulus. When the haptoglobin binding sites are saturated, some free hemoglobin passes into the glomerular filtrate, resulting in hemoglobinuria. Any free hemoglobin present in the plasma may become oxidized to methemoglobin, which breaks down to form heme and globin. Free heme is insoluble at physiologic pH levels but, if bound to albumin and to a β_1-globulin, hemopexin, it maintains its soluble form. Hemopexin is produced by the liver and possesses the ability to bind one-to-one with free heme. This hemopexin-heme complex is removed by the liver parenchyma in the same way as is the hemoglobin-haptoglobin complex. The hemopexin half-life, if unbound, approximates 7 days but, once complexed with heme, it has a half-life of approximately 8 hours. Plasma hemopexin levels, like those of haptoglobin, are reduced in disorders associated with severe intravascular hemolysis, such as sickle cell anemia, thalassemia, and some autoimmune hemolytic anemias.

Chapter 3

Introduction to the Anemias

Anemia refers to a decrease in the total number of circulating red cells, a decrease in the hemoglobin concentration, or a decrease in the hematocrit when compared with a normal group. Such a definition must also take into account the functional ability of the blood to deliver oxygen to deprived tissues.

The symptoms of anemia depend on the degree of reduction in the oxygen-carrying capacity of the blood, the change in the total blood volume, the rate at which these changes occur, the degree of severity of the underlying disease contributing to the anemia, and the power of the cardiovascular and hematopoietic systems to recuperate and compensate. Signs and symptoms in anemic individuals can be classified into three main groups: (1) those due to decreased oxygen transport in which the major physical findings are fatigue, syncope, dyspnea, and angina pectoris; (2) those due to a decrease in blood volume in which the findings are primarily pallor and postural hypotension; and (3) those due to increased cardiac output, among which the principal symptoms are tachycardia and, possibly, the commencement of congestive heart failure.

Other physiologic findings are also seen frequently. In anemia caused by a decreased oxygen-carrying capacity, jaundice, hemoglobinuria, hemoglobinemia, and methemoglobinemia can be found. Depending on the cause of the anemia, the hemoglobin dissociation curve can shift, and alterations in 2,3-disphosphoglycerate levels can be found. Increased cardiovascular output usually en-

sues when the hemoglobin drops below 7 g/dl, and an accelerated heartbeat (tachycardia) is seen when the hemoglobin falls below 5 g/dl. Anemias can be differentiated two ways: by morphologic criteria and by physiologic grouping, each of which will be discussed.

Morphologic Classification of Anemias

The classification of anemias morphologically is based on the red-cell appearance of a standard blood slide and on the red-cell indices calculated from measured hemoglobin, hematocrit, and red-cell count values. Using electrical impedance methods, the mean cell volume (MCV) can be measured directly.

Macrocytic Anemias

The macrocytic anemias include vitamin B_{12} and folate deficiencies, drug-induced macrocytic anemias, and refractory megaloblastic anemia. Bleeding disorders associated with reticulocytosis and liver disease may also show macrocytic characteristics, as may carcinoma of the stomach, idiopathic steatorrhea, and sprue. These anemias usually show increased MCVs (100–160 femtoliters [fl]) and a correspondingly high mean cell hemoglobin (MCH). Most macrocytic anemias are normochromic, having a normal MCH concentration (MCHC) of 31–36 g/dl.

Microcytic Hypochromic Anemias

The physiologic defect in the group of microcytic hypochromic anemias involves decreased hemoglobin production secondary to a wide variety of disorders, including iron deficiency, thalassemia, lead poisoning, sideroblastic anemia, and chronic hemorrhage. Morphologically, the anemia is characterized by reductions in the MCV (<80 fl) and MCHC (<31 g/dl).

Normocytic Normochromic Anemias

Some of the normocytic normochromic anemias are characterized by an overall suppression of red-cell production, and some are characterized by increased red-cell loss through hemorrhage and hemolysis. The normocytic normochromic anemias include a wide range of primary and secondary bone marrow disorders, including hypoplastic anemias resulting from the action of bone marrow suppression by drugs, alcohol intoxication, or infection or from bone marrow replacement (myelophthisic anemia) in cases of tumor or fibrosis, anemia associated with renal disease, acute hemorrhage, leukemia, and hemoglobinopathies. Most of these disorders are characterized by normal red-cell indices (MCV, MCHC, MCH).

Laboratory Investigation of Anemia

The complete blood cell count (CBC) and the reticulocyte count are the key laboratory tests in the diagnosis of anemia. The Council on Foods and Nutrition (1968) defines anemia as a hemoglobin concentration or a hematocrit below the levels shown in Table 3.1.

Usually, a reduction in hemoglobin concentration parallels a reduction in total red-cell number, but exceptions are found. For example, hemodilution results in a falsely decreased hemoglobin concentration and hematocrit, yet these values are not caused by abnormal erythropoiesis. Other conditions manifesting such spurious anemic blood pictures are described in Table 3.2.

The primary decisive point in the investigation of macrocytic anemias is the reticulocyte count. Reticulocytes are immature red cells with a slightly

Table 3.1. Definition of Anemia

Age	Hemoglobin	Hematocrit
6 mos–4 yrs	<11.0 g/dl	<33.0%
4 yrs–puberty	<11.5 g/dl	<34.5%
Postpubertal males	<14.0 g/dl	<42.5%
Postpubertal females	<12.0 g/dl	<36.0%

Source: Data from Council on Foods and Nutrition, Iron deficiency in the United States. JAMA 203:407, 1968.

larger MCV than normal mature cells. On a peripheral blood smear, they appear as macrocytes in the company of increased polychromasia.

However, most cases of macrocytic anemia demonstrate a depressed, or at best a normal, reticulocyte count. In megaloblastic anemias, the disorder is in nuclear maturation. Vitamin B_{12} and folic acid deficiencies are the most typical of these anemias, but chemotherapeutic agents and other drugs can cause similar morphologic changes in the red cells. The laboratory investigation of these disorders traditionally includes radioimmunoassays for vitamin B_{12} and folic acid. The deoxyuridine suppression test can also be used. Additional testing for megaloblastic anemia is directed toward finding a specific cause and can include a Schilling test. A suggested schematic for the laboratory investigation of this group of anemias is shown in Figure 3.1.

As in the investigation of the macrocytic anemias, the first decisive point in the investigation of the normocytic normochromic anemias is the reticulocyte count, which should always be corrected for anemia (see page 274). The reticulocyte is a prime indicator of bone marrow activity and, more specifically, of red-cell production. Normal or decreased reticulocyte counts are present in bone marrow suppression and replacement (by tumors), and a bone marrow examination will clarify this situation: Decreased reticulocyte counts with a normal bone marrow examination indicate some lack of bone marrow response in the presence of anemia.

Anemia associated with renal disease may be related to a circulating erythropoietic inhibitor, a situation suggested by improvement in the hemoglobin and red-cell count following hemodialysis. Increased reticulocyte counts can be seen in cases of gastrointestinal hemorrhage and in acute hemolytic crisis. Laboratory tests useful in determining catabolic hemoglobin products can be carried out and often will

Table 3.2. Conditions Resulting in Spurious Anemic Blood Pictures

Physiologic State	Anemia
Hemodilution or overhydration due to	
Renal disease	
Congestive heart failure	
Hypoalbuminemia associated with	Anemia characterized by a relative increase in plasma volume without a
Liver disease	proportional increase in red-cell mass
Neoplasms	
Malabsorption	
Poor diet	
Hydremia of pregnancy	

shed light on the cause of the disorder. These tests include determinations of serum haptoglobin (Marchand and Galen, 1980), plasma-free hemoglobin, and urinary hemosiderin and a direct antiglobulin test. A suggested scheme for the investigation of this group of anemias is shown in Figure 3.2.

The first series of tests to carry out in the laboratory investigation of a microcytic hypochromic anemia is the serum iron and total iron-binding capacity (TIBC). The iron transport protein, transferrin, is usually measured in terms of the TIBC. In iron-deficiency anemia, the characteristic results are decreased serum iron and an increased TIBC. Ferritin levels can be used as a backup test, reductions in ferritin almost always denoting an iron-deficiency state. Two main problems exist in such testing. First, serum iron undergoes a wide diurnal variation in normal individuals; it is at least one-third higher in the morning than in the afternoon and evening. The TIBC does not exhibit such fluctuations. Second, ferritin values can be raised irrespective of bone marrow–storage iron levels in the presence of inflammation, liver disease, or neoplasms. Once iron deficiency has been established, the cause of the disease should be clarified; hemorrhage and nutritional deficiencies are two common causes.

Anemias due to chronic disease usually produce reduced serum iron and TIBC levels. Such anemias are found commonly in inflammation and in neoplastic disorders. The pathogenesis is unknown.

Thalassemia involves the decreased production of one of the normal globin chains composing the hemoglobin molecule. Serum iron and the TIBC are normal in these disorders, although thalassemia trait can produce an anemia similar to that seen in iron

deficiency. A schematic for the laboratory investigation of microcytic hypochromic anemia is shown in Figure 3.3.

Red-Cell Indices

Red-cell indices are not only useful in the diagnosis of anemias but also provide a built-in automatic control for laboratory variability.

Mean Cell Volume

MCV can be calculated or measured directly. It is defined as the volume of the average red cell expressed in femtoliters. If the mean cell thickness is normal, the MCV bears a linear relationship to the red-cell diameter. Factors required to calculate the MCV are packed red-cell volume (hematocrit) and red-cell count.

$$MCV = \frac{Hematocrit \ (1/1) \times 1,000}{Red\text{-}cell \ count \ (\times 10^{12}/liter)}$$

Calculation example: hematocrit, 45%; red-cell count, 5×10^{12}/liter.

If the hematocrit is 45% (0.45), there are 0.45 ml red cells in 1 ml of whole blood, and if the red-cell count is 5×10^{12}/liter, these cells occupy a total volume of 0.45 fl.

The volume of one red cell (MCV) then is:

$$\frac{0.45 \times 10^9}{5 \times 10^6} = \frac{0.45 \times 10^3 \ fl}{5} = 90 \ fl$$

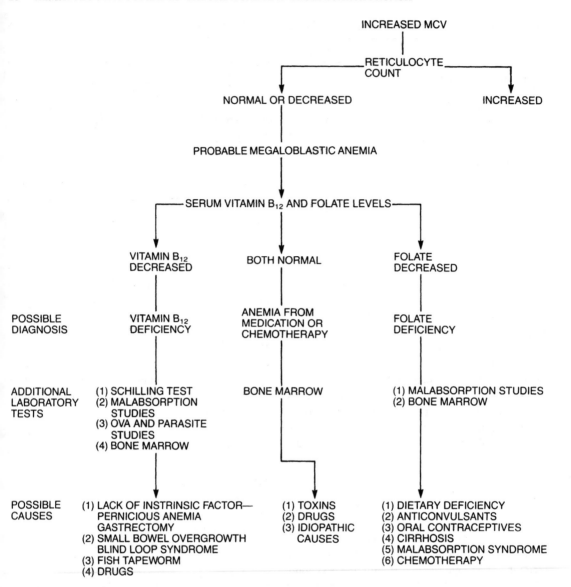

Figure 3.1. The laboratory investigation of macrocytic anemia. (MCV = mean cell volume.)

An abbreviated method of calculating the MCV is to use the formula:

$$\frac{\text{Hematocrit (as a decimal)}}{\text{Red-cell count } (\times 10^{12}/\text{liter})} \times 1{,}000 = \text{MCV}$$

The reference range for MCV is 80–100 fl (method-dependent).

Mean Cell Hemoglobin Concentration

The MCHC value is calculated, not measured directly. It is defined as the ratio of hemoglobin to the volume of packed red cells (hematocrit). The MCHC is, therefore, a measurement of the hemoglobin concentration in the average red cell. The factors required to calculate the

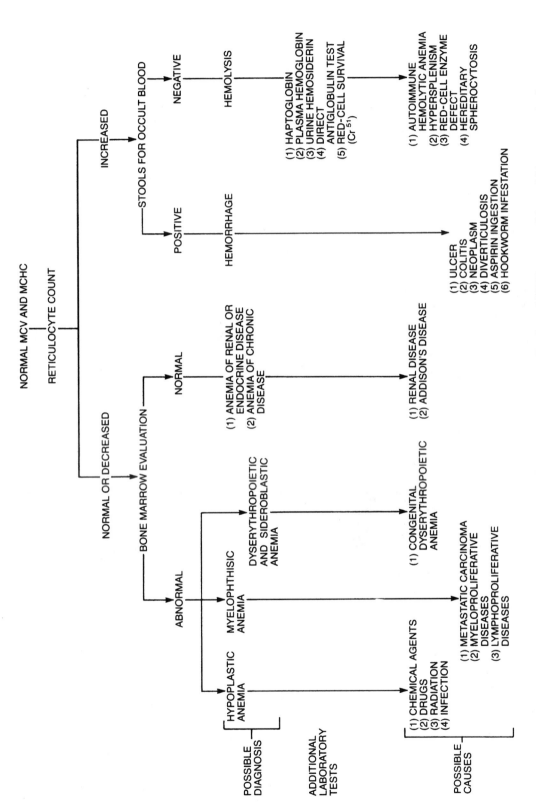

Figure 3.2. The laboratory investigation of normocytic normochromic anemia. (MCV = mean cell volume; MCHC = mean cell hemoglobin concentration.)

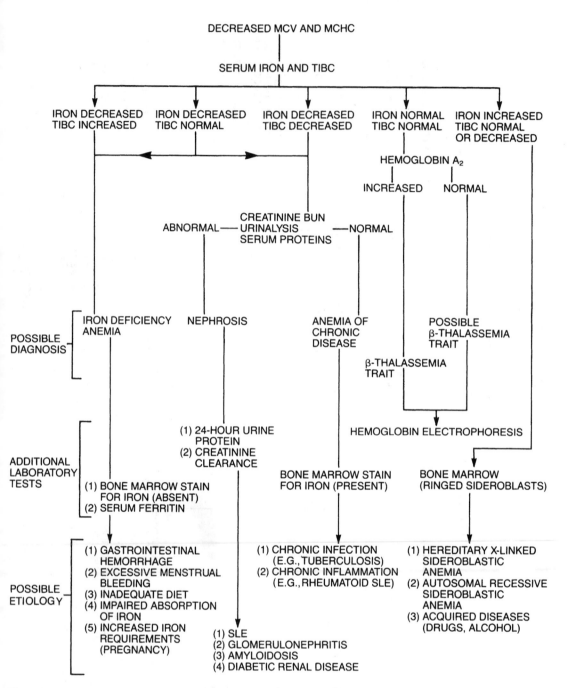

Figure 3.3. The laboratory investigation of microcytic hypochromic anemia. (MCV = mean cell volume; MCHC = mean cell hemoglobin concentration; TIBC = total iron-binding capacity; BUN = blood urea nitrogen; SLE = systemic lupus erythematosus.)

MCHC are packed red-cell volume (hematocrit) and hemoglobin.

$$MCHC = \frac{\text{Hemoglobin (g/liter)}}{\text{Hematocrit (1/1)}}$$

Calculation example: If the hemoglobin is 15 g/dl and the red cells occupy 45% (0.45) of the blood volume, the hemoglobin concentration in the cells is:

$$\frac{15}{45} \times 100 \text{ g/dl} = 33.3 \text{ g/dl} \, (\%)$$

The reference range for MCHC is 31–36% (method-dependent).

Mean Cell Hemoglobin

The MCH value is calculated and is defined as the weight of hemoglobin in the average red cell. If a normocytic red cell is large, the MCH is raised; if it is small, the MCH is reduced. Factors required to calculate the MCH are hemoglobin and red-cell count.

$$MCH = \frac{\text{Hemoglobin (g/dl)}}{\text{Red - cell count } (\times 10^{12}/\text{liter})}$$

Calculation example: If the hemoglobin is 15 g/dl, there is 15/100 g of hemoglobin per milliliter of blood, which is equivalent to 15/100 (1,000 g hemoglobin per liter of blood or 150 g hemoglobin per liter of blood).

If the red-cell count is 5×10^{12}/liter, the average weight of hemoglobin in one red cell is:

$$\frac{150}{5 \times 10^{12}} = 30 \times 10^{-12} \text{ g hemoglobin}$$

An abbreviated method of calculating the MCH is to use the formula:

$$\frac{\text{Hemoglobin (g/dl)}}{\text{Red - cell count } (\times 10^{12}/\text{liter})} \times 10 = MCH$$

The reference range for MCH is 28–32 pg.

Hematologic Rules of Three and Nine

The First Rule of Three

$$\text{Red - cell count (in millions)} \times 10^{12}/\text{liter} \times 3 = \text{hemoglobin (in g/dl)}$$

The first rule of three expresses the normal ratio of hemoglobin to red cells. It applies to all hemoglobinized cells regardless of whether the patient is anemic. Such normalized cells are found in anemias of various causes, so if this rule is found to fit an anemic individual's test results, a great many diseases must be considered. These illnesses include malignancy, acute blood loss, aplastic anemia, and leukemia. If the test results do not fit this rule, the anemia, if present, may be broadly subclassified into that possessing increased numbers of red cells in proportion to the total hemoglobin (i.e., hypochromic microcytic anemia) and that with a disproportionately low red-cell count in relation to the hemoglobin (i.e., macrocytic anemia).

Hypochromia, commonly seen in severe iron-deficiency anemia, can usually be detected on the peripheral blood smear when the hemoglobin is less than 10 g/dl. The valid morphologic interpretation of hypochromia thus is associated with the presence of increased red cells, according to this first rule.

The Second Rule of Three

$$\text{Hemoglobin (in g/dl)} \times 3 = \text{hematocrit (\%)}$$

The second rule of three also is an expression of normal red-cell relationships, and abnormalities of this rule are indicative of pathologic states. For example, moderate to severe iron-deficiency anemia is usually indicated when the hemoglobin is disproportionately lower than the hematocrit, producing an abnormal result when this second rule is applied. The hypochromia of thalassemia frequently does not violate this rule, as there is often agreement between the hemoglobin and the he-matocrit. Consequently, the second rule of three holds in such situations. Thus, this rule is used most often for corroborative rather than diagnostic purposes. Its main use is for checking the validity of the test results as part of a quality-control program (see page 244).

Table 3.3. Abnormal Red-Cell Morphologic Picture

Cause	Morphologic Features
Cell size	Anisocytosis
	Macrocytosis
	Microcytosis
Cell shape	Poikilocytosis
	Spherocytosis
	Elliptocytosis
	Target cells
	Sickle cells
	Schistocytes
	Stomatocytes
	Burr cells
	Acanthocytes
Hemoglobin content and cell color	Hypochromia
	Polychromasia
Cell inclusions	Basophilic stippling
	Pappenheimer bodies
	Howell-Jolly bodies
	Parasitized red cells
	Hemoglobin C crystals
	Hemoglobin H inclusions
	Heinz bodies
Other abnormalities	Rouleaux formation
	Autoagglutination

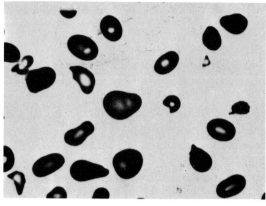

Figure 3.4. Megaloblastic anemia showing macrocytosis and marked anisocytosis (× 875). (Reprinted from JB Henry [ed]. Clinical Diagnosis and Management by Laboratory Methods [17th ed]. Philadelphia: Saunders, 1984. P 606.)

The rule of nine has applications similar to the first rule of three but is more useful in that it allows the separation of red-cell populations into hypochromic microcytic and macrocytic groups on the basis of cell volume, as distinct from mean hemoglobin content.

Abnormal Red-Cell Morphologic Features

Red cells should be examined by staining a well-made slide and searching for abnormalities in size, shape, hemoglobin concentration, and the presence of inclusion bodies. Most of these abnormalities can be graded from 1+ to 4+ to assist in the quantitation of each cell. Table 3.3 lists the more commonly found abnormal erythrocytic morphologic characteristics.

Alterations in Red-Cell Size

Normal. Red cells are usually biconcave discs with a mean cell diameter of between 7.2 and 7.6 μ and a mean average thickness of 1.8 μ.

Anisocytosis. The term anisocytosis denotes large variations in the size of a single red-cell population. The term often is misused and applied to cells that are larger or smaller than normal and to slight, clinically insignificant variations in size. Small fluctuations in red-cell size are normal and not noteworthy. Figure 3.4 depicts megaloblastic anemia, microcytosis, and marked anisocytosis. Table 3.4 shows a standardization of red-cell morphologic characteristics.

The Rule of Nine

$$\text{Red-cell count } (10^{12} / \text{liter}) \times 9 = \text{hematocrit } (\%)$$

If the normal ratio of the red-cell count to the hemoglobin and that of hemoglobin to hematocrit is known, a rule of nine can be calculated that expresses the numeric relationship of the hematocrit to the red-cell count.

This is derived from the two rules of three as follows:

$$\text{Red-cell count} \times 3 = \text{hemoglobin}$$
$$\text{Hemoglobin} \times 3 = \text{hematocrit}$$

That is:

$$\text{Hemoglobin} = \frac{\text{hematocrit}}{3}$$

$$\text{Red-cell count} \times 3 = \text{hemoglobin}$$

That is:

$$\text{Red-cell count} \times 9 = \text{hematocrit}$$

Table 3.4. Standardization of Red-Cell Morphologic Characteristics

Degree	Number of Abnormal Cells															
	Anisocytosis	Macrocytosis	Microcytosis	Poikilocytosis	Elliptocytosis	Spherocytosis	Polychromasia	Acanthrocytosis	Target Cells	Schistocytes	Stomatocytes	Basophilic Stippling	Burr Cells	Hypochromia	Pappenheimer Bodies	Howell-Jolly Bodies
1+	—	10–15%	10–15%	5–10%	1–5%	1–5%	1–5%	1–5%	1–5%	1–5%	1–2%	1–2%	15–20%	0–1%	0–1%	—
2+	15–20%	16–20%	16–20%	11–15%	6–10%	6–10%	6–10%	6–10%	6–10%	6–10%	3–5%	3–5%	3–5%	21–25%	2–3%	2–3%
3+	21–50%	21–25%	21–25%	16–20%	11–25%	11–25%	11–25%	11–25%	11–25%	11–25%	6–10%	6–10%	6–10%	26–30%	4–5%	4–5%
4+	>50%	>25%	>25%	>20%	>25%	>25%	>25%	>25%	>25%	>25%	>10%	>10%	>10%	>30%	>5%	>5%

Table 3.5. Common Staining Reactions of Red-Cell Inclusion Bodies

| Inclusions and Their Nature | Stains | | | | Phase Contrast |
	Supravital	Romanowsky	Iron	Feulgen	
Basophilic stippling (ribonucleoprotein)	+	+	–	–	+
Pappenheimer bodies (trivalent iron in ferritin)	–	+	+	–	–
Howell-Jolly bodies (DNA nuclear remnants)	+	+	–	+	+
Heinz bodies (denatured hemoglobin)	+	–	–	–	+
Hemoglobin H inclusions (α-chain abnormality)	+	+	–	–	+

+ = positive staining reaction; – = no reaction.

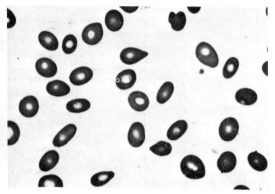

Figure 3.5. Myelofibrosis. Numerous elliptocytes with poikilocytes (teardrop forms). (Reprinted from JB Henry [ed]. Clinical Diagnosis and Management by Laboratory Methods [17th ed]. Philadelphia: Saunders, 1984. P 607.)

Macrocytosis. A macrocyte is a red cell having a fixed diameter in excess of 7.8 μ on a stained blood smear. Usually, the MCV also exceeds 100 fl. Macrocytosis is associated with premature release of bone marrow reticulocytes into the peripheral circulation and is found in acute hemorrhage, hemolytic anemias, vitamin B_{12} or folate deficiency, and chronic pulmonary disease. The macrocytosis present in vitamin B_{12} or folate deficiency results from retarded nuclear chromatin development in cells that possess relatively unaltered RNA cytoplasmic synthesis.

Microcytosis. A microcyte is a red cell having a fixed diameter of less than 7.2 μ on a stained blood smear. In microcytosis, the hemoglobin content of the cell frequently is reduced, the MCHC being less than 31 g/dl and the MCV being less than 80 fl. Microcytes often are present in iron-deficiency anemia and in the thalassemias. Grading of these cells is shown in Table 3.5.

Alterations in Red-Cell Shape

Poikilocytosis. A poikilocyte is classically a pear- or teardrop-shaped red cell that often represents an aged cell ready for erythrofragmentation and phagocytosis (Figure 3.5). The cell displays a single terminal projection, which may be smooth and rounded or have an unfinished jagged appearance. Poikilocytosis can be associated with ineffective erythropoiesis and extramedullary hematopoiesis. It is also particularly notable in the thalassemias, severe iron-deficiency anemia, pernicious anemia, hypersplenism, myeloid metaplasia, and some acquired hemolytic anemias. Poikilocytes are believed to result from forceful extrusion or removal of the red-cell nucleus in extramedullary hematopoiesis or from removal of other rigid inclusion bodies, such as hemosiderin, Howell-Jolly bodies, and Heinz bodies. The protruding portion of the cell is believed to represent a site of minor injury that results in an irreversible protrusion from the cytoplasm.

Spherocytosis. A spherocyte is a red cell with an increased average cell thickness and usually a reduced cell diameter. It appears in fixed blood smears as a small, deeply staining cell lacking normal red-cell central pallor because of its increased thickness. The spheric shape results from a developmental defect that occurs after the erythroblastic stage, during

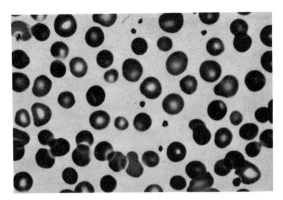

Figure 3.6. Hereditary spherocytosis (× 875). The denser cells are more spheric. Note that they have minimal and eccentric pallor and moderate anisocytosis. (Reprinted from JB Henry [ed]. Clinical Diagnosis and Management by Laboratory Methods [17th ed]. Philadelphia: Saunders, 1984. P 606.)

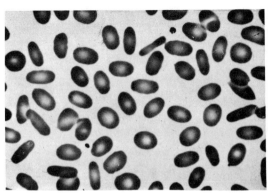

Figure 3.7. Hereditary elliptocytosis (× 875). (Reprinted from JB Henry [ed]. Clinical Diagnosis and Management by Laboratory Methods [17th ed]. Philadelphia: Saunders, 1984. P 607.)

which a normal cell volume is enclosed within a diminished surface area. Normal red cells become thicker as they take up water osmotically but, because the spherocyte already is thicker than normal, it requires less water to hemolyze and therefore is more fragile.

Two types of spherocytes exist: the congenital type found in hereditary spherocytosis (autosomal dominant; Figure 3.6) and the acquired form, associated with contraction and reduction of the surface area of the cell membrane caused by antibody damage, thermal burns, microangiopathic disorders, and uremic syndromes. Microspherocytosis is often seen in ABO erythroblastosis fetalis and, less frequently, in patients with congenital nonspherocytic hemolytic anemia, leukemia, and disorders characterized by splenic stasis.

Red-cell sphering is thus a reflection of intrinsic membrane injury that results in either a direct loss of membrane surface area or formation of a "leaky" membrane. Both of these results greatly increase the demands on adenosine triphosphate to maintain the cellular integrity and prevent osmotic lysis.

Elliptocytosis (Ovalocytosis). Elliptocytes are red cells that vary in shape from elongated forms to true ovals with variable diameters. The cell becomes more elongated as it ages. The hemoglobin content of elliptocytes is normal, and the osmotic fragility

may be normal or increased. The presence of elliptocytes is associated with hereditary elliptocytosis (autosomal dominant) and rarely is seen in normal blood smears, but elliptocytes are seen in varying numbers in almost all anemias. The presence of these cells is believed to reflect a change in the distribution of the cholesterol in the cell membrane, resulting in the accumulation of cholesterol in the opposing polar ends of the cell such that an elongated cell is produced.

Hereditary elliptocytosis may be divided into three clinical types: (1) simple elliptocytosis; (2) elliptocytosis with hemolysis, which is compensated by a hyperactive bone marrow; and (3) elliptocytosis with a hemolytic component. The grading of elliptocytosis is provided in Figure 3.7.

Target Cells (Leptocytes and Codocytes). Two types of target cells are seen. Usually, the red cells are of normal volume but are flat and have a slightly increased diameter, resulting in a decreased cell thickness. These forms appear often as hypochromic cells and are termed *leptocytes*. They are associated with cytoplasmic maturation defects and liver disease (particularly cirrhosis). This type of cell results from a reduction of cellular hemoglobin, which causes incomplete filling of the membrane envelope and promotes a thin, flat cell.

The more commonly recognized target cell possesses redistributed hemoglobin so that

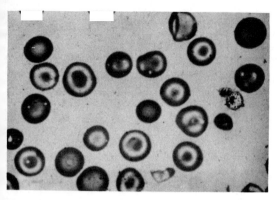

Figure 3.8. Target cells. Note that these cells have an increased diameter (× 875). (Reprinted from JB Henry [ed]. Clinical Diagnosis and Management by Laboratory Methods [17th ed]. Philadelphia: Saunders, 1984. P 608.)

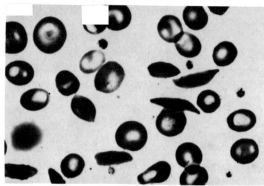

Figure 3.9. Sickle cell anemia. The elongated, pointed cells have greater density in the center than near the edge. (Reprinted from JB Henry [ed]. Clinical Diagnosis and Management by Laboratory Methods [17th ed]. Philadelphia: Saunders, 1984. P 679.)

only the periphery and the central region of the cell appear hemoglobinized. This central disposition of hemoglobin is the result of the cell membrane bulging, so that, on cross-section, the erythrocyte appears to resemble a Mexican hat. These are known as *codocytes*.

Target cells are produced when the intracellular hemoglobin contents are reduced without an accompanying decrease in the total membrane surface area (Figure 3.8). This reflects cholesterol abnormalities between the cell and the plasma and is due to the inhibition of the bile salts of cholesterol esterification. Target cells frequently are found in hemolytic anemias, hemoglobin C disease, thalassemia, iron-deficiency anemia, and liver disease, as well as after splenectomy.

Sickle Cells (Drepanocytes). A sickle cell is a red cell that undergoes bizarre changes in shape when exposed to an atmosphere reduced in oxygen. These morphologic changes take the form of elongations with irregular outlines and sharp terminal projections. Great individual variability among these types of cells is common, the intermediate forms possessing multiple, irregularly spaced spicules. Sickle cells are associated with the presence of hemoglobin S and are seen in sickle cell anemia (Figure 3.9). This cell shape is related to the formation of intracellular "tactoids" of hemoglobin S, which intertwine to form rigid projections along the cell periphery. As these tactoids align themselves into parallel arrays, the typical "holly-leaf" cell evolves. The ultimate alignment results in the classic thin, slightly curved sickle cell.

Most sickle cells reassume their original biconcave shape if reoxygenation occurs. However, a few may remain irreversibly sickled. Red-cell sickling is associated with reversible membrane changes. When sickled, erythrocytes leak potassium and gain sodium (Tosteson and Shea, 1952).

Other hemoglobins have been reported in association with sickling, including hemoglobin C_{HARLEM} (Bookchin and Davis, 1968), hemoglobin $C_{GEORGETOWN}$ (Pierce and Rath, 1963), hemoglobin$_{PORTO-ALEGRE}$ (Boneventura and Riggs, 1967), hemoglobin I (Schwartz, 1957), and hemoglobin Barts (Lie-Injo, 1961).

Schistocytes. Schistocytes are irregularly shaped, triangular, and spiculated red cells and frequently are smaller than mature cells (Figure 3.10). These erythrocytes are believed to be in the process of fragmentation and are removed from the circulation by the reticuloendothelial system. Schistocytes are associated primarily with hemolytic anemia resulting from either intra- or extracorpuscular defects, particularly microangiopathic anemias, disseminated intravascular coagulopathy, and hypersplenism. It is believed that the cells have undergone membrane injury by mechanical stress from artificial cardiac valves, fibrin deposits, invasive carcinomas, blood clots, and other foreign in vivo materials. Less commonly, schistocytes are seen during uremic crises, thermal burns, and some red-cell enzymopathies.

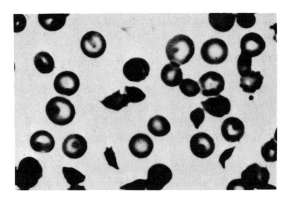

Figure 3.10. Microangiopathic hemolytic anemia showing schistocytes and crenated red cells (× 875). (Reprinted from JB Henry [ed]. Clinical Diagnosis and Management by Laboratory Methods [17th ed]. Philadelphia: Saunders, 1984. P 608.)

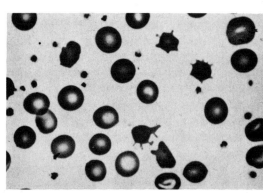

Figure 3.11. Acanthocytes. Note the long spicules, which tend to have bulbous ends (× 875). (Reprinted from JB Henry [ed]. Clinical Diagnosis and Management by Laboratory Methods [17th ed]. Philadelphia: Saunders, 1984. P 608.)

The recognition of these cells is most important, as they always signify pathologic changes in the hematopoietic system.

Stomatocytes. Stomatocytes are red cells characterized by an elliptic or elongated area of central pallor rather than a round one, giving the appearance of a mouth. When viewed from a lateral angle in wet preparations, the cell has a cup-shaped appearance. Stomatocytes are found mainly in three groups of disorders—namely, those characterized by an increase in red-cell sodium and a decrease in potassium, those possessing an Rh$_{null}$ phenotype, and those that do not fit into either of these groups. Stomatocytosis is seen particularly in liver disease (cirrhosis) and in hereditary stomatocytosis (autosomal dominant). This cell variant may be produced as a result of osmotic swelling through cation imbalance and also may be caused by redistribution of membrane phospholipids that results in increased lecithin levels.

Burr Cells. Burr cells are mature red cells similar in appearance to crenated cells, but they have an essentially normal cell volume and are characterized by pointed projections or intracellular vacuoles that usually are regularly spaced around the cell. They differ from acanthocytes in that the projections are more numerous and more uniform in size and are regularly spaced. Rupture of these vacuoles may produce a bihorned or helmet cell. The horned or burrlike projec-

tions are the product of incomplete cuts or similar injury to the cells, most frequently as a result of passage through a fibrin network. Burr cells have been associated with impaired renal function, pyruvic kinase deficiency, and thrombocytopenia. Together with Heinz bodies, they are seen in infants with drug-induced hemolytic anemias as well as in disseminated intravascular coagulopathy and hypersplenism and in patients undergoing chemotherapy.

Acanthocytes. The red cells known as *acanthocytes* possess several irregularly spaced, large, coarse spicules having sharp rather than blunted ends (Figure 3.11). The acanthocyte usually has fewer spicules than a crenated cell and can be distinguished from this artifact also by the irregularity of the projections.

Hereditary acanthocytosis is associated with a deficiency of the low-density β-lipoproteins (abetalipoproteinemia), resulting in the inability of the red cell to maintain a normal biconcave form. Analysis of the red-cell membrane shows abnormal lipid content, an increase in sphingomyelin, and a decrease in phosphatidylcholine. Acquired acanthocytosis usually is associated with the hemolytic anemia of cirrhosis (spur-cell anemia), deficiencies of vitamin E, uremia, retinal degeneration, and hypothyroidism. Acanthocytosis in liver disease, although morphologically indistinguishable from that seen in abetalipoproteinemia, is attributed to a marked increase in the cholesterol

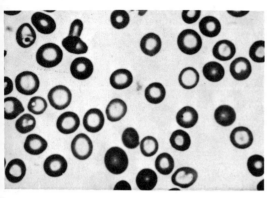

Figure 3.12. Iron-deficiency anemia. Most of the cells are markedly hypochromic and moderately microcytic (× 875). (Reprinted from JB Henry [ed]. Clinical Diagnosis and Management by Laboratory Methods [17th ed]. Philadelphia: Saunders, 1984. P 605.)

content and the cholesterol-to-phospholipid ratio of red-cell membranes. The osmotic fragility of the cell is normal or slightly decreased, whereas both the mechanical fragility and the autohemolysis tests show increased lysis.

Acanthocytes are associated also with the McLeod phenotype (lack of Kell blood group Kx).

Alterations in Hemoglobin Content and Color

Hypochromia. Hypochromic red cells are Romanowsky-stained erythrocytes that, when viewed microscopically, appear to possess greater center pallor than do normocytic cells. This can be attributable either to a lack of hemoglobin and, consequently, a reduction in the MCHC, or to abnormally thin erythrocytes associated with thalassemia and the presence of target cells. Severely hypochromic red cells frequently demonstrate MCHC levels of less than 30% and are associated with iron-deficiency states (Figure 3.12).

Inclusion Bodies

Basophilic Stippling (Punctate Basophilia). Punctate basophilia are red cells throughout which are randomly distributed fine to coarsely granular, blue-black inclusion bodies (Figure 3.13). The granule size is affected by the pH of the buffer used in staining (Romanowsky), a pH of less than 6.4 producing coarser features. These inclusions are artifactual condensations or precipitation of ribosomal RNA and are associated with disordered erythropoiesis and defective hemoglobin synthesis. Included among the causative disorders are sideroblastic anemia, toxic states (lead poisoning), acute hemolytic anemia, severe alcoholism, nuclear maturation defects, and polycythemia vera. In pathologic states, the degree of basophilic stippling does not parallel the severity of the disorder; in lead intoxication, approximately 5% of the red cells will show basophilic stippling by the time clinical symptoms become apparent (Griggs, 1964).

Pappenheimer Bodies (Siderocytes). Pappenheimer bodies (also known as *siderocytes*) stain a faint blue with a Romanowsky dye and represent ferritin aggregates frequently surrounded by a membrane (Diess and Kurth, 1969). These nonrefractive granules usually have a fine texture, can be as large as 2 μ in diameter, and are located near the periphery of the cell rather than being randomly dispersed. Positive identification is possible by staining for iron with Perl's reagent (the Prussian blue reaction).

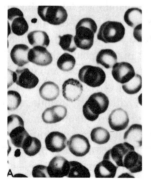
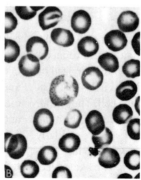

Figure 3.13. Basophilic stippling. One stippled cell is in the center of each field (× 875). (Reprinted from JB Henry [ed]. Clinical Diagnosis and Management by Laboratory Methods [17th ed]. Philadelphia: Saunders, 1984. P 609.)

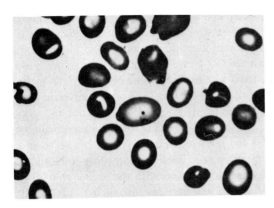

Figure 3.14. Megaloblastic anemia showing Howell-Jolly bodies. The macro-ovalocyte in the center of the field possesses four Howell-Jolly bodies, one in the cell center and three at the lower edge ($\times$ 875). (Reprinted from JB Henry [ed]. Clinical Diagnosis and Management by Laboratory Methods [17th ed]. Philadelphia: Saunders, 1984. P 609.)

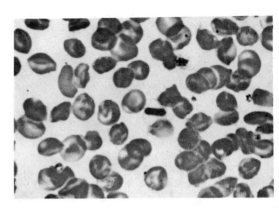

Figure 3.15. Hemoglobin C disease. The center cell possesses a large hemoglobin C crystal that is taking up all the hemoglobin and almost filling the cell. The red-cell membrane is still visible ($\times$ 875). (Reprinted from JB Henry [ed]. Clinical Diagnosis and Management by Laboratory Methods [17th ed]. Philadelphia: Saunders, 1984. P 680.)

Siderocytes are not found in normal blood but are seen in normal bone marrow. They are characteristically increased in hemolytic anemias and infections and following splenectomy. Other disorders in which they are found include sideroblastic anemias, megaloblastic anemias, alcoholism, and leukemia.

The pathophysiology of Pappenheimer bodies is most likely explained by accelerated red-cell mitotic division or impeded hemoglobin synthesis. Normally, iron not yet used in heme synthesis is found in the nucleated red-cell cytoplasm. Usually, this iron is fully consumed in heme production and is not present in mature red cells. When erythrocyte production is greatly enhanced, terminal mitotic divisions are occasionally missed, and incomplete hemoglobin synthesis results in these iron stores being carried over as Pappenheimer bodies or siderocytic granules. When these inclusions are seen in nucleated red cells, the erythrocytes are termed *sideroblasts*.

A second type of sideroblast is found in pathologic conditions. In this cell, the granules form a full or partial ring around the nucleus and are termed *ringed sideroblasts*. These cells are present in hereditary sideroblastic anemia and idiopathic refractory sideroblastic anemia and after various drug therapies.

Howell-Jolly Bodies. Howell-Jolly inclusion bodies appear as purple-violet nonrefractive masses when stained with Romanowsky dyes. They are seen singularly or in groups and often are situated in an eccentric position within the red cell. These inclusions are rounded aggregations of chromatin material staining Feulgen-positive for DNA. Howell-Jolly bodies are believed to originate with abnormal mitosis at the orthochromatic (metarubricyte) stage of erythrocyte development. When a single chromosome becomes detached and fails to be included in the formation of the nucleus, it remains free in the cytoplasm as a nuclear remnant. This predisposition may be a result of chemotherapy, rapid cellular division, or some type of impairment in normal nuclear chromatin function such as is seen in megaloblastic anemia. Howell-Jolly bodies are also seen in postsplenectomy patients and in some acute hemolytic anemias (Figure 3.14).The grading of these inclusion bodies is shown in Table 3.5.

Parasitized Red Cells. Parasites that may be found in red cells include certain spirochetes and leptospires, as well as *Plasmodium, Babesia, Toxoplasma, Trypanosoma, Leishmania,* and *Bartonella* species, microfilaria, and fungi such as *Blastomyces* and *Histoplasma* species. These infestations are reviewed on pages 103–112.

Hemoglobin C Crystals. Hemoglobin C crystals are characteristically tetragonal in shape and are birefringent in the polarizing microscope. They are

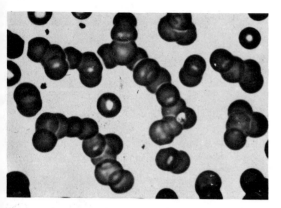

Figure 3.16. Rouleaux formation (× 875). (Reprinted from JB Henry [ed]. Clinical Diagnosis and Management by Laboratory Methods [17th ed]. Philadelphia: Saunders, 1984. P 610.)

found in as many as 10% of circulating cells following splenectomy in patients with homozygous hemoglobin C disease (Figure 3.15) but are rarely seen in patients who do not undergo splenectomy. They also are seen in hemoglobin SC disease, in which the crystals are likely to be elongated and varied (Hyun et al., 1975). Circulating homozygous hemoglobin C red cells contain oxygenated hemoglobin C with little or no hemoglobin F. This hemoglobin inhibits in vitro crystallization of hemoglobin C. Conversely, hemoglobin S accelerates in vitro crystallization of hemoglobin C (Lin et al., 1989).

Hemoglobin H Inclusions. Hemoglobin H inclusion bodies are a β-chain abnormality of the hemoglobin molecule. When the red cells are stained by a supravital stain, they show multiple pale blue, spheric inclusion bodies, varying in size from 0.5 to 1.0 μ. Most of the cells are affected. Hemoglobin H inclusions are unstable, and preparations should be made as soon as possible. The inclusions can be differentiated from reticulocytes by their number in each cell, and they are associated with α-thalassemia.

Heinz Bodies. Heinz bodies are irregular refractile granules 1–2 μ in diameter and often are found at the periphery of the red cell. They can be detected by supravital techniques using brilliant cresyl blue or methyl violet but not by routine Romanowsky stains. They are easily seen as refractile bodies in wet, un-

stained preparations and are believed to be aggregations of denatured globin originally intended for incorporation into a hemoglobin molecule. It should be noted that Heinz-body preparations should never be fixed with methyl alcohol or stained with methyl alcohol–based dyes, as such procedures remove the inclusions from the red cells.

The presence of Heinz bodies in abnormal numbers indicates red-cell injury and can serve as an index of existing anemia. Many drug-induced anemias are associated with the presence of these inclusions, and they can also be found in the thalassemias, unstable hemoglobins, and in intracellular hemoglobin destruction secondary to oxidative damage or red-cell enzymopathies.

Other Abnormalities

Rouleaux Formation. Rouleaux formation is a descriptive term given to red cells that become aligned in aggregates resembling a stack of coins (Figure 3.16). This phenomenon frequently is seen in association with hyperproteinemic disorders such as myeloma and macroglobinemia but can also be found in chronic inflammatory diseases and as an artifact in thick regions of the blood smear.

Polychromia. Polychromatic red cells are those erythrocytes that stain a bluish-red with Romanowsky dyes. Usually, the cells are slightly larger than normal and, when stained with a supravital dye, are revealed to be reticulocytes. The diffuse basophilia seen is produced by the RNA present in the cell. *Polychromasia* is associated with reticulocytosis and bone marrow activity. It can be found in increased levels in any bone marrow–responsive anemia.

Autoagglutination. Red cells may be seen in aggregates of varying sizes in blood smears (Figure 3.17). These aggregates may be the result of the cold autoantibodies seen in cold hemagglutinin disease and paroxysmal cold hemoglobinuria.

Artifacts

Hyperchromia. The state of hyperchromia is physiologically impossible, as it postulates a hemoglobin-supersaturated red cell. Hence, the term should be avoided. Cells that appear to be hyperchromic are

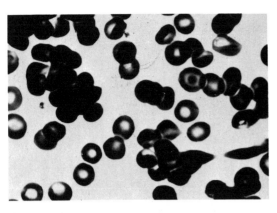

Figure 3.17. Autoagglutination. Blood from an individual with a high-titer cold agglutinin. (Reprinted from JB Henry [ed]. Clinical Diagnosis and Management by Laboratory Methods [17th ed]. Philadelphia: Saunders, 1984. P 610.)

usually large and fully hemoglobinized with no central pallor and usually found at the periphery of the blood smear.

Cabot's Rings. Cabot's rings are blue figure-eight or circular bodies once believed to be related to Howell-Jolly bodies. They currently are thought to be artifacts resulting from damage to the lipoprotein of the cell stroma. Cabot's rings are invisible by phase-contrast microscopy, but they can be stained with Romanowsky dyes.

Crenated Red Cells. When blood smears dry slowly, the red-cell envelope becomes exposed to a hypertonic environment, causing typical seration of the cell. Occasionally, the wrinkling is accompanied by evenly distributed spiny projections, each spicule having a blunt end. Differentiation of these *crenated red cells* from acanthocytes is made by the distribution and morphologic features of the projections. Crenated cells have no clinical significance.

Physiologic Classification of Anemias

See Table 3.6 for a physiologic classification of anemias.

Increased Red-Cell Destruction (Hemolytic Disease)

In hemolytic diseases born of intracellular defects, red cells exhibit a shortened life span because of intrinsic defects in the cell itself. Examples of such disorders include abnormalities in the Embden-Meyerhof and pentose-phosphate glycolytic pathways, quantitative and qualitative disorders of globin synthesis, and abnormalities of the red-cell membrane.

Other hemolytic diseases are the result of extracellular defects, in which the red cells are destroyed because of external factors that cause hemolysis. Included are intracorpuscular parasitic infections (e.g., malaria), antibodies, the action of certain drugs, chemical or physical agents, and abnormal splenic sequestration and activity. These defects also occur in association with lymphomas and other neoplasms.

Increased Blood Loss

Excessive blood loss is an obvious cause of anemia. However, both the speed and degree of blood loss are reflected in laboratory results. Anemia resulting from hemorrhage is divided principally into that caused by acute loss and that caused by chronic loss.

Inadequate Production of Red Cells

Various conditions can result in inadequate production of red cells.

Nutritional Anemias. In nutritional anemias, essential substances required for erythropoiesis are either reduced or lacking. Examples of such substances include iron, vitamin B_{12}, folic acid, proteins, and trace elements such as copper, cobalt, pyridoxine (vitamin B_6), and niacin. Chronic deprivation of vitamin A results in an anemia similar to that of iron deficiency. The MCV and MCHC are reduced, and anisocytosis and poikilocytosis often are present. Despite reduced serum iron levels, liver and bone marrow iron stains are increased, and serum transferrin is usually normal or decreased. The administration of oral iron does not correct the anemia.

Vitamin B_6 deficiency can occasionally be found in patients receiving antituberculous medication.

Table 3.6. Physiologic Classification of Anemias

I. Macrocytic anemias
  A. Nonmegaloblastic
    1. Disorders associated with accelerated erythropoiesis
      a. Hemolytic anemia
      b. Posthemorrhagic anemia
    2. Disorders associated with increased membrane surface area
      a. Hepatic disease
      b. Obstructive jaundice
      c. Postsplenectomy
    3. Myelodysplastic anemia
      a. Aplastic anemia
      b. 5q–/refractory anemia
      c. Acquired sideroblastic anemia
      d. Hereditary dyserythropoietic anemia: Type 1
    4. Alcoholism
    5. Hypothyroidism
    6. Myelophthisic anemia
    7. Chronic obstructive pulmonary disease
  B. Megaloblastic
    1. Vitamin B_{12} deficiency
      a. Dietary deficiency
      b. Lack of intrinsic factor
        (1) Pernicious anemia (congenital and adult)
        (2) Gastric surgery
        (3) Ingestion of caustic materials
      c. Functionally abnormal intrinsic factor
      d. Biological competition
        (1) Small-bowel bacterial overgrowth
        (2) Fish tapeworm disease
      e. Familial selective vitamin B_{12} malabsorption
      f. Chronic pancreatic disease
      g. Zollinger-Ellison syndrome
      h. Hemodialysis
      i. Ileum disease
        (1) Ileal resection and bypass
        (2) Regional enteritis
    2. Folate deficiency
      a. Dietary deficiency
      b. Increased requirements
        (1) Alcoholism and cirrhosis
        (2) Pregnancy
        (3) Infancy
        (4) Diseases associated with rapid cell growth
      c. Congenital folate malabsorption
      d. Drug induced
      e. Intestinal resection
    3. Combined folate and vitamin B_{12} deficiency
      a. Tropical sprue
      b. Gluten-sensitive enteropathy
    4. Inherited disorders of DNA synthesis
      a. Orotic anemia
      b. Lesch-Nyhan syndrome
      c. Thiamine-response megaloblastic anemia
      d. Deficiency of enzymes required for folate metabolism
        (1) N5-methyl-tetrahydrofolate transferase

          (2) Forminimotransferase

          (3) Dihydrofolate reductase

    5. Drug- and toxin-induced

       a. Folate antagonists (methotrexate)

       b. Purine antagonists (6-mercatopurine)

       c. Pyrimidine antagonists (cytosine arabinoside)

       d. Alkylating agents (cyclophosphamide)

       e. Nitrous oxide

       f. Arsenic

       g. Chlordane

    6. Erythroleukemia

II. Microcytic anemias

    1. Disorders of iron metabolism

       a. Iron-deficiency anemia

       b. Anemia of chronic anemia

       c. Atransferrinemia

       d. Shahidi-Nathan-Diamond syndrome

       e. Antibodies to transferrin receptors

    2. Disorders of globin synthesis

       a. Thalassemia

       b. Hemoglobin E trait and disease

       c. Hemoglobin C disease

       d. Unstable hemoglobin disease

    3. Disorders of porphyrin and heme synthesis

       a. Defective δ-aminolevulinic acid synthesis

       b. Vitamin B_6 deficiency

       c. Defective vitamin B_6 metabolism induced by drugs or toxins

       d. Defective ALA synthetase activity

       e. Deficiency of coproporphyrinogen oxidase

       f. Deficiency of heme synthesis

       g. Lead intoxication

III. Normocytic normochromic anemias

    1. Anemia associated with appropriate increased red-cell production

       a. Hemolytic

       b. Posthemorrhagic

    2. Anemia with impaired bone marrow response

       a. Intrinsic bone marrow disease

          (1) Hypoplasia

          (2) Disorders of bone marrow infiltration (leukemia, myeloma, other myelophthisic disorders)

       b. Dyserythropoietic anemia

       c. Myelodysplastic anemia

    3. Decreased erythropoietin secretion

       a. Impaired source (renal insufficiency, liver disease)

       b. Reduced stimulation (anemia of endocrine deficiency)

       c. Protein calorie malnutrition

       d. Anemia of chronic disease

    4. Deficiency of iron

       a. Iron-deficiency anemia

       b. Anemia of chronic disorders

          Anemia of space flights

Such patients develop a microcytic anemia that can be corrected with large doses of pyridoxine.

Copper deficiency produces a microcytic anemia that does not respond to iron therapy. Hypoferremia and neutropenia also are found often. The diagnosis is made by the presence of a low serum ceruloplasmin or copper level.

Zinc deficiency occurs in hemolytic anemias such as thalassemia and sickle cell anemia. Human zinc deficiency may produce impaired wound healing and immunologic abnormalities, but there is little evidence that isolated zinc deficiency produces anemia.

Bone Marrow Atrophy. For a variety of reasons, the bone marrow sometimes ceases or reduces production of red-cell precursors. This aplasia can be directed either solely at the erythrocytic stem cells (pure red-cell aplasia) or at the total hematopoietic system (aplastic anemia), at which point all formed cellular elements are quantitatively reduced. Aplastic anemia is often secondary to the action of chemical or physical agents and is seen as an idiopathic form as well as an inherited characteristic.

Pure red-cell aplasia can result from a carcinoma of the thymus (thymoma), secondary to a variety of chemical and drug exposures, and from exposure to viral infections.

Bone Marrow Infiltrates. Bone marrow infiltrates cause a form of anemia consisting of underproduction of red cells that results from a "crowding out" of erythropoietic tissue in the bone marrow by neoplastic cells. Examples of such disorders include leukemia, lymphoma, myeloma, myelofibrosis, sarcoma, and primary or secondary carcinoma.

Other Causes of Inadequate Red-Cell Production. Anemia is a common finding of *endocrine disorders*, which affect the thyroid gland, adrenal glands, gonads, and pituitary gland. Anemia caused by inadequate red cell production is associated with *chronic renal disease*. This anemia often is a consequence of bone marrow failure resulting from a reduction in erythropoietin production. Examples of *chronic inflammatory diseases* that cause anemia of underproduction include infections, collagen diseases, and granulomatous disorders. Finally, cirrhosis of the liver is a cause of inadequate red-cell production.

Chapter 4

Macrocytic Anemias

As discussed in Chapter 3, the *macrocytic anemias* can be divided into two categories: those that are not megaloblastic and those that demonstrate megaloblastic changes in both the bone marrow and the peripheral blood. The nonmegaloblastic group includes anemias in which the red cell size is increased but there is a normoblastic morphologic appearance. Examples include anemias secondary to alcoholism and certain hemolytic processes.

In this chapter, we are concerned with the megaloblastic macrocytic anemias. The pathophysiology of these anemias is associated with two primary abnormalities: ineffective erythropoiesis and a moderate hemolysis of circulating erythrocytes. The etiologic classification can be divided into three main groups: (1) those anemias due to vitamin B_{12} deficiency, (2) those due to folic acid deficiency, and (3) those that are unresponsive to treatment with either of these essential nutrients and result from a variety of causes.

Biochemistry

Megaloblastic red cells result from impairment of DNA synthesis (Figure 4.1). Such impairment results in arrest at the G_2 stage of mitotic interphase and in the production of macrocytosis, giant metamyelocytes, and neutrophil hypersegmentation (Hoffbrand et al., 1976). Classically, megaloblastic red cells are caused by reductions in the production of the DNA precursor deoxythymidylate (dTMP). This substance is derived from deoxyuridylate (dUMP), the rate of the reaction being controlled by the conversion of 5–10-methylene tetrahydrofolate to dihydrofolate (DHF). This, in turn, is reduced to tetrahydrofolate (THF) by the action of dihydrofolate reductase (DHFR), thus providing an additional supply of THF for the synthesis of 5–10-methylene tetrahydrofolate. Additional THF is provided from 5-methyl tetrafolate during the conversion of homocysteine to methionine. This reaction requires that methyl B_{12} be present as a cofactor. Consequently, megaloblastic cells can arise from either a direct folate deficiency or from a vitamin B_{12} deficiency that leads to a folate deficiency. The disturbance of folate metabolism caused by a deficiency of methyl B_{12} is termed the *folate trap* (Hoffbrand and Walters, 1972) and results in accumulation of 5-methyl tetrafolate that fails to be converted to THF in the folate cycle.

The folate pathway is impaired also by some drugs, particularly those used in cancer chemotherapy. Methotrexate and aminopterin exhibit such inhibitory effects, as they block the action of DHFR on DHF, thereby impairing DNA synthesis.

Laboratory Findings

Megaloblasts are characterized by asynchronous maturation between the nuclear protein and the cytoplasm. This is due to defective DNA synthesis (see preceding discussion) and a normal or relatively normal cytoplasmic development. Such asynchrony results in a classic morphologic triad of

45

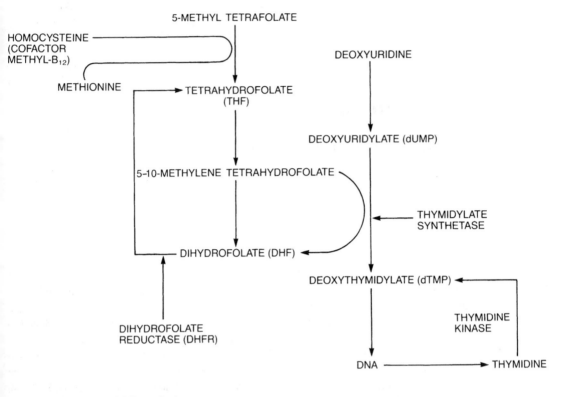

Figure 4.1. Intracellular DNA synthesis.

increased cell size, immaturity of the nuclear protein, and relatively early hemoglobinization of the cell. Additionally, leukocytes frequently exhibit increases in size, particularly the metamyelocytes and band forms, and megakaryocytes often show deficient granulation. Consequently, the platelet count often is decreased.

The mature red cells usually are macrocytic, having a mean cell volume (MCV) in excess of 100 fl. Macro-ovalocytes are also present. Reticulocytes are frequently decreased, reflecting ineffective erythropoiesis. Hemoglobin levels are moderately decreased and can be severely depressed in untreated patients. Hemoglobin levels of less than 7 g/dl are often accompanied by orthochromatic or polychromatic megaloblasts in the peripheral blood.

Besides showing size increases, granulocytes are often seen as multilobulated cells termed *macropolycytes*. The bone marrow is usually cellular and clearly megaloblastic. The myeloid-to-erythroid ratio is reduced from approximately 3:1 to 1:1, and mitotic figures can be seen in metaphase. The megaloblastic hyperplastic bone marrow also includes

large granulocytes. Metabolic and catabolic cell products are present in the blood as well. Bilirubin, iron, lactate dehydrogenase isoenzymes I and II, and muramidase (lysozyme) are increased in the serum, and potassium and uric levels are reduced.

Classification

Vitamin B₁₂ Deficiency

1. Decreased vitamin B_{12} intake
   a. Dietary, usually seen only in true vegetarians
   b. Impaired absorption, such as in pernicious anemia
   c. Malabsorption (familial, drug-induced, sprue, celiac disease, gastrectomy)
   d. Competition from parasites (fish tapeworm [blind loop syndrome]) and bacterial
2. Increased vitamin B_{12} requirements
   a. Pregnancy
   b. Increased cellular proliferation (tumors)
   c. Hyperthyroidism

3. Impaired utilization
   a. Red-cell enzymopathy
   b. Abnormal vitamin B_{12}–binding protein (transcobalamin II [TC II])
   c. Nitrous oxide administration
   d. Lack of transport protein (TC II)

Folate Deficiency

1. Decrease in folate intake
   a. Dietary, usually a lack of green vegetables
   b. Alcoholism
   c. Impaired absorption due to sprue and celiac disease
2. Increased folate requirements
   a. Pregnancy
   b. Increased cellular proliferation (tumors)
   c. Miscellaneous states (homocystinuria, hyperthyroidism)
3. Impaired utilization: folic acid antagonists (methotrexate, aminopterin, dilantin, trimethoprim, pyrimethamine)

Megaloblastic Anemia Unresponsive to Vitamin B_{12}–Folate Therapy

1. Metabolic inhibitors
   a. Drug-induced disorders: purine antagonists (6-mercaptopurine), pyrimidine antagonists (5-fluorouracil), alkylating agents (cyclophosphamide)
2. Hereditary orotic aciduria (inherited disorder of pyrimidine metabolism producing a megaloblastic anemia and increased urinary excretion of orotic acid)
3. Unknown causes
   a. Pyridoxine-responsive megaloblastic anemia
   b. Erythremic myelosis (erythroleukemia or Di Guglielmo syndrome)

Biochemistry

The metabolically active form of folic acid THF is a cofactor, in many reactions, for the transfer of one carbon unit. One of the most important of these reactions is the methylation of deoxyuridylate to thymidylate, an essential step in DNA synthesis.

Vitamin B_{12} serves as a cofactor and is important in purine synthesis, serving to convert newly absorbed N5-methyl-tetrahydrofolate to tetrahydrofolate. It likewise is important in lipid metabolism. Deficiencies of either folate or vitamin B_{12} inhibit DNA synthesis, most severely affecting rapidly dividing cells, particularly erythropoietic precursors. This causes abnormal maturation of these elements, producing a megaloblastic anemia.

The involvement of vitamin B_{12} in lipid metabolism causes an accumulation of abnormal lipids in the central nervous system, contributing often to neurologic abnormalities in pernicious anemia.

Folate is absorbed principally in the proximal jejunum and is converted to N5-methyl-tetrahydrofolate in the intestinal cells. It is transported bound to a serum carrier protein to the liver, which is the main storage site. With normal metabolic requirements, liver storage is limited to a 3- to 4-month supply. Vitamin B_{12} is bound first to R proteins in the stomach and then to intrinsic factor (IF) in the duodenum as R factors, which are degraded by pancreatic enzymes. The B_{12}-IF complex is absorbed selectively in the ileum where there are IF receptors. In the serum, vitamin B_{12} is bound principally to a carrier protein, transcobalamin (TC I). A lesser amount but highly active form is bound to TC II, and a trace is bound to TC III. The transcobalamins are produced by intestinal, hepatic, and hematopoietic cells. Vitamin B_{12} is stored in the liver and other tissues, the total body stores amounting to a 5- to 6-year supply.

Features of Specific Megaloblastic Anemias

Vitamin B_{12} Deficiency

Dietary Deficiency

The dietary form of vitamin B_{12}–deficiency megaloblastic anemia is rare. Only strict vegetarians who avoid all meat, eggs, and milk have been reported to develop this form of anemia (Winawer and Streiff, 1967).

Pernicious Anemia

Pernicious anemia is a megaloblastic disorder associated with a decrease in absorption of vitamin B_{12} caused by gastric atrophy, which, in turn, causes the

Table 4.1. Four Important Human Cobalamins

Cyanocobalamin (vitamin B_{12})
Hydroxocobalamin (analog of cyanocobalamin)
Adenosylcobalamin (functions as an acceptor-donor of hydrogen)
Methylcobalamin (participates in the cobalamin-dependent synthesis of methionine in bacteria and animal cells)

---

gastric parietal cells to cease or decrease their secretion of IF.

Nutritional Requirements. Vitamin B_{12} is the only vitamin exclusively synthesized by microorganisms. It is not produced by animals or in plants. The average diet contains 5–30 µg of the vitamin, of which approximately 1–5 µg is absorbed. Total body stores are between 1 and 5 µg in the adult, and the daily dietary requirement is 2–5 µg, with a daily loss of 0.1% of the total body pool. Consequently, a deficiency will not be apparent for several years following cessation of vitamin B_{12} intake.

Nomenclature and Structure of Vitamin B_{12}. The structure of vitamin B_{12} has two major features: a resemblance to the porphyrin ring and a nucleotide lying nearly perpendicular to the planar group. The porphyrin ring–like moiety contains four pyrrole groups linked to a cobalt atom. These compounds are termed *corroids* (cobalamins) and are synthesized from δ-aminolevulinic acid. Four important cobalamins are listed in Table 4.1.

Intestinal Absorption: Intrinsic Factor. Two mechanisms exist for absorption of vitamin B_{12}. One is inefficient and passive and does not require IF. Only 1% of oral vitamin is absorbed by this mechanism. The second is efficient and active, occurring in the ileum and requiring IF. This is an alkali-stable glycoprotein possessing the ability to bind with cobalamin with high affinity. This glycoprotein is secreted by the parietal cells of the gastric mucosa, its secretion being enhanced by the presence of histamine and gastrin. IF levels usually parallel hydrochloric acid secretion.

Bound vitamin alters the configuration of the molecule, making it more resistant to proteolytic digestion. Gastric juice contains several vitamin B_{12}–binding proteins. There are two main types, their classification depending on their electrophoretic mobility—S (slow) protein and R (rapid) protein.

R proteins are found in serum, leukocytes, saliva, gastric juice, and most body cells. They are known also as *TC I* and *TC III* and are believed to be the prime vehicle in transporting vitamin B_{12} and in preventing loss of cobalamins in the urine.

TC II is an S protein whose function is also to bind vitamin B_{12}. However, TC II takes up the vitamin before TC I, and the TC II–vitamin B_{12} complex is removed from the plasma within hours. By comparison, the TC I–vitamin B_{12} complex is cleared slowly from the plasma, with a half-life on the order of 9–12 days. TC II levels often are decreased in myeloproliferative diseases and, occasionally, in pernicious anemia.

Autoimmune Aspects. There is documented evidence that pernicious anemia develops as a result of a genetically determined autoimmune disease (Chanarin and James, 1974). Antibodies against parietal cells (>80%) and against IF (>55%) are commonly present in individuals with pernicious anemia (Ungar, 1968; Chanarin, 1969). These antibodies are known as either *blocking* or *binding* antibodies.

Blocking antibodies are the most common type, and they prevent vitamin B_{12} from forming a complex with IF. Binding antibodies usually are present together with blocking antibodies. This form can be subdivided into those that bind equally well with IF or the IF–vitamin B_{12} complex and those that have a greater affinity for the IF–vitamin B_{12} complex than for pure IF. Parietal cell antibodies, although frequently present in patients with pernicious anemia, are not diagnostic of the disease. Normal subjects—particularly women over 55, patients with simple atrophic gastritis, and some individuals with thyroid disease—produce these antibodies. In contrast, the presence of circulating IF antibodies is diagnostic of pernicious anemia and is uniformly lacking in patients with atrophic gastritis.

Clinical and Laboratory Features. The onset of the disease is gradual. The disorder affects either gender, particularly individuals in the 40- to 80-year-old group. Northern European peoples, especially Scandinavians, appear to have the highest incidence. The main clinical features include glossitis, achlorhydria after histamine stimulation, weakness, anorexia, and complaints of minor neurologic disturbances. When the anemia is severe, the patient's skin possesses a lemon-yellow tint: the sclerae may be yellowish, and some mild icterus may be seen.

The peripheral blood picture shows an increase in the MCV (frequently >110 fl), a normal mean cell hemoglobin concentration (MCHC) (unless a coexisting iron deficiency is present), and a slightly raised mean cell hemoglobin (MCH) level. The hemoglobin is often 6–10 g/dl, and the red-cell count is reduced to 2×10^{12}/liter. There is marked anisocytosis, poikilocytosis, and basophilic stippling. Leukopenia and thrombocytopenia are commonly found, especially in untreated cases. The leukopenia, due primarily to a granulocytopenia, often is accompanied by a "shift to the right," in which many of the granulocytes exhibit hypersegmentation and appear as giant cells, termed *macropolycytes*.

The bone marrow is hyperplastic, and the predominant cell is the megaloblast at all stages of maturation. Granulocytes are characteristically large at all stages of development. Megakaryocytes are commonly seen, with bizarre nuclei possessing unattached nuclear lobes. A variety of nonspecific chromosomal abnormalities have been described in bone marrow cells. Individual chromosomes may be elongated, and the frequency of randomly distributed gaps and breaks is increased. On occasion, hypodiploidy has been reported.

Biochemically, there are low concentrations of vitamin B_{12} in the serum, increased excretion of methylmalonic acid in the urine, and a reduction in the excretion of radioactive vitamin B_{12} in the urine on performance of the Schilling test. This test depends on saturating the capacity of the serum to bind vitamin B_{12} so that the tagged vitamin will be excreted in the urine (see later).

The deoxyuridine (dU) suppression test (Herbert et al., 1973) can also be used to distinguish between vitamin B_{12} and folate deficiencies. If dU is added to aspirated bone marrow cultures, it becomes incorporated into DNA. This normally suppresses the rate of incorporation of ^{3}H-thymidine into these cells. When the dU test is carried out on patients with megaloblastic anemia, the incorporation of the dU into DNA is impaired and can be measured by the relative increase in incorporation of ^{3}H-thymidine. This abnormality is corrected by the addition of folic acid in either vitamin B_{12} or folate deficiencies or by the addition of vitamin B_{12} in vitamin B_{12} deficiencies. The dU suppression test is corrected when treatment has returned the bone marrow morphologic features and the serum and red-cell vitamin levels to normal. However, the test remains abnormal in lymphocytes for as long as 84 days after successful therapy because of the relatively long life span and low turnover of these cells in vivo and their delayed response to treatment.

The Schilling test has classically been used to distinguish among IF deficiency (pernicious anemia–postgastrectomy state), malabsorption, and blind loop syndrome as the cause of vitamin B_{12} deficiency. The test is carried out in three stages. First, a loading dose of vitamin B_{12} is given intramuscularly, and this is followed by an oral dose of radiolabeled vitamin B_{12}. The urinary excretion of labeled vitamin B_{12} over 24 hours is then measured and should exceed 7% of the total in normal individuals.

The second step is to repeat the test if the results appear low, this time with the addition of an oral dose of IF.

Finally, if the results are still low, blind loop syndrome should be suspected, and the test repeated with IF after 3–5 days of an oral broad-spectrum antibiotic. Correction of the first phase of the test by the oral IF and oral broad-spectrum antibiotic is consistent with blind loop syndrome. If all testing, including the use of IF and antibiotics, produces abnormal results, the diagnosis is malabsorption syndrome.

Other common nonspecific findings in pernicious anemia include increased serum bilirubin, lactic dehydrogenase, and iron levels, and decreased serum haptoglobin, alkaline phosphatase, and uric acid concentration.

Malabsorption of Vitamin B_{12}

Disordered absorption of vitamin B_{12} may be due to tropical sprue, celiac disease, or familial selective malabsorption syndrome. Tropical sprue is an intestinal malabsorption disorder resulting in a depletion of both vitamin B_{12} and folate. Celiac disease (idiopathic steatorrhea) is caused by a sensitivity to gluten, producing abnormal small-bowel mucosa that results in malabsorption of vita-

min B_{12}. Like tropical sprue, folate is also implicated in this disorder and, consequently, the presence of megaloblasts is a nonspecific finding and
does not differentiate these disorders. Other malabsorption disorders include regional enteritis,
anatomic abnormalities resulting from surgery, di-
verticulitis, and the ingestion of drugs such as
neomycin, para-aminosalicylic acid, and colchicine.

Competition for Vitamin B_{12}

Competition for vitamin B_{12} can occur in blind loop
syndrome and following ingestion of the fish tapeworm. Blind loop syndrome can follow partial gastrectomy and involves the formation of a cul-de-sac
into which bile and pancreatic secretions are emp-
tied. If this takes place, bacterial overgrowth commonly results, with a concomitant reduction of
vitamin B_{12} caused by bacterial uptake.

Fish tapeworm, a parasite acquired by the ingestion of raw tainted fish, produces a megaloblastic
anemia because of the parasite's ability to absorb
vitamin B_{12}.

Increased Requirements

Disorders characterized by increased metabolic demands for vitamin B_{12} can produce megaloblastic
hematologic pictures. They include pregnancy and
hyperthyroidism and disorders associated with rapid
cellular proliferation (neoplasms and so on).

Impaired Utilization

Defective transportation of vitamin B_{12} because of a
congenital deficiency of TC II is a rare condition
that produces a severe and potentially fatal disorder.
Acquired deficiency of this transport protein, as
well as an abnormally structured molecule that is
unable to bind with vitamin B_{12}, has also been described. Exposure to nitrous oxide for periods of 24
hours can produce megaloblastic effects resulting
from the active cobalt-containing coenzymes of vitamin B_{12} that are oxidized to a nonfunctional form
(Cullen et al., 1979).

Increased serum vitamin B_{12} levels often are
caused by an increase in serum transcobalamins,
frequently associated with myeloproliferative disorders (chronic myeloid leukemia, polycythemia
vera, etc.).

Folate Deficiency

The clinical findings in folate deficiency closely resemble those in vitamin B_{12} deficiency, the one exception being the absence or the rare finding of
neurologic disturbances. In humans, folic acid is absorbed more readily from the upper than from the
lower jejunum. Such absorption is rapid, a rise usually being detected within minutes and a folate peak
within 1 or 2 hours after ingestion.

Dietary Deficiency

Dietary deficiency of folates is found principally in
Southeast Asia and Africa but can also occur when
vegetables are allowed to cook for long periods, destroying folates (Hoffbrand, 1971a). This deficiency
can also be found in infants.

Deficient intake is seen in chronic alcoholics, because these individuals generally consume a diet
low in folate. In alcoholics, megaloblastosis may
ensue from malabsorption of folate and inadequate
storage resulting from cirrhosis of the liver (Halsted
et al., 1967).

Malabsorption of Folic Acid

Impaired absorption of folic acid resulting from disorders of the jejunal mucosa, such as in tropical
sprue and celiac disease, also produces a megaloblastic anemia. The laboratory abnormalities in
anemia from this cause include increase in stool fat,
defective D-xylose absorption, and reductions in
serum carotene and vitamin A levels.

Increased Requirements

Physiologic Causes. Pregnancy is the most common cause of folate deficiency, resulting from the
increased physiologic demands on the mother. In
infancy, folate demands are 4–10 times those of an
adult, based on body weight (Sullivan et al., 1966).

Cellular Proliferation. Folate is required as a
coenzyme for reactions involving purine and
pyrimidine synthesis. Consequently, folate
turnover is increased whenever cell turnover is increased. As folate is not reused as efficiently as
iron, a deficiency ultimately results. These excessive demands are seen principally in hemolytic

anemias, myelosclerosis, malignant disease, and inflammatory disease.

Chronic hemolytic anemias, such as sickle cell anemia, thalassemia, congenital spherocytosis, autoimmune hemolytic anemia, and paroxysmal nocturnal hemoglobinuria, have been implicated in folate depletion (Hoffbrand, 1971b). Folate deficiency and megaloblastosis have also been reported in 66% of patients with myelofibrosis (Hoffbrand and Chanarin, 1968) because of excessive turnover of primitive hematopoietic cells in the bone marrow and at extramedullary sites. Depressions of serum folate are seen in leukemia, lymphoma, myeloma, and other neoplastic disorders, although in such situations it is rare for a severe megaloblastic anemia to develop.

Impaired Utilization Caused by Antifolate Drugs

Drugs used in the treatment of malignant diseases, bacterial infections, and malaria can inhibit folate metabolism and DNA synthesis and consequently produce a megaloblastic response if the deficiency is sufficiently severe. These drugs act principally as DHFR inhibitors and ultimately interfere with the production of THF synthesis. Methotrexate and aminopterin are examples of such powerful inhibitors. Other drugs inhibiting DHFR include the antimalarial agents pyrimethamine and trimethoprim.

Megaloblastic Anemia Unresponsive to Vitamin B_{12}–Folate Therapy

Metabolic Inhibitors

Megaloblastosis occasionally fails to respond to specific therapy in three general groups of disorders: (1) those that ensue after therapy with antimetabolites that interfere with folate synthesis (see preceding discussion), (2) those associated with inborn errors of metabolism, and (3) refractory megaloblastic anemia.

Antifolate drugs such as methotrexate and aminopterin were discussed earlier, but three other megaloblastic anemia–inducing medications also exist. *Purine antagonists,* such as 6-mercaptopurine, thioguanine, and azathioprine, inhibit RNA and DNA synthesis, causing bone marrow depression with resultant leukopenia, anemia, and thrombocytopenia. Before this hypoplasia is evident, the marrow exhibits a mild megaloblastosis despite normal serum folate and vitamin B_{12} levels. Such a reaction generally is unresponsive to treatment with either folate or vitamin B_{12}.

Pyrimidine inhibitors function either by blocking methylation of dUMP (see Figure 4.1) or by blocking de novo synthesis of the pyrimidine ring.

Chemotherapeutic drugs that act in the blocking of dUMP include 5-fluoro-2-deoxyuridine and 5-fluorouracil, and those that act by interfering with pyrimidine ring synthesis include 6-azauridine.

Other commonly used megaloblastic anemia–producing drugs include cytosine arabinoside (inhibition of ribonucleotide reductase) and hydroxyurea.

Inborn Errors of Metabolism

Hereditary orotic aciduria is a rare disease of pyrimidine metabolism exhibiting a refractory megaloblastic anemia and an increased urinary excretion of orotic acid.

Erythroleukemia (Di Guglielmo Syndrome)

Megaloblasts are seen in erythroleukemia, which is described on page 148.

Chapter 5

Microcytic Hypochromic Anemias

This chapter discusses the microcytic hypochromic anemias. Microcytic red cells can be arbitrarily classified as those erythrocytes with mean cell volumes (MCVs) of less than 80 fl. Microcytic anemias include a wide variety of disorders, including those secondary to nutritional deficiencies caused by alterations of heme synthesis, and the thalassemias, which are anemias resulting from abnormal globin synthesis. The thalassemias are discussed in Chapter 7.

Iron-Deficiency Anemia

The main source of iron for hemoglobin metabolism is obtained by recycling hemoglobin from effete red cells. The amount of iron lost by excretion is balanced by the dietary intake of ferric salts. Prior to absorption, ferric iron is reduced to the ferrous state with gastric acid and then absorbed by the upper and middle portions of the small intestine. If the dietary intake of ferric iron is reduced, as it is in the newborn period, or if ferric iron is not absorbed in sufficient quantities, a microcytic hypochromic anemia will develop once all the body reserves of iron are depleted.

Inadequate intake of iron is also seen in childhood. During periods of rapid growth, the diet may provide insufficient iron. Other factors, such as intestinal parasites, may contribute to this iron deficiency. In adults, the most common cause of iron deficiency is hemorrhage, particularly in men. In women, iron deficiency is commonly due to men-

struation and blood losses that occurred in past pregnancies and were never replaced.

Iron-deficiency anemia can be defined as the final stage in the progressive depletion of the body's iron stores. In the early stages of the anemia, iron stores in the reticuloendothelial cells of the bone marrow are often reduced or even absent, but the serum iron and transferrin saturation in the peripheral blood are normal. Anemia is absent at this juncture, because at this stage the iron stores have been sufficient to provide normal iron transportation in the metabolism of hemoglobin.

The next physiologic stage is the absence of iron stores and a reduction in the serum iron and transferrin saturation. This takes place in the absence of a demonstrable anemia and reflects the delicate balance of the iron transport system in meeting hemoglobin requirements. The final stage in the cycle is an overt iron deficiency, exhibiting lack of iron stores, low serum iron and transferrin saturation, and a microcytic hypochromic anemia that is reflected in reduced values for MCV and the mean cell hemoglobin concentration (MCHC). In addition, there are abnormal red-cell morphologic features.

The clinical manifestations of the anemia can be divided into two groups: those related to decreases in oxygen-carrying capacity and those related to depressions of hemoglobin concentration. Symptoms include fatigue and pallor and, on occasion, an unusual craving to eat ice, dirt, and clay known as *pica*. Other findings include histamine-fast achlorhydria and a flattening or concavity of the nails (koilonychia).

Table 5.1. Laboratory Results in the Various Stages of Iron-Deficiency Anemia

Test	Stage 1 Depletion of Iron Stores	Stage 2 Impaired Erythropoiesis	Stage 3 Anemic Phase
Bone marrow iron stores	Decreased	Decreased or absent	Lack of iron
Serum ferritin	Often decreased	Often decreased	Decreased
Total serum iron-binding capacity	Normal	Increased	Increased
Serum iron	Normal	Often decreased	Decreased
FEP	Normal	Increased	Increased
MCV	Normal	Normal or decreased	Decreased
MCHC	Normal	Normal	Decreased
MCH	Normal	Normal or decreased	Decreased
Hemoglobin	Normal	Normal	Decreased

FEP = free erythrocyte protoporphyrin; MCV = mean cell volume; MCHC = mean cell hemoglobin concentration; MCH = mean cell hemoglobin.

Laboratory Tests

The best way to evaluate the presence or lack of iron in tissues is by staining with iron sections prepared in a neutral fixative without decalcification and cut to a thickness of 1–2 μ in methacrylate. Smears are problematic in that they always entail artificial precipitation of iron, which is difficult to evaluate because the cells storing the iron are usually located in the thicker part of the smear. Paraffin sections are too thick to evaluate with accuracy, and they require decalcification, which removes substantial amounts of iron (Block, 1980).

The staining of iron in tissue, albeit the best method of diagnosing iron deficiency, does not lend itself to routine laboratory use. A three-step diagnostic system has been proposed that uses the serum ferritin and MCV as a screen, followed by serum iron level and total iron-binding capacity (TIBC) in some patients, and by the erythrocyte sedimentation rate in a few individuals (Beck and Cornwell, 1981). This system was found to have 96% agreement with bone marrow iron stores.

The major laboratory changes and the stages in the progression of an iron-deficiency anemia are shown in Tables 5.1 and 5.2.

Depletion of Iron Stores (Stage 1)

Iron reserves begin to fall during the early stages of iron deficiency. Serum ferritin is decreased when early iron deficiency is uncomplicated by other dis-

orders, but hemoglobin levels are usually stable and do not reflect anemia as long as any iron stores remain. The serum ferritin level, then, is the best indicator in the detection of early iron-deficiency anemia. The level decreases parallel with iron stores. When serum ferritin is low or lacking, iron stores are completely depleted. However, the reverse does not always hold true, as normal ferritin levels can be found in an existing iron deficiency complicated by bacterial infections, parasitic infestations, tissue necrosis, or malignancy. In such situations, a bone marrow stain for iron is the best indicator and usually is diagnostic (Hersko et al., 1981).

Impaired Erythropoiesis (Stage 2)

As the iron deficiency progresses, iron is drawn from the serum for erythropoiesis. Serum iron levels fall, and transferrin (TIBC) synthesis is stimulated. The ratio of these two measurements (the transferrin saturation) is more sensitive than either the serum iron or the TIBC alone. The specificity of the assay is decreased by the changes in serum iron that can occur with even transient infection or tissue injury.

Free erythrocyte protoporphyrin (FEP) increases when restrictions in the supply of iron lead to impaired heme synthesis. FEP has a sensitivity similar to transferrin saturation but is a more stable analyte. Transferrin saturation can change in hours, whereas FEP levels change only after several weeks of iron deprivation to erythroid tissues. Moreover, FEP levels return to normal more slowly than does trans-

Table 5.2. Relationship of Common Laboratory Tests to Some Anemias

Test	Disorder					
	Stage 3 Iron Deficiency	Folate Deficiency	Vitamin B$_{12}$ Deficiency	Chronic Infection	β-Thalassemia Trait	Lead Poisoning
Bone marrow iron stores	D	N	N	N/I	N	N
Serum ferritin	D	N	N	N/I	N	N
Transferrin saturation	D	N	N/D	N/I	N	N
FEP	I	N	N	N	N	I
MCV	D	I	I	D/N	D	D
MCHC	D	N	N	N/D	N/D	N/D
MCH	D	I	I	N/D	D	N/D
Hemoglobin	D	D	D	D	N/D	D

FEP = free erythrocyte protoporphyrin; MCV = mean cell volume; MCHC = mean cell hemoglobin concentration; MCH = mean cell hemoglobin; D = decreased; N = normal; I = increased; N/D = normal or decreased; N/I = normal or increased.

ferrin saturation after iron therapy (Cook and Finch, 1979). FEP may also provide a sharper separation between iron-deficient children and normal children, and it appears to be a better guide to the adequacy of iron replacement therapy (Thomas et al., 1977). When therapy is effective, the FEP level falls but, as the test is not specific for iron deficiency, caution should be used in its interpretation. FEP is reduced in lead poisoning as well.

During this second stage of iron deficiency, red-cell indices may begin to change, but anemia still is not present. Of the routine red-cell indices, the mean cell hemoglobin (MCH) appears to be the most sensitive to decreases in iron levels (Hersko et al., 1981; Knight et al., 1982), but it does not revert to normal until the iron reserves are restored.

Anemic Phase (Stage 3)

Hemoglobin levels are clinically insensitive to and nonspecific for early iron-deficiency states. Reductions in values can result from many types of anemias and should only be interpreted together with other tests of erythropoietic function. Serum ferritin can aid in distinguishing true iron deficiency from other anemias, as a low ferritin level almost always can be attributed to the disease.

Bone marrow iron detected by routine iron stains appears to be the most definitive test but is used less often because of the procedure involved in specimen collection. Table 5.2 shows the relationship of the common laboratory tests to the anemias.

The morphologic observations in severe iron deficiency usually are well defined. The microcytic hypochromic anemia is generally more pronounced than in other chronic disorders, as is the degree of severity of anisocytosis and poikilocytosis. However, differentiation between iron-deficiency anemia and thalassemia is usually subtle and is outlined in Table 5.3.

Other hematologic findings in iron-deficiency anemia include low or normal reticulocyte counts, lack of nucleated red cells, and normal leukocyte and platelet counts. Serum iron levels are often less than 40 μg/dl, and ferritin levels are usually less than 10 ng/dl. The bone marrow shows a normoblastic hyperplasia with poorly defined normoblasts that often exhibit ragged cellular outlines.

Aside from dietary insufficiency, other disorders that can produce an iron-deficiency anemia include chronic blood loss and malabsorption syndrome.

Many factors influence serum iron concentrations and TIBC. Day-to-day variation is marked in healthy persons. Diurnal variation causes serum iron levels to be distinctly lower in the afternoon than in the morning and quite low in the evening (10–20 μg/dl in healthy persons). Many individuals with iron deficiency have normal values of serum iron and TIBC (Hamilton et al., 1950).

Table 5.3. Morphologic Differentiation Between Iron-Deficiency Anemia and Thalassemia

Disorder	Anisocytosis and Poikilocytosis	Stippled Cells	Target Cells
Iron-deficiency anemia	1+ to 3+	0	Occasional
Thalassemia	3+	3+	3+

Causes of Iron-Deficiency Anemia

Chronic blood loss is the most common cause of iron-deficiency anemia. Of the many etiologic factors causing this state, gastrointestinal bleeding is by far the most common in men, and menstrual blood loss is the most frequently seen cause in women (Hallberg, 1979).

The lesions causing *gastrointestinal bleeding* include hemorrhoids, duodenal and gastric ulcers, esophageal hemorrhage, ulcerative colitis, and gastric neoplasms. Iron depletion that occurs in chronic hemorrhage can be estimated by assuming a loss of 0.5 mg iron for every milliliter of blood lost. Consequently, a consistent loss of 3–4 ml blood per day will result in a slow depletion of approximately 2 mg iron, which can, if not balanced by dietary intake, result in a negative iron balance and anemia. The laboratory findings are extremely variable and relate to the severity and length of the hemorrhagic episodes. However, if bleeding takes place over a long time, hematologic results are those described earlier for iron-deficiency anemia.

Excessive menstrual flow is the most common single cause of iron deficiency in women. In healthy normal women, menstrual flow averages approximately 35 ml each period, the upper limit being approximately 80 ml.

Hereditary hemorrhagic telangiectasia is an uncommon disorder characterized by recurrent bleeding from the nose and gastrointestinal tract.

During *pregnancy,* there is a major loss of the body's iron stores. Each pregnancy results in the average loss of 680 mg iron, the equivalent of approximately 1,300 ml whole blood.

Sideroblastic Anemia

Sideroblastic anemia is a term used to describe a dyshematopoietic anemia in which defective hemoglobin formation is associated with excessive accumulation of iron granules in developing immature red cells. When this heme synthesis is defective and iron uptake is normal, the iron accumulates in the mitochondria of the cells if there is insufficient protoporphyrin in the cell.

This group of anemias is characterized by the presence of ringed sideroblasts and increased iron deposits in the tissues. Sideroblastic anemia may be hereditary or acquired. The acquired form may be primary, in which there is no associated disease, or secondary, in which diseases such as carcinoma or rheumatoid arthritis are present. A reversible form of the anemia may develop in alcoholics, in patients receiving treatment with certain drugs, and in individuals with malabsorption due to celiac disease. A secondary sideroblastic anemia may accompany blood disorders such as polycythemia, myelosclerosis, leukemia, and myeloma, and may also be seen in Di Guglielmo syndrome. A classification of the sideroblastic anemias is presented in Table 5.4.

Hereditary Sideroblastic Anemia

Hereditary sideroblastic anemia usually occurs in men. Physical findings include a mild hepatosplenomegaly with increased iron stores in the liver. Other signs of iron overload include skin pigmentation and, on occasion, disturbances of cardiac function. The disease affects the heme synthesis pathway and is similar to that described later under Secondary Sideroblastic Anemia.

The hematologic picture includes a severe anemia that frequently is microcytic and hypochromic. (Table 5.5 shows the principal hematologic characteristics of the major sideroblastic anemias.) Red-cell morphologic features include pronounced anisocytosis, poikilocytosis, basophilic stippling, and the presence of target cells. Leukocytes and platelets are normal. The bone marrow shows a normoblastic erythroid hyperplasia, and there are usu-

Table 5.4. Classification of Sideroblastic Anemias

Refractory	Hereditary	X-linked sideroblastic anemia
	Acquired	Primary idiopathic sideroblastic anemia
		Secondary idiopathic sideroblastic anemia
		Associated with hematologic disease (hemolytic anemia, leukemia, myeloma, myeloproliferative disorders, etc.)
		Associated with nonhematologic disease (infections, uremia, metastatic carcinoma, rheumatoid arthritis, hypothyroidism, etc.)
Reversible	Acquired	Associated with toxins and drugs (alcohol, lead, isoniazid, chloramphenicol, phenacetin, etc.)

ally excessive hemosiderin stores. Ringed sideroblasts are present in up to 40% of the normoblasts. The predominant cell is either the polychromatic or the orthochromatic normoblast. Hyperferremia, with an increase in transferrin saturation, increased plasma iron turnover, and reduced red-cell iron use, together with reductions in protoporphyrins, are commonly found features.

Hereditary sideroblastic anemia has been associated with bleeding secondary to reduced platelet adenosine triphosphate release (Soslan and Brodsky, 1989).

In addition to the X-linked inheritance form, several families have been reported in which sideroblastic anemia occurred in an autosomal hereditary form (Kasturi et al., 1982).

Idiopathic Sideroblastic Anemia

Idiopathic sideroblastic anemia is a fairly uncommon disorder seen in individuals who are usually older than 66 years (Kushner, 1971). It differs from the true hereditary form of the disease in that it does not present with a microcytic blood picture, more often exhibiting a normocytic hypochromic anemia or even a macrocytic hypochromic anemia. One characteristic morphologic feature of this form of anemia is the presence of many stippled hypochromic erythrocytes. Leukocytes and platelets may be within normal limits or may occasionally be reduced in numbers.

The bone marrow shows a normoblastic erythroid hyperplasia that stains negatively with periodic acid–Schiff (PAS), but megaloblastic changes can sometimes be seen and are corrected by the administration of folic acid. These PAS-negative cells are one useful feature in separating this disorder from erythroleukemia, which usually contains PAS-positive blocks in the erythrocytes together with megaloblastic changes. Ringed sideroblasts may be present, typically occurring at all stages of the red-cell development, along with increased hemosiderins. Transferrin saturation and ferritin levels often are increased, as are iron stores in the liver.

Table 5.5. Principal Hematologic Characteristics of the Major Sideroblastic Anemias

	Hereditary	**Secondary to Drugs**	**Idiopathic**
Mean cell volume	Decreased	Decreased	Normal or increased
Bone marrow	Normoblastic	Normoblastic	Normoblastic
	Erythroid	Erythroid	Erythroid
	Hyperplasia	Hyperplasia	Hyperplasia
			Megaloblastic changes may be present
Ringed sideroblasts	Present at the polychromatic or orthochromatic normoblastic stages	Present usually at the polychromatic or orthochromatic normoblastic stages	Present at all stages of red-cell immaturity
Cause	Heme synthesis defect	Heme synthesis defect	Heme, DNA, and RNA synthesis defects

Secondary Sideroblastic Anemia

Secondary sideroblastic anemia has been associated with other disorders such as lead poisoning, myeloma, leukemia, pernicious anemia, and myeloproliferative diseases, and with drugs such as chemotherapeutic agents and alcohol. Etiologically, the anemia secondary to drug ingestion results from the reduction of aminolevulinic acid (ALA) synthetase activity by either influencing pyridoxal-5-phosphate availability or by inhibiting pyridoxal-5-catalyzed reactions. These medications, which are primarily antituberculous, as well as chloramphenicol and alcohol, are associated with the presence of many ringed sideroblasts. Discontinuing the medication usually reverses the blood picture.

The peripheral blood is usually dimorphic and microcytic. Bone marrow changes are similar to those in the hereditary form of the anemia, and ringed sideroblasts are frequently confined to the more mature nucleated red cells.

Lead Poisoning

Lead poisoning is now a relatively rare disorder found primarily in young children. It results from the ingestion of lead-based paints. Lead fills no physiologic purpose, but, once ingested, it passes to the blood and bone marrow and causes severe anemia.

Three basic mechanisms occur in lead-induced red-cell injury: (1) impaired globulin synthesis, (2) an impaired red-cell membrane, and (3) defective heme synthesis. Lead accumulates in the normoblastic mitochondria and results in disturbances of cellular enzymes and in the disruption of heme synthesis (Goldberg, 1968). Enzymatic inhibition within the red cell depends on the lead concentration, the most sensitive activity occurring in ALA-dehydrase (ALA-D), which converts ALA to porphobilinogen. As a consequence, urinary ALA is greatly increased, whereas porphobilinogen levels are usually normal. Reduced ALA-D activity in red cells is the most sensitive index of lead poisoning, but it may be too sensitive a test to use for investigating occupational exposure.

The blood picture presents a mild microcytic hypochromic anemia. In children, the anemia often is more severe because of an accompanying iron-deficiency anemia. The reticulocyte count is increased, reflecting bone marrow hyperplasia, and marked red-cell basophilic stippling frequently is present. This stippling is not proportional to the severity of the anemia and cannot be used as a guide to the intensity of lead exposure.

The bone marrow shows a normoblastic erythroid hyperplasia and, as in the other sideroblastic anemias, ringed sideroblasts are confined to the later stages of erythroid maturation.

Biochemically, there is an increase in the red-cell protoporphyrin level and a reduction in red-cell enzymes associated with the heme synthesis pathway (ALA-D, heme synthetase, etc.). Urine ALA (see earlier discussion) consequently is greatly increased, as are coproporphyrin and porphobilinogen levels. Excretion of lead is frequently unremarkable unless the patient has been treated with chelating agents such as ethylenediaminetetraacetic acid.

Pyrimidine-5'-Nucleotidase Deficiency

Pyrimidine-5'-nucleotidase (P5'N) is an enzyme involved in the catabolism of RNA. It catalyzes the dephosphorylation of pyrimidine-5-monophosphate to its respective nucleotides and inorganic phosphate. A congenital deficiency of P5'N is associated with hemolytic anemia characterized by the presence of basophilic stippling and the accumulation of pyrimidine nucleotides in the red cells. Acquired deficiency of P5'N occurs in occupational lead overload and in normal red cells exposed to low lead concentrations. Decreased P5'N activity has been demonstrated in several cases of lymphoproliferative and myeloproliferative disorders, in erythroblastopenia of childhood, and in β-thalassemia trait (Liebermann and Gordon-Smith 1980; Vives et al., 1984; Beutler and Hartman, 1985; David et al., 1989).

Chapter 6

Normocytic Normochromic Anemias

The normocytic normochromic anemias include those in which the red-cell indices are usually within the normal range, but they differ from both the macrocytic and the microcytic hypochromic anemias in that they are a heterogeneous group. In general, these disorders can be physiologically grouped according to the classification shown in Table 6.1.

Anemia Associated with Bone Marrow Response

Acute Blood-Loss Anemia

Acute blood-loss anemia varies in severity, making an estimation of the actual blood loss very difficult. The determination of the blood volume is probably the most valuable indicator, but it may be misleading if the patient is in shock or still hemorrhaging.

Hematologically, hemorrhage is characterized by a normocytic normochromic anemia and a mild reticulocytosis, which produces some macrocytosis. Concomitantly, polychromasia is often present, together with leukocytosis and thrombocytosis. A reticuloctye response is usually observed 3–5 days after the hemorrhage and reaches a peak at approximately 6–11 days after the hemorrhage.

During or immediately after the hemorrhage, the platelet count, fibrinogen, and activated partial thromboplastin–time results may be decreased. These abnormalities, however, tend to revert to nor-

mal shortly after bleeding stops, the platelet count frequently rebounding to levels as high as 1 million. A neutrophilic leukocytosis also is found approximately 2–5 hours after bleeding; counts as high as 35,000 have been reported (Lee, 1993).

Hemolytic Anemia

Hemolytic anemias are characterized by a decreased red-cell life span due to a variety of causative factors. These anemias are discussed in Chapters 8 and 9.

Intrinsic Bone Marrow Disease

Pancytopenia

Pancytopenia refers to a reduction of erythrocytes, leukocytes, and thrombocytes and results from a number of different disorders. The mechanisms leading to these reduced states include ineffective hematopoiesis with cell death in the bone marrow, the production of defective cells that then are removed promptly from the circulation by the reticuloendothelial system, and sequestration of such cells or their destruction by complement or antibody action.

Some of the diseases that exhibit pancytopenia include aleukemic leukemia, myeloma, lymphoma, myeloid metaplasia, storage reticulosis, pernicious anemia, paroxysmal nocturnal hemoglobinuria

Table 6.1. Causes of Normocytic Normochromic Anemias

Group	Examples
Associated with bone marrow response	Acute blood loss
	Hemolytic anemia
Associated with defective bone marrow response	Intrinsic bone marrow disease (hypoplasia or aplasia, myelophthisic anemia, bone marrow infiltration, leukemia, myeloma)
	Dyserythropoietic anemia
Depression of erythropoietin production	Impaired source (renal insufficiency, anemia of liver disease)
	Reduced stimulus; anemia of endocrine disorders
	Anemia of chronic disorders

(PNH), and aplastic anemia. All these disorders, except aplastic anemia, are discussed elsewhere in the text.

Acquired Aplastic Anemia

Aplastic anemia is not a single disorder. The term describes a condition in which there is inadequate hematopoietic activity and, finally, a cessation of this activity by the bone marrow. It has been defined as a syndrome of peripheral blood destruction. *Aplastic anemia* is associated with hypocellularity of the hematopoietic tissue in both intramedullary and extramedullary sites without bone marrow fibrosis or invasion by malignant cells (Geary and Testa, 1979).

The cause of aplastic anemia is uncertain, though two possible causes have been theorized: the incapacity of a common stem cell to reproduce (stem-cell deficiency) and the lack of a suitable bone marrow environment that provides for the continuing nourishment of the primitive cells (microenvironment deficiency; Boggs and Boggs, 1976). The anemia can be subdivided into two principal classifications: acquired and congenital (Table 6.2).

The list of agents suspected to be associated with aplastic anemia is extensive. Certain agents will induce either a temporary or a prolonged marrow injury, and they include benzene and its derivatives, cytotoxic drugs used in chemotherapy, and some poisons, such as organic arsenicals. A less predictive marrow reaction to chloramphenicol, pyrazolones, sulfonamides, and gold compounds has been reported (Williams et al., 1973).

Ionizing radiation produces bone marrow injury and can induce changes that lead to chronic bone marrow hypoplasia and pancytopenia. Dose and time relationships are most important in this form of injury. If radiation exposure is not very intense and is of short duration, stem-cell regeneration can occur (George and Depratti, 1979). Similar hypoplasia can occur secondary to infections such as hepatitis and tuberculosis (Hagler et al., 1975).

Peripheral blood results show reductions in all formed elements. Hemoglobin levels reflect the severe reductions in total red cells. Besides being quantitatively abnormal, the red cells exhibit anisocytosis, poikilocytosis, and often a macrocytosis. There usually is no polychromasia, nucleated red cells, or basophilic stippling, and this parallels the expected reticulocytopenia found. The thrombocytopenia is severe and platelets, if found, appear small. A concomitant increase in bleeding time and poor clot retraction also are present. Leukopenia, principally caused by a neutropenia, occurs and can be as severe as 0.5×10^9/liter. Leukocyte morphologic features are unremarkable. Serum iron is elevated and iron-binding proteins are saturated. Erythropoietin levels are markedly increased and, in children with the disorder, hemoglobin F levels also may be increased.

The hematologic diagnosis depends on the bone marrow, which is usually very hypocellular or even aplastic. Occasionally, cellular fragments are seen, especially when bone marrow sections are cut. In some patients, there may be a lymphocytosis, which may be associated with an autoimmune process. The dyserythropoietic aspects of this disorder, as suggested by the presence of distorted red cells, are prominent (Lewis, 1975). Macrophagic iron stores can be demonstrated, especially in hypertransfused patients.

Table 6.2. Classification of Aplastic Anemia

Acquired	Congenital
Chemical and physical agents	Fanconi's anemia
Viral infections	Pure red-cell aplasia
Idiopathic causes	

Congenital Aplastic Anemia

Fanconi's Anemia

Fanconi's anemia is a rare hereditary disorder characterized by bone marrow hypoplasia and a variety of congenital anomalies that include skeletal and chromosomal instability and an increased incidence of neoplasms (Prindull and Tillmann, 1979). The laboratory results reveal a normocytic anemia, though occasionally a macrocytic picture develops. The relative reticuloctye level is increased, but there is an absolute reticulocytopenia. Immature leukocytes and nucleated red cells sometimes are present in the peripheral blood, and a moderate leukopenia, principally resulting from a neutropenia, is present. Unlike in aplastic anemia, increased levels of hemoglobin F are usually seen. The bone marrow may be normocellular early in the disease, with a mild plasmacytosis, but ultimately it becomes hypocellular.

Pure Red-Cell Aplasia

Pure red-cell aplasia is characterized by a selective decrease in red-cell precursors in the presence of normal production of both leukocytes and platelets. The acquired form of pure red-cell aplasia can be associated with a variety of diseases, including hemolytic anemias, infections, and various neoplasms. Drug therapy can also be involved.

The congenital form of red-cell aplasia is termed *Diamond-Blackfan syndrome*. The cause of this disorder is unknown, but it is characterized by a slowly progressive anemia, beginning in infancy, in which the only abnormalities are in erythroid production of the bone marrow. The severe anemia is normocytic and normochromic and, as in the other aplastic anemias, there is a severe reticulocytopenia and a lack of polychromasia or stippling. Leukocytes and platelet production appear normal, and so there are no hemorrhages seen in the congenital aplasias. Erythropoietin levels are increased in both the serum and the urine.

Pure red-cell aplasia has also been reported in chronic myeloid leukemia.

Myelophthisic Anemias

The myelophthisic anemias are considered as individual disorders and are discussed further in Chapter 13. The term describes the hematologic consequences of bone marrow infiltration and is a generalization that includes idiopathic myelofibrosis and other diseases that produce both nucleated erythrocytes and immature granulocytes in the peripheral blood, as in leukemia and multiple myeloma.

Dyserythropoietic Anemias

The dyserythropoietic anemias are considered as individual disorders in Chapters 5 and 7. *Dyserythropoietic anemia* is a term used to describe qualitative disturbances of erythropoiesis. The classification comprises thalassemia, iron-deficiency anemia, sideroblastic anemia, megaloblastic anemia, and erythroleukemia, as well as a poorly defined rare group of anemias known as *congenital dyserythropoietic anemia* (CDA), discussed in the following paragraphs. CDA is characterized by bizarre red-cell changes and is a refractory anemia. Three subgroups are recognized.

CDA Type 1

CDA type 1 is extremely rare and is believed to be transmitted as an autosomal recessive trait. The anemia usually is detected at birth and can cause neonatal jaundice. It often produces a mild macrocytic blood picture together with prominent anisocytosis, poikilocytosis, and basophilic stippling. The bone marrow exhibits binucleate erythrocytic cells and occasional megaloblastic cells, in conjunction with an erythroid hyperplasia. Ringed sideroblasts are usually absent. Leukopoiesis and thrombopoiesis are normal (Heimpel, 1977).

CDA Type 2

CDA type 2 is known also as *hereditary erythroblastic multinuclearity with positive acidified serum* (HEMPAS). It is the most common of the CDAs and is inherited as an autosomal recessive disorder. Heterozygotes are normal, with the one exception of increased binding of anti-i to their cells.

The principal laboratory findings are of a normocytic anemia that can be severe, especially if present in infancy. Peripheral blood smears show anisocytosis, poikilocytosis, and basophilic stippling. The bone marrow shows a normoblastic erythroid hyperplasia, with up to 40% of the nucleated red cells at the polychromatic and orthochromatic stages showing two nuclei. In contrast to individuals with CDA type 1, megaloblastosis is not seen in this disorder. Gaucher-like cells containing birefringent, needlelike crystalline inclusions may be present.

The serologic findings resemble those of PNH in that the cells are susceptible to hemolysis in acidified normal serum. This test is particularly important in the recognition of CDA type 2. Approximately 30% of normal sera will produce lysis of HEMPAS red cells in acidified serum, but, in contrast to PNH, lysis will not occur when the patient's own serum is used. The causative IgM antibody is termed *anti-HEMPAS* and is present normally in serum.

Other serologic abnormalities found in HEMPAS are a high agglutination titer with anti-i, unusual susceptibility to lysis by anti-i and anti-I, and a negative sucrose lysis test. The cause of the disease remains unknown, but there is evidence to suggest a red-cell membrane defect in early erythroid precursors (Anselstetter et al., 1977; Vainchenker et al., 1979).

The red-cell abnormality in HEMPAS gives rise to marked ineffective erythropoiesis (Verwilghen, 1976). If the disease presents in childhood, skeletal abnormalities occur and may give rise to the so-called hair-on-end radiologic appearance (McCann et al., 1980).

CDA Type 3

CDA type 3 is a rare normocytic anemia that is inherited in an autosomal dominant manner. The peripheral blood shows marked anisocytosis, poikilocytosis, stippled cells, and occasional macrocytes. Many of the erythroid precursors in the bone marrow show marked multinuclearity with giant normoblasts having up to 12 nuclei. Lobulations and karyorrhexis are commonly seen. Neither ringed sideroblasts nor red cells that stain

positively for periodic acid–Schiff are seen, in contrast to the findings in erythroleukemia. The acidified serum test (Ham's) is negative, and strong agglutination and lysis are obtained with anti-i (Gouldsmit, 1977).

Anemia Associated with Depression of Erythropoietin Production

Anemia of Renal Disease

Both acute and chronic renal disease are generally accompanied by alterations in erythrokinetics. Some patients present with bone marrow failure caused by reduced erythropoietin production, whereas in other patients a change in a hemolytic component occurs.

The anemia is usually normocytic and normochromic but, if severe, a mild macrocytosis and anisocytosis may be present. Usually only mild anisocytosis is seen, but when renal function is severely impaired, burr cells, helmet cells, and other schistocytic fragments can be detected. The number of reticulocytes is usually decreased, but both the osmotic and mechanical fragility of the red cells is normal.

The bone marrow usually shows a mild normoblastic erythroid hyperplasia but, in acute renal failure, erythroid hypoplasia can occur. Serum iron levels are variable but are normal in the milder phases of the disease.

Anemia of Liver Disease

The anemia associated with liver disease is primarily one that demonstrates a macrocytic blood picture, although in the uncomplicated form, the anemia may be normocytic and normochromic.

Many causative factors have been implicated in the anemia of liver disease, including sideroblastosis and iron deficiency. The anemia is usually mild and shows classic "thin macrocytes," target cells, and a reticulocytosis. A mild thrombocytopenia is present in approximately half of the patients with cirrhosis. The bone marrow can reveal an erythroid hyperplasia but may possess normal cellularity and large erythroid precursors. Macronormoblasts may be seen that possess a normal nuclear structure and cytoplasm.

Anemia of Endocrine Disorders

Hormones from the pituitary and thyroid glands, the adrenal cortex, and the gonads assist in the regulation of erythropoiesis through their influence on protein synthesis. Hypoplasia may result from pituitary deficiency caused by a loss of adenohypophyseal hormones, producing a normocytic normochromic anemia. Hypoplastic anemia may exist in individuals with hypothyroid states, producing a mild normocytic normochromic picture with a reticulocytopenia. On occasion, the anemia is hypochromic if there is a coexisting iron deficiency.

Anemias of Chronic Infections and Inflammatory Disorders

Anemia of chronic infections has a multifactorial origin. In general, the anemia develops during the first few months of the primary disease and does not progress in severity after that time. The peripheral blood picture is normocytic and normochromic, although a hypochromic anemia can develop over a long period, reflecting the use of iron stores. Anisocytosis is present, but poikilocytosis rarely is seen. The concentration of free protoporphyrin in the red cells tends to increase in patients with chronic disorders, and increased levels of serum copper occur. This hypercupremia precedes the development of anemia and, as the infection subsides, the copper content of the blood returns to normal more rapidly than does the serum iron level.

Normocytic normochromic anemias have been reported secondary to a wide range of chronic noninfectious inflammatory disorders, including rheumatoid arthritis, rheumatic fever, systemic lupus erythematosus, trauma, and thermal injury (Weinstein, 1959). Malignant disorders such as leukemia, Hodgkin's disease, and multiple myeloma can exhibit similar anemic pictures, but these diseases may produce variations in red-cell morphologic features, depending on the degree of the bone marrow invasion.

Vitamin B₂ (Riboflavin)

Normocytic normochromic anemia can be produced by deprivation of riboflavin or the administration of riboflavin antagonists. The anemia is characterized by and associated with erythroid hypoplasia of the bone marrow and a reticulocytopenia. Occasionally, vacuolated normoblasts are seen in severe deficiencies. Plasma iron transport and reduced red-cell iron incorporation are present. Leukocytes and platelets remain normal.

Naturally occurring riboflavin deficiency is associated mostly with other nutritional deficiencies, the principal clinical findings being angular stomatitis and seborrheic dermatitis (Horwitt, 1980).

Nicotinic Acid (Niacin)

Most scientific data have involved the effect of nicotinic acid on dogs. The clinical effect is the production of a macrocytic hypochromic or normocytic normochromic anemia. Because nicotinic acid is involved principally in the synthesis of peritoneal nucleotide (nicotinamide adenine dinucleotide and nicotinamide adenine dinucleotide phosphate) and in cell respiration, it is believed that a lack of it may interfere with the respiration of immature red cells (Lee, 1993).

Chapter 7

The Thalassemias

The thalassemias are a heterogeneous group of inherited disorders characterized by one or more defects in the synthesis of the normal globin chains of hemoglobin (Hb). The disorders are genetically classified as β, βδ, and α forms, depending on the identity of the hemoglobin chain gene or genes involved. In α-thalassemias, the defect resides in the α-chain synthesis, whereas in β-thalassemias, the abnormality is in the β chain, thus reducing the amount of Hb A in each red cell. In the βδ-thalassemias, there is a simultaneous suppression of β- and δ-chain synthesis and therefore a reduction in the individual red-cell content of both Hb A and Hb A_2. The two main forms of this type of thalassemia are Hb F thalassemia and Hb Lepore thalassemia.

The reduced production of globin chains caused by this group of genetic disorders results not only in reduced amounts of hemoglobin but also in an imbalance of the globin chains. This leads to the production of tetramers containing the surplus chains—for instance, $β_4$ tetramers in α-thalassemia and $α_4$ tetramers in β-thalassemia. These tetramers are useless for delivering oxygen and are unstable, which leads to red-cell hemolysis.

The clinical manifestations of the thalassemias vary considerably and can be classified into thalassemia major, thalassemia intermedia, thalassemia minor, and thalassemia minima. The distinction between the major and intermediate forms is based on the age of onset, the course of the disease, and the severity of the clinical manifestations.

The geographic distribution of the disorder is mainly around the Mediterranean Sea, but it is also found in Southeast Asia, the Middle East, and the Orient.

The molecular defect and expected hemoglobin levels are summarized in Tables 7.1 and 7.2. Briefly, in the β°-thalassemias, β-chain synthesis is lacking, despite the presence of intact β genes. In β°-thalassemia, β-chain synthesis is reduced, whereas in δ-thalassemia, a different deletion involving both genes occurs. In α°-thalassemia (α-thalassemia-1 trait), the disorder results from the deletion of both α-globin genes on the chromosome, which leads to a lack of α-chain synthesis. The α⁺-thalassemia is due to various deletions that result in the lack of one or more α-globin genes, which ultimately reduces the production of messenger RNA.

α-Thalassemia caused by Hb Constant Spring is due to an abnormality in the α-globin gene, resulting in an elongated α chain comprised of 31 extra amino acids and a retarded chain synthesis.

Hb Lepore consists of normal α chains combined with an abnormal chain consisting of the N-terminal ends of the δ chain fused to the C-terminal ends of the β chains (Baglioni, 1965). This hybrid is believed to be the product of a δβ-fusion gene arising from a crossover between misaligned δ and β-globin structural genes on different chromosomes.

Almost one-third of American blacks have some type of deletional α-thalassemia. Gene-mapping studies show that 27% of the black population has a single gene deletion (α-thalassemia, α-thalassemia-2) and that nearly 3% are homozygous for α-thalassemia-2 (have one α locus deleted on both chromosomes).

65

Table 7.1. General Classification of the α-Thalassemias

Syndrome	Genotype	Principal Clinical Features, Hemoglobin (Hb) Pattern, Molecular Defect, and Blood Picture
α°-Thalassemia (α-thalassemia-1 trait)	–/–	Hydrops fetalis, fetal or neonatal death, erythroblastosis, moderate to severe anemia Hb Bart's >80% Hb H and Hb Portland Deletion of both α-chain genes
Hb H disease	–/–α	Chronic hemolytic anemia with anisocytosis, hypochromia, target cells, and Hb H inclusions Hb Bart's 20–40% in the newborn Hb H 5–30% and Hb Bart's trace after first year
α⁺-Thalassemia (α-thalassemia-2 trait; α-thalassemia minor)	–/αα –α/–α ααᶜˢ/ααᶜˢ –/αᶜˢαᶜˢ	Little or no anemia; slight microcytosis Hb Bart's 2–10% in the newborn; no abnormality seen after the first year Hb Constant Spring 5–6% in the homozygous type and 0.5–1.0% in the heterozygous type Deletion of one α-chain gene or α-chain mutation produces Hb H when combined with α-thalassemia-1 trait
Silent carrier (heterozygous α-thalassemia-2 trait)	–α/αα	No clinical or hematologic features Hb Bart's 1–2% in the newborn No abnormality seen after the first year Deletion of one α chain

αᶜˢ = Hb Constant Spring.
Source: Data adapted from MM Wintrobe, GR Lee, et al. Clinical Hematology (8th ed). Philadelphia: Lea & Febiger, 1981.

α-Thalassemia

The α-thalassemias produce a wide spectrum of clinical features. The most severe form of the disorder is the Bart's Hb (Hb Bart's)–hydrops fetalis syndrome, which results in stillbirth and is associated with complete suppression of α-globin synthesis. Hb H disease is a milder disorder characterized by slight to moderate anemia and the presence of an abnormal β_4 tetramer (Hb H). α-Thalassemia trait usually is associated with a lack of clinical manifestations.

α°-Thalassemia (Hydrops Fetalis, α-Thalassemia-1 Trait)

α°-Thalassemia is seen widely in Southeast Asia and is due to a defect in α-chain synthesis, whereby δ and β chains are produced that form tetramers δ_4 (Hb Bart's) and β_4 (Hb H). Hb Bart's has a high oxygen affinity and lacks the Bohr effect. Consequently, it cannot supply oxygen to the tissues. Hb H is unstable and results in reduced red-cell survival and hemolysis. Neonates with such hemoglobin

makeup are usually stillborn or die soon after birth. The clinical picture is that of a premature, pale, hydropic infant, mainly of Chinese or Thai ancestry, with a severe anemia and peripheral blood showing anisocytosis, poikilocytosis, hypochromia, and nucleated red cells. There is a massive splenomegaly. The hemoglobin consists of almost 100% Hb Bart's or 90–95% Hb Bart's and 5–10% Hb H. Both parents have hematologic findings of α-thalassemia. Starch-gel hemoglobin electrophoresis shows a fast-moving band, principally Hb Bart's. Hb A, Hb A_2, and Hb F are not detected.

Hemoglobin H Disease

Hb H disease is a chronic hemolytic anemia caused by double heterozygosity for two α-thalassemia genes, one causing a severe deficiency and the other a mild deficiency of α chains. This disorder, like hydrops fetalis, is more commonly seen in Southeast Asia.

Four variants have been identified: (1) that associated with deletion of three of the four α-globin

Table 7.2. General Classification of the β-Thalassemias

Syndrome	Genotype	Principal Clinical Features, Hemoglobin (Hb) Pattern, Molecular Defect, and Blood Picture
β°-Thalassemia, homozygous state (thalassemia major)	β°/β°	No Hb A Hb A$_2$ 1.0–5.9% Hb F >94% Usually a lack of β-chain mRNA
β°-Thalassemia, heterozygous state (thalassemia minor)	β°/β	Hb A ~94% Hb A$_2$ 3.5–8.0% Hb F 1–5%
β⁺-Thalassemia, homozygous state (thalassemia major)	β⁺/β⁺	Hb A variable but reduced Hb A$_2$ 2.4–8.7% Hb F 20–80% Thalassemia intermedia usually presents with Hb A$_2$ levels of 5.4–10.0% and Hb F levels of 30–73%; there is diminished β-chain mRNA
β⁺-Thalassemia, heterozygous state (thalassemia minor)	β⁺/β	Hb A >90% Hb A$_2$ 3.5–8.0% Hb F 1–5% Diminished β-chain mRNA
δβ°-Thalassemia, homozygous state (thalassemia intermedia)	δβ°/δβ°	No Hb A Hb A$_2$ 0.3–2.4% Hb F >97% No β- and δβ-chain mRNA β-genes deleted
δβ°-Thalassemia, heterozygous state (thalassemia minor)	δβ°/δβ	Hb A >90% Hb A$_2$ 2.5–3.0% Hb F 5–20%
Hb Lepore, homozygous state (thalassemia major)	δβ^LEPORE/δβ^LEPORE	No Hb A and Hb A$_2$ Hb F ~75% Hb Lepore ~25% δβ–fusion gene; likely unstable δβ-mRNA Decreased synthesis of non-α chains
Hb Lepore, heterozygous state (thalassemia minor)	δβ^LEPORE/δβ	Hb A present but variably reduced Hb A$_2$ 1.2–2.6% Hb F 1–14% Hb Lepore 5–15%

mRNA = messenger RNA.
Source: Data adapted from GR Lee, TC Bithell, TC Foerster, et al. Clinical Hematology (8th ed). Philadelphia: Lea & Febiger, 1981.

genes (Kan et al., 1975); (2) that identified with the double heterozygosity for α-thalassemia-1 trait and Hb Constant Spring (Weatherall and Clegg, 1975); (3) that characterized by double heterozygosity for α-thalassemia-1 trait (Orkin and Old, 1979) and nondeletion α-thalassemia; and (4) a homozygous nondeletion gene (Pressley et al., 1980). Because of the insufficient production of α chains, the β chains combine with one another to form Hb H (β$_4$). This hemoglobin is unstable, and its precipitation intracellularly results in shortened cell survival and a chronic hemolytic anemia. At birth, infants show a typical thalassemic picture. Hemoglobin levels usually range from 9 to 12 g/liter, and the red-cell morphologic examination shows severe hypochromia, macrocytosis, target cells, and polychromasia. Nucleated red cells are rare. Basophilic stippling usually is present, and the reticulocyte levels often are normal except during a hemolytic crisis.

Hemoglobin electrophoresis is variable, but typically Hb Bart's level is 20–40% in the newborn, decreasing as the patient ages in a reciprocal manner to the increase in Hb H. This results from the switch from α-chain production to β-chain synthesis. The hemoglobin is identified by its fast migration on cellulose acetate in alkaline pH buffers.

Hb A_2 levels are slightly reduced, and Hb F is within normal limits. Hb H inclusions can be identified when peripheral blood is incubated with 1% brilliant cresyl blue, with 5–90% of the cells containing multiple inclusions. These spherical, bright green inclusions are mainly arranged peripherally and consist of precipitated Hb H. They are formed by the redox action of the dye on the abnormal hemoglobin. Care should be taken not to confuse Hb H inclusions with normal reticulocytes.

Other laboratory tests show increases in unconjugated bilirubin of 2–5 mg/dl, shortened red-cell survival, and moderate bone marrow erythroid hyperplasia. Typically, iron overload is not seen, probably because of the lack of affinity of Hb H for haptoglobin. The pathophysiology of the disorder is due to several factors, including ineffective oxygen transportation, iron depletion, ineffective erythropoiesis, defective synthesis of hemoglobin, and hemolytic anemia.

Hb H is also seen in association with other hematologic disorders, including erythroleukemia, myeloproliferative disease, and refractory sideroblastic anemia.

α^+-Thalassemia (α-Thalassemia Minor)

α^+-Thalassemia demonstrates a deletion of two of the α-globin genes, which produces a fairly benign disease with little or no anemia. α^+-Thalassemia is common among Thai and Chinese people and is less common among Greeks, Italians, Sephardic Jews, and American blacks. The red-cell morphologic characteristics are usually unremarkable except for some microcytosis. Hb H inclusions are rare, and the reticulocyte count is normal or slightly increased. Other laboratory test results include decreased osmotic fragility, normal plasma iron, decreased Hb A_2 (1–2%), and normal Hb F levels. The disorder is usually diagnosed in infancy, the typical finding being slightly increased levels of Hb Bart's of between 2 and 10%. After the first year of life, the blood picture is relatively normal, a diagnosis being made only through the use of gene mapping or by measuring the relative rates of α- and β-chain synthesis (Zaizov et al., 1973).

Hb Constant Spring is an α-thalassemia. The α chains of this hemoglobin variant contain an additional 31 amino acids, which produce an elongated chain that is synthesized at a slower-than-normal rate. Thereby, a relative deficiency of α chains is produced that, when combined with α-thalassemia-1 trait, results in Hb H disease. The disorder, like most α-thalassemias, is found primarily in Southeast Asia.

Silent Carrier (Heterozygous α-Thalassemia-2)

The silent carrier variant does not produce any clinical or hematologic abnormalities. Presumptive normal parents and children of Hb H individuals may be silent carriers, but this can be confirmed only by gene mapping.

β-Thalassemia

Like the α-thalassemias, β-thalassemias produce a wide range of clinical and hematologic findings. These disorders show decreased rates of β-chain synthesis and, consequently, reduced amounts of normal Hb A in the erythrocytes. β-Thalassemias are found mainly in the Mediterranean, the Middle East, India, and throughout Southeast Asia. Individuals with homozygous β-thalassemia often survive childhood but usually show tissue siderosis that results in cardiac failure as well as liver disease, skeletal deformity, and splenomegaly.

β^0-Thalassemia: Thalassemia Major (Cooley's Anemia)

β^0-Thalassemia is not clinically expressed during the first few months of life, but soon after a progressive pallor associated with anemia develops. Growth retardation continues throughout life. Abdominal enlargement occurs as a result of hepatosplenomegaly. Infections are frequent findings, and mental retardation, leg ulcers, chronic lassitude, and a distinctive mongoloid-appearing face (thalassemic facies) develops.

The laboratory features include a severe microcytic anemia, with marked anisocytosis, poikilocytosis, and hypochromia, and numerous target cells. A moderate reticulocytosis, the presence of nucleated red cells in the peripheral blood, and basophilic stippling also are common findings. A slight leukocytosis and thrombocytosis are seen. Plasma hemoglobin and serum iron are increased. Serum transferrin often is fully saturated, and haptoglobin and the red-cell half-life are decreased. The osmotic fragility is strikingly decreased, some cells showing increased osmotic resistance even in distilled water.

The bone marrow shows a normoblastic erythroid hyperplasia and increased iron stores. Occasionally, ringed sideroblasts are seen. Iron kinetics indicate the presence of markedly ineffective erythropoiesis. Hb F levels in excess of 94% are found, and increased Hb A$_2$ levels of 3.5–8.0% are seen.

β°-Thalassemia: Thalassemia Minor

In the heterozygous state of thalassemia minor, the clinical and laboratory findings are unimpressive. The hematologic features may reveal a mild anemia and reticulocytosis. The peripheral blood morphologic examination shows microcytosis, hypochromia, anisocytosis, poikilocytosis, basophilic stippling, and characteristic target cells. Nucleated red cells are usually not seen. Like thalassemia major, the osmotic fragility is decreased markedly in proportion to the number of target cells present. Red-cell free protoporphyrin levels are within normal limits. The bone marrow is normal or can exhibit a mild erythroid hyperplasia due to a slight degree of ineffective erythropoiesis. Red-cell survival is normal. Hemoglobin electrophoresis can show mildly elevated levels of Hb A$_2$ and Hb F.

Thalassemia Minima

Thalassemia minima is a condition in which the impairment of β-chain synthesis is so mild as to produce normal laboratory results and only very small clinical changes. "Silent" β-thalassemia genes have been identified in Greek and black patients. This form of the syndrome is implied in a normal parent of a child with thalassemia intermedia if the other parent has a high Hb A$_2$ thalassemia minor.

Thalassemia Intermedia

Thalassemia intermedia is produced by the homozygous state of some β-thalassemia alleles. This is especially true of homozygous β^+-thalassemia in black patients. The doubly heterozygous state for the β° and $\delta\beta^\circ$ genes have been described in Greeks, Italians, Orientals, and blacks. The signs and symptoms of thalassemia intermedia are comparable to those of thalassemia major but are less important. Patients usually do not require transfusions, and growth and development during childhood are normal. The laboratory features include hemoglobin concentrations of 6–9 g/dl, and peripheral blood smears show anisocytosis, hypochromia, target cells, basophilic stippling, and nucleated red cells. Bone marrow hyperplasia is prominent.

Other Rare Thalassemias

$\beta\delta$-Thalassemia

The term $\beta\delta$-thalassemia applies to those syndromes characterized by a simultaneous decrease in or lack of β and δ chains. Because there is a deficiency of β chains, the $\beta\delta$-thalassemias affect production of Hb A in a way similar to the β-thalassemia mutants. In contrast to the β-thalassemias, however, heterozygotes for $\beta\delta$-thalassemia have normal levels of Hb A$_2$. Two types of $\beta\delta$-thalassemias have been described: Lepore thalassemia and Hb F thalassemia.

Hb Lepore thalassemia is characterized by a decreased synthesis of non-α chains, resulting in the production of a fusion gene. This hybrid fusion gene ($\delta\beta$) can be expressed in either the heterozygous or the homozygous form. Hb Lepore has the same electrophoretic mobility as does Hb S and does not separate from Hb A on citrate agar electrophoresis. Clinically, the peripheral blood findings are similar to those of heterozygous β-thalassemia. In addition to the finding of the abnormal hemoglobin, electrophoresis reveals low or normal Hb A$_2$ levels and a slight elevation of Hb F in the heterozygous form, and approximately 75% Hb F levels in the homozygous state. Hb S can be differentiated from Hb Lepore by either the solubility test or the sickling test. The disorder is found most commonly in persons of Mediterranean ancestry, although it has been reported in most ethnic groups.

A number of Hb Lepores have been described that differ in the number of amino acids composing the β and δ chains in the Lepore molecule. Lepore may occur with other hemoglobinopathies such as

Table 7.3. Differentiation Between Iron-Deficiency Anemia and Thalassemia Trait in a Mildly Anemic Individual

Laboratory Tests	β-Thalassemia Trait	Iron-Deficiency Anemia
Serum iron	N	D
Total iron-binding capacity	N	I
% Iron saturation	N	D
Hb A$_2$	I	D
Hb F	I	N
Mean cell volume: red-cell ratio	<13	>13
Red-cell protoporphyrins	N	I
Serum ferritin	N	D

N = normal; D = decreased; I = increased.

Hb S, Hb C, or thalassemia with varying clinical severity. The heterozygous state does not cause anemia, jaundice, or splenomegaly; a mild microcytosis is seen.

Heterozygotes for Hb F thalassemia show the typical hematologic picture of thalassemia trait, normal levels of Hb A$_2$, and Hb F levels of 5–15%. The homozygotes have only Hb F present, with a complete lack of Hb A and Hb A$_2$. Combinations of Hb F thalassemia with Hb S or Hb E produce no Hb A (Patrick et al., 1975).

δ-Thalassemia

The δ chain takes part in the formation of only the minor hemoglobin component, Hb A$_2$; thus, no hematologic abnormalities are found in individuals who carry a δ-thalassemia mutant.

Hereditary Persistence of Fetal Hemoglobin

Hereditary persistence of fetal hemoglobin (HPFH) is found principally in American blacks and in Greeks. Unlike thalassemia, there is a failure of globin synthesis and imbalance of the α–non-α synthetic chain ratio. The various types of HPFH are classified by the type of Hb F present ($\gamma^A\gamma^G$, γ, or γ^G alone). HPFH is characterized by the persistence of fetal hemoglobin in adult life in the absence of other abnormalities. In association with β-chain structural variants, such as Hb S, HPFH produces hemoglobin electrophoretic findings similar to those found in Hb S/β°-thalassemia or homozygous sickle cell anemia, but with an unusually high level of Hb F, no Hb A, 65–85% Hb S, and

15–35% Hb F. Clinically, however, this disorder is benign, with no anemia, hemolysis, hypochromia, or sickle cell crises. The benign nature of the disorder is most likely related to the fact that the Hb F is evenly distributed among the red cells and appears to inhibit sickling of Hb S (Bunn et al., 1977a).

Thalassemia trait is sometimes difficult to distinguish from iron-deficiency anemia by laboratory methods. Table 7.3 details the common differentiating features of the disorders.

Sickle Cell Thalassemia

Sickle cell thalassemia occurs in parts of Africa and in the Mediterranean area, particularly in Greece and Italy. The clinical results of carrying one gene for Hb S and one gene for β-thalassemia depend mainly on the type of β-thalassemia gene. Where a normal β chain is not synthesized, the hemoglobin pattern consists of Hb S with an increase in Hb F and Hb A$_2$. The associated clinical findings are similar to those of sickle cell anemia, with severe anemia and recurrent sickle crises. In those cases in which the β-thalassemia only partly depresses β-chain synthesis, the hemoglobin consists of approximately 70% Hb S and 10–25% Hb A. The symptoms are less severe than in sickle cell anemia, with only a mild anemia and few sickle crises.

Hemoglobin C Thalassemia

Hb C thalassemia is a mild hemolytic disorder associated with splenomegaly. The hemoglobin pattern is variable, depending on whether the thalassemia gene is of the β$^+$ or β$^-$ type. Hb C thalassemia is found mainly in North Africa but has been reported in American blacks. When Hb A is produced, the hemolytic disorder is very mild and may be detected only during pregnancy as a refractory anemia or with folic acid deficiency.

Hemoglobin E Thalassemia

Hb E thalassemia is found principally in Southeast Asia. Hb E is synthesized at a reduced rate and produces the clinical phenotype of a mild form of β-thalassemia. Consequently, when it is inherited with a β-thalassemia gene, there is a marked deficit of β chains producing the clinical picture of severe β-thalassemia.

Hb E thalassemia, in its most severe form, presents a clinical picture similar to Cooley's anemia, with marked anemia, growth retardation, bone deformity, a tendency to infections, iron loading, splenomegaly, and hypersplenism. The hematologic features are similar to homozygous β-thalassemia, except that on electrophoresis, Hb E, Hb F, and Hb A_2 are present, but Hb A is absent.

Chapter 8

Introduction to the Hemolytic Anemias

Basic Mechanisms and Physiology of Hemolysis

Red cells normally have a life span of approximately 120 days. As the cells age, glycolysis slows down and enzymatic activity diminishes, as do adenosine triphosphate (ATP) levels and potassium and cell membrane lipids. However, the slowing of glycolysis can be accelerated if abnormalities are present, leading to cellular death, which involves the internal structure or membrane of the cell. The term *hemolysis* is usually applied to a situation in which there is premature red-cell destruction. In most of these situations, the red cells are removed from the circulation by the reticuloendothelial (RE) system (spleen or liver) and are broken down within these organs. The resulting hemoglobin (Hb) is catabolized within the sequestering organ and is either reused or excreted according to the defect encountered. Such a process is known as *extravascular lysis* and is the most common mechanism of cell death.

A second method of red-cell lysis involves the destruction of the red cell within the circulation. When this occurs, free hemoglobin is liberated directly into the plasma and is catabolized only when it is taken up by the liver or excreted through the kidneys. This is known as *intravascular lysis*.

Hemolytic anemias are disorders involving the in vivo premature destruction of red cells. Several methods of classification are in use. As already described, the site of cellular lysis can be either extravascular or intravascular, but the mechanism causing the actual cell breakdown can be subdivided into two broad groups: those that arise from within the cell itself, the so-called intracorpuscular defects, and those that arise from an initiating event that takes place outside the cell, the extracorpuscular defects. A second principal classification has been used that differentiates these disorders into the inherited anemias and the acquired anemias.

Irrespective of the classification and sites of red-cell destruction, all hemolytic anemias are marked by signs of an increased rate of hemoglobin catabolism, usually with signs of increased erythropoiesis. The main indicators of accelerated hemoglobin catabolism are jaundice, hemoglobinuria and hemosiderinuria, hemoglobinemia, reductions of plasma haptoglobin, anemia, and possibly, methemalbuminemia. These indicators can be present to a wide degree, depending on the cause and the duration of the disease or crisis. If the hemolysis is principally extravascular, most of the liberated hemoglobin becomes converted to bilirubin, as previously described on page 22. This conversion liberates 1 mol of iron, carbon monoxide, and bilirubin for each mole of heme that is catabolized, resulting in an increased unconjugated serum bilirubin level. If the hemolysis is acute, conjugated serum bilirubin may also be elevated.

Acute hemolysis, independent of cause, results in the reduction of plasma haptoglobin. Plasma haptoglobin is an α_2-globulin that possesses the ability to bind free hemoglobin, thus preventing its excretion through the urinary tract. The resulting hemoglobin-haptoglobin complex is removed by the RE system (liver). Consequently, the presence of free hemoglobin in the plasma substantially reduces the level of haptoglobin until a point is reached at which there is no haptoglobin. At this point, free plasma hemoglobin can be detected. Thus, if the rate of hemolysis is so brisk that it exceeds the ability of the liver to produce haptoglobin, hemoglobinemia is found. Plasma normally possesses sufficient haptoglobin to bind 100–150 mg of hemoglobin per deciliter. During hemolysis, an approximation of the level of free plasma hemoglobin may be made by macroscopic examination of the specimen. At a plasma hemoglobin of approximately 25 mg/dl, the sample appears faintly pink, and at between 50 and 100 mg/dl, it is a distinct reddish color.

The excretion of hemoglobin results mainly from its dissociation into half molecules known as *dimers*. Each dimer has a molecular weight of nearly 32,000 d or half that of the intact molecule. Normal glomerular filtration prevents these dimers from appearing in the urine, and usually the plasma hemoglobin level must exceed 30 mg/dl before hemoglobinuria is seen. After filtration by the kidneys, the protein components of the molecule are catabolized, leaving residual iron. This stimulates the production of apoferritin from the liver, and both ferritin complexes and hemosiderin are slowly excreted in the urine and partially reabsorbed into the blood.

If hemolysis is rapid, this mechanism produces iron accumulations in the proximal tubule cells of the kidney, and some of these cells are excreted in the urine. These cells and free hemosiderin can be detected in the laboratory by staining the urine deposit for iron using the Prussian blue reaction (Perl's stain).

In the case of an acute crisis, hemoglobinemia that persists for more than an hour can produce an oxidation product of hemoglobin termed *methemoglobin*. The process by which this occurs involves the affinity of oxidized heme for albumin, and it produces a brown coloration. Plasma also contains an oxidized heme-binding protein (β_{1B}-globulin) termed *hemopexin*, which binds heme with greater affinity than albumin. The resulting heme-hemopexin complex is removed from the circulation in a manner similar to that of the hemoglobin-haptoglobin complex.

Classification of Hemolytic Anemias

As discussed previously, the classification of hemolytic anemias is complex and can overlap. The following general classifications are based on the disease mechanisms and are shown in Table 8.1.

Inherited Intracorpuscular Defects

Defective Red-Cell Membrane

Hereditary Spherocytosis. Hereditary spherocytosis, a common autosomal dominant disorder, is found principally in northern Europeans. Clinically, it is characterized by jaundice, anemia, chronic cholecystitis, and hemolytic episodes. The findings are usually observed during early childhood. Nonsplenectomized patients have been reported to have relative iron-deficiency anemia because of expansion of erythropoiesis caused by the anemia (Zanella et al., 1989).

The laboratory features are fairly nonspecific and reflect the chronic hemolytic nature of the disorder. The normocytic anemia can vary in severity, with hemoglobin levels between 9 and 12 g/dl. The mean cell volume (MCV) can be normal, decreased, or increased, according to the cell thickness. The mean cell diameter is always reduced, reflecting the presence of small, biconvex microspherocytes that are thicker than normal cells. The mean cell hemoglobin concentration (MCHC) is usually increased because of the spherocytic nature of the erythrocytes. Reticulocytes are often increased in parallel with the normoblastic erythroid hyperplasia of the bone marrow. Besides the presence of micro-spherocytes, the red-cell morphologic features include polychromasia and anisocytosis.

The direct antiglobulin test results are negative, unless secondary sensitization is also present. Both osmotic and mechanical fragility tests are abnormal and demonstrate increased fragility. A leukopenia may be present during an aplastic crisis, but usually the total white cell count and platelet count are normal. The autohemolysis test, with and without glucose added, can be useful in confirming the diagnosis, as can the acidified glycerol lysis test (Zanella et al., 1980). The latter procedure, although showing absolute sensitivity, appears to be poorly reproducible because of the critical importance of the pH of the reagents used, and it has been suggested that it be replaced by a new technique, the "pink" test, which avoids this problem (Vettoro et al., 1984).

The physiologic defect is related to increased permeability of the erythrocyte membrane to the

Table 8.1. General Classification of the Hemolytic Anemias

Inherited intracorpuscular defects		
Based on defective red- cell membrane		Hereditary spherocytosis Hereditary elliptocytosis Hereditary stomatocytosis Acanthocytosis

Based on abnormalities
of glucose metabolism
	Decreased enzyme levels	Pentose-phosphate shunt: G6PD deficiency
		Embden-Meyerhof pathway
		    Pyruvate kinase deficiency
		    Glucose-phosphate isomerase deficiency
		    Triosephosphate isomerase deficiency

	Increased enzyme levels	δ-Aminolevulinic acid synthetase
Based on abnormal hemoglobin (Hb) chains		Sickle cell anemia Hb C disease Hb E disease Unstable hemoglobins, etc. Methemoglobinemia
Based on impaired synthesis of Hb chains		Thalassemias
Acquired intracorpuscular defects		
Based on membrane abnormal- ities or injuries		Paroxysmal nocturnal hemoglobinuria
Based on hemoglobin molecular abnormalities		Hb H disease Hb Kaellicker Hb A_2 and Hb F Methemoglobinemia
Acquired extravascular defects		
Based on immune disorders	Isoantibodies	Erythroblastosis fetalis associated with anti-D, anti-K, others
	Transfusion reactions	Most commonly associated with anti-A, anti-B, anti-D, anti-Jk[a], anti-K, anti-Fy[a], and others

	Autoimmune disease	Warm-reacting antibodies
		    Primary
		    Secondary to other disorders (e.g., lymphoma,
		        systemic lupus erythematosus)
		Cold-reacting antibodies
		    Idiopathic (e.g., paroxysmal cold hemoglobinuria)
		    Secondary to other diseases (e.g., pneumonia, lymphoma)

Based on nonimmune disorders	Physical trauma or agents, or both	Thermal injury Hypoxia Microangiopathic hemolytic disease Infectious agents Chemical toxins Drugs
	Mechanical trauma	Artificial prostheses (e.g., heart valves, Teflon patches)

	Poorly defined mechanisms	Hemolysis seen in association with other diseases
		    (e.g., malignant tumors, acute and chronic infections,
		    renal disease, splenic malfunctions, liver disease)

	Acquired defects altering heme solubility, synthesis, or intracellular enzymes	Chemical toxins Heavy metals Naphthalene Phenylhydrazine Oxidative compounds

G6PD = glucose-6-phosphate dehydrogenase.

passive influx of sodium ions. The cell compensates for this leakage by increasing the rate of active transport of sodium out of the cell, resulting in increased use of glucose and ATP. Lipid depletion of the cell membrane also occurs secondary to this abnormality. It is believed to be caused by the increased metabolic activity required for the electrolyte pump, which results in increased phospholipid turnover and a reduction of membrane lipids. Other evidence suggests that the membrane defect involves the microfilament structure of spectrin, associated with impaired spectrin phosphorylation (Valentine, 1977; Lux, 1979).

The sum of the biochemical changes results in the production of a rigid biconvex microspherocytic red cell that becomes easily trapped in the microcirculation, especially in the spleen. It has also been demonstrated that the red cells of hereditary spherocytosis possess approximately half the normal number of Rh CD antigen sites (Szymanski, 1989).

Hereditary Elliptocytosis. Like hereditary spherocytosis, hereditary elliptocytosis is inherited as an autosomal dominant trait and is widespread throughout the world. Clinically, the disease exhibits findings similar to those seen in other chronic hemolytic anemias, although the symptoms are usually mild and the laboratory findings, except for the presence of elliptic red cells, are relatively normal.

The disease is characterized in the newborn by a scanty number of elliptocytes, which are seen in increasing numbers as the child ages. These cells show a membrane defect opposite that seen in hereditary spherocytosis—that is, the cell membrane is abnormally permeable to sodium efflux. During incubation of elliptocytes, there is a loss of intracellular sodium and a reduction of red-cell ATP and 2,3-diphosphoglycerate activity. Additionally, there are accumulations of cholesterol at each pole of the cell, and Hb appears to be unevenly concentrated.

The peripheral blood picture shows elliptic red cells accompanied by varying degrees of anisocytosis, poikilocytosis, polychromasia, and reticulocytosis. The anemia is frequently mild, with Hb levels between 10 and 12 g/dl. Red-cell survival is often normal, with only 10–15% of patients showing decreased cell survival. The osmotic fragility test results are usually normal too, whereas the autohemolysis test results are abnormal. The autohemolysis is corrected by the addition of glucose and ATP. The direct antiglobulin test results are negative.

The defective cells, like those in hereditary spherocytosis, become trapped in the spleen and consequently are removed from the circulation. Elliptocytes are found in other disorders, including thalassemia, iron-deficiency anemia, megaloblastic anemia, and myelophthisic anemia.

Hereditary Stomatocytosis. Stomatocytes are bowl-shaped red cells that possess a slitlike appearance when viewed by light microscopy. The appearance of these cells is associated with three principal disorders: (1) those characterized by increases in intracellular sodium and decreases in intracellular potassium, (2) those characterized by a lack of Rh antigens (Rh_{null}), and (3) those not associated with either cation imbalance or surface antigen loss.

The stomatocytes associated with defective cation movement are believed to be caused by passive membrane leaks and increased cation pumping. If sodium gain exceeds potassium loss, the total number of cations of the cell increases, and there is a corresponding gain of cell water. This results in macrocytic erythrocytes that possess reduced MCHC values and increased osmotic fragility (Mentzer, 1975). If potassium loss either exceeds or is equivalent to sodium gain, the cation and intracellular water content are decreased, leading to increased MCHC values and decreased osmotic fragility (Wiley, 1975). The increase in cation-membrane activity results in increased glucose consumption and lactate production. Stomatocytic cell membrane lipid content is variable, but lipid metabolism is not increased as it is in hereditary elliptocytosis.

Rh_{null} disease exhibits stomatocytes associated with a shortened life span and a membrane abnormality resulting in increased potassium permeability. This is due to a 35–40% increase in the number of pump sites per cell (Lauf and Joiner, 1976).

Hereditary stomatocytosis is an autosomal dominant disorder characterized by the presence of large numbers of stomatocytes. In most cases, the anemia is mild, and hemolytic symptoms are either lacking or minimal. Associated with the anemia is a variable reticulocytosis and macrocytosis. Increased serum bilirubin and decreased haptoglobin levels are seen only if the disease is severe, and then increased osmotic fragility may be demonstrated. Autohemolysis usually is increased and is corrected by both glucose and ATP.

The Rh_{null} variety of stomatocytosis usually produces a mild normocytic normochromic hemolytic anemia with a mild reticulocytosis. The autohemolysis and osmotic fragility test results are both positive. Adult red cells agglutinate with anti-i as well as anti-I and, by definition, they do not agglutinate with any anti-rhesus antisera. Consequently, the genotype of such cells is amorphic for Rh antigens lacking all determinants (- - -/- - -, or Rh_{null}).

Acanthocytosis. Acanthocytes are erythrocytes that possess several irregularly spaced, large, coarse spicules, having sharp rather than blunted ends. These cells are found in two principal clinical states: abetalipoproteinemia and severe liver disease. The acanthocytes seen in abetalipoproteinemia differ from those seen in liver disease in that, when incubated in normal serum, they do not revert to a normal shape.

Abetalipoproteinemia is a rare disorder characterized by a hypolipidemia, acanthocytosis, malabsorption of fat, and neurologic damage. The primary defect is the abnormal synthesis of apolipoprotein B, which causes both low-density lipoproteins and very low-density lipoproteins and chylomicrons to be absent from the serum. This produces deficient metabolic activity involving these proteins. The plasma cholesterol level is sharply decreased, but that of the acanthocyte appears normal or slightly increased. Red-cell lecithin levels are reduced, and sphingomyelin levels are increased.

The acanthocyte appears to possess normal glycolytic mechanisms and normal cation permeability. There is an association between acanthocytes and the McLeod blood group system, the McLeod phenotype being characterized by weak Kell antigens, a lack of Kx antigen, and acanthocytic red-cell morphology.

The laboratory findings include a mild normocytic normochromic anemia. Reticulocytosis may be present, depending on the anemia and bone marrow response. Morphologically, large numbers of acanthocytes are seen. The osmotic fragility test results usually are normal, but the mechanical fragility test results often reveal increased fragility. Red-cell sedimentation rates are decreased irrespective of the degree of anemia because of the cells' inability to produce rouleaux formation. The bone marrow is normal but occasionally shows a mild erythroid hyperplasia. The direct antiglobulin test results are negative.

Other Red-Cell Membrane Disorders. Several other rare hemolytic anemias associated with defective erythrocyte membranes have been reported. Such disorders include familial lecithin-cholesterol acyltransferase deficiency, high phosphatidylcholine hemolytic anemia, and hereditary pyropoikilocytosis.

Abnormal Glycolysis Involving the Pentose-Phosphate Shunt

Glucose-6-Phosphate Dehydrogenase Deficiency. Glucose-6-phosphate dehydrogenase (G6PD) is an intracellular erythrocytic enzyme that catalyzes the initial step of the pentose-phosphate shunt. A deficiency of this enzyme results in a reduced ability within the cell to withstand oxidizing challenges, which is expressed as a hemolytic anemia. This reduction is principally due to a decrease in reduced glutathione, which protects the red cell from peroxide changes. If peroxide damage takes place, Hb is degraded, reducing the precipitation of Hb (as Heinz bodies) and resulting in the ultimate lysis of the cell. Many G6PD variants are known. The disorder is sex-linked, with full expression in affected males and partial expression in females. Distribution of G6PD deficiency occurs worldwide, the highest incidence being in the black population. The deficiency also is found in Italian, Greek, Asian, American Indian, and Jewish populations.

The principal deficiency states are manifested as favism in Mediterranean populations; drug-induced hemolysis in black and Mediterranean populations; congenital nonspherocytic anemia in Oriental, European, and Mediterranean populations; and hemolysis induced by viral and bacterial infections, which may occur in any G6PD-deficient population.

Favism is a severe, acute hemolytic anemia resulting from the ingestion of or contact with the fava bean. Hemolytic episodes have occurred in sensitive males who inhale the pollen of the bean. All patients with favism have G6PD deficiency, but not all G6PD-deficient individuals are sensitive to the bean. The disorder is most common in boys

Table 8.2. Examples of Drugs that Induce Hemolysis in G6PD Deficiency

Antimalarials	Primaquine, quinacrine hydrochloride, quinine, and others
Sulfonamides	Sulfanilamide, sulfisoxazole, sulfacetamide, and others
Nitrofurans	Nitrofurantoin, nitrofurazone, furazoline,and others
Antipyretics	Acetylsalicylic acid, acetanilid, acetophenetidin, and others
Sulfones	Sulfoxone, thiazolsulfone, diaminodiphenyl sulfone
Others	Methylene blue, phenylhydrazine, chloramphenicol, fava beans, naphthalene

G6PD = glucose-6-phosphate dehydrogenase.
Source: Data from WJ Stuckey, Jr. Hemolytic anemia and erythrocyte glucose-6-phosphate dehydrogenase deficiency. Am J Med Sci 251:104, 1966.

younger than 12 years and occurs primarily in the spring.

Clinically, severe hemolysis is found, with hemoglobinuria and Heinz bodies present during the acute phase. These inclusion bodies consist of denatured protein that distorts the cell membrane, resulting in a loss of cellular elasticity. As a result, the cells are trapped by the liver and spleen and are removed from the circulation.

Drug-induced hemolytic anemia is found principally in G6PD-deficient black and Mediterranean people and, infrequently, in the population of Southeast Asia. There are, however, large numbers of patients who develop drug-induced hemolysis but have no G6PD deficiency. Hemolysis is caused by a wide variety of oxidizing drugs (Table 8.2). Evidence of acute hemolysis appears within 24 hours after administration of the offending agent, and hemoglobinemia and hemoglobinuria usually are seen. Within 48–96 hours after the drug is discontinued, hemolysis ceases. The extent of the cell destruction appears to be dose-dependent and self-limiting. Older red cells are more susceptible to lysis because of their lowered enzyme levels. The diagnostic tests include a direct assay for G6PD and the formation of Heinz bodies after staining with methyl violet or after in vitro stimulation with acetylphenylhydrazine. Both the glutathione stability test and the methemoglobin reductase test produce positive results.

Congenital nonspherocytic hemolytic anemia may result from a deficiency of several red-cell enzymes, including G6PD, pyruvate kinase, glutathione reductase, diphosphoglyceromutase, adenosine triphosphatase, triosephosphate isomerase, hexokinase, and glutathione.

Those individuals who have a G6PD deficiency, in addition to being sensitive to hemolytic drugs, show spontaneous hemolysis. Such patients have a chronic, moderately severe anemia, with nonspherocytic red cells and jaundice, which is usually apparent during childhood. Reticulocytosis sometimes is present; when this occurs, the MCV is increased proportionally.

Hemolysis induced by viral or bacterial agents often occurs in G6PD-deficient individuals. A variety of agents have been implicated, including *Escherichia coli* (Burka and Weaver, 1966), *Salmonella* species (Rattazzi et al., 1971), *Streptococcus* species (Mengel and Metz, 1967), and *Rickettsiae* species (Whelton and Donadio, 1968). Other chronic systemic diseases associated with hemolysis in G6PD-deficient individuals include viral hepatitis, pneumococcal pneumonia, diabetic acidosis, rheumatoid arthritis, renal failure, and malaria.

Recently, a case of severe hemolytic anemia with agranulocytosis has been described in a patient who had a normal G6PD activity and was on dapsone therapy. Hemolytic anemia and methemoglobinemia often are found secondary to dapsone therapy, irrespective of G6PD levels (Figueiredo et al., 1989).

Abnormal Glycolysis Involving the Embden-Meyerhof Pathway

Pyruvate Kinase Deficiency. A deficiency of the glycolytic enzyme pyruvate kinase is probably the most common cause of congenital nonspherocytic hemolytic anemia (Beutler, 1979). The deficiency results in impaired generation of ATP, thereby inhibiting the electrolyte pump and producing red-cell membrane abnormalities.

The disorder is found worldwide, although it appears to be most common in northern Europe. The mode of inheritance is autosomal recessive, homozygotes usually having a hemolytic anemia and splenomegaly, whereas heterozygotes are asymptomatic. The clinical expression of the deficiency is variable, ranging from severe neonatal jaundice to a fully compensated hemolytic anemia. The normocytic normochromic anemia is more severe than that seen in hereditary spherocytosis. Macrocytes may be present during a hemolytic crisis, reflecting bone marrow hyperplasia and reticulocytosis. The peripheral blood morphologic examination shows polychromasia, anisocytosis, poikilocytosis, and nucleated red cells. The osmotic fragility is normal, but the autohemolysis test often shows a moderate degree of lysis that is poorly corrected by the addition of glucose or ATP. The diagnostic test is the pyruvate kinase assay.

Glucose Phosphate Isomerase Deficiency. Glucose phosphate isomerase is inherited in an autosomal recessive mode. The disorder does not possess any clinical or hematologic features that distinguish it from other red-cell enzymopathies. The deficiency is characterized by a moderately severe hemolytic anemia that may be complicated by an aplastic crisis (Van Biervliet, 1975). The peripheral red-cell morphologic examination frequently shows nucleated red cells and moderate anisocytosis, poikilocytosis, polychromasia, and reticulocytosis. Autohemolysis is increased and can be partially corrected by glucose and ATP. The definitive diagnosis can best be made by specific enzyme assay.

Triosephosphate Isomerase Deficiency. Triosephosphate isomerase deficiency is a fatal disorder involving multiple tissues and causing a severe hemolytic anemia. The deficiency is autosomal recessive in inheritance and is first detected early in infancy. Neurologic involvement, cardiac arrhythmias, and hemolytic anemia usually result in death before the age of 5 years.

The peripheral blood smear contains small numbers of acanthocytelike cells. The autohemolysis test results are abnormal and are corrected by ATP but not by glucose. In this regard, triosephosphate isomerase deficiency resembles hereditary spherocytosis. The osmotic fragility test result is flattened, containing populations of both osmotically fragile and resistant cells.

Other Enzyme Defects. In addition to G6PD, pyruvate kinase, glucose phosphate isomerase, and

Table 8.3. Hemoglobin Chains and Amino Acids

Chain	Number of Amino Acids
α	141
β	146
γ	146
δ	146

triosephosphate isomerase deficiencies, a depletion of other enzymes involved in the glycolytic pathway can result in hemolytic disease. These enzymopathies are very rare but can include deficiencies of hexokinase, aldolase, and diphosphoglycerate mutase (Beutler, 1979).

Hemoglobinopathies

A hemoglobinopathy is a disorder in which production of normal adult hemoglobin is partially or completely suppressed or partially or completely replaced by production of one or more variant hemoglobins. The protein hemoglobin is composed of four heme groups and globin and has a molecular weight of 64,458 d. The heme complex is composed of an iron atom centrally placed in a protoporphyrin ring, and the globin consists of two pairs of polypeptide chains (see page 19). These chains differ in numbers and types of amino acids. For example, the α chain has 141 amino acids and the β, γ, and δ chains possess 146 amino acids. The γ and δ chains differ in composition, the γ chain having 39 different amino acid substitutions and the δ chain being composed of 10 different substitutions, compared with the β chain. Consequently, normal globin is made up of 574 amino acid moieties, derived from two α and two β chains. In total, 17 different amino acids are involved in the structure (Table 8.3).

The designation of the hemoglobin molecule reflects the type of globin chains present. In the normal situation, in which the α and β chains are present, the form $\alpha_2\beta_2$ is used to denote Hb A (adult), whereas during fetal development, Hb F ($\alpha_2\gamma_2$) predominates. Here γ chains replace the β chains. Hb A_2 also is present normally in individuals in small amounts and is characterized by δ-chain replacement of the β chains.

Abnormal hemoglobins result from mutations in the hemoglobin gene. Most arise from single substitutions of amino acids, the remaining being prod-

Table 8.4. Genetic Makeup of the Common Hemoglobins

Hemoglobin	Polypeptide Chain Abnormality
A	$\alpha_2{}^A\beta_2{}^A$
A_2	$\alpha_2{}^A\delta_2{}^A$
F	$\alpha_2{}^A\gamma_2{}^F$
S	$\alpha_2{}^A\beta_2{}^S$
C	$\alpha_2{}^A\beta_2{}^C$

Source: Data from RM Schmidt, EM Brosious. Basic Laboratory Methods of Hemoglobinopathy Detection (pub. no. 77-8266). Atlanta: US Department of Health, Education, and Welfare, 1976.

ucts of deletions, globin chain fusions, or elongated subunits. Examples of these forms are shown in Table 8.4. Table 8.5 differentiates the gene abnormalities in the common hemoglobins.

The type of shorthand formulation depicted in Table 8.4 shows more clearly the structurally defective globin chains. For example, Hb C possesses two normal α chains and two abnormal β chains, written as β^c. The drawback of such notations is that the exact substitution or deletions are not specified.

Abnormal Hbs are assigned a common name and a scientific designation. The common name usually denotes the place of discovery, whereas the scientific notation indicates the structural aberration. Thus, $\beta6(A3)Glu{\rightarrow}Val$ represents Hb S and indicates that valine has been substituted for glutamic acid at the sixth position, the third amino acid in the A helix of the β chain. Likewise, $\beta6(A3)Glu{\rightarrow}Val; \beta3(E17)Asp{\rightarrow}Lys$ represents Hb C Harlem. Here two substitutions are present, the first being exactly as in Hb S and the second substitution occurring at the seventy-third position of the β chain, the seventeenth amino acid of the E helix, in which

aspartic acid has been substituted for lysine. Generally, these hemoglobins are written as follows:

$$\text{Hb S } (\alpha\beta^{6Glu{\rightarrow}Val}) \text{ and } (\alpha_2\beta_2{}^{6Glu{\rightarrow}Val\ 73\ Asp{\rightarrow}Lys})$$

The development of human hemoglobins is shown on page 15. The ϵ chain is normally present only in very early embryonic life and soon is replaced by the γ chain and, eventually, by the β and δ chains in the adult. There probably are two kinds of embryonic hemoblobin, Gower I (ϵ_4) and Gower II ($\alpha_2\epsilon_2$). Hb F is the major oxygen carrier in fetal life and contains two α chains and two γ chains. After birth, the proportion of Hb F decreases and, by the first year, it represents only a minor component of the total hemoglobin.

The common clinical human hemoglobin variants are shown in Table 8.6. Disorders due to the presence of sickle hemoglobin constitute the most important group.

There are more than 400 hemoglobin variants, most of which differ by a single point mutation. Point mutations can change the charge of the protein significantly, the difference being electrophoretically detected. Standard hemoglobin electrophoresis is carried out on cellulose acetate at pH 8.6 using hemolysate containing intact hemoglobin. Cellulose acetate electrophoresis separates hemoglobin variants based on charge, although many variants have similar charges and migrate to the same location. Therefore, hemoglobin variants identified on cellulose acetate electrophoresis should be confirmed by citrate agar electrophoresis at pH 6.2. Citrate agar contains negatively charged agaropectin, which binds to the surface of amino acids of the globin chain. Mutations that cause substitutions on these surfaces, such as Hb S and Hb C, have a greater affinity for agaropectin binding than those that cause internal substitutions. Increased

Table 8.5. Molecular Basis of the Common Hemoglobin (Hb) Variants

Mechanism	Involved Chain	Examples
Single amino acid substitution	α	Hb I and others
	β	Hb S, Hb C, Hb D, and others
	γ	Hb F and others
	δ	Hb A and others
Two amino acid substitutions	α	Hb J Singapore
	β	Hb C Harlem
Amino acid deletions	β	Hb Gun Hill
Fusion hemoglobins	$\delta\beta$	Hb Lepore
	$\gamma\beta$	Hb Kenya
Elongated subunits	α	Hb Constant Spring

Table 8.6. Clinically Important
Hemoglobin (Hb) Variants

Variant	Globin Chain Substitution
Hb S	$(\alpha_2\beta_2^{6GLU \to VAL})$
Hb C	$(\alpha_2\beta_2^{6GLU \to LYS})$
Hb D	$(\alpha_2\beta_2^{121GLU \to GLN})$
Hb E	$(\alpha_2\beta_2^{26GLU \to LYS})$
Hb G Accra	$(\alpha_2\beta_2^{73ASP \to ASN})$
Hb C Harlem	$(\alpha_2\beta_2^{6GLU \to VAL\ 73ASP \to ASN})$
Hb I	$(\alpha_2^{16LYS \to GLU}\beta_2)$
Hb H	β_4
Hb O Arab	$(\alpha_2\beta_2^{121GLU \to LYS})$

GLU = glutamic acid; VAL = valine; LYS = lysine; GLN = glutamine; ASP = aspartic acid; ASN = asparagine.

agaropectin binding results in an increased electrophoretic mobility. Thus, acid electrophoresis differentiates hemoglobins by charge and location of the substitution, and the comparison of the migration pattern on cellulose acetate with citrate agar allows for identification of most common hemoglobin variants.

Sickle Cell Anemia. The two main features of sickle cell anemia are its hemolytic tendencies, caused by a reduced red-cell life span, and the propensity of the red cell to take an elongated form in reduced oxygen tension, thereby impeding the microcirculation and leading to stasis. Sickle cell anemia is inherited as an autosomal dominant disorder and is seen only in its homozygous form (Hb SS). Hb S is found commonly in blacks and their descendants, most frequently in people from equatorial Africa. It also is seen, though less commonly, in the populations of the Mediterranean area and India (Brittenham et al., 1974).

Hb S differs from normal Hb A only in the single substitution of valine for glutamic acid in the sixth position of the β chain. This single substitution induces a major alteration in the configuration and stability of the molecule, causing drastic shape changes and loss of flexibility. Low oxygen tension, acidosis, and dehydration can polymerize the Hb S molecule to form "tactoid" rodlike structures that impart to the cell its characteristic elongated sickle or oat-leaf morphologic form.

When Hb S is combined with oxygen, it possesses essentially the same solubility as Hb A. However, in the deoxygenated state, the β chains open or rotate, allowing the substituted valine to interact with the valine that occupies the first position of the β chain, forming an intramolecular bond and producing a bulge in the otherwise straight configurations of this part of the β chain. This protrusion projects down and away from the mass of the hemoglobin tetramer. In the deoxygenated state, these protrusions from the β chain are capable of interacting with a complementary site in the α-chain portion of neighboring hemoglobin molecules. They then enter into a hydrophobic type of bonding arrangement, thereby connecting the two molecules together by joining the β portions of one molecule to the α region of its neighbor. As this continues, "stacking" takes place intracellularly, and eventually stacks of joined molecules begin to intertwine and form thin, rodlike structures that are seen as microfilaments. Under electron microscopy, these filaments are seen to be composed of six helically intertwined bundles of molecules that ultimately align themselves in a parallel formation, stretching the cell membrane and resulting in a typical sickle cell.

The actual sickling process is usually reversible in 10–15 seconds on reoxygenation of the intracellular hemoglobin. Ligand bonding with oxygen will change the positions of the β chains, drawing them closer together. When this occurs, the valine-valine bump no longer fits into the neighboring α-chain site, and the stacking phenomenon described earlier is reversed (Patrick et al., 1975). This allows the red cell to take on its normal shape. However, repeated sickling induces sufficient membrane damage to some susceptible cells that the rigidity and sickle shape persist, even after the cell has been reoxygenated (Bunn et al., 1977b).

Sickling also depends on the degree of intracellular Hb S concentration present. Individuals who are heterozygous for the disease (sickle cell trait Hb AS) have sufficient Hb A to act as a protective mechanism and thereby avoid hemolytic crises. Similarly, this mechanism can be seen in the true homozygous sickle cell anemia, in which increased levels of Hb F appear to be protective. The more Hb F that is present, the less likely it is that a cell will sickle. Individuals who have both sickle cell anemia and hereditary persistence of fetal hemoglobin (HBFH) will show far fewer symptoms than those with usual sickle cell anemia. The clinical manifestations of the sickle cell disorders are determined by the amount of Hb S present, the type and amount of other coexisting hemoglobins, and the presence of other red-cell abnormalities. C peptide levels in the disease have been found to be reduced (Saad et al., 1989) and, consequently, lead to inadequate insulin secretion by the pancreas or an independent genetic abnormality in linkage disequilibrium with the β_s gene.

Clinically, sickle cell anemia produces a chronic hemolytic process characterized by hepatosplenomegaly, hematuria, chronic infections, leg ulcers, and vaso-occlusive crises. The peripheral blood picture is of a normocytic normochromic anemia, with a hemoglobin level of 5–9 g/dl. A proportional decrease in the hematocrit and red-cell count also is seen. The blood smear shows moderate numbers of sickled cells, target cells, basophilic stippling, Howell-Jolly bodies, and nucleated red cells. The reticulocyte count is elevated between 10 and 15%, particularly during and following hemolytic episodes. The total leukocyte count shows a moderate leukocytosis with a mild leftward shift, caused by the redistribution of these cells from the marginal to the circulating granulocyte pool. Platelets may be moderately decreased during an infarction but may be increased during remission.

The bone marrow shows a marked normoblastic erythroid hyperplasia, and active marrow present in the bone is usually yellow and fatty. During an aplastic crisis, a maturation arrest of the red-cell precursors is sometimes seen. Iron deposits are increased, signifying iron overload resulting from hypertransfusion. Haptoglobin levels are reduced or absent, depending on the severity of the hemolytic crisis, and unconjugated bilirubin levels are elevated. The erythrocyte sedimentation rate is decreased disproportionately to the anemia because of the inability of the erythrocytes to make rouleaux formations. This produces a normal sedimentation rate in the presence of moderate anemia.

The diagnostic laboratory tests include the separation of Hb S by electrophoresis, a positive solubility test for Hb S and, occasionally, the demonstration of small increases in Hb F. In addition, high-performance liquid chromatography has been recommended as an additional test in the diagnosis of hemoglobinopathies and thalassemias. The reported advantages of this method include increased sensitivity, resolution, and speed (Rogers et al., 1985).

Hemoglobin electrophoresis using cellulose acetate with a pH 8.6 buffer separates most of the common Hbs (Figure 8.1). However, Hb S migrates

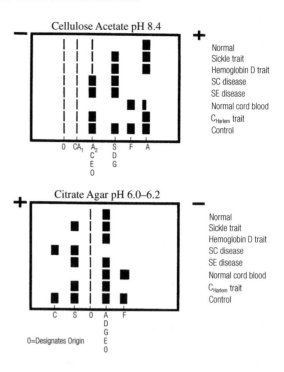

Figure 8.1. Hemoglobin electrophoresis. Comparison of various hemoglobin samples on cellulose acetate and citrate agar, showing relative mobilities. (Reprinted with permission from JB Henry [ed]. Clinical Diagnosis and Management by Laboratory Methods [17th ed]. Philadelphia: Saunders, 1984. P 676.)

in the same position (between Hb C and Hb A) as other abnormal Hbs, as shown in Table 8.7.

Separation of Hb S from Hb D and Hb G Philadelphia can be made by electrophoresis on citrate agar at pH 6.2 (see Figure 8.1), Hb S moving toward the anode while both Hb D and Hb G Philadelphia move slowly toward the cathode. In addition, Hb S produces a positive sickle cell test, whereas Hb D and Hb G do not sickle. However, hemoglobins that have the $\beta6Glu{\rightarrow}Val$ substitution (Hb C Georgetown and Hb S Memphis) also exhibit the sickling phenomenon. Hemoglobin solubility is another useful test in screening for Hb S. Decreased solubility of deoxygenated Hb S produces a turbid solution when blood is added to a reducing agent, and this differentiates Hb S from nonsickling hemoglobin variants. The test is nonspecific, as other sickling hemoglobins such as Hb C Georgetown, Hb I, and Hb Bart's also precipitate. Table 8.8 shows hemoglobins with reduced solubility that may sickle, polymerize, or aggregate.

Table 8.7. Examples of Abnormal Hemoglobins Possessing Similar Electrophoretic Mobilities to Hemoglobin S on Cellulose Acetate, pH 8.6

Hemoglobin	Chain Abnormality	Comments, Distribution, and Levels Found in Heterozygotes
D	β	American blacks, Middle East, India, 35–40%
Shiminoseki	α	Japan, 20%
Zürich	β	Unstable hemoglobin, whites, 20%
Lepore	δβ fusion	<20%
D Ibadan	β	Blacks, 20%
G Philadelphia	α	Migrates slightly faster than Hb S
P	β	Blacks, 50%
Sabine	β	Unstable hemoglobin, whites 7–10%
Hasharon	α	Ashkenazi Jews, 15–20%
Memphis	α	Blacks, 50%
L Ferrara	α	Italy, Jews

Source: Data from RM Schmidt, EM Brosious. Basic Laboratory Methods of Hemoglobinopathy Detection (pub. no.77-8266). Atlanta: US Department of Health, Education, and Welfare, 1976.

Table 8.8. Hemoglobins (Hbs) with Reduced Solubility That May Sickle, Polymerize, or Aggregate

Hemoglobin Type	Residue Changed	Comments
Single-Mutant Variants		
S	$\beta^{6GLU \rightarrow VAL}$	Common variant sickles because of the formation of hydrophobic bonds of the hemoglobin molecule; the red-cell membrane then assumes the typical elongated shape
C	$\beta^{6GLU \rightarrow LYS}$	Paracrystallization: common variant; crystal formation believed to be related to the decreased intermolecular distance, water loss, and membrane alterations
Porte Alegre	$\beta^{9SER \rightarrow CYS}$	Abnormal polymerization: abnormal disulfite bonding
Ypsi	$\beta^{99ASP \rightarrow TYR}$	Abnormal polymerization: increased oxygen affinity and mild polycythemia
Double-Mutant Variants		
C Georgetown	$\beta^{6GLU \rightarrow VAL}$ $\beta^{73ASP \rightarrow ASN}$	Sickles by hydrophobic bonding
C Harlem	$\beta^{6GLU \rightarrow VAL}$ $\beta^{73ASP \rightarrow ASN}$	Sickles by hydrophobic bonding; differences between Hb C Harlem and Hb C Georgetown unclear
Hemoglobins Without α Chains		
Bart's	No substitutions; δ_4	Sickles in high concentrations; mechanism unknown

GLU = glutamic acid; VAL = valine; LYS = lysine; SER = serine; CYS = cysteine; ASP = aspartic acid; TYR = tyrosine; ASN = asparagine.
Source: Data from CW Patrick, G Stamatoyannopoulos. Genetics: Hematology [workshop]. Chicago: American Society of Clinical Pathologists, 1975.

Table 8.9. Quantitative Hemoglobins (Hbs) in Hemoglobinopathies and Thalassemias

Disorder	Defect	% Hb A	% Hb Variant	% Hb A$_2$	% Hb F
Normal adult	—	>95	0	<3.5	<2
Normal infant	—	20–40	0	0–1	60–80
Hb S trait	Mutation of 1 β gene	60	40	<4.5	<2
Hb C trait	Mutation of 1 β gene	60	40	*	<2
Hb E trait	Mutation of 1 β gene	70	30	*	<2
Hb D trait	Mutation of 1 β gene	60	40	<3.5	<2
Hb O Arab trait	Mutation of 1 β gene	60–70	30–40	*	<2
Hb G Philadelphia trait					
With 1 α gene	Mutation of 1 α gene	75	25	<3.5	<2
With 2 α genes	Mutation of 2 α genes	70	30	<3.5	<2
With 3 α genes	Mutation of 3 α genes	65	45	<3.5	<2
Hb Köln	Mutation of 1 β gene	70–80	20–25	<3.5	<10
Sickle cell disease	Mutation of 2 β genes	0	>85	<6	<10
Hb S/β+-thalassemia	Combination	5–30	>50	Variable	1–20
Hb S°-thalassemia	Combination	0	75–90	Variable	5–20
Hb S/δβ°-thalassemia	Combination	0	75–90	Variable	10–25
Hb S/α-thalassemia	Mutation of 1 β and deletion of 1–2 α genes	65–75	25–35	<4.5	<2
Hb S/HPFH	Combination	0	65–85	Variable	15–45
Hb SC disease	Combination	0	Approx. equal	*	<10
Hb C disease	Mutation of 2 β genes	0	>85	*	<10
Hb C/β+-thalassemia	Combination	5–30	>50	*	1–20
Hb E disease	Mutation of 2 β genes	0	>85	*	<10
Hb E/β°-thalassemia	Combination	0	60–85	*	15–40

HPFH = hereditary persistence of fetal hemoglobin.
*Hb A$_2$ cannot be measured in the presence of these abnormal hemoglobins.

Sickle Cell Trait. Sickle cell trait is the expression of the heterozygous state of Hb S. The disorder is rarely associated with clinical or hematologic findings. There is no anemia, and the red-cell morphologic appearance is normal. Sickle cell trait is found in approximately 8.5% of American blacks; most individuals under nonstress conditions possess Hb S in concentrations of 35–50%.

The laboratory findings are clear-cut. Electrophoretic patterns are usually diagnostic unless the individual has received recent transfusions of normal blood. Unless this has occurred, Hb A is between 50 and 65% and Hb S levels are between 35 and 50%.

One distinguishing feature of sickle cell trait and sickle cell anemia is their association with infections by *Plasmodium falciparum*. Apparently, the presence of Hb S within the red cell of carriers inhibits trophozoite multiplication rates. As the developing parasite reduces the intracellular oxygen tensions, increasing amounts of deoxyhemoglobin accumulate. Ultimately, the sickling process begins killing the developing trophozoite.

Hemoglobin SC Disease. Hb SC disease results from the inheritance of an Hb S gene and an Hb C gene. On electrophoresis, Hb S and Hb C are present in equal proportions, and there is no Hb A or Hb F.

Clinically, the disease is less severe than sickle cell anemia. The most common symptoms are abdominal and skeletal pain. Moderate splenomegaly often is seen, together with an increased incidence of infection.

The laboratory diagnosis depends on the electrophoresis results. Anemia is mild and frequently is not seen. The peripheral blood shows no obvious abnormalities, with the possible exception of increased target cells and the presence of occasional Hb C crystals. Sickling may also be demonstrated.

Other Sickle Cell Syndromes. Besides sickle cell anemia, sickle cell trait, and Hb SC disease, other rare sickling syndromes have been documented. They include Hb SD disease, Hb SE disease, Hb SO Arab, Hb S–HPFH, Hb C Harlem trait, and Hb S thalassemia (α and β) (Milner, 1974).

Table 8.10. Classification of the Unstable Hemoglobins

Degree of Severity	Hemoglobin Examples
Severe hemolytic disease	Hammersmith, Bristol, Savannah, Bibba, etc.
Moderate hemolytic disease	Atlanta, Genova, Newcastle, Sabine, Santa Ana, Madrid, etc.
Mild hemolytic disease	Gun Hill, Seal Rock, Cranston, Constant Spring, Köln, Sidney, Zürich, Duane, Shepherds Bush, Ann Arbor, Leiden, Lyon, Freiburg, etc.
Asymptomatic disease	Hopkins II, Manitoba, Tacoma, Sögn, etc.

Hemoglobin C Disease. Hb C disease is the second most frequently encountered hemoglobin variant in most areas of the United States. The disorder is mild and, like sickle cell anemia, is inherited as an autosomal recessive characteristic. The abnormality results from the substitution of glutamic acid by lysine in the sixth position of the β chain. As the glutamic acid residues carry a net negative charge and the lysine carries a net positive charge, in effect such a substitution represents a double-charge change. The positive charge now conferred by the lysine in the outside position of the molecule retards the electrophoretic mobility of the Hb C molecules, causing them to remain closer to the cathodal zone of the electrophoretic field at pH 8.6–8.8. The molecular change is represented by $\alpha_2\beta_2^{6Glu\rightarrow Lys}$.

The disease is characterized by a moderate hemolytic anemia and splenomegaly. Occasional fragmented red cells and microspherocytes are seen in the peripheral blood. Target cells are also present and mainly responsible for the decreased osmotic fragility (increased red-cell resistance) test results. The red-cell life span is usually reduced to 30–50 days. The bone marrow shows a mild normocytic hyperplasia that varies in severity according to the degree of anemia. On occasion, intraerythrocytic crystals of Hb C may be seen, particularly in moist blood preparations.

The differential diagnosis is made by hemoglobin electrophoresis. At alkaline pH values on cellulose acetate, Hb C migrates with Hb A_2, Hb E, and Hb O Arab, but can be separated using citrate agar electrophoresis at acid pH levels (see Figure 8.1).

Hb C trait is found in individuals who are heterozygous for Hb A and Hb C. Such people are usually asymptomatic, and the disorder is considered a benign condition, with the possible exception of some crises described in association with pregnancy (Patrick et al., 1975). The peripheral blood picture is relatively normal except for increased numbers of target cells. Electrophoretic patterns show 28–44% Hb C, the remainder of the Hb being Hb A. See Table 8.9.

Other Hemoglobinopathies. *Hb D disease* is characterized by a mild hemolytic anemia and splenomegaly (Ozsoylu, 1976). The presence of Hb D should be suspected when electrophoresis reveals a typical pattern for sickle cell trait, when efforts to demonstrate sickling are unsuccessful, and when the ferrosolubility test is normal.

Hemoglobin electrophoresis shows mainly Hb D $(\alpha_2\beta_2^{121Glu\rightarrow Gln})$ with normal levels of Hb A_2 and Hb F. Hb D disease can be differentiated from Hb D-β^0-thalassemia by the presence of Hb A_2 and Hb F and by the relative lack of microcytes and target cells (Schneider and Veda, 1968).

Hb D migrates with Hb S on cellulose acetate electrophoresis in alkaline buffers, but it can be separated by using either agar gel or starch at acidic pH levels. Differentiation can also be accomplished with solubility tests, Hb D being negative and Hb S being positive. Although Hb D has been described in several different geographic locations and involves several types of amino acid substitutions, the most common form is the result of a substitution at the one hundred and twenty-first position of the β chain, at which point glutamic acid is replaced by glycine. This hemoglobin is known by several names, including Hb D Punjab, Hb D Los Angeles, Hb D Cyprus, and Hb D Portugal. Its frequency rate is approximately 0.4% in American blacks and 2–3% in the Sikhs of India (Vella and Lehmann, 1974). Hb D, unlike Hb S, does not sickle or aggregate.

Individuals heterozygous for Hb D (Hb D trait) are completely asymptomatic and do not demonstrate any morphologic abnormalities.

Hb SD disease is a rare disorder in which the mild clinical and hematologic findings resemble

Table 8.11. Mechanisms of Some of the Unstable Hemoglobins

Mechanism	Unstable Hemoglobin
Amino acid substitution in the vicinity of the heme pocket	Hammersmith, Zürich, Sabine, Bristol, etc.
Disruption of the secondary structure	Duarte, Madrid, etc.
Substitution in the interior of the subunit	Sögn, Bristol, Shepherds Bush, Ann Arbor, etc.
Amino acid deletions	Leiden, Lyon, Freiberg, Gun Hill, etc.
Elongated subunit	Constant Spring, Seal Rock, Cranston, etc.

mild sickle cell anemia. Again, the definitive diagnosis is made by the presence of both Hb S and Hb D on citrate agar electrophoresis.

Hb E ($\alpha_2\beta_2^{26Glu \rightarrow Lys}$) is the second most common Hb variant worldwide. The gene frequency exceeds 10% in the Orient (Bunn and Schechter, 1983). It has also been reported in black populations (Nelson and Davey, 1984a). The heterozygote state (Hb AE) is common and asymptomatic. Diagnosis of this variant is made by electrophoresis, using either cellulose acetate or agar gel; approximately 30% Hb E typically is found.

The homozygous state does not produce anemia. In most cases, there is a microcytosis (65–70 fl) that may be difficult to interpret because of a concomitant iron-deficiency anemia; the exception is in women, some of whom show minimal anemia (Hb ~11.5 g/dl). Target cells are present, and a decreased osmotic fragility test result usually is found. Hb E occurs at a frequency of 50–60% at the junction of Thailand, Laos, and Cambodia. Mutation and gene interaction account for more than 60 different clinical symptoms. Of these, homozygous β-thalassemia and Hb E β-thalassemia are the most common and produce the most severe clinical syndromes compatible with live births. Hb E β-thalassemia disease is more frequent than homozygous β-thalassemia in Southeast Asia because of the higher frequency of Hb E.

Hb O Arab ($\alpha_2\beta_2^{121Glu \rightarrow Lys}$) has been found in black, Arab, and Sudanese populations (Ramot, 1960; Javid, 1973). On cellulose acetate, this Hb migrates like Hb C, but on agar gel electrophoresis its mobility is similar to Hb S. The homozygous state is characterized by a mild hemolytic anemia and the presence of numerous target cells.

Hb G Philadelphia occurs mainly in American and African blacks. Physical and hematologic findings are normal in heterozygotes. Sickling is not seen in Hb G Philadelphia double heterozygotes. Such individuals appear healthy.

Other β-chain variations—Hb J Amiens and Hb Villejuif—have been described in association with polycythemia vera.

Unstable Hemoglobins. The unstable hemoglobins are those that become denatured and form intracellular Heinz bodies.

Unstable hemoglobin disease can be subdivided as shown in Table 8.10. Of the more than 80 different unstable hemoglobins known, there are nearly four times as many β-chain examples as there are α-chain variants. The instability of most of these variants can be attributed to one of the following mechanisms: amino acid substitution in the vicinity of the heme pocket, disruption of the secondary structure, substitution in the interior of the subunit, amino acid deletions, and elongated subunits. Examples of such mechanisms are illustrated in Table 8.11.

Unstable hemoglobin disease exhibits an autosomal dominant pattern of inheritance. Consequently, affected individuals are heterozygotes. The anemia produces a wide variety of effects of clinical severity, ranging from a severe hemolytic anemia to an asymp-tomatic picture. The most common unstable variant is Hb Köln, which produces a mild compensated hemolytic anemia, particularly after splenectomy. When the disease is severe, it is usually present with anemia during early childhood. On occasion, such hemolysis is enhanced by viral or bacterial infections or following exposure to an oxidant agent such as a sulfonamide.

Hemoglobinuria and many Heinz bodies are common findings. Methemalbumin associated with cyanosis also is present. Heinz bodies are aggregates of precipitated unstable hemoglobin that accumulates in the center of the cell. As they move to the periphery, the Heinz bodies form larger aggregates

Table 8.12. Some Causative Agents Implicated in Acquired Methemoglobinemia

	Group	Agent
Direct oxidants	Therapeutic agents	Amyl nitrite, ethyl nitrite, ammonium nitrate, silver nitrate, nitroglycerin, etc.
	Domestic and indus- trial agents	Nitrate-rich well water, nitrate-rich foods, nitrous gases, etc.
Indirect agents	Sulfonamides	Sulfamethizole, sulfanilamide, sulfathiazole, etc.
	Analine dyes	Marking ink, dyed blankets, laundry markings, red wax crayons, etc.
	Miscellaneous agents	Acetanilid, nitrobenzenes, nitrotoluenes, phenacetin, etc.

that become visible by light microscopy. At the periphery of the cell, these aggregations form an intimate relationship with the inner aspect of the cell membrane through the formation of hydrophobic bonds. The Heinz bodies are rigid and tend to alter the cell membrane integrity, which affects its passage through the spleen. When this takes place, the red cell is retained in the spleen, and the inclusion body is removed or "pitted" from it with minimal hemoglobin loss. Eventually, the cell is also removed from the circulation if the reduction of its surface area to its volume becomes sufficiently great. As a result of this splenic activity and the removal of the precipitated unstable hemoglobin from the circulation, electrophoresis often reveals that levels of 8–30% of the total hemoglobin belong to the unstable variant.

The laboratory findings are similar to those of other forms of chronic hemolysis. They include a variable reticulocytosis, bilirubinemia, and decreased serum haptoglobins. Because the precipitated hemoglobin takes up supravital stain, cells containing Heinz bodies may be mistaken for reticulocytes, so care should be taken when estimating the number of reticulocytes. When stained by a Romanowsky stain, the peripheral blood smear is usually normal, although an occasional mild hypochromia is seen. The definitive diagnostic test is the presence of Heinz bodies, which may be detected using crystal violet or new methylene blue (see page 308). To demonstrate these inclusions adequately, it may be necessary to incubate the cells with an oxidant, such as acetylphenylhydrazine.

Hemoglobin electrophoresis may be helpful in detecting the abnormality, but because of the relatively small amount of abnormal hemoglobin present, together with the lack of a specific marker, this technique may fail to yield definitive results. Other useful laboratory tests include the heat denaturation test and the isopropanol precipitation test.

Hemoglobins Associated with Abnormal Oxygen Affinity: Methemoglobinemia

Some hemoglobinopathies result in cyanosis and other abnormal pigmentation and are associated with decreased arterial oxygen saturation. Methemoglobin is found in the red cell in three instances: (1) when the rate of heme oxidation is increased, (2) when methemoglobin reduction is limited by reduced nicotinamide adenine dinucleotide (NAD) phosphate–methemoglobin reductase deficiency, and (3) when a structural abnormality in the globin moiety stabilizes hemoglobin in the oxidized state.

Acquired Methemoglobinemia. Acquired methemoglobinemia can result from oxidative stress. Many drugs are potentially capable of inducing the formation of methemoglobin, which results in globin denaturation and Heinz body formation, as well as increased hemolysis. Some of these drugs are listed in Table 8.12. These agents can be subdivided into two groups: those that act directly and those that act indirectly on hemoglobin.

Drugs that are capable of oxidizing hemoglobin directly include many nitrites and nitrates, particularly when they are ingested or absorbed through the skin in burn patients. Well water rich in nitrates has been implicated in methemoglobinemia in children and in hemodialysis patients, and foods high in nitrates have also been recognized as precipitative causes (Smith and Olson, 1973). Methemoglobinemia can cause a reduced antioxidant potential in some because of low levels of reduced glutathione. Such individuals, when exposed to normal or small doses of offending agents, exhibit hemolysis, the most frequent example being in G6PD deficiency. The indirect mechanism by which drugs and chemicals produce methemoglobinemia is not well defined.

Table 8.13. Some High-Affinity Hemoglobins Associated with Polycythemia

Name	Amino Acid Substitution	Electrophoresis		Ethnic Origin
α-Chain variants				
Chapel Hill	$\alpha_2^{74ASP \to GLY}$	—	Slow	—
Chesapeake	$\alpha_2^{92ARG \to LEU}$	Normal	Fast	American, white
J Capetown	$\alpha^{92ARG \to GLN}$	—	Fast	Cape black
β-Chain variants				
Malmo	$\beta^{97HIS \to GLY}$	Normal	Normal	Swedish American
Yakima	$\beta^{99ASP \to HIS}$	—	Slow	Scandinavian American
Ypsilanti	$\beta^{99ASP \to TYR}$	—	Slow	American, black
San Diego	$\beta^{109VAL \to MET}$	Normal	Normal	Filipino
Little Rock	$\beta^{143HIS \to GLY}$	Fast	Normal	Lithuanian American
Syracuse	$\beta^{143HIS \to PRO}$	Normal	Normal	American, white
Bethesda	$\beta^{145TYR \to HIS}$	Fast	Normal	Chinese American
Hiroshima	$\beta^{146HIS \to ASP}$	Slow	Fast	Japanese
York	$\beta^{146HIS \to PRO}$	Fast	Normal	American, white
Zurich	$\beta^{63HIS \to ARG}$	Unstable	—	—
Gun Hill	β^{91-95*}	Unstable	—	—
Köln	$\beta^{98VAL \to MET}$	Unstable	—	—
Ypsilanti	$\beta^{99ASP \to TYR}$	—	—	—

ASP = aspartic acid; GLY = glycine; ARG = arginine; LEU = leucine; GLN = glutamine; HIS = histidine; TYR = tyrosine; VAL = valine; MET = methione; PRO = proline.
*Leu, His, Cys, Asp, and Lys deleted.

Table 8.14. Hemoglobins with Decreased Oxygen Affinity

Name	Amino Acid Substitution	Other Major Property
Seattle	$\beta^{70ALA \to ASP}$	—
Kansas	$\beta^{102ASN \to THR}$	Increased dissociation
Hammersmith	$\beta^{42PHE \to SER}$	Unstable
Beth Israel	$\beta^{102ASN \to SER}$	—
Bristol	$\beta^{67VAL \to ASP}$	Unstable

ALA = aminolevulinic acid; ASP = aspartic acid; ASN = asparagine; THR = threonine; PHE = phoeline; SER = serine; VAL = valine.

Hemoglobins with increased oxygen affinity bind oxygen more easily and release it to the tissues more slowly. This results in tissue anoxia and an increased compensating hemoglobin with a polycythemic blood picture. Those hemoglobins with decreased oxygen affinity release hemoglobin more easily to the tissues, producing a normal to decreased hemoglobin concentration. Some aromatic compounds such as acetanilid, sulfonamides, and a wide range of analine dyes have been implicated in the reaction (Nathan et al., 1977).

The clinical features vary but are usually mild. They include cyanosis, fatigue, and tachycardia. The diagnostic laboratory test is the quantitation of methemoglobin by spectrophotometric methods, the pigment having characteristic absorption bands at 630 nm. See Tables 8.13 and 8.14.

Congenital Methemoglobinemia. Congenital methemoglobinemia includes the following disorders.

NAD-methemoglobin reductase deficiency, a rare form of methemoglobinemia, is inherited by an autosomal recessive route. Individuals with this deficiency have variable cyanosis but no associated symptoms or physical findings, although some may

Table 8.15. The M Hemoglobins

Name	Amino Acid Substitution	Oxygen Affinity	Heat Labile	Present at Birth
M Boston	$\alpha_2^{58\text{HIS}\rightarrow\text{TYR}}\beta_2$	Reduced	No	Yes
M Iwate	$\alpha_2^{87\text{HIS}\rightarrow\text{TYR}}\beta_2$	Reduced	No	Yes
M Saskatoon	$\alpha_2\beta_2^{63\text{HIS}\rightarrow\text{TYR}}$	Nearly normal	Yes	No
M Hyde Park	$\alpha_2\beta_2^{92\text{HIS}\rightarrow\text{TYR}}$	Nearly normal	Yes	No
M Milwaukee	$\alpha_2\beta_2^{67\text{VAL}\rightarrow\text{GLU}}$	Normal	Yes	No

HIS = histidine; TYR = tyrosine; VAL = valine; GLU = glutamic acid.

have mild polycythemia. Untreated individuals usually have 15–30% methemoglobin.

Hb M disorders are associated with the five variants of the abnormal Hb M: In four of the variants, tyrosine is substituted for a heme-linked histidine of the α or β chain. The other variant, Hb M Milwaukee, involves the substitution of glutamic acid for valine at the sixty-seventh position of the β chain. Such changes stabilize the heme moieties in the ferric form, and this changes the absorption spectrum and gives the hemoglobin a brown color.

Heterozygotes are usually asymptomatic, although cyanosis is a common feature. Hb M Saskatoon and Hb M Hyde Park produce mild hemolysis because of their unstable nature. The M hemoglobins are shown in Table 8.15.

Acquired intracorpuscular defects include membrane injury—*paroxysmal nocturnal hemoglobinuria*—which is a unique chronic hemolytic anemia resulting from an acquired defect of the red-cell membrane. An intrinsic abnormality in paroxysmal nocturnal hemoglobinuria (PNH) is in the production of erythroid cells susceptible to lysis by complement and by their low or complete lack of acetylcholinesterase activity.

There is general agreement that PNH results from the expansion of an abnormal hematopoietic clone that has developed through a somatic mutation. In most patients, the abnormal clone coexists with residual normal hematopoiesis, whereas in some patients it constitutes most of the hematopoietic tissue (Rotoli and Luzzatto, 1989).

Three different cell populations possessing different sensitivities to hemolysis in acidic media have been demonstrated (Rosse, 1980). Cells that are only mildly affected are designated *PNH I,* cells that are moderately sensitive to lysis are

termed *PNH II,* and cells markedly sensitive to lysis are known as *PNH III.* When complement is activated, the same amount of the responsible antibody and complement fractions (C1, C2, and C4) is attached to the red-cell membrane of both normal and PNH I cells. However, the amount of C3 is proportionally increased on PNH I and PNH II cells relative to normal cells, causing increased hemolysis. The red-cell membrane defect also leads to an abnormally low acetylcholinesterase level, especially in PNH III cells. The cause of the disorder is unknown, although it has been considered to be related to the myeloproliferative group of diseases.

Most patients exhibit symptoms of chronic hemolysis without the classic symptom of hemoglobinuria. Approximately 25% demonstrate hemoglobinuria, although in most cases this symptom is not seen at night. Complications include bone marrow aplasia, thrombosis, and infection.

The laboratory findings usually show a variable anemia with no characteristic morphologic changes. A mild reticulocytosis may be present, together with a moderate bone marrow erythroid hyperplasia in those patients who do not exhibit the aplastic phase. Iron stores are frequently reduced or completely absent. Bone marrow chromosomes may show some abnormalities but are not specific for the disorder.

The peripheral leukocyte count is reduced because of the presence of a granulocytopenia. Neutrophil alkaline phosphatase levels are reduced or absent, as is leukocyte acetylcholinesterase. The urine may contain variable amounts of free hemoglobin or may be normal (see previous discussion). Hb F levels may be increased. The red-cell osmotic fragility is normal unless the disease is complicated by an iron deficiency, which will be manifested by decreased fragility. Both the direct and indirect antiglobulin tests produce negative results.

The plasma reflects the level of hemoglobin catabolism associated with the hemolytic crisis. Bilirubin, free hemoglobin, and methemalbumin levels are increased, whereas serum haptoglobins are greatly reduced or absent. The diagnosis depends on the demonstration of complement-sensitive red cells. The acid serum and Ham's test results usually are positive, as are the sucrose lysis test and Crosby test (thrombin test). False-positive results can be produced in the Ham's test in hereditary erythroblastic multinuclearity with positive acidified serum (HEMPAS) or in the presence of spherocytosis derived from any cause. However, HEMPAS cells can be differentiated from those of PNH in that not all normal sera produce acid hemolysis of HEMPAS cells, hemolysis does not occur in the patient's morning serum, and the reaction to the sucrose lysis test is negative. The sucrose lysis test can yield false-positive results in megaloblastic anemias and in some autoimmune hemolytic anemias.

Chapter 9

Hemolytic Anemias: Extracorpuscular Defects

Red-Cell Isoimmune Antibodies

Isoimmune and autoimmune hemolytic anemias result in red-cell destruction by the interaction of IgM antibodies, which causes intravascular lysis, or by the action of IgG antibodies, which results in extravascular sequestration. The isoimmune anemias result from sensitization to specific blood group antigens, usually following a blood transfusion or as a sequela to hemolytic disease of the newborn (HDN; erythroblastosis fetalis).

Blood Transfusion Reactions

Sensitization resulting from the transfusion of incompatible blood produces a wide variety of clinical and laboratory findings. The clinical features include chills, rigors, lumbar pain, fever, jaundice, hypotension, and oliguria leading to anuria. Typical laboratory test results are those of hemoglobinemia, hemoglobinuria, reduced serum haptoglobin levels, bilirubinemia, and abnormal kidney function test results. All these results, however, can vary in degree and depend on both the rate of hemolysis and the time elapsed between the transfusion and the laboratory testing. For example, hemoglobinemia and hemoglobinuria may be found a few hours after a reaction but, in severe cases, there often is a peak in approximately 24 hours. Blood urea nitrogen and creatinine levels can also be abnormal within 24 hours, but they may take a week to become mildly elevated if the hemolysis is not brisk. It is also common to find a positive direct antiglobulin test result and, on occasion, a positive but weaker indirect antiglobulin test result. Figure 9.1 illustrates the relative laboratory abnormalities found.

Most reactions due to IgM red-cell antibodies are dramatic and severe and begin after the transfusion of relatively small volumes of blood. The antibodies responsible for this type of reaction usually are those that can cause rapid activation of large quantities of complement. As soon as the incompatible blood is infused, antigen-antibody complexes are formed and complement becomes activated. This type of blood transfusion reaction is caused mainly by antibodies of the ABO blood group. The degree of cell destruction is proportional to the quantity of A or B antigen on the transfused red cells, the amount of antibodies in the patient's plasma, and the volume of incompatible blood transfused. Total destruction of the transfused cell is likely to occur in a short time when the patient possesses high-titered, avid, complement-binding antibodies that combine with the transfused red cells. These antibodies are easily detected by routine laboratory procedures, and so transfusion reactions of this type rarely occur.

Hemolytic reactions involving extravascular cell destruction principally involve IgG antibodies. When transfused blood is incompatible with an antibody in the patient's plasma that is unable to bind complement or can bind complement only minimally, red-cell destruction will be less severe than that seen when intravascular destruction occurs. These reactions principally involve antibodies to the

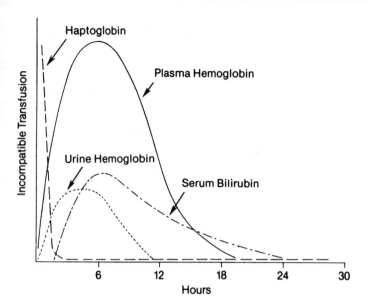

Figure 9.1. Common laboratory test results following a hemolytic transfusion reaction. (Reprinted with permission from DW Huestis, J Bove, S Busch. Practical Blood Transfusion [3rd ed]. Boston: Little, Brown, 1981. P 251.)

rhesus (Rh), Kell, Kidd, and Duffy antigens. The antibodies so produced coat the red cells, which then are destroyed extravascularly through phagocytosis in the reticuloendothelial (RE) system of the spleen. Complement-activated antibodies responsible for positive direct antiglobulin test results are similarly destroyed in the liver. The laboratory and clinical features of this type of hemolysis are similar to those seen in intravascular destruction, although in general the findings are less severe. Fever and chills are the most common clinical findings but, unlike those resulting from intravascular hemolysis, these symptoms may not occur until some time after the transfusion is completed. The laboratory results reflecting hemoglobin catabolism can also be delayed and are usually milder than those in intravascular hemolysis. Table 9.1 details the main differences between intravascular and extravascular hemolysis.

Hemolytic Disease of the Newborn

Isoimmune hemolytic anemia occurring in the newborn results from the transplacental passage of maternal antifetal erythrocyte antibody. This process is most commonly the result of incompatibility between mother and fetus of either the ABO or the Rh blood group, but it can also occur from the involvement of other blood group systems that produce IgG antibodies. Such systems include the Kell, Duffy, and Kidd blood groups.

In HDN, fetal red cells that possess antigens foreign to the mother are transferred across the placenta into the maternal circulation. If the mother lacks that antigen, IgG antibodies will be produced against these foreign antigens (fetal cells), the antibodies will gain access to the fetal circulation by passive transfer back across the placenta, and they will ultimately hemolyze the fetal red cells.

It should be noted that for a hemolytic anemia to occur, the antibodies produced must be small enough to cross the placenta. Consequently, IgM antibodies are not involved in such a process (molecular weight, 900,000 d); only IgG molecules are small enough to pass across the placenta and destroy the fetal cells.

ABO Disease

Anti-A and anti-B cause the most common form of HDN. Clinically, most cases are mild and often go unrecognized and undetected unless an indirect antiglobulin test on the cord serum is performed and both a direct antiglobulin test is carried out and eluates are separatted from fetal red cells. The direct antiglobulin test result is frequently negative or weakly positive, and this finding distinguishes it from Rh disease. The main laboratory features are of a mild bilirubinemia 24 hours after birth and the finding of immune anti-A or anti-B in the cord serum. On occasion, an eluate prepared from fetal

Table 9.1. Principal Differences Between Intravascular and Extravascular Hemolysis

	Intravascular Lysis	Extravascular Lysis
Antibody system most often involved	ABO	Rh, Duffy, Kell, Kidd
Speed of reaction and hemolysis	Rapid, often onset occurs before the transfusion is complete	Slower, sometimes takes place days after the transfusion
Severity of the reaction	Severe	Less severe, sometimes mild
Complement involvement	Strong	Weak or none
Hemoglobinemia	Strong	Weak or none
Hemoglobinuria	Often	Present, but less strong
Bilirubinemia	Mild or none	Moderate to strong
Bleeding following disseminated intravascular coagulation	Yes	Rarely present
Renal failure	Common	Less common

red cells will show anti-A or anti-B specificity. The peripheral blood shows a moderate degree of anisocytosis, the presence of microspherocytes, and a mild reticulocytosis with some polychromatic normoblasts.

In general, disease caused by ABO antibodies also differs from disease caused by Rh and other blood group antibodies in that infants from the first pregnancy can be affected.

Rh Disease

Hemolytic disease caused by blood group incompatibility usually is more severe clinically than is that seen in ABO disease. This form of anemia generally does not affect the firstborn child unless the mother already possesses alloantibodies derived from sensitization from previous transfusions.

The disorder, although not as common as ABO disease, most often produces clinical disease and can result from antibodies of most of the known antigens of the system. The most common antibody found is anti-D, alone or in combination with anti-C or anti-E. Unlike ABO disease, Rh disease can be predicted by a precise medical history of affected infants, by the presence of a rising titer of immune Rh antibodies during gestation, or by spectrophotometric analysis of amniotic fluid.

The laboratory diagnosis of the disease depends primarily on the presence of a strong positive direct antiglobulin test using the infant's cord cells. The presence of an immune Rh antibody in the maternal serum as a consequence of a previous pregnancy cannot be excluded. If the maternal genotype includes C

or E, it may act as a protective influence on the infant. The potency of the D antigen varies, depending on the cell genotype. R_2(cDE) cells react more strongly to anti-D than do R_1(CDe) cells, and infants who have an R_2 phenotype are more likely to be severely affected because of their genetic composition.

Laboratory tests that can be useful in the prediction of severe HDN include sequential titers of maternal antibody and the spectrophotometric analysis of amniotic fluid. In general, antibody titers are only moderately helpful in the prediction of the disease. Titer determinations suffer from a lack of precision, particularly when carried out by different technologists. Irrespective of the techniques used, the titer should be controlled by a parallel titration of a previously obtained serum that has been frozen and stored. Alterations of titer are not clinically significant unless they exceed at least a one-tube difference—that is, the titer must show a fourfold increase to be considered significant.

The spectrophotometric analysis of amniotic fluid basically measures the amniotic bilirubin level. The presence of bilirubin leads to an abnormal elevation of optical density (OD) at 450 nm. The difference in OD between the baseline and the peak elevation is known as δOD. The normal value of the δOD varies with gestational age and, consequently, the result can be interpreted only if the normal (baseline) value is known. Figure 9.2 illustrates a typical spectrophotometric pattern of amniotic fluid at 450 nm.

The spectral analysis of amniotic fluid bilirubin can be correlated with the severity of the disease, using the Liley curve (Liley, 1963; Figure 9.3). This nomogram plots the δOD at 450 nm against the ges-

Figure 9.2. The difference between points A and B is the δ optical density at 450 nm (δOD$_{450}$). Liley curve used for the measurement of amniotic fluid bilirubin. The *XY* line represents the expected OD of the amniotic fluid in the absence of bilirubin. The *AB* line represents the OD deviation from the expected curve at 450 nm, which is caused by the presence of bilirubin.

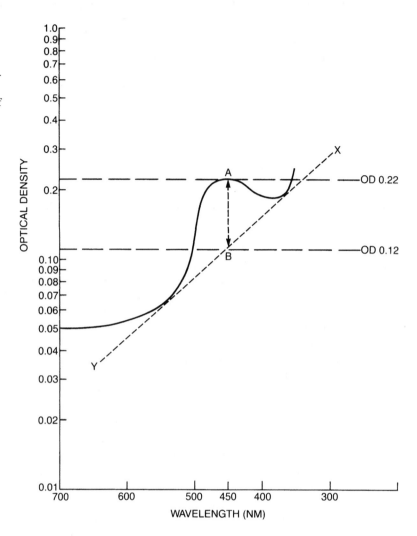

tational age. The chart is divided into three zones. Fetuses with values falling into the upper zone before the thirty-second week of gestation require intrauterine transfusion to survive. The midzone value indicates the need for repeated analysis and early delivery. Values in the low zone point to a good outcome when delivery is planned at or near term. The upper-zone values represent fetuses with severe hemolysis, and the midzone values require repeated analysis and close monitoring.

Other main differences that distinguish Rh from ABO disease include the presence of jaundice and bilirubinemia within the first 24 hours of life and the fact that firstborn infants rarely are affected.

The causative antibody in this type of hemolytic anemia is produced by the maternal immune system as a result of a challenge from the foreign fetal cells. For it to be effective, this antibody must be small enough to be passively transferred back across the placental barrier to the fetus. This limits the involved type of immunoglobulin to the IgG forms and thereby restricts some blood group systems from being causative agents in Rh disease. Thus, in theory, any blood group system that can produce IgG molecules and possesses sufficient antibody avidity has the potential to cause anemia. Other than ABO and Rh blood groups, HDN can be caused by maternal-fetal incompatibility due to Kidd, Duffy, and Kell blood groups as well as other rarer groups. The sole exception to this rule is the Lewis system. Lewis antibodies do

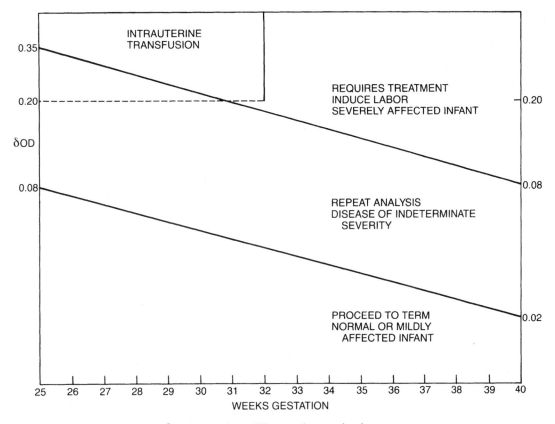

Figure 9.3. Liley curve relating the δ optical density at 450 nm to the gestational age.

not cause HDN because all fetal cells are Lewis-negative and because most Lewis antibodies are IgM forms.

Table 9.2 shows the principal differences between ABO and Rh hemolytic diseases.

Autoimmune Hemolytic Anemias

Warm-Antibody Type

Warm-antibody is the most common type of autoimmune hemolytic anemia, and this classification is reserved for those cases in which the autoantibody is optimally reactive at 37°C. The term *autoimmune hemolytic anemia* (AIHA) is used to denote individuals possessing warm-reacting autoantibodies. The cause of AIHA is unknown, although it is associated with various disorders, including lymphomas, systemic lupus erythematosus, and other autoimmune disorders.

The clinical features are similar to those in other acute hemolytic processes, the major findings being pallor, jaundice, and splenomegaly. The peripheral blood picture often presents normal mean cell hemoglobin (MCH) and variable mean cell volume (MCV) values. Anisocytosis, polychromasia, and reticulocytosis are commonly found, and spherocytes, schistocytes, and nucleated red cells may also be present.

The bone marrow exhibits a normocytic normochromic hyperplasia. Catabolic products of hemoglobin are usually demonstrated, including bilirubinemia, increases in urinary urobilinogen, and an increase in serum lactate dehydrogenase (LDH) levels. The most common laboratory test result is a positive direct antiglobulin test. Using monospecific antisera, approximately 30% of all cases demonstrate red-cell coating with IgG molecules, 50% demonstrate IgG and complement, and the remainder demonstrate complement only. This component is primarily a split product of C3 known as *C3b*.

Table 9.2. Principal Differences Between ABO and Rh Diseases

	ABO Disease	Rh Disease
Prediction of disease	No	Possible by amniocentesis and by rising maternal titers
Firstborn affected	Yes	No, unless mother is already sensitized by prior transfusion or by previous pregnancy
Clinical presentation	Usually mild	Can be severe and, if not treated, can be fatal
Anemia	Mild	May be severe
Peripheral blood	Microspherocytosis	Many immature nucleated red cells, polychromasia, and reticulocytes often present; spherocytes uncommon
Bilirubinemia	If present, usually delayed	Within first 24 hrs
Serologic characteristics	IgG form of anti-A or anti-B present in the maternal serum; cord cells may show anti-A or anti-B eluate; direct antiglobulin test on cord cells often negative or weakly positive	Anti-Rh detected in the maternal serum; direct antiglobulin test on cord cells often strongly positive; cord cell eluates often reveal presence of anti-Rh

Human serum contains C3b inactivator, which functions in cleaving the C3b component into two additional fractions: $C3c(\beta_{1A}$-globulin) and $C3d(\alpha_{2D}$-globulin). It is the C3b inactivator that is responsible for the binding of C3d to the red-cell surface and its subsequent detection by the direct antiglobulin test. Removal of complement-coated red cells is, however, not mediated by C3d fragments, this being accomplished by the specific binding of C3b to the red cells that attach to C3b receptor sites on the phagocytic liver cells.

When red cells are sensitized with IgM and complement fractions, frank intravascular hemolysis often occurs, but cell removal also takes place by sequestration in the liver with phagocytic ingestion. In addition, sequestration can occur with later return to the circulation. These recirculated sensitized red cells may survive normally. The determining factors in such red-cell survival are the rate and extent of complement sensitization, the nature of the antibody that causes complement sensitization, the number of antigenic sites on the red cell, the biological activity of the components involved, and the efficiency of the RE system.

Red cells sensitized by IgG are destroyed mainly in the spleen. Although the liver is a much larger organ, it has been shown that the spleen is approximately 100 times more efficient at removing sensitized red cells (Mollison, 1983). In general, there

appears to be a direct relationship between the amount of IgG on the red cells and the amount of red-cell destruction (Lalezari, 1976).

Red cells sensitized by IgM alone rarely occur. IgM antibodies usually activate complement, and this promotes intravascular hemolysis or red-cell removal extravascularly through C3b-macrophage interaction.

Warm-reacting AIHA is associated with a wide variety of specific antibodies, the most common belonging to the Rh blood group. Table 9.3 lists those known to be associated with AIHA.

Of the Rh antibodies known to cause AIHA, the majority have clear-cut specificity against one or more of the five major antigens, the most common being anti-e. However, some Rh antibodies may be detected only by using rare Rh cells. Thus, using red cells that possess a normal complement of Rh antigens, D-deleted red cells (D−−, etc.), and Rh_{null} cells, it can be shown that autoantibodies in AIHA often can be divided into one of three groups. One group reacts with cells of normal Rh phenotype (anti-nl), another group reacts with partially deleted cells but not with deleted cells (anti-pdl), and a third group reacts with all three cell types (anti-dl). Some autoanti-dl antibodies have been shown to have anti-Wr[a] or anti-En[a] specificity, whereas other anti-dl autoantibodies have been shown to contain anti-U or anti-LW specificity (Issitt, 1974). The reactions are shown in Table 9.4.

Table 9.3. Antibodies Associated with Auto-immune Hemolytic Anemia

System	Antibody
Rh	Anti-D, anti-C, anti-E, anti-c, anti-e, anti-pdl, anti-nl, anti-dl, anti-LW
Kell	Anti-K
Kidd	Anti-Jk[a]
MN	Anti-U
En	Anti-En[a]
Xg	Anti-Xg[a]

On occasion, specific antibodies may be eluted from red cells lacking the corresponding antigen. Anti-E has been eluted from E-negative cells and reabsorbed onto E-positive cells. Such an antibody is said to *mimic anti-E* (Issitt and Pavone, 1978).

Cold-Antibody Type

Some antibodies react most efficiently with red cells at temperatures of less than 37°C and may agglutinate optimally at temperatures ranging from 4–25°C. These so-called cold autoantibodies give rise to two principal disorders: cold hemagglutinin disease (CHD) and paroxysmal cold hemoglobinuria (PCH).

CHD is the most common type of cold autoimmune hemolytic anemia. It can occur as an acute or a chronic form. In the acute form, it often is associated with *Mycoplasma pneumoniae* and infectious mononucleosis. Individuals with CHD generally are elderly and present with a chronic hemolytic anemia of mild to moderate intensity. Antibody specificity frequently is anti-I and, less

commonly, anti-i, which is seen particularly in association with infectious mononucleosis.

On rare occasions, anti-Pr is found, as are anti-IA and anti-IB. Classically, cold-reacting antibodies do not react at 37°C and usually do not produce hemolytic reactions. However, the cold-reacting antibodies seen in CHD are distinguished by their wide thermal amplitude (they react best in the cold but also react at 30°C) and by an extremely high titer. Additionally, these IgM antibodies bind complement, with the result that C3d is fixed on the red-cell surface.

As shown in Table 9.5, occasionally anti-i also can cause CHD. It is believed that proliferation of the marrow and reduced transit times of red cells through the marrow, from the initial precursor cell state to the released red-cell state, cause an increase in the amount of i antigen to which antibody-producing cells are exposed. This then results in the production of autoanti-i. It is apparent that there is sufficient i antigen on the cells of patients with CHD for hemolysis to occur.

Cold agglutinins belonging to the I system are assigned I specificity when they react more strongly with adult red cells than with cells from a newborn. Conversely, anti-i specificity is assigned when the agglutination reaction is stronger with cord cells than with adult cells. Usually, normal adult sera contain low levels of anti-I, reacting only in the cold and not causing any pathologic reactions. However, the anti-I antibodies demonstrated in CHD possess the characteristics shown in Table 9.6.

The laboratory findings reflect the severity of the anemia and a corresponding reticulocytosis. Peripheral blood smears are difficult to obtain if the autoantibody is sufficiently avid and of high titer. In such cases, the slides should be prewarmed to avoid red-cell agglutination. Likewise, cell counts are frequently erroneous, especially when carried out by a

Table 9.4. Reactions of Autoantibodies in the Rh System

	Antibody Specificity			
Red-Cell Phenotype	**Anti-nl**	**Anti-pdl**	**Anti-dl**	**Anti-LW**
Normal Rh phenotype (e.g., R_2R_2)	+	+	+	+
Normal Rh phenotype but LW-negative	+	+	+	−
Partially deleted cells (e.g., D– –)	−	+	+	+
Rh_{null}	−	−	+	−

+ = positive reaction; − = no reaction.

Table 9.5. Autoantibodies Causing Cold Hemagglutinin Disease

System	Antibodies
I	Anti-I, anti-i, anti-IH
P	Anti-P (paroxysmal cold hemoglobinuria)
Sp-Pr	Anti-Sp$_1$ (Pr$_2$), anti-Pr$_1$, anti-Pr$_a$
Others	Anti-A, anti-B

volume-displacement method (e.g., the Coulter method) in which the blood is subjected to cold isotonic diluents. When this occurs, red-cell agglutination takes place, producing erroneously high MCV data and affecting all other red-cell indices.

The serologic findings, as previously detailed, show extremely high titers of a cold agglutinin often having anti-I specificity. Complement levels are frequently reduced during the hemolytic crisis, and the direct antiglobulin test results are positive when using a serum containing anticomplement components.

PCH is a disorder characterized by acute intermittent attacks of hemoglobinuria after exposure to the cold. The agglutinin responsible for this disease is the Donath-Landsteiner (D-L) antibody. It is a biphasic autohemolysin capable of attaching to the patient's cells only at low temperatures. When exposed to the cold, antigen-antibody complexes are formed and, as the cells return to a normal temperature, these complexes bind complement and produce a hemolytic crisis. The disease has been associated with syphilis, viral disorders, and bacterial infections (Burkart and Hay, 1979; Walach et al., 1981; Lau and Sererat, 1983).

The specificity of the D-L antibody is an IgG autoanti-P. The laboratory findings include the presence of spherocytes, reticulocytosis, and erythrophagocytosis (Hernandez and Steane, 1984). Hemoglobinuria is a common feature. The direct antiglobulin test result may be positive with anti-

IgG serum if the cells are washed at 4–12°C, but it is negative if they are washed with warmer saline. The indirect antiglobulin test result is positive. A positive Donath-Landsteiner test result is diagnostic for this disorder.

Combined Cold- and Warm-Antibody Type

Most patients with AIHA can be classified as having warm-antibody type disease, cold-antibody type disease, CHD, or PCH, depending on the laboratory findings. However, approximately 8% of all AIHA patients have been found to possess serologic features characteristic of both warm and cold AIHA (Shulman et al., 1985). This form of AIHA demonstrates characteristic serologic features, including the presence of both IgG and C3d on the red cells and the presence of both IgG warm autoantibodies and high–thermal amplitude cold autohemagglutinins in the serum. There appears to be an association between combined cold- and warm-antibody AIHA and systemic lupus erythematosus in at least two reported studies (Sokol et al., 1983; Shulman et al., 1985). This variant of AIHA appears to respond well to corticosteroid therapy.

Drug-Induced Hemolytic Anemia

Many drugs lead to the formation of antibodies, either against the drug itself or against intrinsic red-cell antigens. For substances to act as immunogens, they usually have to be of a molecular weight in excess of 5,000 d. To induce an immune response, a drug must first bind irreversibly to some tissue protein. Once conjugated, the hapten-protein complex can induce the formation of specific antibodies against the drug. These antibodies can cause a positive direct antiglobulin test result. Four basic mechanisms for producing a positive test result are

Table 9.6. Differences Between Anti-I in Cold Hemagglutinin Disease (CHD) and Normal Anti-I

Differences	Anti-I in CHD	Normal Anti-I
Titer	Usually >1:1,000; as high as 1:10,000 at 4°C	<1:32 at 4°C
Albumin as a titer fortifier	Titer enhanced	Titer not enhanced
Thermal range	4–30°C; may fix complement at 37°C	4–25°C
Specificity	May react well with i cord cells	Usually negative with cord cells
Nature of the antibody	Monoclonal	Polyclonal

Table 9.7. Drugs Reported to Cause Autoimmune Hemolytic Anemia

Mechanism	Drug
Immune complex adsorption (innocent bystander type)	Stibophen, quinidine, para-aminosalicylic acid, quinine, phenacetin, chlorinated hydrocarbons (insecticides), sulfonamides, antihistamines, isonicotinic acid hydrazide, chlorpromazine, aminopyrine, dipyrone, L-phenylalanine mustard, sulfonylurea, insulin, rifampicin, tetracycline, dipyrone, acetaminophen
Drug adsorption	Penicillin, cephalosporins, carbromal, chlorpromazine, methadone
Modified red-cell membrane	Cephalothin
Unknown mechanism	α-Methyldopa, L-dopa, ibuprofen, procainamide

Source: Reprinted with permission from G Garratty. Immune hemolytic anemia II. Drug-induced immune hemolytic anemia. Adv Immunohematol Oxnard Spectra Biol 3, 1975.

known: (1) immune complex adsorption, (2) drugs absorbed onto red cells, (3) a modified red-cell membrane, and (4) unknown mechanisms.

Immune Complex Adsorption

Drugs causing immune complex adsorption are not bound firmly to red cells, and washing in saline easily removes them. However, these drugs have a high affinity for their specific antibodies, forming antigen-antibody complexes in the plasma. The complexes attach nonspecifically to red cells, frequently activating complement. This produces a positive direct antiglobulin test result caused either by the bound immunoglobulin–drug complex reacting with complement or by complement attachment alone. The finding of complement on only the red cells demonstrates that the immune complex may have become dissociated from the cells, allowing it the freedom to reattach to other cells and in such a way as to enhance the complement activation cycle. Among the common characteristics of this group of drugs are acute intravascular hemolysis with hemoglobinuria and hemoglobinemia and IgM antibody formation. Only a small amount of drug may cause the reaction, and red cells often are sensitized by complement only. In vitro reactions are obvious only when the patient's serum, drug, and red cells are incubated together. The drugs causing this immune complex adsorption phenomenon are shown in Table 9.7.

Drugs Adsorbed onto Red Cells (Hapten)

Some drugs bind firmly to the red-cell membrane. When this immune reaction occurs, an an-

tibody is produced that reacts with the bound drug. The end result is a cell sensitized with IgG. Complement is usually not involved, and intravascular hemolysis does not take place. Cell destruction occurs extravascularly in the RE system in a manner similar to sensitization of cells by Rh (IgG). The principal clinical feature of this form of drug-induced hemolytic anemia is hemolysis, which develops only in patients who receive extremely large doses of medication This hemolysis is subacute in onset but may be life-threatening if the cause of the anemia is not recognized and the drug discontinued. Like the immune complex form of the anemia, the direct antiglobulin test result is strongly positive because of IgG sensitization.

Modified Red-Cell Membrane

The cephalosporins are the only drugs believed to react by modifying the red-cell membrane. The membrane is modified in such a way that the cell takes up proteins nonimmunologically. As many different proteins can be bound to cephalothin-treated red cells, the number of positive direct antiglobulin test results obtained will depend on how well the antiglobulin serum detects these proteins.

Unknown Mechanisms

An autoimmune hemolytic anemia caused by α-methyldopa and L-dopa has been described (Carstairs and Breckenridge, 1966). The mechanism of the anemia is not clear, but autoantibodies are pro-

Table 9.8. Examples of Microangiopathic Hemolytic Anemias and Their Causes

Microangiopathic Hemolytic Anemia	Cause
Abnormalities of the heart and great vessels	Heart valve prostheses, cardiac valve disease, etc.
Small-vessel disease	Hemolytic uremic syndrome, thrombotic thrombocytopenic purpura, disseminated intravascular coagulation, etc.
Associated with immune mechanisms	Lupus erythematosus, acute glomerulonephritis, etc.
Hemangiomas	Giant hemangioma, etc.
Pregnancy	Eclampsia, postpartum period, hemolytic uremic syndrome
Disseminated carcinoma	—
Malignant hypertension	—
Pulmonary hypertension	—

duced that react with intrinsic red-cell antigens. The serologic characteristics cannot be distinguished from those of warm autoimmune hemolytic anemia (see page 95). The patient's serum will react with normal cells in the absence of the drug. Very often the antibody can be shown to have specificity associated with the Rh blood group system.

The clinical and laboratory features of this form of anemia include a positive direct antiglobulin test that is usually dose-dependent; the test result usually becomes positive after 3–6 months of treatment. The patient's red cells usually are sensitized with IgG antibody only. The positive direct antiglobulin test result gradually reverts to negative once the drug is stopped, but this can take considerable time. Hematologic data improve within the first week or two following the last ingestion of the drug.

Physical and Thermal Injury

Microangiopathic Hemolytic Anemia

The term *microangiopathic hemolytic anemia* is used to designate any hemolytic anemia that results from red-cell fragmentation that occurs in association with small-vessel disease. A classification of such anemias is shown in Table 9.8. The disorder is generally associated with deposition of fibrin within the microvasculature or with severe hypertension. The blood changes are characteristic, showing many fragmented and distorted red cells (schistocytes), including helmet cells, triangular red cells, and pincer cells. Microspherocytes are seen commonly, in conjunction with a moderate thrombocytopenia and intravascular hemolysis. In severe or chronic anemia, hemoglobinuria and hemosiderinuria can be found.

Hemolytic Anemia Resulting from Burns

Acute hemolysis can be produced after thermal injury. The laboratory features include the presence of schistocytes and spherocytes in the peripheral blood. Hemoglobinuria is present in moderately affected individuals, the degree of hemolysis being related to the severity of the burns. The defect is believed to be caused by the irreversible denaturation of the red-cell membrane protein spectrin.

Heinz Body Anemia (Unstable Hemoglobin Disease)

Heinz body anemia, or unstable hemoglobin disease, is a hemolytic anemia inherited as an autosomal dominant characteristic, the most common form being that caused by the presence of hemoglobin Köln. A wide variety of abnormal unstable hemoglobins are associated with the disorder, most of which produce only a mild anemia and the intracellular precipitation of denatured hemoglobin as Heinz bodies (see page 40).

Lead interferes with the cation pump (Franklin, 1972), possibly inhibiting membrane adenosine triphosphatase (Dacie, 1967). The pathogenesis of copper hemolysis may relate to oxidation of intracellular reduced glutathione, hemoglobin, and reduced nicotinamide adenine dinucleotide phosphate

(NADPH), and the inhibition of glucose-6-phosphate dehydrogenase (G6PD) by copper.

Chlorates and oxidative drugs have been known to produce methemoglobinemia, Heinz bodies, and hemolytic anemia. Although it is presumed that the oxidative mechanism may be similar to that seen in G6PD deficiencies, no cases have been described in patients deficient in this enzyme.

March Hemoglobinuria

March hemoglobinuria is the development of hemoglobinuria after exercise, especially walking or running. Physically, the patient is normal and splenomegaly and hepatomegaly are not found. The blood may show some mild reticulocytosis, but morphologically it is normal. Schistocytes are not seen.

Plasma hemoglobin levels may be elevated, with a decrease in serum haptoglobin. The urine shows marked hemoglobinuria and, often, hemoglobin casts.

Nonoxidizing Drugs and Chemicals

Many chemicals have been implicated in the causation of hemolytic anemia, among them arsenic hydride, lead, copper, and chlorates. Arsenic hydride may interfere with sulfhydryl groups in the cell membrane and cause a hemolytic crisis.

Normal red cells generally are not subject to oxidative denaturation by drugs. This is because the cells maintain their reducing enzymes that scavenge reduced products of oxygen, superoxide dismutase, catalase, glutathione peroxidase, NADPH, methemoglobin reductase, membrane-associated vitamin E, vitamin C, intracellular glutathione, and reduced pyridine nucleotides.

In drug-induced oxidative damage, all or some mechanisms available for maintaining the reducing environment are mobilized. This depends in part on the site of oxidative denaturation or the biochemical behavior of the drug. Major changes may occur in red-cell hemoglobin, membrane proteins and phospholipids, and cellular metabolism.

Red cells do not typically undergo oxidative changes to their proteins or lipids unless the oxidant drug turnover exceeds the reducing capacity of the cell or unless the scavenging system is compromised by genetic, acquired, or environmental factors. In addition, these oxidative changes occur if genetic disorders related to cell structure or function are present. In vivo oxidative denaturation of red cells is rare, usually being seen in drug overdose or in individuals having congenital or acquired anomalies.

Chapter 10

Hematoparasites: Parasitic and Bacterial Infections

Malaria (*Plasmodium*)

The malarial plasmodia are protozoa belonging to the class Sporozoa. Four species are pathogenic to humans: *Plasmodium falciparum, P. vivax, P. malariae,* and *P. ovale.*

Life Cycle

The parasitic infection is acquired from the bite of certain species of mosquito of the genus *Anopheles.* When the female mosquito bites an infected individual, she acquires both male and female gametocytes, which develop to form many spindle-shaped male microgametocytes and female macrogametocytes. After fertilization of the macrogametocyte by the microgametocyte, a zygote is formed, which ultimately becomes elongated and active. This zygote, or *ookinete,* penetrates the mosquito's stomach wall and develops into an oocyst that produces a number of thin sporozoites. These organisms find their way into the salivary glands of the mosquito and become injected into the human circulation during an insect bite.

The sporozoites so introduced into a bitten individual invade the parenchymal cells of the liver, wherein they undergo asexual division and finally become liberated back into the circulation as merozoites and invade the red cells. Once the merozoites become intracellular, a process known as *schizogony* occurs, which results in the formation of 4–36 new parasites in each infected cell. This phase takes 48–72 hours to occur. At the end of schizogony, the infected red cell ruptures, liberating the merozoites, which then infect new red cells. The stages seen in the red cells are trophozoites (growing forms), schizonts (dividing forms), and gametocytes (sexual forms).

P. falciparum is the causative agent of malignant tertian malaria, a disease that is almost entirely confined to tropic and subtropic areas. Clinically, falciparum malaria can be differentiated from other forms of malaria in several ways. Morphologically, the gametocytes are sausage-shaped, in contrast to the ovoid or spheric gametocytes of the other species. Schizogony does not occur in the peripheral blood, and consequently only the trophozoites and gametocytes ordinarily are seen. Double or triple infections of the red cells are fairly common, which results in heavily parasitized cells. The young trophozoites are minute rings and, in *P. falciparum* infections, two small chromatin dots often are seen in these rings. Infected red cells that retain their original size may develop a few of these irregular, red, rodlike inclusions called *Maurer's dots.* Morphologically, gametocytes appear crescent-shaped with pointed or rounded ends.

P. malariae is the causative agent of quartan malaria, a disease that occurs in subtropic and temperate areas and is relatively rarer than either *P. vivax* or *P. falciparum.* The ring forms of *P. malariae* are morphologically similar to those of *P. vivax.* As the parasite grows, it exhibits little ameboid activity and tends to assume an elongated form. The infected red cell is not enlarged but, as the parasite grows, it nearly fills the cell prior to schizogony. Gametocytes of *P. malariae* are difficult to distinguish from the growing trophozoites but, when they mature, they may be slightly larger than the mature trophozoites and tend to be oval-shaped. The fully developed schizont normally contains eight merozoites that surround the pigment situated at the center, the so-called daisy form.

P. vivax is the most common malarial parasite in most parts of the world. This species is found almost everywhere that malaria is endemic and is the causative agent for benign tertian malaria. The young trophozoite is ring-shaped and very mobile, its diameter being approximately one-third that of a red cell. Between 6 and 24 hours after the start of the cycle, the trophozoites are nearly half the size of the cell, which itself is enlarged and may contain a number of fine red granules termed *Schüffner's dots*. These inclusions will always be seen in a red cell that has been infected longer than 15–20 hours and are diagnostic of either *P. vivax* or *P. ovale* infections. The parasite continues to increase in size and to fill the infected red cell, which by this time may be as large as 10–12 μ. At approximately 40 hours after infection, the trophozoite ceases its ameboid activity and becomes compact, producing up to 24 nuclear masses during schizogony. This cell division results in the production of the merozoites, which ultimately become liberated from the ruptured red cell.

P. ovale commonly is found in tropical Africa and also is seen in South America and Asia. Morphologically, the parasite is difficult to distinguish from *P. vivax*, although *P. ovale* appears less ameboid than *P. vivax*, and pigmentation is scanty. Typically, 4–12 merozoites are seen in schizogony. The infected red cells are enlarged and pale and show the presence of Schüffner's dots. The margins of these cells often appear ragged, and the cells are distinctly elongated, ovoid, or irregular in shape. The most important distinguishing features of *Plasmodium* species are shown in Table 10.1.

Laboratory Findings

Hematologic findings in malaria include a variable anemia, an occasional reduced red-cell life span or none, increased osmotic fragility, and a reduction in or total lack of haptoglobin. Hemolysis is the result of the red-cell invasion by the parasite, the cells being either intravascularly lysed when the merozoites are liberated or extravascularly lysed through splenic sequestration. Occasionally, an immune mechanism also is involved, IgG antibody against the parasite forms, and there is nonspecific attachment of the immune complexes to the red-cell membrane. This causes complement activation and subsequent phagocytosis, resulting in a positive direct antiglobulin test result owing to the presence of IgG or C3d or both (Fleming, 1981).

The most serious aspect of malarial infection follows the erythrocyte invasion by *P. falciparum*. Although occurring only rarely, an acute hemolytic crisis can take place, with chills, fever, hemoglobinemia, methemoglobinemia, hemoglobinuria, and bilirubinemia, together with renal shutdown. Such an extreme clinical reaction is termed *blackwater fever*.

In examining a blood smear for the presence of malaria, one should always report the species of parasite, as the clinical handling of patients as well as therapy may vary. For the study of parasitic morphologic characteristics, a stained thin blood smear is recommended. However, in some situations, the organisms may not be seen, and thick smears should be scanned, allowing for a more rapid examination of a larger volume of blood. Using this technique, the morphologic appearance of the parasites usually is altered, and there are no accompanying red cells because of the use of a hemolyzed sample.

Thick smears are best examined in the center area. If species characteristics are unclear, more typical organisms often are found in the thinner area. For routine purposes, at least 100 oil-immersion thick-smear fields should be examined before a negative result is reported.

Four components of the malarial parasite should be identified before species identification is established: (1) cytoplasm, (2) chromatin, (3) pigment granules, and (4) parasitic outline. Artifacts such as cellular debris, stain precipitate, bacteria, yeasts, molds, and platelets may be confused with the parasite. In thin blood smears, the appearance of the infected red cell and the parasite are the principal facts used in determining the exact species. Attention should be given to the size of the red cell, the presence or absence of red-cell stippling and, if *P. ovale* is suspected, the shape of the red cell. Although occasionally *P. vivax* parasites may be found in oval red cells, this shape is more commonly associated with *P. ovale* infections. Both *P. vivax* and *P. ovale* are seen in macrocytes, but the degree of red-cell enlargement is more often greater with *P. vivax*. Furthermore, trophozoites and schizonts are smaller in *P. ovale* than in *P. vivax,* and they occupy less of the red-cell area.

The appearance of the parasite may vary in several respects. Parasites in thick smears are usually more compact and smaller than in thin smears and appear more densely stained. The growth stages— trophozoites, schizonts, and gametocytes—cannot be differentiated by gender. Because the trophozoite and schizont stages of *P. falciparum* develop in capillaries, only the rings and gametocytes ordinarily are found. For this reason, falciparum malaria is diagnosed more easily from thick preparations than are other malarial species. The rings often appear as fine delicate structures and may easily be overlooked.

Frequently, only small red chromatin dots are seen, and careful focusing is required to observe the pale blue, fine cytoplasm of the rings. As the rings grow, the cytoplasm of *P. falciparum* stains a light or pale blue and contains coarse black pigment granules, in contrast to the densely staining organisms of *P. malariae*. Rings are found most often in acute cases of falciparum malaria, whereas the gametocytes are more typical of the chronic infection. Although in thick smears they are typically crescent-shaped, the gametocytes may also be ovoid or rounded in outline.

Of the remaining three species, only *P. vivax* and *P. malariae* can be distinguished in thick blood preparations, the parasites of *P. ovale* being identified only by the examination of thin blood smears. In general, differentiation of *P. vivax* and *P. malariae* is based on the appearance of the parasite, although evidence of Schüffner's stippling around the *P. vivax* parasite is a distinctive feature. The most difficult stage on which to base species identification is the immature schizont. The schizonts of *P. vivax* become round, more regular in outline, and denser in appearance than the trophozoites, and consequently they resemble the corresponding forms of *P. malariae*. Fortunately, species differentiation can be made on the basis of the other stages that are usually present.

The most distinctive stage for species identification is the mature schizont, because the number of merozoites formed is characteristic of the species.

Mature schizonts of *P. malariae* are often seen, but those of *P. vivax* are less common. Gametocytes of *P. vivax* and *P. malariae* are similar in morphologic appearance and cannot readily be distinguished as to species. However, it is unlikely that only gametocytes are seen, and the specific diagnosis should be made on the morphologic features of the asexual stages present. Gametocytes of both species usually appear as large chromatin masses surrounded by pigment granules. Sometimes a small area of blue cytoplasm is visible around the chromatin, but more often only chromatin and pigment are seen. Frequently, the entire parasite appears reddish.

In the differential diagnosis, several morphologic features should be emphasized. If only a few ring forms are seen, a diagnosis of malaria, species undetermined, should be made, as there are insufficient differences in ring forms alone to make a reliable specific diagnosis. However, if many small delicate rings are present in the absence of older stages, a diagnosis of *P. falciparum* can be established. The growth range seen also is of value; it is broader with *P. vivax* than with other species. In smears of *P. malariae* infections, most of the parasites are in a similar trophozoite developmental stage of maturation. Occasionally, mixed infections occur, with one species usually predominating.

The optimal time for obtaining blood smears is about midway between chills. At this time circulating forms will be sufficiently developed to permit an easier species identification. Smears taken just before the chill may contain mature asexual stages of *P. vivax, P. ovale,* and *P. malariae,* which are the most readily identified forms of those species, but the smears may be devoid of *P. falciparum* parasites, which complete their asexual cycle in the internal organs. Smears taken during the chill are apt to contain only young ring forms, which are difficult to identify as to species.

Factors Affecting Parasitization of Red Cells

P. vivax is not found in populations in which the amorphic Duffy blood group Fy$^{(a-b-)}$ is present. Young red cells appear to be invaded principally by *P. vivax* and *P. ovale* and only to a lesser extent by *P. falciparum*. This is believed to result from the fact that sialoglycopeptide receptors on the red-cell membrane are needed for *P. falciparum* mediation. Parasitic invasion is decreased in cells containing hemoglobin

Table 10.1. Main Morphologic and Clinical Features of *Plasmodium*

Characteristic	*P. falciparum*	*P. malariae*	*P. vivax*	*P. ovale*
Incubation period	8–11 days	18–40 days	10–17 days	10–17 days
Fever periodicity pattern	36–48 hrs	72 hrs	48 hrs	48 hrs
Red-cell size	Normal	Normal	Markedly enlarged; round	Markedly enlarged; oval
Red-cell inclusions	Rare Maurer's dots	None	Common Schüffner's dots	Common Schüffner's dots
Completion of growth cycle in peripheral blood	36–48 hrs	72 hrs	48 hrs	48 hrs
Can produce relapse years later	No	Unknown	Yes	Unknown
Early trophozoites	Very delicate ring	Compact ring	Delicate ring	Delicate ring
Developing trophozoites				
Size	Small	Small	Small	Small
Shape	Compact	Compact, often band form	Very irregular shape	Compact
Vacuoles	Inconspicuous	Inconspicuous	Prominent	Inconspicuous
Chromatin	Chromatin dots present	Chromatin dots present	Chromatin dots present	Large, irregular chromatin clumps
Pigment	Coarse black aggregated pigment	Coarse dark brown pigment	Fine yellow-brown pigment	Coarse dark yellow-brown pigment
Distribution	Present in two clumps	Present as scattered clumps and rods	Present as scattered fine particles	Present as scattered coarse particles
Immature schizonts				
Size	Almost fills the red cell	Almost fills the red cell	Almost fills the red cell	Almost fills the red cell
Shape	Compact	Compact	Somewhat ameboid	Compact
Chromatin	Many irregular masses	Few irregular masses	Many irregular masses	Few irregular masses
Pigment	Scattered	Scattered	Scattered	Scattered
Mature schizonts				
Size	Nearly fills the red cell	Nearly fills the red cell	Fills the red cell	Fills 75% of the red cell
Shape	Segmented	Segmented, daisy-head shape	Segmented	Segmented
Merozoites	8–32 small organisms	6–12 large organisms	14–24 medium organisms	6–12 large organisms
Pigment	Aggregated in center, black	Aggregated in center, dark brown	Aggregated in center, yellow-brown	Aggregated in center, dark yellow-brown
Microgametocytes				
Numbers in blood	Many	Scanty	Many	Scanty
Size	Larger than the red cell	Smaller than the red cell	Fills the red cell	Fills the red cell
Shape	Kidney-shaped, blunted round ends	Round, compact	Round or oval, compact	Round, compact

Table 10.1. (*continued*)

Characteristic	*P. falciparum*	*P. malariae*	*P. vivax*	*P. ovale*
Cytoplasm	Red-blue	Pale blue	Pale blue	Pale blue
Pigment	Dark granules throughout	Abundant brown granules throughout	Abundant brown granules throughout	Abundant brown granules throughout
Chromatin	Fine granules scattered throughout	Fibrils in skein with surrounding unstained area	Fibrils in skein with surrounding unstained area	Fibrils in skein with surrounding unstained area
Macrogametocytes				
Numbers in blood	Many	Scanty	Many	Scanty
Size	Larger than the red cell	Smaller than the red cell	Fills the red cell	Fills the red cell
Shape	Crescent, sharply rounded or pointed bands	Round, compact	Round or oval, compact	Round, compact
Cytoplasm	Dark blue	Dark blue	Dark blue	Dark blue
Chromatin	Compact masses near center	Compact peripheral masses	Compact peripheral masses	Compact peripheral masses
Pigment	Black granules around nucleus	Small, dark masses around periphery	Small, dark masses around periphery	Small, dark masses around periphery

(Hb) S but not in those containing Hb C and Hb E nor in those containing high levels of Hb F. However, the growth and replication of the parasites within the cells are reduced in the presence of elevated levels of Hb F, by the presence of Hb S at low oxygen tension, and in homozygous Hb C disease. Red cells of individuals with thalassemia and glucose-6-phosphate dehydrogenase deficiency often do not allow replication of *P. falciparum,* possibly because of their sensitivity to oxidant stress (Pasvol and Weatherall, 1980).

The relationship of arthropod to parasite is essentially one of the vector; that is, the parasite does not pass through a sexual cycle in the tick, the tick passing the parasite to its offspring, which in turn transfers it to a new mammalian host.

Hemolytic Anemia Caused by Other Infections

Bartonella bacilliformis

This flagellated bacillus is transmitted by the sandfly and is the causative organism of Carrión's disease, and acute hemolytic anemia found principally in Peru (Reynafarje and Ramos, 1961).

The first stage of the disease, Oroya fever, runs an acute course with high fever. Untreated, it can be fatal within 2–3 weeks in approximately 30% of cases. The second stage, verruga peruana, occurs 3–4 months after the primary infection and represents the chronic form. This stage is characterized by nodular and verruciform skin lesions.

The organism is a small delicate rod, 1–2 μ in length and 0.2–0.5 μ in breadth. Less commonly, it is coccoid and is stained by routine Romanowsky dyes. *Bartonella* organisms occur in red cells and monocytes and may appear as V- or Y-shaped rods.

Babesia

Babesia is a sporozoan parasite that usually infects domestic and wild animals, causing fever and jaundice. Infections of humans are very rare and are characterized by a gradual onset of malaise followed by fever, chills, and weakness. Hepatosplenomegaly and a hemolytic anemia are present, with accompanying bilirubinemia and hemoglobinuria and increases in transaminase levels (Ruebush et al., 1977). Unlike most sporozoea, *Babesia* multiply by binary fission in human red cells and in the organs of hard ticks.

The organism measures 0.9–2.0 μ and infects the red cells. It appears as a pleomorphic ringlike structure, somewhat similar to that of the ring stages of

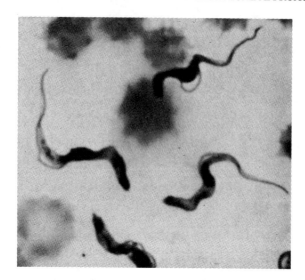

Figure 10.1. *Trypanosoma gambiense.* (Reprinted with permission from EK Markell, M Voge. Medical Parasitology [5th ed]. Philadelphia: Saunders, 1981. P 40.)

Plasmodium. As reproduction or schizogony commences, the parasite enlarges, displaying a prominent red-staining nucleus and a clump of blue cytoplasm. There usually is a small unstained vacuole that may, at times, increase to up to 2–4 μ in diameter as the parasite enlarges. As schizogony begins, the nuclear chromatin dot separates into fragments, usually no more than four. Often, strands of blue cytoplasm connect the four organisms, establishing a tetrad form (Healy, 1982). One can distinguish *Babesia* species from *Plasmodium* species by the absence of gametocytes and enlarged red cells.

Serologic diagnosis of suspected *Babesia* infection can be made on the basis of an indirect immunofluorescence test (Chisholm, 1978). The organism is transmitted by the bite of nymphal stages of the hard tick *Ixodes dammini* (Spielman, 1979; Bruckner et al., 1985).

Other Bacterial Infections

Hemolytic anemia can result from infections with a variety of different bacteria, including *Clostridium perfringens, Salmonella,* and *Escherichia coli* (Gombert et al., 1982).

Trypanosomes

Trypanosomes are protozoa belonging to the hemoflagellates. Humans can be infected by four species of trypanosomes: *Trypanosoma gambiense, T. rhodesiense, T. cruzi,* and *T. rangeli.* The narrow-bodied forms found in the blood are mobile and have central nuclei. At the forward-moving end, there is a flagellum that extends back alongside the body and forms the outer edge of an undulating membrane.

T. gambiense (Figure 10.1) is the causative organism of African sleeping sickness, which occurs mainly in Gambia or West Africa. The organism is pleomorphic, displaying a variety of forms ranging from a slender organism with a long free flagellum to a shorter, thicker form without a free flagellum.

T. rhodesiense, the cause of Rhodesian or East African sleeping sickness, is morphologically indistinguishable from *T. gambiense.* Infection occurs after the bite of an infected tsetse fly and is followed by an incubation period of up to several weeks. After this time, examination of a peripheral blood smear often will reveal presence of the parasites. Diagnosis depends on such a demonstration and may be enhanced by scanning thick blood smears.

T. cruzi (Figure 10.2) is found in the southern regions of the United States, in Mexico, and in Central and South America. This organism is the causative agent of Chagas' disease, the symptoms of which are anemia, edema, lymphadenopathy, and hepatosplenomegaly. The parasite is transmitted by the assassin bug *Triatoma.* Morphologically, it is shorter than the other trypanosomes, being 15–20 μ long. Other distinguishing features include a larger flagellum and a clearly visible kinetoplast.

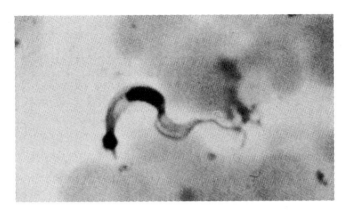

Figure 10.2. *Trypanosoma cruzi.* (Reprinted with permission from EK Markell, M Voge, Medical Parasitology [5th ed]. Philadelphia: Saunders, 1981. P 107.)

T. rangeli is found principally in Central and South America. It is transmitted by the bite of the reduviid bug *Rhodnius prolixus.* The parasites are approximately 30 μ long, with a nucleus anterior to the middle of the body and a small kinetoplast (Markell and Voge, 1981).

Leishmania

Leishmania is a genus of protozoa that, like trypanosomes, are blood flagellates. Three species occur in humans: *Leishmania donovani, L. tropica,* and *L. brasiliensis.* They are morphologically indistinguishable from one another. The parasites are transmitted by small sandflies and are round or oval organisms 2–6 μ long, with a nucleus and a kinetoplast but no external flagellum. Leishma-niae are found intracellularly within monocytes, which may rupture easily. Consequently, the parasite may be demonstrated extracellularly around the broken cell.

L. donovani (Figure 10.3) is the causative agent of visceral leishmaniasis or kala-azar, seen in India and other Southeast Asian countries, as well as in Central Africa. Bone marrow examination reveals many parasites, and buffy-coat preparations from venous blood may help to concentrate the organisms. Splenic imprints appear to be the most effective method of determining the presence of the parasites, which also infest the liver, lymph nodes, intestines, and skin.

During the active phase of kala-azar, the red-cell life span is reduced. At this time, a patient's antibody titers are increased and the red cells are often agglutinated by anticomplement and anti–non-γ-

Figure 10.3. *Leishmania donovani.* Organism in splenic impression obtained from infected hamster. (Reprinted with permission from EK Markell, M Voge. Medical Parasitology [5th ed]. Philadelphia: Saunders, 1981. P 122.)

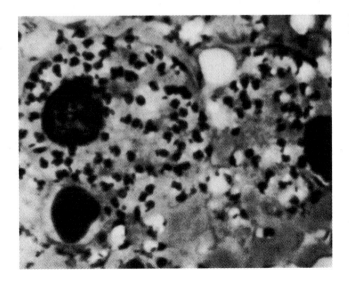

Table 10.2. Distribution and Common Features of the Filariae

Species	Geographic Distribution	Principal Vector	Periodicity	Sheath	Other Features
Wuchereria bancrofti	Tropics and subtropics	Mosquito	Mainly at night	Yes	Larvae sheathed
Loa loa	Tropics and West Indies	*Chrysops*	Diurnal	Yes	Nuclei seen in the tail region; PAS-positive granules present Larvae sheathed
Dipetalonema perstans	Africa, Central and South America	Midges and gnats	None	No	Larvae unsheathed

PAS = periodic acid–Schiff.

globulin sera. Erythrocyte destruction takes place largely in the spleen, and it is believed that an autoimmune mechanism is responsible for the anemia that is found (Woodruff et al., 1972).

L. tropica is the causative agent of Oriental sore, producing a boil-like infectious lesion in the skin that finally becomes ulcerated.

L. brasiliensis causes South American cutaneous leishmaniasis, which produces ulcers without boils that involve the face and mucous membranes.

Leishmaniae sometimes are morphologically difficult to differentiate from fungi but can be sep-arated by their negative reaction to the periodic acid–Schiff (PAS) stain for glycogen.

Filariae

The filariae are long threadlike nematodes (Table 10.2). Five species are known to infect humans, producing microfilariae that appear in the blood. These larvae have elongated bodies (250–300 μ long) that contain a large number of distinct nuclei. The cylindric body is bluntly rounded anteriorly,

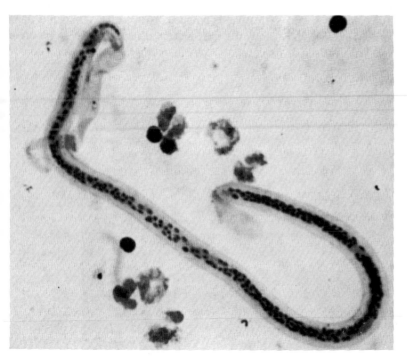

Figure 10.4. Microfilaria of *Wuchereria bancrofti.* (Reprinted with permission from EK Markell, M Voge. Medical Parasitology [5th ed]. Philadelphia: Saunders, 1981. P 144.)

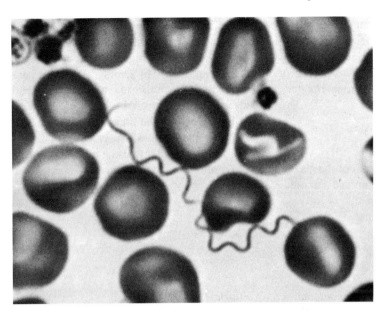

Figure 10.5. *Borrelia hermsii.* (Reprinted with permission from EK Markell, M Voge, Medical Parasitology [5th ed]. Philadelphia: Saunders, 1981. P 1143.)

and posteriorly it tapers to a point. Nuclei are not seen in the tail region except in *Loa loa.*

Wuchereria bancrofti (Figure 10.4) is the causative agent of Bancroft's filaria. The larvae or microfilariae appear to be sheathed by a thin eggshell surrounding the embryo as it circulates in the blood. The parasite is distributed widely throughout the tropics and subtropics and is transmitted by mosquitos. In most parts of the world where filariasis is endemic, it produces periodic night infections. It is rarely seen during daytime hours. The parasite frequently produces fever and lymphadenopathy. The organism lodges in the lymphatic system and affects the limbs, breast, and scrotum.

Loa loa is the causative agent of loiasis. The site of infestation is mainly the skin, within which the parasites appear mobile, producing transient swellings. The filariae frequently penetrate the eye and can be seen crossing the conjunctiva. Adult male *Loa loa* are 2.0–3.5 cm long, and the females are up to 7 cm long. The microfilariae are sheathed, measuring 250–300 μ long and 6–8 μ wide. Morphologically, these filariae can be differentiated from *W. bancrofti* by the presence of nuclei extending to the tail. PAS-positive granules are present between the body and the sheath.

Dipetalonema perstans is a filaria whose larvae are unsheathed. The parasite is commonly found in humans and apes in Africa, as well as in Central and South America. The adult worms live deep in connective tissue, and their unsheathed larvae are found in the peripheral blood. Periodicity is not a feature of this infection.

The laboratory diagnosis of filariasis rests on the demonstration of the microfilariae in the blood. Specimens obtained randomly may be used to detect *D. perstans,* but the nocturnal habits of *W. bancrofti* necessitate the collection of blood during the night, the best time being between 10 PM and 2 AM. If specimens are collected in ethylenediaminetetraacetic acid anticoagulant and stored at 37°C, microfilariae can be kept mobile for several hours. A concentrate can be made by lightly centrifuging blood and examining the buffy coat and related red-cell area for the presence of the parasites. Alternatively, the concentrate can be made by saponin lysis of the red cells, centrifugation, or membrane filtration.

Spirochetes

Borreliae (Figure 10.5) are loosely coiled spirochetes that measure 10–20 μ in length. The organism is the causative agent of relapsing fever and is transmitted by the human body louse. During the acute phase of the disease, borrelia organisms can be demonstrated in Romanowsky-stained blood smears.

Leptospirae are tightly coiled spirochetes that measure 6–20 μ long and usually have hooked ends. The organism is transmitted through human drinking water contaminated by the urine of the water rat or through rat bites. The parasite can be demonstrated in the blood only during the first few days of the disease, usually by dark-field examination. The spirochete is highly mobile and is the causative agent of Weil's disease (*Leptospira icterohaemorrhagiae*).

Toxoplasma gondii

Toxoplasma gondii is a sporozoan of the coccidian group and is widespread in humans and domestic animals. The trophozoites are rarely seen in infections but can be demonstrated in the mesenteric lymph nodes and in other organs of the cat. Diagnosis is usually established by serologic tests. The parasite is arc-shaped. When spread out in smears of body fluids and in touch preparations, it is 4–7 μ long and 2–4 μ thick. Some of the organisms contain 1–5 small PAS-positive granules. The parasite is phagocytosed by monocytes and is transmitted either in utero from the mother to the fetus or orally at a later time through the feces of contaminated animals.

Chapter 11

Leukopoiesis

Embryonic hematopoiesis produces all three formed elements of the blood (see page 1), including the colony-forming units that are precursors to T and B lymphocytes, neutrophils, monocytes, and eosinophils. The classification of leukocytes can be physiologic or morphologic. Their physiologic role can be broadly divided into two groups: phagocytic leukocytes (granulocytes and monocytes) and leukocytes concerned primarily with antibody production and cellular immunity (lymphocytes and plasma cells). Morphologically, leukocytes can be subdivided by two main criteria: their nuclear shape and the presence or lack of cytoplasmic granules.

Granulocytes

Maturation

Normal granulocytic production takes place in the bone marrow, where the cells undergo an orderly dispersion from this organ to the blood and then to various tissues throughout the body. Granulocytic maturation takes place in six defined morphologic stages: (1) blast cell, (2) progranulocyte, (3) granulocyte, (4) metagranulocyte, (5) band, and (6) the segmented or polymorphonuclear stage. Table 11.1 details these features. Like the maturation of the erythroid cells, immature leukocytes become smaller as they mature, slowly reversing the nucleus-to-cytoplasm ratio. Similarly, cytoplasmic basophilia, an index of RNA presence, is seen most abundantly in the myeloblast. The promyelocyte usually has a large amount of granulation that progressively diminishes until the metamyelocyte stage, at which point the granulation remains constant until the cell matures.

In the granulocytic series, specifically staining granules are not seen until the myelocyte matures, at which point, on occasion, both basophilic and eosinophilic granules are present within the same cell. As maturation progresses, the eosinophilic or basophilic granules possess more pronounced staining characteristics. Nucleoli are seen only in the myeloblast, but fading remnants occasionally are present in the promyelocyte cell.

As the cells mature, the chromatin becomes progressively more coarse and deeply stained and fewer chromosomal structures are visible. The nucleus becomes relatively smaller until, at the metamyelocyte stage, it begins to become flattened, indented, and band-shaped. Finally, the band becomes segmented at the final stage of maturation.

Identification of leukocytes follows a scheme similar to that of red-cell precursors (page 10).

Myeloblast

Cell size	2–3 times that of a mature red cell (15–22 μ).
Cell shape	Round
Cytoplasm	Nucleus-to-cytoplasm ratio: 4:1
	Staining: deeply basophilic
	Granules: none present
	Vacuoles: none present
	Perinuclear halo: none present

Table 11.1. Main Morphologic Features of Granulocytic Maturation

Morphologic Features	Myeloblast	Promyelocyte	Myelocyte	Metamyelocyte	Band	Segmented Cell
Cell size	Large, progressively smaller to the mature segmental form					
Cytoplasm						
Basophilia	4+	1+	±	0	0	0
Azurophilic granules	0/+	3+	2+	1+	1+	1+
Specifically staining granules	0	0	3+	2+	2+	2+
Nucleus						
Nucleoli	3+	1+	0	0	0	0
Chromatin	Immature and dispersed			Progressively more coarse with less chromosomal structure visible; more deeply stained		
Size	Large			Progressively smaller and finally segmented		
Shape	Round	Round	Round	Indented	Band	Segmented
Capacity for cell division	Yes	Yes	Yes	No	No	No

± = weak; 0/+ = occasional; 0 = none present/no cell division; 1+ = few/scanty; 2+ = moderate; 3+ = many; 4+ = marked.

Nucleus	Position: centrally placed
	Shape: round
	Staining: stains evenly with a characteristic reticular network; chromatin aggregations not normally present; nuclear membrane smooth and even; no condensation of chromatin near the inner surface of the nucleus, as is found frequently in the lymphoblast
	Nucleoli: 2–6 present normally
Main points of recognition	Primary differentiation based on number and distribution of the accompanying cell, although one good criterion is nucleoli number, the myeloblast commonly having 3–4 cells, whereas the lymphoblast usually has 1–2 nucleoli

Promyelocyte

Cell size	3–4 times that of a mature red cell (22–30 μ)
Cell shape	Round
Cytoplasm	Nucleus-to-cytoplasm ratio: 2:1
	Staining: less basophilic than the myeloblast
	Granules: contains few to many blue-purple moderate-sized granules
	Vacuoles: none present
	Perinuclear halo: none present
Nucleus	Position: centrally or eccentrically placed
	Shape: oval or round
	Staining: chromatin pattern possibly coarser than in the myeloblast, although still fine-textured
	Nucleoli: may still be present in the cell in varying stages of clarity; some nucleoli seen fading in the more mature promyelocyte
Main points of recognition	Larger than the myeloblast and may show some myeloid cytoplasmic granulation and presence of nucleoli, depending on its age; helpful to view this cell as possessing some of the morphologic characteristics of both its

precursor cell and its progeny, the myelocyte

Myelocyte

Cell size	Up to twice the size of a mature red cell (<15 μ)
Cell shape	Round
Cytoplasm	Nucleus-to-cytoplasm ratio: 3:1–3:2
	Staining: pink-blue
	Granules: contains few to moderate number of nonspecifically or specifically staining granules of varying size, scattered over the entire cell
	Neutrophilic myelocyte: Cytoplasmic granules finer in texture and size, staining a red-blue with standard stains
	Eosinophilic myelocyte: Cytoplasmic granules large, spheric, orange-brown bodies, more numerous than in the neutrophilic myelocyte and often mixed with neutrophilic granulation
	Basophilic myelocyte: Cytoplasmic granules generally larger than in the eosinophilic myelocyte and less numerous; these inclusions very prominent and stain a deep blue-black with standard stains
	Vacuoles: none present usually
	Perinuclear halo: may be present, especially in the neutrophilic myelocyte
Nucleus	Position: centrally or eccentrically placed
	Shape: round or occasionally flattened on one side
	Staining: chromatin pattern coarser than in the promyelocyte, with aggregation of nuclear protein present
	Nucleoli: none present
Main points of recognition	Classic criteria for differentiation: absence of nucleoli, decreased nucleus-to-cytoplasm ratio, and presence of typical cytoplasmic granulation
	Basophilic myelocytes: Characteristic sparse blue-black cytoplasmic

granulation, generally somewhat smaller cells

Metamyelocytes

Cell size	Up to twice the size of a mature red cell (<15 μ)
Cell shape	Round
Cytoplasm	Nucleus-to-cytoplasm ratio: 7:3–1:1
	Staining: pink-blue
	Granules: characteristic, depending on the cell lineage
	Neutrophilic metamyelocyte: Numerous fine red-blue granules
	Eosinophilic metamyelocyte: Medium-sized, bright orange, more numerous granules than in the precursor cell
	Basophilic metamyelocyte: Relatively sparse granules but still more numerous than in the myelocyte and appear as well-defined deep blue-black structures
	Vacuoles: none present usually
	Perinuclear halo: none present
Nucleus	Position: centrally or eccentrically placed
	Shape: typically kidney-shaped but may be only slightly indented or flattened
	Staining: chromatin pattern coarser than the myelocyte and stains a deep blue-black
	Nucleoli: none present
Main points of recognition	Smaller cell size; fine, abundant granulation; characteristic nuclear shape

Band

Cell size	Up to 1.5 times the size of a mature red cell (<12 μ)
Cell shape	Round
Cytoplasm	Nucleus-to-cytoplasm ratio: 1:1–1:2.
	Staining: pink-blue
	Granules: characteristic granulation similar to that found in the metamyelocyte
	Vacuoles: occasional
	Perinuclear halo: none present

Nucleus	Position: centrally or eccentrically placed
	Shape: may be band-shaped or deeply indented, with or without constrictions forming rudimentary lobes. For cell to be classified at this stage of maturation, nucleus should show a band of chromatin connecting the nuclear bridge. If a filament is present, cell is classified as a polymorphonuclear cell
	Staining: coarse chromatin structure staining homogeneously blue-black
	Nucleoli: none present
Main points of recognition	For all 3 cell lines (neutrophilic, eosinophilic, and basophilic bands), classic nuclear shape, as described previously

Polymorphonuclear Neutrophil (Segmented Neutrophil)

Cell size	Up to 1.5 times the size of a mature red cell (<12 μ)
Cell shape	Round
Cytoplasm	Nucleus-to-cytoplasm ratio: 1:3–1:5
	Staining: pink-blue
	Granules: abundant fine azurophilic granules scattered over the cell
	Vacuoles: occasional
	Perinuclear halo: none present
Nucleus	As found in the neutrophil, except normally fewer lobes present (frequently only 2)
Main points of recognition	Typical lobulated nucleus and pink-blue finely granulated cytoplasm

Eosinophil

Cell size	Slightly smaller than the neutrophil (<10 μ)
Cell shape	Round
Cytoplasm	As found in the neutrophil, except full complement of large (approximately 1 μ), round, orange granules are scattered over entire cytoplasm

Table 11.2. Granulocytic Maturation Compartments

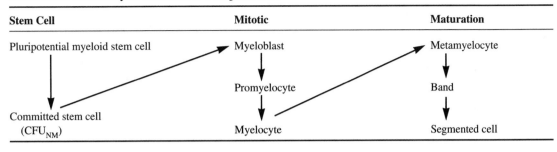

Stem Cell	Mitotic	Maturation
Pluripotential myeloid stem cell	Myeloblast	Metamyelocyte
	Promyelocyte	Band
Committed stem cell (CFU$_{NM}$)	Myelocyte	Segmented cell

Nucleus	As found in the neutrophil, except normally fewer lobes present (frequently only 2)	
Main points of recognition	Slightly smaller than the neutrophil; possesses fewer nuclear lobes; has abundant large, orange, cytoplasmic granules	

Basophil

Cell size	Slightly smaller than the neutrophil (<10 μ)
Cell shape	Round
Cytoplasm	As found in the neutrophil and eosinophil, except fewer granules than are seen in the eosinophil; water-soluble inclusions that stain blue-black and consequently tend to wash out when stained
Nucleus	As found in the neutrophil, except appears less coarse and has 2–4 lobes
Main points of recognition	Easily identified by specifically staining cytoplasmic granules

Normal Kinetics

Granulocytes maintain the property of mitotic division up to the myelocytic stage of maturation (Bond, 1959), after which development proceeds without further proliferation. Those early cells, therefore, constitute the mitotic compartment, and the more mature cells (the metamyelocyte and the band and segmented cells) constitute the maturation compartment. Table 11.2 shows the granulocytic maturation compartments.

With the use of tritiated thymidine as a nuclear DNA marker, it is possible to estimate the transit time of these cells through the mitotic and maturation compartments. Table 11.3 illustrates the approximate time that each cell remains in transit for each specific compartment.

Once the granulocyte has matured, it becomes distributed into one of two pools: the circulating granulocytic pool (CGP) or the marginal granulocytic pool (MGP). In this latter pool, the cells marginate along the capillary walls and venules and, by the process of diapedesis, they migrate in constant equilibrium, reflecting constant cell production and destruction to and from the CGP (Figure 11.1).

When a physiologic need arises for these cells, those within the MGP migrate to the source of infection in the tissues and then are replaced by cells from the CGP; in turn, these cells are replenished

Table 11.3. Granulocytic Transit Time (Using ^{3}H-TdR label)

Compartment	Cell	Transit Time (hrs)
Mitotic	Blast	15
	Promyelocyte	24
	Myelocyte	104
Maturation	Metamyelocyte	40
	Band	66
	Segmented	95
Equilibrium	CGP↔MGP	7

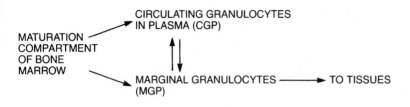

Figure 11.1. Normal granulocytic equilibrium.

by those from the maturation compartment in the bone marrow. Cells are removed from the CGP randomly; their half-life in this pool approximates 7 hours.

Release

The exact mechanisms leading to increased granulocytic release and the subsequent increase in cell production are unclear, but it has been postulated that recruitment of the pluripotential stem cell is modified by a hematopoietic inductive microenvironment (HIM), which aids in the conversion of the resting cell to a committed stem cell. This microenvironment, or colony-stimulating factor, may result from the interaction of fat cells, phagocytic cells, and epithelial cells (Dexter et al., 1977) and may be affected by cyclic nucleotides (Oshita et al., 1977). However, once the commitment to a given cell line occurs, the system may be enhanced or even modified by specific proteins, such as erythropoietin (Chervenick and LoBuglio, 1975; Cline et al., 1977). The actual release of granulocytes is thought to take place in one of two ways: A slow release is believed to be under the control of the colony-stimulating factors, allowing cellular release into the mitotic compartment, and a fast release, controlling the stored granulocytes' release from the bone marrow, is believed to be under the influence of a neutrophil-releasing factor (Broxmeyer et al., 1974). However, the exact regulation and performance of granulocytic release is still theoretical, the experimental models having involved either tissue culture or animal experimentation.

If not used in an inflammatory exudate, those granulocytes that arrive in the circulation and enter the tissues are eliminated within a few days in the bronchial secretions, saliva, gastrointestinal tract, and urine.

Function

Granulocytes function mainly as the first line of defense against microorganisms. Monocytes and macrophages share this role, providing a means of final removal of microorganisms. They also clear aged and damaged cells from the body. For these events to take place, phagocytes have to accumulate in sufficient numbers and must attach to, engulf, and dispose of these waste materials.

Granulocytes spend approximately 1 day in the circulation before migrating through the endothelial walls and being disposed of in the tissues. This continuous physiologic interaction results in nearly one-tenth of the total blood neutrophil pool emigrating from the CGP each hour. The fate of these cells is unclear, but they do not appear to reenter the blood in significant numbers. A dynamic interaction also exists between endothelium and neutrophils in the MGP, but it is uncertain whether these neutrophils actually adhere to the endothelium.

These normal physiologic interactions are greatly changed in acute inflammation. The mechanisms appear to undergo several distinct changes: initial adhesion, maintained adherence, diapedesis, and extravascular migration (Mayrovitz et al., 1977). Increased neutrophilic adherence to endothelium is recognized as a hallmark of the acute inflammatory response and sometimes occurs when other signs of inflammation are lacking (Harlan, 1985).

Inflammatory lesions release specific leukotoxins, which function by increasing capillary permeability, thereby aiding in the local migration and accumulation of the cells. The exact role of leukotoxins is unclear, but receptors on the surface of the lesion initiate phagocytic ingestion, with the attachment of the cell to the lesion depending on opsonization. This process is activated by low-molecular-weight C3 and C5 fragments of complement, as well as by specific bacterial peptides. Once phagocytic ingestion occurs, the cell membrane engulfs the foreign material, which, in turn, is enveloped by surface membranes that form distinct phagocytic vacuoles (phagosomes). Lysosomal granules then become attached and release antibacterial and digestive enzymes into the phagosomes. Bacterial membranes are destroyed by the peroxidation of hydrogen peroxide in the presence of tyrosine-derived iodine. This process is associated with an increase in energy production, primarily from glycolysis from the Embden-Meyerhof and hexose-phosphate pathways (Sbarra et al., 1977).

Glycolysis is accompanied also by an increase in lactate production, an increased synthesis of membrane lipids, and a large increase in oxygen consumption—the so-called respiratory burst. The oxidative bactericidal function is initiated by the presence of myeloperoxidase (MPO) in the neutrophil granules. If MPO is reduced or lacking in the cell, large increases in hydrogen peroxide and halides are required to destroy the organisms effectively (Table 11.4).

Besides aerobic killing of ingested organisms, granulocytes and macrophages use anaerobic conditions to destroy bacteria. Such conditions include acid production and the effects of lysozyme, lactoferrin, and cationic proteins.

After partial digestion, the intraphagosomal pH becomes acidic and destroys organisms such as pneumococci. Lysozyme, a low-molecular-weight protein found in neutrophil granules, is capable of hydrolyzing some bacterial cell walls, causing death. Most organisms are resistant to this lytic action but may become susceptible after exposure to hydrogen peroxide, complement, or antibodies. Lactoferrin, which also is present in specific granules, functions by inhibiting bacterial growth by binding essential cell nutrients, such as iron, at low pH levels. Cationic proteins that are present are believed to possess bactericidal properties.

Cellular digestion results from the release of acidic hydrolytic enzymes into the phagosomes from the primary lysosome. Neutrophilic granules also release a wide variety of other enzymes, including ribonuclease, deoxyribonuclease, hyaluronidase, histamine, vitamin B_{12}–binding proteins, and lysozyme.

The vitamin B_{12}–binding proteins (*transcobalamins*) are composed of three globulins, the best studied being transcobalamin III (TC III), which is thought to be formed by the neutrophilic granules. It also is believed to be the main transport mechanism of vitamin B_{12} to the liver. The functions of

Table 11.4. Effect of the Removal of Myeloperoxidase in Antimicrobial Activity

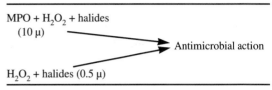

TC I and TC II are unclear, but they too may possess bactericidal properties. Increases in TC I are seen in chronic myeloid leukemia and myeloid metaplasia, whereas reductions of this protein are found in aplastic anemia and leukopenia.

Lysozyme is present in both primary and secondary granules of neutrophils and in monocytes. Increased serum and urinary levels are associated primarily with acute myeloid leukemia, particularly the M1 and M5 forms. Lysozyme levels are believed to reflect granulocytic turnover.

Granulocytic Antigens and Antibodies

Alloantibodies and autoantibodies to granulocyte antigens are important in several diseases and in transfusion medicine. Alloantibodies to antigens specific to neutrophils are etiologic factors in alloimmune neonatal neutropenia and in febrile and pulmonary transfusion reactions. Neutrophilic alloantibodies that define eight separate genetic loci have been identified. The most common antigen seen is NA 1, which has been shown to reside on the FcR111 immunoglobulin receptor (CD 16); the antithetic antigen NA 2 represents an isoform of FcR111. It is believed that a congenital deficiency of FcR111 may cause impaired granulocytic function. Detection of alloantibodies to neutrophilic antigens still remains difficult; procedures for this include agglutination, immunofluorescence, enzyme-linked immunosorbent assay, radioimmunoassay, and immunocytochemical reactions. Identification of granulocytic alloantibodies rarely is important, except in cases of transfusion reactions or transplantation rejection.

Eosinophils

The morphologic features of eosinophils were described on page 116. The main characteristic of the cell is the presence of large, refractile, orange-stained secondary granules that can be recognized as early as the myelocytic stage of development. The inclusions are composed of a double-layered membrane and an electron-dense crystalline core containing strong peroxidase activity. Eosinophil lysosomes are similar in content to those of neutrophils, except that they do not possess lysozyme. The cell is rich in arylsulfatase as well as a zinc-rich major basic protein (MBP) and eosinophilic cationic protein (ECP).

The mature eosinophil has a tissue life span of 8–12 days and a peripheral blood half-life of 4–5 hours. There is evidence, however, of recirculation of eosinophils between the blood and the tissues (Butterworth and David, 1981).

The phagocytic action of eosinophils is less intense than that of neutrophils, despite the fact that more hydrogen peroxide is produced by the cells' physiologic makeup. Eosinophils respond to chemotactic stimulation, and immune complexes and complement are released from the tissue-bound cell.

When phagocytosis occurs, it usually is associated with degranulation. Besides this activity, eosinophils are believed to be associated with the inactivation of substances resulting from hypersensitivity reactions (arylsulfatases) and with the destruction of parasites in the larvae stage. This latter role might be attributable to cell membrane receptor attachment to antibody-sensitized larvae, followed by release of the MBP and ECP, which damages the parasite (Beeson and Bass, 1977).

Basophils

Basophils are the least common leukocytes normally seen in the blood. Their principal morphologic feature is the presence of sparse, large, blue-black secondary granules that can be identified at the myelocytic stage of maturation. These histamine- and heparin-rich granules are released during degranulation. This release is associated with IgE binding to the cell. The remaining cellular chemistry is similar to that of neutrophils, except that nonspecific esterases and alkaline phosphatase are not demonstrable.

Like all the granulocytes, basophils can become motile and are attracted by chemotoxins such as complement. Phagocytosis is poor, but the cells possess pinocytic properties and thus can transport exogenous materials to the cytoplasmic granules.

The cell is believed to be involved in cell-mediated hypersensitivity reactions and local inflammatory responses, as well as in anaphylaxis (Church and Holgate, 1980).

Monocytes and Macrophages

Maturation and Kinetics

Monocytes are derived from the bone marrow and are believed to be the precursors of fixed and free tissue macrophages. The cells mature more rapidly in the bone marrow than do granulocytes, occupying approximately 55 hours of transit time. Once liberated in the peripheral blood, monocytes remain for another 12 hours before migrating to the tissues by diapedesis, at which point they mature further, forming macrophages (Table 11.5). Like neutrophils, monocytes must first adhere to the endothelium before emigrating from the blood to extravascular sites. Complement activation in vivo induces a transient monocytopenia, but it is likely that the cell behaves like a neutrophil by undergoing aggregation and margination. The process by which adherent monocytes perform diapedesis across intact endothelium also appears similar to that observed in neutrophils. The transformation of the monocyte to a macrophage takes place with an accompanying increase in cell size, the loss of peroxidase granules, and the production of large amounts of lysosomes filled with acid hydrolases. These changes are associated with an increase in mitochondria and an increased dependence for energy obtained from the tricarboxylic acid cycle. Consequently, monocytes are rich in lysozyme and nonspecific esterase and possess only small amounts of peroxidase.

Morphologically, the monocyte is recognized first at the promonocytic stage of maturity. Identification follows a scheme similar to that outlined in the discussion of erythrocyte maturation and identification (see page 10).

Promonocyte

Cell size	2–3 times that of a mature red cell (14–21 μ)
Cell shape	Round or oval
Cytoplasm	Nucleus-to-cytoplasm ratio: 2:1–1:1

Table 11.5. Monocyte-Macrophage Transit Time (Using ^{3}H-TdR Label)

Cell	Transit Time (hrs)	Compartment
Promyelocyte	55	Bone marrow
Monocyte	12	Blood
Macrophage	Unknown; likely several months	Tissue (lung, spleen, liver, lymph nodes, gastrointestinal tract, peritoneum)

Source: Data adapted from G Meuret, G Hoffman. Monocyte kinetic studies in normal and disease states. Br J Haematol 1973;24:275.

	Staining: dull blue, ground-glass appearance
	Granules: many fine dustlike azurophilic granules present
	Vacuoles: occasionally present
	Perinuclear halo: none present
Nucleus	Position: centrally placed
	Shape: oval or indented
	Staining: stains lightly, illustrating a fine reticular chromatin pattern
	Nucleoli: 1–5 present normally
Main points of recognition	Resemblance to a mature monocyte in size, shape, and cytoplasmic characteristics, but with immature nuclear chromatin and nucleoli

Monocyte

Cell size	2–3 times that of a mature red cell (14–21 μ)
Cell shape	Round or sometimes oval
Cytoplasm	Nucleus-to-cytoplasm ratio: approximately 1:1
	Staining: dull blue, ground-glass appearance
	Granules: small, irregularly distributed areas of dense azurophilic granulation seen occasionally
	Vacuoles: occasionally present
	Perinuclear halo: none present
Nucleus	Position: centrally or eccentrically placed
	Shape: frequently indented or horseshoe-shaped; can also be lobulated; similar to that of a mature neutrophil
	Staining: open, loose chromatin structure; often a sharp segregation of chromatin and parachromatin, with chromatin distributed in a linear arrangement of delicate strands that give the nucleus a stringy appearance; nuclear membrane delicate but clear
	Nucleoli: none present
Main points of recognition	Ground-glass smoky cytoplasm and indented nuclear shape

Function

Little is known about the exact release mechanism of the monocyte, but the cell migrates by diapedesis and physiologically and morphologically becomes a macrophage once in the tissues. Two forms of macrophages are recognized. The fixed macrophages attach to collagen or reticular fibers and appear similar to fibroblasts. This fixed cell is abundant particularly in connective tissue, spleen, liver, and lymph nodes and becomes motile or "free" only after inflammatory lesion stimulation. The exact mechanism of phagocytic activity is unclear, but it is believed to be qualitatively similar to that of neutrophils.

Several differences do exist in the cellular biochemistry: Neutrophils require more oxygen, generate more superoxide, and release more peroxide than do monocytes. The energy requirements differ from those of neutrophils. The monocyte obtains up to 70% of its consumed oxygen from the mitochondrial respiratory chain by anaerobic glycolysis (Axline, 1970). One exception to this, however, is the alveolar macrophage, which depends on aerobic glycolysis for metabolism (Reiss and Roos, 1978).

Both the monocyte and the macrophage possess similar functions—defense reactions against microorganisms, removal of damaged or dying cells and cell debris, interaction with lymphoid cells, and stimulation of granulopoiesis (Territo and Cline, 1975).

Phagocytosis is believed to occur in four distinct stages: (1) the attachment phase, which requires that specific opsonizing immunoglobulins be present on the surface of the cell to be phagocytized; (2) the ingestion phase, which occurs by pseudopodal extension and engulfment to form a phagosome; (3) secondary lysosomal formation, which occurs by phagosomal fusion with primary lysosomes that inject acid hydrolases into the secondary lysosomes to initiate the digestion phase, reflecting cytolysis; and (4) the disposal of degraded material by a process known as *exocytosis*. The removal of damaged cellular material is particularly obvious in the role of disposing of effete red cells. The iron recovered from these cells forms a complex with macrophagic apoferritin to form ferritin, which is stored in membrane-bound aggregates within the cell, awaiting final exit and movement to other storage sites by transferrin transportation.

After antigenic stimulation, the activation of macrophages and lymphocytes is carried out through a series of cellular interactions, which result in the release of many biologically active mediators. The sequential release of lymphokines and monokines from antigen-active cells is known as the *interleukin cascade*. Following antigen activation, lymphocytes release substances that potentiate cellular mobilization through altered vessel permeability; as a consequence, macrophages, neutrophils, basophils, eosinophils, and other lymphocytes accumulate at the antigenic site. Once there, their random movement may be inhibited by lymphokines, and their activation may occur. This leads to enhanced phagocytosis as well as to the release of various monokines. Interleukin 1, a monokine released by activated macrophages, further potentiates the T-lymphocyte response by promoting activation of T cells, which are then stimulated to produce lymphokines (interferon, interleukin 2) that recruit, activate, and cause cellular proliferation of many other cells. Antibody synthesis by B lymphocytes may also be modulated directly by production of helper or suppressor lymphokines produced by stimulated T cells. Lymphokines are potent immunoregulatory factors that modulate the activity of macrophages, monocytes, and lymphocytes. B lymphocytes are thought to produce lymphokines that act as growth and differentiation factors for other B cells. Additionally, it is believed that the lymphokine interleukin 3 influences proliferation and development of hematopoietic cells and plays a role in the regulation of lymphocyte differentiation and growth (Inle et al., 1982).

The monocyte and macrophage appear to be essential for lymphocyte transformation. In addition, it is believed that these cells contribute to antibody response by trapping antigen by pinocytosis or phagocytosis and converting this material into more antigenic forms that can be stored or transmitted to immunologically competent cells. Once this takes place, antibody production becomes stimulated (Nelson, 1976). The monocyte and macrophage also play a role in delayed hypersensitivity. The introduction of antigen into a sensitized animal promotes lymphocytes to release chemotactic substances to monocytes, thus recruiting monocytes to the area. An example of this is provided by skin-testing procedures.

Interferon production is carried out by monocytes and by peritoneal- and alveolar-trapped macrophages. Little is known about the mechanism of this production, but other phagocytic granulocytes have also been shown to produce this antiviral agent, although in smaller quantities (Stecher, 1970).

Lymphocytes

Lymphopoiesis

Lymphocytes are mononuclear cells whose cytoplasm does not contain specifically staining granules. In postnatal mammals, the bone marrow and thymus are the primary lymphopoietic organs. These tissues supply undifferentiated cells that, when appropriately stimulated, become immunocompetent. Normally, lymphopoiesis takes place in peripheral lymphatic tissue, the secondary lymphopoietic areas (Figure 11.2). Cellular proliferation in such regions usually depends on antigen stimulation, in contrast to the antigen-independent lymphocyte production that arises from the primary lymphopoietic organs.

The production, release, and recirculation of lymphocytes are such that multiple populations of lymphocytes of varying morphologic characteristics are found at any one time in the peripheral blood. Identification of these subpopulations cannot be

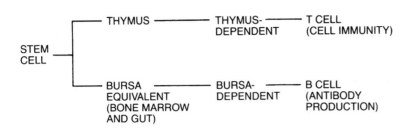

Figure 11.2. Lymphopoiesis.

made from a simple Romanowsky-stained blood smear alone; differences in the physical properties of the cell are involved, including cell membrane susceptibility to enzymes, differences in the cells' ability to adhere to plastic and glass, and differences in antigenic determinants.

The pluripotential stem cell of the bone marrow is capable of giving rise to pre-T cells and pre-B cells, but the exact nature of the kinetics and maturation is not entirely clear. It is believed that these stem cells migrate from the bone marrow to the thymus to become immunologically competent T lymphocytes. Some cells migrate to peripheral lymphoid structures and become antibody-producing B lymphocytes, eventually evolving into plasma cells that produce humoral antibodies.

Peripheral blood lymphocytes emigrate to extravascular lymphoid tissue or sites of inflammation. Tissue lymphocytes reenter the circulation after passage through the lymphatics, lymph nodes, and thoracic duct. This dynamic process allows for constant surveillance of extravascular tissue by these immunocompetent cells, a task that is assisted by the ability of lymphocytes to recognize specialized endothelium, the area known as the *high-endothelium venule* (HEV). Lymphocytes adhere to the HEV through microvilli that attach to shallow pits on the luminal surface of the endothelium. Migration is believed to take place in a manner similar to that of neutrophils—that is, by an interendothelial route (Yamaguchi and Schoefl, 1983).

B Cells

B-cell differentiation can be divided into two stages. The initial phase involves the antigen-independent generation of diversity, whereas the second stage is regulated by antigen-triggering interactions and macrophages occurring in the secondary lymphoid organs. The first recognizable B cell is known as the *large pre-B cell*. It is characterized by the presence of IgM within the cell cytoplasm, the cell surface being totally devoid of any membrane immunoglobulins. This large cell undergoes rapid mitosis and produces a small pre-B cell having a long life span. It is this cell that produces B lymphocytes (bursa and bone marrow–derived) with surface IgMs and receptor sites for Fc, C3b, and C3d. B cells interact with antigen in the presence of T cells and macrophages and transform into plasma cells, which have the capability to produce immunoglobulins. The B lymphocyte also is responsible for humoral immunity, the cell actively producing antibodies against encapsulated pyogenic bacteria and other foreign material.

T Cells

Differentiated lymphocytes involved in immune functions are termed *T cells* (thymus derived). Precursors of these cells are present in embryonic hematopoiesis, in the yolk sac, in the liver, and in adult bone marrow. When they migrate to the thymus, these cells are influenced by thymopoietin, a polypeptide that aids in the proliferation and maturation of the cells (Storrie et al., 1976). This lymphocyte differentiation is usually accompanied by surface changes that lead to the development of various antigens.

T cells are believed to be capable of transformation when exposed to certain antigens, including phytohemagglutinin, pokeweed mitogen, and staphylococcal endotoxin. Such stimulation is nonspecific in nature in that there does not need to be prior sensitization of the lymphocytes to the antigen (Miale, 1982). Specific antigen stimulation results only when the lymphocytes have been sensitized to antigens such as tuberculin, diphtheria toxoid, and penicillin.

Besides mediating delayed hypersensitivity reactions, T cells may act as helper T cells, enhancing antibody production by B lymphocytes, or they may act as suppressor T cells, inhibiting antibody production by B cells. Suppressor T cells have receptor sites for the Fc portion of the IgG molecule, whereas helper T cells exhibit receptor sites for the Fc portion of the IgM molecule. The major markers on human T cells are the receptors for sheep red blood cells (SRBCs; Lay, et al., 1971) and the presence of THY-1 antigen (Raff, 1971). The SRBCs usually are detected by rosetting, and the THY-I antigen is demonstrated by either direct antibody-mediated cytotoxicity or indirect fluorescence. A number of other cell markers used to detect T cells, B cells, and monocytes are summarized in Table 11.6.

Another function of T cells is to produce lymphokines. These substances are capable of destroying target cells, either directly or indirectly, by exerting cytotoxic effects, promoting complement activation, and attracting macrophages. Examples of such lymphokines include lymphotoxin, migration inhibition factor, transfer factor, interferon, chemotactic factor, and lymphocyte-transforming factor.

Lymphotoxins are derived from specifically sensitized lymphocytes. Once stimulated, the lymphocyte releases the lymphotoxins into the surrounding medium around the target tumor cell, disrupting its membrane and so destroying the cell.

Migration inhibition factor is produced by T cells that inhibit the migration of macrophages. Such action causes macrophages to become attracted to the site of the reaction.

Transfer factor is produced by the T cell for a specific antigen and, once made, it can stimulate other noncommitted lymphocytes to undergo blastic transformation, but only when exposed to the specific antigen.

Interferon acts as an antiviral agent, chemotactic factor is believed to direct macrophage movement, and the lymphocyte-transforming factor is believed to be capable of blastogenic stimulation.

Null Cells

A third type of lymphocyte, the null cell, has been described. It possesses none of the characteristics of either T or B cells. Null cells are found in leukemia and lymphomas and are believed to be im-

mature lymphocytes that, because of their age, have not yet acquired B- or T-cell characteristics (Table 11.7; Shevach et al., 1974).

Maturation

Lymphoblast

Cell size	Similar to that of the myeloblast (15–22 μ)
Cell shape	Round
Cytoplasm	Nucleus-to-cytoplasm ratio: 4:1
	Staining: deeply basophilic
	Granules: none present
	Vacuoles: none present
	Perinuclear halo: none present
Nucleus	Position: centrally placed
	Shape: round
	Staining: similar to that of the myeloblast, but often possessing a slightly coarser reticulum
	Nucleoli: 1–2 present normally; appear more prominent than in the myeloblast
Main points of recognition	Difficult to distinguish from other blast cells; number of nucleoli and relative size of the cell, together with the type of accompanying cell, should be assessed before a conclusion is reached

Prolymphocyte

Cell size	2–3 times that of a mature red cell (15–22 μ)
Cell shape	Round
Cytoplasm	Nucleus-to-cytoplasm ratio: 3:1
	Staining: deeply basophilic
	Granules: scanty azurophilic granules occasionally present
	Vacuoles: none present
	Perinuclear halo: none present
Nucleus	Position: centrally placed
	Shape: round
	Staining: appears coarser than that of the lymphoblast
	Nucleoli: may contain one to two nucleoli

Table 11.6. Leukocyte Antigen Markers

Cells	Cluster Designation	Cells Identified
T and NK lymphocytes	CD 1	Common thymocytes
	CD 2	Pan T, some NK cells
	CD 3	Pan T, TcR complex
	CD 4	Helper-inducer subset
	CD 5	Pan T, anomalous on CLL
	CD 6	Pan T
	CD 7	Early T, many NK, some AML
	CD 8	Cytotoxic/suppressor subset, some NK cells
	CD 25	IL-2R–activated T cells
	CD w29	Inducer of B-cell function; B cells, monocytes
	CD 38	Activated T and B, plasma cells
	CD w45R	Inducer of cytotoxic/suppressor cells, B cells, monocytes
	HNK-1	NK cells, some suppressor T cells
	CD 56	NK cells, may be expressed in both AML and ALL
B lymphocytes	HLA-DR	Pan B, activated T and NK cells, monocytes, granulocytes
	CD 10	Early B cells, some T-ALL cells
	CD 19	Pan B cells
	CD 20	Pan B cells
	CD 21	B-subset, C3dR
	CD 22	Pan B cells
	CD 24	Pan B cells
	Surface Ig	Mature B cells, plasma Ig bound to Fc receptor on some lymphocytes, granulocytes, and monocytes
	PCA-1, PC-1	Some plasma cells weakly expressed on monocytes, granulocytes, hairy-cell leukemia, Waldenström's disease
Granulocytes and monocytes	CD 11b	C3biR on granulocytes, monocytes, and some Ts/C
	CD 11c	Monocytes, granulocytes, NK cells, hairy-cell leukemia
	CD 13	Monocytes
	CD 14	Monocytes
	CD 15	Granulocytes, monocytes, some T lymphomas, Reed-Sternberg cells
	CD 16	Fc receptor for IgG, granulocytes, NK cells, monocytes
	CD 33	
Other	CD 30	Activated T, B, and Reed-Sternberg cells
	CD 34	Immature precursors, many leukemias
	CD 41a	Megakaryocyte, platelets
	CD 42b	Megakaryocyte, platelets
	Factor VIII–related	Megakaryocyte, platelets
	Antigen, CD 45	Pan-leukocytes
	Glycophorin	Red cells and precursors
	TdT	Early B cells, thymic T cells

NK = natural killer cells; CLL = chronic lymphocytic leukemia; AML = acute myeloid leukemia; IL-2R = interleukin-2R; ALL = acute lymphocytic leukemia; T-ALL = T-cell lymphocytic leukemia.

Table 11.7. Characteristics of B and T Cells

Characteristics	B Cells	T Cells
Origin	Bone marrow	Bone marrow
Life span	Days	Years
Functions		
Cell-mediated immunity	Weak	4+
Humoral activity	4+	4+
Antibody production	4+	–
Immunologic memory	Uncertain	Yes
Phytohemagglutinin response	No	Yes

4+ = strongly positive; – = negative.

Main points of recognition	Increased volume of cytoplasm and presence of occasional azurophilic granules, which provide a fine distinction between this cell and the lymphoblast

Large Lymphocyte

Cell size	Up to twice the size of a mature red cell (15 μ)
Cell shape	Round
Cytoplasm	Nucleus-to-cytoplasm ratio: 3:2
	Staining: hyaline blue
	Granules: most often no granules, though sometimes a small number of fine azurophilic granules present
	Vacuoles: none present
	Perinuclear halo: none present
Nucleus	Position: centrally or eccentrically placed
	Shape: round
	Staining: intense, showing coarse reticulum masses and chromatin aggregations
	Nucleoli: seen rarely
Main points of recognition	Clear, pale blue cytoplasm, lumpy chromatin, and usually round nucleus, which differentiate this cell from a monocyte

Small Lymphocyte

Cell size	Approximately that of a mature red cell
Cell shape	Round
Cytoplasm	Nucleus-to-cytoplasm ratio: >9:1
	Staining: rim of pale blue cytoplasm present normally, but more basophilic cytoplasm seen occasionally
	Granules: sparse, fine azurophilic granules sometimes present
	Vacuoles: none present
	Perinuclear halo: none present
Nucleus	Position: centrally placed
	Shape: round
	Staining: intense, exhibiting dense chromatin aggregates
	Nucleoli: none present

Main points of recognition	Amount and color of cytoplasm and presence of occasional granules, which serve to distinguish this cell from basophilic and poly-chromatic normoblasts

Variant Lymphocytes (Reactive or Atypical Lymphocytes)

Cell size	2–3 times that of a mature red cell (15–22 μ)
Cell shape	Round or irregular
Cytoplasm	Nucleus-to-cytoplasm ratio: 4:1–1:1
	Staining: muddy, deeply basophilic blue
	Granules: none present usually, but rare fine azurophilic granules present occasionally
	Vacuoles: true vacuoles not seen, but cytoplasmic texture can appear foamy with many small vacuole-like structures
	Perinuclear halo: wide halo present often, surrounding the nucleus and giving the appearance of a very intense band of basophilia at the cell periphery; occasionally, a ballerina-skirt appearance, with bands of cytoplasmic basophilia radiating from the nucleus
Nucleus	Position: centrally or eccentrically placed
	Shape: possibly oval, kidney-shaped, round, or lobulated
	Staining: nuclear chromatin stains as dense, coarse network with deeply staining aggregates
	Nucleoli: nucleoli present occasionally
Main points of recognition	Characteristic foamy basophilic cytoplasm with a wide perinuclear halo and, on occasion, a ballerina-skirt striated appearance; not always easy to identify, as this cell can be confused with a monocytoid or an immature lymphoid cell

Plasmablast

Cell size	2–3 times that of a mature red cell (15–23 μ)

Cell shape	Irregular or oval
Cytoplasm	Nucleus-to-cytoplasm ratio: 2:1–1:1
	Staining: basophilic with rare azurophilic patches
	Granules: none present
	Vacuoles: fine foamlike texture seen occasionally; true vacuolation not present
	Perinuclear halo: present in some cells
Nucleus	Position: eccentrically placed frequently
	Shape: round or oval
	Staining: fairly open chromatin structure but usually stains more intensely than the correspondingly aged lymphocytic cell
	Nucleoli: multiple nucleoli possible
Main points of recognition	Cell size, eccentrically placed nucleus, and perinuclear halo characteristic of the plasma cell group; also immature nuclear chromatin, particularly if nucleoli are visible

Proplasmacyte

Cell size	Approximately the same or a little smaller than the plasmablast (12–23 μ)
Cell shape	Usually oval or round
Cytoplasm	Nucleus-to-cytoplasm ratio: 2:1–1:1
	Staining: intensely basophilic
	Granules: none present
	Vacuoles: none usually visible
	Perinuclear halo: seen often
Nucleus	Position: eccentrically placed
	Shape: round or oval
	Staining: similar to the plasmablast, but often exhibiting coarser, densely staining chromatin aggregates
	Nucleoli: nucleoli occasionally visible
Main points of recognition	Similar morphologically to its precursor cell, the main differences being an increase in the amount of the basophilic cytoplasm and a slightly coarser, more deeply staining nuclear chromatin; nucleoli, if seen, generally are less prominent than in the plasmablast

Plasma Cell

Cell size	Up to twice that of a normal red cell (7–15 μ)
Cell shape	Usually oval, but sometimes round
Cytoplasm	Nucleus-to-cytoplasm ratio: approximately 1:1–1:2
	Staining: intensely basophilic and foamy
	Granules: occasional scanty acidophilic inclusions visible (Russell bodies)
	Vacuoles: none present
	Perinuclear halo: large, well-defined halo
Nucleus	Position: usually eccentrically placed
	Shape: round
	Staining: dense, occasionally exhibiting cartwheel-like striations radiating from the center
	Nucleoli: none present
Main points of recognition	Classic features of oval cell shape, eccentrically placed mature nucleus, deeply basophilic cytoplasm, and clear perinuclear halo

Chapter 12

Leukocytic Disorders

Granulocytic Cells

Three main factors influence the concentration of granulocytes: (1) the rate of input from the storage pool to the circulating granulocytic pool (CGP), (2) the proportion of circulating cells compared with marginated cells, and (3) the rate at which these cells leave the blood.

Neutrophilia can be brought about by both pathologic and nonpathologic mechanisms. For instance, vigorous exercise or the administration of epinephrine decreases the number of cells in the marginal pool and, consequently, neutrophilia is produced by releasing the cells into the circulation. Such a change occurs without either a change in bone marrow output or an alteration in the rate at which the cells exit the blood. A similar mechanism that leads to neutropenia is activated during anesthesia: The cells from the blood marginate without any change in either production or destruction outputs.

The kinetics of granulocytes after an infection are illustrated by an increase in the flow of cells from the circulatory pool to the marginal pool and tissues. This is followed by an increased flow of cells from the bone marrow to the blood. Such increases often exceed the outgoing migration of cells to the tissues and result in increased numbers of granulocytes in the blood. Figure 12.1 illustrates such a mechanism in acute infection.

In acute infections, in which large numbers of granulocytes are in demand, the bone marrow storage pool can become exhausted even in the face of increased production. When this takes place (in overwhelming infections), neutropenia is seen, which often signifies a poor prognosis. In chronic infections, a steady state may develop in which granulocyte production and release may equal the flow from the CGP to the marginal granulocytic pool (MGP) and from there to the tissues. Such an increase in cell kinetics is seen in chronic neutrophilia caused by polycythemia vera and in Hodgkin's disease. The kinetics of chronic infection are shown in Figure 12.2; the kinetics of an inflammatory state are shown in Figure 12.3.

Neutropenia can be caused not only by an acute infection but also by a defective bone marrow production rate that results in inadequate input of cells to the CGP. In such situations, the bone marrow mitotic pool is unable to meet the physiologic demands, and this results in a reduced or absent storage pool. The appearance of increased numbers of bands in inflammatory conditions is due to the fact that the bone marrow in the normal state contains more bands than segmented neutrophils. Usually, segmented neutrophils are released from the bone marrow to the blood in preference to bands but, when the demand for cellular release is accelerated, the storage pool of neutrophils is exhausted first, and the proportion of released bands increases. This mechanism results in increased numbers of bands in the peripheral blood.

Neutrophilia

Neutrophilia may be caused by many organisms, as shown in Table 12.1. In acute infections, total

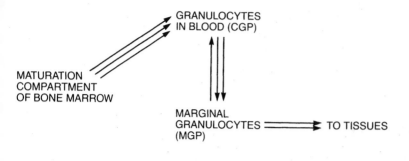

Figure 12.1. Granulocytic kinetics in acute infection. (CGP = circulating granulocytic pool; MGP = marginal granulocytic pool.)

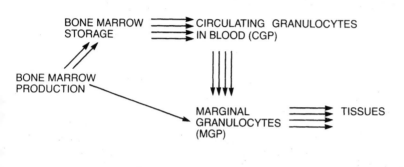

Figure 12.2. Granulocytic kinetics in chronic infections. (CGP = circulating granulocytic pool; MGP = marginal granulocytic pool.)

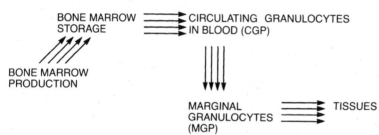

Figure 12.3. Granulocytic kinetics in inflammation. (CGP = circulating granulocytic pool; MGP = marginal granulocytic pool.)

leukocyte counts can reach 40×10^9/liter, but they are more often between 15 and 20×10^9/liter. Other causes of neutrophilia besides microbiological ones are shown in Table 12.2.

Neutropenia

Neutropenia can result from a variety of pathologic situations, among them overwhelming acute infections resulting from bacteria, viruses, *Rickettsia* species, protozoa, and nonmicrobiological agents. It can be defined as a reduction of the absolute neutrophil count to less than 2×10^9/liter. The principal causes of neutropenia are shown in Table 12.3. Neonatal neutropenia has been associated with maternal hypertension, and can produce an increased risk of nosocomial infections (Koenig and Christensen, 1989).

Infection

The laboratory findings of infection vary. The cells seen in the peripheral blood resulting from the marginal pool release have normal morphologic features, but those released from the bone marrow usually show significant immaturity. Examples of such immaturity include bands, metamyelocytes, and myelocytes. Often, toxic granulation, cytoplasmic vacuolation, and Döhle bodies are also seen, and these morphologic characteristics represent important features delineating infectious states. Other changes seen in the granulocytes include an increase in granulocyte-derived peroxidase and alkaline phosphatase activity and an increase in neutrophils that stain positively for nitroblue-tetrazolium (NBT).

Toxic granulation is seen often in the granulocytes when infection is present. The azurophilic granules are coarse, stain more intensely, and are

Table 12.1. Common Bacteriologic Causes of Neutrophilia

Organism	Examples
Cocci	*Staphylococcus, Streptococcus, Pneumococcus, Gonococcus, Meningococcus*
Bacilli	*Escherichia coli, Pseudomonas aeruginosa, Corynebacterium diphtheriae*
Parasites	Liver fluke
Fungi	*Actinomyces*
Spirochetes	*Leptospira icterohaemorrhagiae*
Viruses	Rabies, herpes zoster
Rickettsia	Typhus

Table 12.2. Principal Causes of Neutrophilia Other than Microbiological Causes

Cause	Examples
Inflammation	Surgery, burns, myocardial infarction, rheumatic fever, rheumatoid arthritis
Intoxication	Uremia, drug and chemical poisoning
Hemorrhage	—
Acute hemolysis	—
Neoplasms	Liver, gastrointestinal tract, bone marrow
Physiologic causes	Vigorous exercise, emotional problems, neonatal disease, pregnancy
Myeloproliferative causes	Chronic myeloid leukemia, polycythemia vera
Pharmacologic causes	Epinephrine, cigarette smoking, vaccines, corticosteroids
Acute febrile conditions	
Neutrophilic conditions	
Dermatosis	
(Sweet's syndrome)	

strongly peroxidase-reactive. It is possible that such changes are induced in vivo in already-formed neutrophils and represent phagosomes or autophagic vacuoles. The granules associated with Alder's anomaly and with the Chédiak-Higashi syndrome are frequently confused with toxic granulation.

Döhle bodies are round, oval, or spindle-shaped structures, 1–4 μ in length. There may be three or four inclusions situated at the periphery of the granulocytes. Döhle bodies stain gray-blue with Romanowsky dyes and are believed to be part of the vestigial cytoplasm left from earlier cellular stages. These inclusions are found in toxic conditions such as scarlet fever, septicemia, pneumonia, burns, measles, and exposure to cytotoxic drugs. Differentiating between Döhle bodies and May-Hegglin bodies may be difficult. Döhle bodies are not permanent structures, whereas those found in the May-Hegglin anomaly are inherited as an autosomal dominant trait.

The NBT test is a procedure that measures intracellular activity during phagocytosis. During such activity, the reduced form of nicotinamide adenine dinucleotide (NADH) oxidase is produced, and this is detected by the reduction of colorless NBT to form dark blue intracellular formazan deposits. In afebrile individuals, 3–10% of all mature granules elicit such a reaction (Simmons, 1980). Increases in NBT-positive neutrophils are seen in bacterial meningitis, candidiasis, septicemia, and other acute bacterial infections. However, other febrile diseases do not routinely produce positive results unless the original test is modified (Miller et al., 1976).

Phosphatases are enzymes that liberate orthophosphoric acid from alcohol or phenolic monoesters. The alkaline phosphatases are distinguished from acid phosphatases not only by their pH requirements but also by other features, which include their activation by magnesium ions and their resistance to inhibition by fluorides. Leukocyte alkaline phosphatase activity reflects intracellular metabolic activity, and it is believed that this is controlled by a gene on chromosome 21. The enzyme activity often is greatly increased in leukocy-

Table 12.3. Principal Causes of Neutropenia

Cause	Examples
Gram-negative bacterial infections	Typhoid, paratyphoid
Viral infections	Influenza, measles, hepatitis B
Rickettsial infections	Rocky Mountain spotted fever, typhus
Protozoal infections	Malaria, leishmaniasis
Acute overwhelming infections	Severe infections
Physical agents and drugs	Radiation, benzene, antimetabolites, antibiotics, antihistamines
Hematologic conditions	Pernicious anemia, aplastic anemia, leukemia, Hodgkin's disease, myeloma
Immunoneutropenic conditions	Lupus erythematosus, rheumatoid arthritis, infectious mononucleosis
Immunodeficiency	Agammaglobulinemia, dysgammaglobulinemia
Pediatric conditions	Chronic granulocytopenia of childhood, hereditary neutropenia
Miscellaneous conditions	Cyclic neutropenia, copper deficiency

tosis, particularly when associated with bacterial infections, and is useful in distinguishing leukemoid states from leukemia and polycythemia vera from erythrocytosis.

Myeloperoxidase is present in azurophilic granules of the granulocytes and, less commonly, in monocytes. The enzymes consist of a protein moiety attached to a prosthetic iron-porphyrin complex. In the presence of hydrogen peroxide, they catalyze the oxidation of many substances, including phenols, some amino acids, and some aromatic acids. The cytochemical demonstration of peroxidases depends on the use of an oxidizable substrate having brightly colored oxidation products. The distribution of peroxidases in the granules of myelogenous cells is well established. In acute bacterial infections, especially when toxic granulation is present, the reaction appears more pronounced.

Agranulocytosis

Besides the microbiological agents that cause neutropenia, a wide variety of drugs and medications are known to induce an acute reaction that leads to agranulocytosis. This is manifested as severe neutropenia that nearly always is associated with eosinopenia and basopenia. Drug-induced agranulocytosis interferes with granulocytic production by cytolytic mechanisms (alkylating agents, mitotic inhibitors, etc.) and by metabolic interference with DNA synthesis (cytosine arabinoside, 6-mercaptopurine, methotrexate, etc.). Additionally, an idiopathic form of neutropenia that can persist for years and results from the administration of phenylbutone and chloramphenicol is well-known (Table 12.4).

Eosinophilia

Eosinophilia is defined as an absolute increase in the total number of circulating eosinophils. A wide range of disorders is known to be responsible for such an increase; these are listed in Table 12.5. Many organs, principally the lungs, central nervous system, and skin, frequently are infiltrated by mature eosinophils, leading to severe organ dysfunction due to eosinophilic cytoplasmic protein accumulation.

Allergic disorders are often characterized by eosinophilia caused by the release of eosinophilic chemotactic factors from basophil degranulation (see page 120). The degree of eosinophilia may reach 34×10^9/liter in bronchial asthma. Dermatologic disorders such as atopic dermatitis and eczema, as well as pemphigus, also are associated frequently with an absolute increase in eosinophils.

Eosinophilia can be caused by parasitic infections, particularly parasites that invade tissues, such as *Trichinella spiralis,* and visceral larva migrans. Intestinal parasitism is associated with eosinophilia less often, though it is found, albeit less prominently, in individuals infected with *Strongyloides, Ascaris,* and *Taenia* species. Lymphoproliferative diseases such as lymphoma often produce eosinophilias of greater than 20% (Harris, 1979). More moderate increases are seen in Löffler's syndrome and in a wide range of infectious diseases.

Table 12.4. Common Drugs that Cause Agranulocytosis

Drug Group	Examples
Analgesics, sedatives, and anti-inflammatory agents	Phenacetin, barbiturates, aminopyrine, dipyrone
Tranquilizers	Chlorpromazine
Antibacterial agents	Sulfonamides, chloramphenicol, methicillin
Antithyroid agents	Thiouracil
Anticonvulsants	Phenytoin

Table 12.5. Principal Causes of Eosinophilia

Cause	Examples
Allergy	Asthma, hay fever, drug sensitivity
Dermatoses	Pemphigus, dermatitis, herpetiformis
Parasitic conditions	Tissue parasites (visceral larva migrans filariasis, malaria, toxoplasmosis), intestinal parasites (tapeworm)
Hematologic disease	Lymphoma, Hodgkin's disease, chronic myeloid leukemia, other myeloproliferative disorders
Infection	Recovery from an acute infection, tuberculosis, brucellosis
Poisoning	Pilocarpine, phosphorus, camphor
Miscellaneous conditions	Löffler's syndrome, pulmonary infiltration with eosinophilia, tropical eosinophilia

Eosinopenia

Eosinopenia consists of a decrease in the absolute number of circulating eosinophils to less than 0.04×10^9/liter. Such decreases are impossible to detect with any degree of accuracy if manual eosinophil counts are carried out and can be determined reliably only by using an automated cytochemical flow-through apparatus such as the H6000 H1, H2, or the Hemalog-D90 (Miles [Technicon] Inc, Tarrytown, NY). Reductions in total circulating eosinophils are due to migration of these cells into inflammatory sites. Eosinopenia is seen also in Cushing's syndrome and after administration of corticosteroids (Nelson and Morris, 1984).

Basophilia

Basophilia is seen most frequently in myeloproliferative disorders, particularly in chronic myeloid leukemia and myeloid metaplasia. It is found less commonly in a variety of conditions such as infections, chronic hemolytic anemia, and stress (Table 12.6). Like eosinophilia, basophilia can be identified reliably only by using automated flow-through methods that count large numbers of cells.

Basopenia

Basopenia is defined as a decrease in the circulating absolute basophil count to less than 0.01×10^9/liter. Again, because of the level of the count, basopenia can be determined only by using automated methods and counting a large volume of blood cells. Reductions in basophils can be seen in hyperthyroidism (Gilbert and Ornstein, 1975), in acute infection, and after long-term treatment with adrenal glucocorticoids. Like eosinophils, basophils exhibit diurnal variation, lower levels being found in the morning and increased levels during the night (Nelson and Morris, 1984).

Monocytosis

The primary causes of monocytosis are listed in Table 12.7. In bacterial infections, particularly in tuberculosis and subacute bacterial endocarditis caused by *Streptococcus viridans,* the monocyto-

Table 12.6. Principal Causes of Basophilia

Cause	Examples
Inflammation	Infection, varicella, variola
Hypothyroidism	Myxedema, antithyroid therapy
Immunologic conditions	Foreign protein injection, nephrosis
Hematologic conditions	Chronic hemolysis, Hodgkin's disease, chronic myeloid leukemia, polycythemia vera

Table 12.7. Principal Causes of Monocytosis

Cause	Examples
Bacteria and other microorganisms	Tuberculosis, streptococcal infection, *Treponema pallidum, Plasmodium, Trypanosoma, Rickettsia*
Hematologic disease	Myeloproliferative disorders, myeloma, lymphoma, histiocytosis
Malignancy	Ovary, stomach, breast
Collagen vascular diseases	Lupus erythematosus, arthritis
Chronic inflammatory disorders	Ulcerative colitis, regional enteritis

Table 12.8. Principal Causes of Lymphocytosis

Cause	Examples
Acute viral infections	Infectious mononucleosis, mumps, chickenpox, hepatitis B
Chronic infections	Brucellosis, syphilis, tuberculosis
Hematologic disorders	Chronic and acute lymphocytic leukemia, lymphosarcoma, non-Hodgkin's lymphoma

sis may be moderate. An absolute level exceeding 0.8×10^9/liter is considered to be increased and sometimes is present during the recovery stage of an acute infection and in myeloproliferative disease, such as acute monocytic leukemia (types M4 and M5).

Monocytopenia

The term *monocytopenia* is reserved for absolute monocyte counts of less than 0.2×10^9/liter. As for the eosinopenias and basopenias, little is known concerning the clinical value of such situations, mainly because of the small number of cells counted in normal differential counts. However, using the H6000 H1, H2, or the Hemalog D90, it is possible to count much larger numbers of cells and, with the use of such an apparatus, monocytopenia has been reported in hairy-cell leukemia

(Seshadri et al., 1976) and during prednisone therapy (Rinehart et al., 1975).

Lymphocytic Cells

Lymphocytosis

Lymphocytosis can be defined as an absolute increase of lymphocytes to more than 4.0×10^9/liter in adults and more than 8.8×10^9/liter in children. The principal causes of lymphocytosis are shown in Table 12.8. The most common of the disorders producing lymphocytic increases is acute viral disease, particularly that caused by the Epstein-Barr virus (EBV), the causative agent of infectious mononucleosis. This disorder more frequently involves young adults and classically presents with variant lymphocytes as well as an absolute and relative lymphocytosis (see page 126).

Table 12.9. Principal Causes of Lymphopenia

Cause	Examples
Physiologic	Stress, exercise, hemorrhage
Pharmacologic	Corticosteroids, cytotoxic agents, irradiation
Pathologic	Immunologic deficiencies, acute infections, liver disease

Lymphocytopenia

Lymphocytopenia is defined as an absolute lymphocyte count of less than 1.5×10^9/liter in adults and 3.0×10^9/liter in children. The principal causes of lymphocytopenia are immunodeficiencies that often are due to impaired lymphopoiesis, but decreases can also be found in acute infections (Shillitoe, 1950), disseminated lupus erythematosus, Hodgkin's disease, and acute radiation syndrome (Miale, 1982; Table 12.9).

Functional Disorders of Granulocytes, Macrophages, and Immunodeficiencies

Quantitative Granulocytic Disorders

Infantile Genetic Agranulocytosis

Infantile genetic agranulocytosis is a fatal disorder inherited as an autosomal recessive characteristic with severe agranulocytosis. The main laboratory findings are a neutropenia (usually less than 0.5×10^9/liter) and mature granulocytes in the peripheral blood. The bone marrow shows variable cellularity, commonly with a maturation arrest at the myelocyte stage of development, although mature eosinophils and basophils are present. The cause of the disorder is unclear, although it has been suggested that the defect is due to abnormal cell production rather than increased cell destruction (Olofsson et al., 1976).

Cyclic Neutropenia

Cyclic neutropenia is believed to be inherited as an autosomal dominant disorder characterized by mild infections and fever and a relative neutropenia, lymphocytosis, and monocytosis. These cell changes occur at approximately 3-week intervals and last between 3 and 10 days. The bone marrow examination shows lack of granulocytic precursors during the time of crisis, possibly because of a failure of cell production at the pluripotential stem-cell level.

Chronic Granulomatous Disease

Chronic granulomatous disease (CGD) is congenital and is inherited either as a sex-linked or an autosomal recessive disorder. It is characterized by recurrent bacterial infections with *Staphylococcus aureus* and Enterobacteriaceae species and the inability of neutrophils and monocytes to kill certain ingested bacteria. Specific infections of the skin, bone, lungs, liver, and lymph nodes result in generalized lymphadenopathy and hepatosplenomegaly (Gabig, 1980).

Phagocytes from patients with CGD display none of the manifestations of the respiratory burst following phagocytosis or other stimuli that activate the burst in normal situations. Pneumococci and streptococci produce hydrogen peroxide but lack the enzyme catalase that destroys the peroxide. These organisms are killed normally by CGD neutrophils in vitro, and it is believed that the lack of hydrogen peroxide production by phagocytes is responsible for their killing defect. Organisms that do not excrete hydrogen peroxide, such as *S. aureus* and Enterobacteriaceae species, are not killed by CGD phagocytes unless an exogenous source of hydrogen peroxide is provided to the phagolysosome in vitro.

The laboratory findings include elevated immunoglobulin levels, increased numbers of bone marrow plasma cells, and elevated absolute and relative peripheral blood neutrophils. The diagnostic test is the NBT. Affected leukocytes fail to reduce the dye at a normal rate and, consequently, blue-black formazan deposits are found intracellularly.

CGD, like other inherited disorders, is actually a group of closely related abnormalities, each caused by a defect affecting a different element of a single

Table 12.10. Inherited Neutrophilic Dysfunctions

Disorder	Dysfunction	Inheritance	Laboratory Tests
CR3 deficiency	Lack of complement receptors on neutrophils and monocytes; decreased adherence and phagocytosis	Autosomal recessive	Flow cytometry for CR3(CD11b) antigen on neutrophil surface
Specific granule deficiency	Failure to synthesize specific neutrophil granules, causing severe bacterial infections	Autosomal recessive	Leukocytes possess bilobed nuclei with clefts; lack of specific granules
Chédiak-Higashi syndrome	Defective chemotaxis and lysosomal granules; fusion of cytoplasmic granules in leukocytes, causing infections and neurologic abnormalities	Autosomal recessive	Giant granules in neutrophils, monocytes, and lymphocytes
Chronic granulomatous disease	Defective oxidative bacterial killing in neutrophils and monocytes; deficiency of cytochrome b558	X-linked; 66% autosomal recessive; 34% autosomal dominant	NBT test; oxidative burst analysis by flow cytometry
Myeloperoxidase deficiency	Defective oxidative bacterial killing in vitro	Autosomal recessive	Leukocyte myeloperoxidase stain
G6PD deficiency	Defective oxidative burst, lack of NADH and NADPH	X-linked	Red-cell G6PD

NBT = nitroblue tetrazolium; G6PD = glucose-6-phosphate dehydrogenase; NADH = reduced nicotinamide adenine dinucleotide; NADPH = reduced nicotinamide adenine dinucleotide phosphate.

biochemical system. These groups of disorders can be classified based on subordinate clinical and laboratory criteria that distinguish among the individual components of the group (Table 12.10). Two major criteria are used—the mode of inheritance and the presence or absence of cytochrome b558 in the affected leukocytes. On this basis, CGD can be classified into three main types; X-linked, autosomal recessive cytochrome b558–negative, and autosomal recessive cytochrome b558–positive (Bobior and Woodman, 1990).

Myeloperoxidase Deficiency

A deficiency of myeloperoxidase from the azurophilic granules of the neutrophils is a rare autosomal recessive disorder that seldom results in infection. The disease is characterized by a pronounced delay in the killing of both catalase-positive and catalase-negative intracellular bacteria. All other aspects of phagocytic function are normal or, in the case of the respiratory burst, supranormal. Neutrophils and monocytes appear to be affected, although eosinophils show normal activity (Kitahara and Eyre, 1981; d'Onofrio and Mango, 1984).

Storage Disorders of Monocytes and Macrophages

Gaucher's Disease

Gaucher's disease is a rare familial autosomal recessive disorder found most commonly in Ashkenazi Jews. The disease has been divided into three principal forms: type 1, the chronic adult nonneuropathic form; type 2, the acute infantile neuropathic form; and type 3, the subacute juvenile neuropathic form (Peters et al., 1977; Nishimura and Barranger, 1980; Soffer et al., 1980). Gaucher's disease is characterized by hepatosplenomegaly, skin pigmentation, and bone lesions, as well as progressive spasticity and mental retardation. The disorder is caused by deficient activity of β-glucocerebrosidase, which cleaves glucose from glucosyl ceramide in normal individuals. A reduction of this enzyme results in the accumulation of glucosyl ceramide in reticuloendothelial cells, producing Gaucher's cells. These histiocytes may be present in the spleen, liver, bone marrow, and lymph nodes. Morphologically, they are round or oval cells 20–70 μ in diameter. The cytoplasm occupies 60–80% of the cell, is fibrillar in form, and stains best with eosin, but does not stain with Sudan III or the oil red-O stain for fat. In Romanowsky-stained smears, the cytoplasm is pale blue-gray. The fibrillar pattern is demonstrated best with Mallory's aniline blue dye. The nucleus is moderately condensed and usually eccentrically placed within the cell.

Besides the presence of these abnormal storage cells in the bone marrow, the laboratory findings often demonstrate a moderate normocytic anemia with little or no evidence of bone marrow response, such as polychromasia or reticulocytosis. Leukopenia and thrombocytopenia are present, and serum acid phosphatase levels are increased. The diagnosis usually is made by the recognition of Gaucher's cells in bone marrow smears or sections.

Niemann-Pick Disease

Niemann-Pick disease is a disorder of young children, characterized by tissue infiltration of foamy storage cells. The disease probably includes five different but related conditions, the most common of which is the classic infantile or A form. Like Gaucher's disease, the clinical manifestations are of mental retardation and hepatosplenomegaly but also include growth retardation and bone changes. Niemann-Pick disease is found most frequently in Ashkenazi Jews and is characterized by increased levels of phosphorylcholine ceramide (sphingomyelin) in the tissue. The metabolic defect is a deficiency of sphingomyelinase, which hydrolyzes phosphorylcholine ceramide to phosphorylcholine and ceramide.

The peripheral blood usually shows a microcytic anemia and thrombocytopenia secondary to hypersplenism. The total leukocyte count is variable. Lymphocytes and monocytes frequently show discrete vacuolation. Serum acid phosphatase levels are normal. The diagnosis may be based on the clinical history and on the presence of large histiocytic cells in the bone marrow and spleen, as well as on the sphingomyelinase activity in specimens of solid tissue.

Niemann-Pick cells are 20–80 μ in diameter and contain an extremely foamy cytoplasm that stains with Sudan black B and oil red-O stain. The nucleus often is polyploid, and frequently two nuclei are present. These foamy, globular cytoplasmic inclusions are composed of sphingomyelin and stain blue-green with Romanowsky stain.

Sea-Blue Histiocytosis

Sea-blue histiocytosis, a storage reticulosis, can be found as both an autosomal recessive and an acquired disorder. Tissue lipid analyses have shown an increase in phospholipid, sphingomyelin, and total lipid in the spleen and bone marrow. The most marked clinical feature is hepatosplenomegaly, but macular abnormalities of the eye, pulmonary infiltrates, skin pigmentation, and neurologic abnormalities also are seen.

Morphologically, typical sea-blue histiocytes are present that vary in diameter from 20 to 60 μ and contain a single eccentric nucleus. The nucleus is of block chromatin and possesses a medium-sized, easily discernible nucleolus. The cytoplasm is packed with sea-blue or blue-green granules when stained by a Romanowsky dye. These granules are variable in size, shape, and staining intensity and frequently obscure the nucleus.

Sea-blue histiocytes are found scattered throughout the bone marrow, spleen, and liver. Their presence is the principal diagnostic feature of the disease.

Table 12.11 shows the cytochemical reactions of the more common storage reticuloses. Table 12.12 summarizes the principal biochemical defects in the major lipidoses.

Morphologic Abnormalities in Leukocytes

Nuclear Abnormalities

Hypersegmentation

The nucleus of a mature polymorphonuclear neutrophil normally contains two to five lobes. In hypersegmented states, such a cell often contains six to 10 lobes. Such cells are rarely seen in healthy individuals but are found most often in the peripheral blood in the presence of either folic acid or vitamin B_{12} deficiency. When these cells are present, they are abnormally large, being between 16 and 25 μ in diameter. Usually associated with these macropolycytes are giant bands and metamyelocytes.

Rieder Cells

In leukemia, occasional irregularities are found in the nuclear outline of both myeloblasts and lym-

Table 12.11. Cytochemical Reactions of the More Common Storage Reticuloses

Stain	Gaucher's Disease	Niemann-Pick Disease	Sea-Blue Histiocytosis
Romanowsky	Colorless	Blue-green	Blue-green
Periodic acid–Schiff	Positive	Variable	Positive
Oil red-O	Usually negative	Positive	Positive
Sudan black B	Weakly positive	Positive	Positive
Acid phosphatase	Positive	Negative	Negative
Acid-fast	Negative	Positive	Positive
Hematoxylin and eosin	Colorless	Green-yellow	Brown-yellow

Table 12.12. Chemical Abnormalities in the Common Lipidoses

	Gaucher's Disease	Niemann-Pick Disease
Enzyme deficiency	β-Glucosidase	Sphingomyelinase
Substrate accumulated	Glucocerebroside	Sphingomyelin

phocytes. Normally, these cells have a round or oval nuclear outline, but when the nucleus becomes cleft or deeply indented by a slitlike aperture, the cell is termed a *Rieder cell*. This anomaly is thought to represent asynchronism of nuclear and cytoplasmic maturation, whereby the nucleus is highly differentiated but the cytoplasm is immature.

Nuclear Appendages

Gender-specific, drumstick-shaped nuclear structures can be found in up to 7% of neutrophils in normal women. These structures must be differentiated from small clumps or racquets of chromatin material that are found in both men and women. The principal distinguishing feature is that these gender-specific structures morphologically possess a thin, threadlike chromatin neck, in contrast to the thicker neck seen in the racquet chromatin. The drumstick is approximately 1.5 μ in diameter and has a dense, bulbous end. No more than one structure has ever been found in a cell.

Cytoplasmic Abnormalities

Alder's Anomaly (Alder-Reilly Anomaly)

Alder's anomaly, or *Alder-Reilly anomaly*, is an autosomal recessive characteristic manifested by the presence of clusters of nonspecific azurophilic granules in the cytoplasm of all leukocytes. Nuclear maturation is normal in such situations, the anomaly being attributed to mucopolysaccharides and sphingomyelin stored in the granules because of a lysosomal deficiency of a hydroxylase. When all the leukocytes are affected, it is common to find cells in which the nucleus is obscured by the dense granulation. This is particularly common in basophils. The anomaly may be associated with Hurler's syndrome (gargoylism).

Toxic Granulation

Toxic granulation was discussed previously on page 130. The abnormality relates to the presence of peroxidase-positive granules in neutrophils and other granulocytes in infections.

Döhle Bodies

Döhle bodies were discussed previously on page 131. The inclusions are found in granulocytes in many toxic conditions, such as scarlet fever and septicemia.

May-Hegglin Anomaly

The *May-Hegglin anomaly* is a rare autosomal dominant trait associated with mild hemorrhage, giant platelets, and thrombocytopenia. The inclusion bodies, which measure 2–5 μ, are similar morphologically to Döhle bodies and appear as structures that stain negatively for periodic acid–Schiff and peroxidase but stain as pale blue spindles with Romanowsky stains. These spindles are present in all mature granulocytes. May-Hegglin inclusions are RNA material believed to be derived from the endoplasmic reticulum.

Other laboratory findings in this anomaly include abnormal clot retraction, positive tourniquet tests, and reduced platelet survival. Platelet aggregation is normal.

Chédiak-Higashi Syndrome

Chédiak-Higashi syndrome, a rare autosomal recessive disorder, is characterized by large numbers of specific green-gray granules, varying in size up to 4 µ in diameter. These inclusions are peroxidase-positive and are present principally in neutrophils, eosinophils, basophils, and monocytes. Those seen in monocytes are believed to represent phagocytosed material. Large azurophilic-staining granules can also be seen in lymphocytes and plasma cells.

The anomaly is seen in children with severe, chronic, and often fatal infections and frequently is associated with albinism. Other laboratory results include abnormal platelet aggregation, prolonged bleeding time, normal platelet counts, and shortened red-cell and granulocytic survival. Pancytopenia also is seen, especially as the disease progresses.

The accelerated phase of the disorder is characterized by lymphocytic proliferation in the liver, spleen, and bone marrow.

Pelger-Huët Anomaly

The *Pelger-Huët anomaly* is benign, inherited as a non-sex-linked dominant trait, and characterized by decreased segmentation of the granulocytes and chromatin condensation in all stages of maturation. Cell cytoplasmic maturation is normal. The shift to the left takes two distinct morphologic forms: (1) the so-called heterozygous form of the anomaly, in which the granulocytic nucleus appears as spectacles, and (2) the homozygous form, in which the nucleus is round and regular in outline. Pelger-Huët cells function normally and are able to phagocytize microorganisms (Skendzel and Hoffman, 1962). Identification is best accomplished using the following criteria: (1) 70–90% of the neutrophils are bilobed; (2) fewer than 10% of the neutrophils have three lobes; and (3) no neutrophil has more than three lobes.

A second, *pseudo-* or *acquired* form of the Pelger-Huët anomaly exists that is seen most often in chronic myelocytic leukemia. However, it can also be present in acute leukemia, myeloid metaplasia, chronic lymphocytic leukemia, non-Hodgkin's lymphoma, Hodgkin's disease, and other disorders. When present, pseudo–Pelger-Huët cells tend to appear late in the disease and often after bouts of chemotherapy. Most of the cells appear morphologically similar to the homozygous form, possessing a round, centrally placed nucleus.

Care should be taken in the differentiation of Pelger-Huët cells, as they can be mistaken for bands or metamyelocytes and, consequently, an incorrect impression of a left shift may result.

Auer Bodies

Auer bodies are rodlike inclusions found in the cytoplasm of myeloblasts, promyelocytes, and monoblasts. They stain a vivid azurophilic color with Romanowsky dyes and are between 1 and 6 µ long and usually less than 1.5 µ wide. Cytochemically, Auer bodies are peroxidase-positive, sudanophilic, RNA-positive, acid phosphatase-positive, and AS-D chloroacetate–positive structures. They produce negative reactions for glycogen, DNA, and alkaline phosphatase. Auer bodies are found in acute myeloid leukemia and during blastic crisis in chronic myeloid leukemia, as well as in erythroleukemia (Sondergaard-Petersen, 1975).

Jordans' Anomaly

Jordans' anomaly is characterized by the presence of many large sudanophilic inclusions in the cytoplasm of all granulocytes and monocytes. Routine Romanowsky-stained blood smears show only vacuolation of the involved cells, as the lipid constituents of the inclusions are removed during the fixation and staining involving methyl alcohol (Jordans, 1953).

Other Leukocytic Disorders

Infectious Mononucleosis

Infectious mononucleosis is a self-limiting lymphoproliferative disorder caused by EBV. The virus infects B lymphocytes, which appear to be the only

Table 12.13. Antibodies Formed Following Epstein-Barr Virus Infections

Antibodies	First Detected	Period of Persistence	Comments
VCA IgG	2 wks	Life	Past infection
VCA IgM	Onset	4–8 wks	Acute infection
Early membrane	Onset	Life	In carrier states
EA-D	3–4 wks	Transient	—
EA-R	2–8 wks	1 yr	Burkitt's lymphoma
EBNA	2–4 wks	Life	Absence of EBNA and presence of VCA in acute infections

VCA = viral capsid antigen; EA-D = early antigen, diffuse; EA-R = early antigen, restricted; EBNA = Epstein-Barr nuclear antigen.

lymphoid cells with receptors for this agent. The B cells, containing EBV nuclear antigen, are found only in the acute phase of the disease, and both these cells and EBV-specific killer T cells disappear once this phase has passed.

Infectious mononucleosis is found principally in young adults and occurs only in individuals who do not have anti-EBV, as the presence of the antibody confers lifelong immunity. There are three major causes of infectious mononucleosis syndrome. EBV accounts for 60% of the cases in young children and more than 90% of the cases in young adults. The heterophil antibody of the Paul-Bunnell type is displayed in 90% of the cases in young adults. Cytomegalovirus (CMV) accounts for nearly 5% of the cases, and *Toxoplasma gondii* is seen in approximately 1% of cases. The remaining cases are due to herpes simplex virus type 2, varicella, viral hepatitis, adenovirus, rubella, and drug toxicity syndromes.

Patients who develop infectious mononucleosis due to CMV are heterophil-negative. Clinically, affected individuals exhibit malaise, sore throat, headaches, splenomegaly, and lymphadenopathy. The peripheral blood shows a slight leukocytosis, peaking at 2–3 weeks after the initial exposure. The predominant cell seen is the T lymphocyte, which constitutes approximately 60% (or 5.0×10^9/liter) of the cells commonly found. The diagnostic cell seen in the peripheral blood is the variant lymphocyte described on page 126. Leukocyte alkaline phosphatase staining is reduced, and the degree of anemia and thrombocytopenia can vary. The anemia is often hemolytic in nature and results from the presence of a strong auto-anti-i antibody. In a minority of individuals, liver function tests are abnormal.

Serologic tests are the key laboratory procedures aiding in the diagnosis (Table 12.13). The first antibodies to appear are the IgM forms of anti–viral capsid antigen (anti-VCA), which can be detected during the incubation phase of the disease. These antibodies peak within 2 weeks and then rapidly disappear in 4–8 weeks (Schmitz and Scherer, 1972). The IgG form of anti-VCA is detected soon after the IgM form, peaks 2–3 weeks later than the IgM antibodies, and persists for life. Antibodies to Epstein-Barr nuclear antigen (EBNA) are found several weeks after the initial onset of the disease; like IgG, anti-VCA persists throughout life (Henle et al., 1974). A majority of individuals also transiently exhibit antibodies to the diffuse component of the EBV early antigen (anti-EA-D), which is detectable 3–4 weeks after exposure. A titer of less than 1:10 for antibodies to VCA indicates susceptibility to the disease. High titers usually indicate immunity. A fourfold rise in titer between acute and convalescent serum is not common in infectious mononucleosis, because anti-VCA titers usually are near peak levels when first examined. A single titer of 1:640 or greater strongly suggests an active or recent infection and is diagnostic if the IgM anti-VCA level also is raised. Persistently high titers (1:160 or greater) are commonly seen in chronic, active EBV disease (see Table 12.13).

Titers of antibodies to early antigen (anti-EA) of at least 1:20 strongly suggest a current or recent infection. EA is a complex of at least two distinct components, diffuse (D) and restricted (R) parts. Elevated anti-EA-D titers appear transiently in approximately 85% of individuals with infectious mononucleosis. Anti-EA-D titers also are increased

Table 12.14. Reactions of Different Animal Species' Red Cells with Heterophil Antibodies

Red Cells	Infectious Mononucleosis Antibodies	Forssman Antibodies	Serum Sickness Antibodies
Sheep	+	+	+
Horse	+	+	+
Ox	+	−	+
Guinea pig	−	+	+

Table 12.15. Absorption Patterns of Heterophil Antibodies of Infectious Mononucleosis

Antibody	Absorbed by Guinea Pig Cells	Absorbed by Ox Cells
Infectious mononucleosis	Incomplete absorption	Complete absorption
Serum sickness	Complete absorption	Complete absorption
Forssman	Complete absorption	Partial absorption

Table 12.16. Interpretation of Results of Epstein-Barr Virus (EBV) Tests

Clinical State	EBV Capsid Antibody IgM	EBV EA Antibody	EBV Capsid Antibody IgG	EBNA Antibodies
Noninfected	Negative <1:10	Negative <1:10	Negative <1:10	Negative <1:10
Acute primary infection	Positive >1:10	Positive >1:10	Positive >1:20	Negative <1:2
Old nonreactive infection	Negative <1:10	Negative <1:10	Positive >1:20	Positive >1:2
Reactivated infections	Variable	Positive >1:10	Positive >1:10	Positive >1:2

EA = early antigen; EBNA = Epstein-Barr nuclear antigen.

in nasopharyngeal carcinoma. Anti-EA-R titers often are increased in Burkitt's lymphoma

Besides the detection of antibodies to various fragments of EBV, serologic tests for heterophil antibodies usually produce positive results. The heterophil antibody in normal serum is directed against the *Forssman antigen,* which is widely distributed in nature. Table 12.14 shows the reactions of the heterophil antibody of infectious mononucleosis, the Forssman antibody, and of serum sickness with cells of various animal species. Separation of these heterophil antibodies can be accomplished using ox cells and guinea pig kidney cells. The IgM form of the antibody usually appears between the fifth and tenth days of illness, rises to its highest level in the second to third week and, in some cases, persists for years. Although the presence of these antibodies is relatively specific for infectious mononucleosis, it has been observed that they fail to develop in

5–10% of adult patients (Henle et al., 1974). Heterophil antibodies may be found in a variety of other hematologic disorders, including lymphoma, leukemia, and histiocytic medullary reticulosis (Davson et al., 1981). Antibodies to EBV-VCA develop in all patients with Burkitt's lymphoma, nasopharyngeal carcinoma, and EBV infectious mononucleosis. In addition, high EBV antibody titers often are associated with Hodgkin's disease, lymphocytic leukemia, systemic lupus erythematosus, sarcoidosis, and Izumi fever (Evans, 1971; Takada, 1973).

The laboratory diagnosis depends on the demonstration of antibodies to EBV and heterophil antibodies that are unabsorbed by guinea pig kidney and are completely absorbed by beef cells. Table 12.15 details this absorption pattern.

In infectious mononucleosis, the titer level is not indicative of the severity of the disease, nor does it parallel the morphologic changes seen in the peripheral blood (Table 12.16).

Cytomegalovirus Mononucleosis

CMV mononucleosis is the most common cause of heterophil-negative infectious mononucleosis and is due to CMV infection. Clinically, a fever and malaise and, occasionally, a rubellalike rash are found. On occasion, splenomegaly is present, but hepatomegaly is not seen. Leukocytosis is characteristic, with an absolute lymphocytosis. Morphologically, lymphocytes appear as variant cells. Liver function tests often are abnormal, and increased titers of nonspecific cold agglutinins and antinuclear antibodies may be detected. The heterophil test result is always negative, and antibodies to EBV are not seen. Diagnosis can be made by demonstrating antibodies to CMV by complement fixation, by indirect hemagglutination methods (Jordan et al., 1973), or by direct latex agglutination.

Chapter 13

Hematologic Neoplasms

Classification of Hematologic Neoplasms

A broad general classification of hematologic neoplasms is shown in Table 13.1. From this, it can be seen that the leukemias are subdivided into two principal groups—myeloid and lymphocytic. Each group is subclassified as chronic or acute. The lymphomas are, in turn, divided into two categories—Hodgkin's disease and non-Hodgkin's lymphomas (NHLs). In addition, miscellaneous disorders that do not fall into these divisions include other myeloproliferative and lymphoproliferative disorders as well as the paraproteinemias.

Leukemia is a disorder characterized by the replacement of normal bone marrow with uncontrolled proliferating hematopoietic cells and a concomitant increase of peripheral blood leukocytes that reflect such cellular immaturity. The terms *acute* and *chronic* are usually used to denote the clinical course of the disease, but they are also used as general terms suggesting the predominant degree of cell immaturity seen. In the acute form, the principal cells are poorly differentiated and are less mature than those seen in the chronic leukemias. The lymphomas are not always associated with bone marrow abnormalities and mainly show abnormal lymphocytic and lymphoidlike cellular proliferation of the lymph nodes and reticuloendothelial organs. The term *myeloproliferation* is used to denote any bone marrow proliferation of granulocytic or granulocyte-derived cells. Such disorders include polycythemia, myelofibrosis, thrombocythemia, and other granulocytic proliferative diseases.

Leukemia

Leukemia may be defined as a neoplastic disorder involving blood-forming cells. Uncontrolled proliferation of these cells results in overcrowding of the bone marrow to the exclusion of red-cell and platelet production and in the expression of extreme leukocytosis, anemia, and thrombocytopenia in the peripheral blood. The traditional classification of leukemia is shown in Table 13.2, and the French-American-British (FAB) classification of acute leukemia is shown in Tables 13.3 and 13.4.

Etiology

The etiology of human leukemia still is not clearly understood, although certain predisposing factors associated with its development are well established. Among them are an inherited host susceptibility, exposure to physical or chemical agents capable of causing chromosomal damage, and virally induced transformation of susceptible stem cells. It is likely that several, if not all, of these factors must be present in order for leukemia to manifest itself.

Hereditary characteristics play an important role in the etiology of the disease. It is known that the incidence of leukemia in siblings is approximately fourfold that in unrelated children (Miller, 1968a) and that there is a high prevalence of the disease in patients with Down's syndrome and Fanconi's anemia (Miller, 1968b). Down's syndrome produces a

Table 13.1. General Classification of Hematologic Neoplasms

Group	Examples
Leukemia	Myeloid, lymphocytic
Lymphoma	Hodgkin's disease, non-Hodgkin's lymphoma
Myeloproliferative tumors	Idiopathic myelofibrosis, polycythemia vera, idiopathic thrombocytosis
Other tumors	Hairy-cell leukemia, mast cell leukemia
Immune-related defects	Myeloma, macroglobulinemia, heavy-chain disease

Table 13.2. Traditional Classification of Leukemia

Type	Example
Stem cell	—
Lymphocytic	Acute lymphocytic, chronic lymphocytic
Granulocytic	Acute myelocytic, chronic myelocytic, acute progranulocytic
Monocytic	Acute monocytic
Myelomonocytic	Acute myelomonocytic
Erythremic myelosis	—
Megakaryocytic	—

Table 13.3. French-American-British Classification of Acute Myeloid Leukemia

Predominant Component	Leukemia	Principal Characteristics
Granulocytic	M1	Myeloblastic without maturation; >3% blasts; delicate nuclear chromatin; rare Auer bodies; peroxidase-positive
	M2	Myeloblastic without maturation; cells mature beyond the promyelocyte stage; >50% blasts and promyelocytes; in older cells, often abundant cytoplasm, azurophilic granules, and Auer bodies
	M3	Promyelocytic; most cells heavily granulated; Auer bodies common; variant type characterized by lack of granulation and presence of bilobed, multilobed, or reniform nuclei
Monocytic	M4	Myelomonocytic; characteristic monocyte nucleus and cytoplasm present; >20% monocytes; >20% myeloblasts and promyelocytes
	M5a	Monocytic; cells mainly monoblasts; lacy chromatin pattern and one or more nucleoli in nucleus; abundant granular cytoplasm; Auer bodies rare
	M5b	Monocytic; cells mainly differentiated; monoblasts, promonocytes, and monocytes predominate; Auer bodies rare
Erythroid	M6	Erythroleukemia (Di Guglielmo syndrome); >50% abnormal erythroid series cells, or <30% normal erythroid series cells and 10% abnormal erythroid series cells and >30% myeloblasts and promyelocytes; occasional Auer bodies and abnormal megakaryocytes present; nucleated red cells sometimes show megaloblastoid changes and possess glycogen blocks that stain by the PAS reaction
Megakaryocyte	M7	Bone marrow megakaryocytes increased; micromegakaryocytes and nuclear hypolobulation common; angular undifferentiated blasts that possess a high nucleus-to-cytoplasm ratio; cytoplasm occasionally vacuolated; variable number of nucleoli found

PAS = periodic acid–Schiff.

Sources: Data from JM Bennett, et al. Proposals for the classification of acute leukemias. Br J Haematol 33:451, 1976; JM Bennett, et al. Proposals for the classification of the myelodysplastic syndromes. Br J Haematol 51:189, 1982; and HM Golomb, et al. "Microgranular" acute promyelocytic leukemia: a distinct clinical, ultrastructure and cytogenic entity. Blood 55:25, 1980.

Table 13.4. French-American-British Classification of Acute Lymphocytic Leukemia

Predominant Component	Leukemia	Principal Characteristics
Acute lymphocytic (childhood)	L1	Small cells are present that possess homogeneous chromatin, regular nuclear shape, rare nucleoli, and moderately basophilic cytoplasm. Many cells react with anti–null acute lymphocytic leukemia serum. Approximately 25% possess T-cell markers. There is a high terminal transferase activity. In a few cases, the Ph[1] chromosome is seen.
Acute lymphocytic (adult)	L2	Large cells are present, with variable chromatin and an irregular nuclear shape (often cleft). One to two nucleoli are present with a moderate amount of cytoplasm and a variable degree of basophilia. Approximately 50% of the cells are positive with anti–null acute lymphocytic leukemia serum. Approximately 25% have T-cell markers and a high terminal transferase activity. The Ph[1] chromosome is seen in some cases.
Burkitt's type	L3	Large cells are present, with finely stippled chromatin and a round to oval nuclear shape. One to three nucleoli are present. The moderate amount of cytoplasm shows intense basophilia. The cells are negative with anti–null acute lymphocytic leukemia serum. All cells possess B-cell markers.

Sources: Data from JM Bennett, et al. Proposals for the classification of acute leukemias. Br J Haematol 33:451, 1976; and JM Bennett, et al. The morphological classification of acute lymphoblastic leukemia: concordance among observers and clinical correlation. Br J Haematol 47:553, 1981.

chromosomal aberration (trisomy 21), and the cytogenetically abnormal cells of affected individuals may be basically unstable and liable to further leukogenic chromosomal changes (Gunz, 1973).

Exposure to radiation is known to be a factor in any individual's predisposition to acquire leukemia. A small but definite group of patients receiving nodal irradiation for Hodgkin's disease develops acute myeloid leukemia (Potolsky et al., 1982), and there is a definite correlation between the disease and individuals exposed to nuclear explosions (Brill et al., 1962). The survivors of the atomic bomb explosions in Japan provide the clearest evidence of such an association, particularly with acute and chronic myeloid leukemia and, to a lesser extent, with acute lymphoblastic leukemia.

Chronic exposure to toxins and chemicals is also a known causative factor in the formation of leukemic cells. The incidence of acute leukemia is known to be increased in individuals exposed to benzene and benzol derivatives and, in general, this incidence appears relative to the length of the exposure. Alkylating drugs, such as busulfan, chlorambucil, and cyclophosphamide, are also associated with a high incidence of acute myeloid leukemia.

Viruses are known to cause leukemia in some animals, but the evidence for direct viral causation in human acute leukemia is only just becoming available with the discovery of a human leukemia virus that is implicated in the acquired immunodeficiency syndrome (AIDS). The leukemia virus in lower primates is RNA C-type virus, which replicates with the aid of an RNA-directed DNA polymerase. Several workers have reported on the similarity between this and the reverse transcriptase in leukemic cells of patients with acute myeloid leukemia (Gallagher et al., 1975). The widely encountered Epstein-Barr DNA virus of the herpes family is incriminated on the basis of both serologic studies in patients with Burkitt's lymphoma and the self-limiting lymphoid proliferation in infectious mononucleosis.

Acute Leukemia

The traditional classification of leukemia is subject to inconsistent and sometimes subjective morphologic criteria and is limited by a lack of cytochemical markers. The FAB classification separates myeloid and nonmyeloid leukemias and subdivides each group on the basis of Romanowsky-stained blood and bone marrow smears.

The original FAB classification (Bennett et al., 1976) of the acute lymphocytic leukemias has been modified (Bennett et al., 1981). A reclassification of acute myeloid leukemia (type M3) has been proposed (Golomb et al., 1980; Bennett et al., 1980), and a revised set of morphologic criteria has been published (Bennett et al., 1982) that differentiates blasts into two groups: type 1 blasts lacking cytoplasmic granules and type 2 blasts possessing small numbers of primary granules.

Acute Myeloid Leukemia

Acute myeloid leukemia appears suddenly, typically with fever, body pains, rigors, and often a sore throat. There is a progressive hypochromic anemia and a tendency to hemorrhage from the mucous membranes. This bleeding is due to thrombocytopenia. The lymph nodes are usually not enlarged, but moderate hepatosplenomegaly and sternal tenderness are present. Many of these presenting manifestations are directly attributable to a combination of the expanding tumor mass and the failure of normal hematopoiesis.

The laboratory features characteristic of acute myeloid leukemia are anemia, moderate leukocytosis, and thrombocytopenia, in addition to morphologic evidence of leukemic invasion of the bone marrow and peripheral blood. Hyperuricemia and hyper- and hypocalcemia are common laboratory findings. In the peripheral blood, one usually finds an increased leukocyte count of $15–50 \times 10^9$/liter, the majority of the cells being myeloblasts.

Occasionally, Reider cells (blastic cells possessing indented or bilobed nuclei) may be seen. Auer bodies may also be present in the cytoplasm of myeloblasts and promyelocytes. These inclusions are derivatives of azurophilic granules and stain with Sudan black B, peroxidase, and chloroacetate esterase methods. Auer bodies are found in most cases of acute myeloid leukemia and in some cases of types M4 and M6 leukemia.

Moderately severe anemia is often characterized by polychromasia and other related evidence of attempted bone marrow regeneration, such as reticulocytosis and the presence of nucleated red cells in the peripheral blood. The general picture in acute myeloid leukemia is of a severe iron-deficiency anemia and a progressive thrombocytopenia. Diagnosis and differentiation between acute myeloid leukemia and iron-deficiency anemia is most frequently accomplished by the careful study of both the peripheral blood and the bone marrow. A more detailed morphologic, cytochemical, and chromosomal description and the subclassification of acute myeloid leukemia follows.

Type M1 (Myeloblastic Leukemia without Maturation).   The M1 type of acute myeloid leukemia usually reveals a predominantly immature blastic picture with lack of cellular maturation. Cytochemical stains are helpful in differentiating this leukemia from the acute lymphocytic form. The blastic cells are nongranular and usually contain one or more distinct nucleoli. More than 3% of these cells are peroxidase-positive, and a few blastic cells contain some azurophilic granules and Auer bodies. Differentiation between types M1 and M2 leukemia sometimes is difficult.

Acute myeloid leukemia has been reported in association with Sweet's syndrome (Sweet, 1964), a disorder characterized by pyrexia, neutrophilia, erythematous plaques, a dense dermal infiltrate of mature neutrophils, and a rapid response to corticosteroid therapy. This acute febrile neutrophilic dermatosis has also been described in association with chronic myeloid leukemia (Cohen and Kurzrock, 1989).

Type M2 (Myeloblastic Leukemia with Maturation).   The principal feature that distinguishes type M2 acute leukemia from type M1 leukemia is the maturation of immature cells beyond the promyelocyte stage of development in the former. More than 30% of the cells are blasts (both type 1 and type 2). Pseudo–Pelger-Huët cells are sometimes seen, as are poorly granulated mature neutrophils. The leukemic cells are frequently nucleolated and contain varying amounts of cytoplasm with heavy azurophilic granulation and usually single Auer bodies. The chromosomal translocation t(8;21) has been reported in the M2 type of acute leukemia (Catovsky, 1981). Common chromosomal abnormalities in acute leukemia are listed in Table 13.5.

Type M3 (Promyelocytic Leukemia).   Type M3 acute leukemia is characterized predominantly by

Table 13.5. Common Chromosomal Abnormalities in Acute Leukemia

Disease	Chromosomal Abnormalities
Acute myeloid leukemia	
M1	t(9;22)(q34;q11)
M2	t(8;21)(q22;q22)
M3	t(15;17)(q22;q11)
M4	Abnormalities involving chromosome 11
M5	t(9;11)(p21–22;q23)
M4 with eosinophilia	inv(16)(p13;q22);del(16)(q22)
M2,M4 with basophilia	t(6;9)(p23;q34)
M1,M2,M4,M7 with normal or elevated platelets	inv(3)(q21;q26)
Acute lymphocytic leukemia	
Early B lineage	t(9;22)(q34;q11);6q–;t/de112p
Early B lineage hyperdiploid	+21; +6; +12; +14; +10; +4; +8; +18
Pre–B-cell lineage	t(1;19)(q23;p13);t(1;11)(p32;q23)
Biphenotype (early B-cell lineage, monocytic)	t(4;11)(q21;q23)
L1 or L2	t(10;14)(q24;q11);t(11;14)(p13;q11)t(9;22)(q34;q11)
L3 (B-ALL)	t(8;14) or t(8;22) or t(2;8)
T-cell lineage	Abnormalities involving chromosome 11(q23) or 14; (6q–, 9q–)

B-ALL = B-cell acute lymphocytic leukemia.

the presence of promyelocytes demonstrating heavy cytoplasmic granulation. The nucleus varies greatly in size and shape and is frequently bilobed in outline. Some cells contain bundles of Auer bodies randomly distributed in the cytoplasm. A variant form of type M3 leukemia that shows minimal cytoplasmic granulation also exists (Bennett et al., 1980; Golomb et al., 1980). This variant is characterized by the presence of multiple Auer bodies and bilobed or multilobed nuclei. It is of some importance that the M3 form of acute leukemia be recognized, as a high proportion of individuals exhibit disseminated intravascular coagulation. A chromosomal translocation t(15;17) has been associated with this type of acute leukemia (Testa et al., 1978). Transformation to type M3 leukemia has been reported in a patient in whom chronic myeloid leukemia previously was diagnosed. In addition to the Philadelphia chromosome (Ph[1]) aberration, an isochromosome 17q[i(17q)] was noted. There was no t(15;17) (van der Merwe et al., 1986).

Type M4 (Myelomonocytic Leukemia). The M4 type of acute leukemia characteristically reveals granulocytic and monocytic differentiation in varying proportions in both the bone marrow and the pe-

ripheral blood. Type M4 leukemia resembles the M2 form except that in type M4, monocytes and promonocytes constitute more than 20% of all cells. Promonocytes may be difficult to distinguish from promyelocytes unless cytochemical stains are used. Rarely, Auer bodies are present. Clinically, the symptoms resemble those of the other acute leukemias. Blood changes show a progressive hypochromic anemia, often with a hemolytic component. The leukocyte count may be increased to 50 × 10⁹/liter, but it might also be normal.

Type M5 (Monocytic Leukemia). The differentiation of type M5 leukemia should be based on both the Romanowsky-stained smear and cytochemical methods. Two variants are recognized. The M5a type is poorly differentiated and shows large blastic cells in the bone marrow and, occasionally, in the peripheral blood. These blasts exhibit a lacy chromatin pattern and up to three prominent nucleoli. The cytoplasm is abundant and frequently basophilic, containing occasional azurophilic granules and pseudopodia.

The M5b type of monocytic leukemia is well differentiated, and monoblasts, promonocytes, and monocytes are seen. The predominant cell in the bone marrow is the promonocyte, which has a large cerebriform nucleus with occasional nucleoli. The cytoplasm is less basophilic than the monoblast, having a gray ground-glass texture and possessing fine azurophilic granules scattered throughout the cell. Rarely, Auer bodies are present.

Monocytic leukemia has been associated with elevated serum lysozyme (muramidase) and intracellular lysozymes. Basophilic differentiation is relatively common in patients with leukemia or myeloproliferative disease but has been reported as well in a patient with M5 leukemia having a t(9;11)(p22,q23) chromosomal abnormality (Kubota et al., 1980).

Type M6 (Erythroleukemia, Di Guglielmo Syndrome).   Type M6 leukemia shows abnormal proliferation of both erythroid and granulocytic precursors. The erythroid component usually exceeds 50% of all nucleated cells and demonstrates bizarre morphologic features that include multilobulation of the nucleus, multiple nuclei, megaloblastic changes in chromatin structure, and occasional giant forms. Nucleoli usually are large, and mitotic figures are often seen. Cytoplasmic vacuolation is present occasionally. Nucleated red cells are seen frequently in the peripheral blood, some of which possess glycogen blocks stained by the periodic acid–Schiff (PAS) reaction. Immature granulocytes, especially myeloblasts and promyelocytes, commonly are seen in the blood and bone marrow. Auer bodies also are seen, as are abnormal megakaryocytes (Allen et al., 1989).

Type M7 (Megakaryocytic Leukemia).   Until recently, M7 leukemia was believed to be uncommon. It now is considered to account for 8–10% of all acute leukemias (Huang et al., 1984). The M7 type produces cytologic findings similar to L2 and M1 blasts. M7 leukemia occurs in children and can be classified into two groups, one that includes children with Down's syndrome in whom myelofibrosis and megakaryocytic dysplasia is present, and another that includes children in whom acute megakaryocytic leukemia has been diagnosed morphologically, by ultrastructural demonstration of platelet peroxide, or immunophenotypically. The diagnosis of M7 leukemia is made by bone marrow examination.

Megakaryoblasts may be difficult to recognize morphologically. Primitive M7 blasts typically are small and have a high nucleus-to-cytoplasm ratio and a basophilic cytoplasm similar to that of lymphoblasts. More differentiated forms may be larger and exhibit cytoplasmic granules and cytoplasmic budding. Up to six nucleoli may be present, and these might be rounded or lobulated with acidophilic, finely dispersed strands of chromatin. Auer rods are not seen, but mature micromegakaryocytes and bizarre dysplastic megakaryocytes might be.

The blasts typically stain negatively for myeloperoxidase, chloroacetate esterase, and usually α-naphthyl butyrate esterase but may be positive for PAS, α-naphthyl acetate esterase, and acid phosphatase. A similar cytochemical profile is seen in erythroleukemia. Immunophenotypically, the cells generally are negative for pan–T-cell and pan–B-cell markers, terminal deoxynucleotidyl transferase, and the myeloid OKM1 antigen (Bennett et al., 1985).

Polyclonal and monoclonal markers to specific surface proteins on megakaryocytes can be used in the diagnosis. The most promising antigens are the glycoprotein Ib complex (Ib plus 1X), glycoprotein IIb/IIIa, and the von Willebrand protein (factor VIII antigen or factor VIII–related antigen) (Windebank et al., 1989; Moscinski et al., 1989).

Acute Lymphocytic Leukemia

Acute lymphocytic leukemia is the most common form of acute leukemia. Clinically, pyrexia, limb pain, headaches, and rigors generally are found. Nodal enlargement may not be significant in the early stages of the disease, but cervical nodes may rapidly swell in the later stages.

The peripheral blood picture reveals a characteristic leukocytosis of between 10 and 100×10^9/liter, the predominant cell being the lymphoblast. These cells may be confused morphologically with those seen in acute myeloid leukemia; they are described more fully later. The number of red cells declines progressively, and a moderate anemia is present. Red-cell regeneration is evidenced by the presence of polychromasia, reticulocytosis, and nucleated red cells. The mature cells show marked anisocytosis and poikilocytosis, and it is common to find a moderate thrombocytopenia. The hematologic diagnosis is made by careful examination of blood and bone marrow smears. A more detailed morphologic, cytochemical, immunologic, and chromosomal description and the subclassification of acute lymphocytic leukemia follow.

Type L1 (Childhood). Type L1 acute lymphocytic leukemia is characterized by a uniformity of the lymphoid elements, the cells being relatively small. Nuclear chromatin varies from being finely dispersed to irregularly clumped, but it is homogeneous in a given individual. Nuclear shape is regular, but indentation or clefts may be seen. The nucleolus may be difficult to distinguish, and the scanty cytoplasm appears less basophilic than in the L2 type of leukemia (Ching-Hai et al., 1989).

Type L2 (Adult). In type L2 acute lymphocytic leukemia, the predominant cells are more than twice the size of a normal small lymphocyte. Cell size is markedly heterogenic in a given patient, and clefts and nuclear indentation are commonly seen. Nucleoli vary in number and often are large and distinct. The amount of cytoplasm and the degree of basophilia are inconsistent.

Type L3 (Burkitt's Type). The cells seen in type L3 acute lymphocytic leukemia are morphologically similar to those seen in Burkitt's lymphoma. They are homogeneous in appearance and are large, possessing dense but finely stippled nuclear chromatin with one or more distinct nucleoli. The vacuolated cytoplasm is moderately abundant and basophilic.

The larger cell forms associated with the L3 group may require additional cytochemical testing to separate them from the M1 forms of acute myeloid leukemia. The cells seen in acute lymphocytic leukemia may occasionally demonstrate some scattered azurophilic granules, which usually are acid phosphatase–positive and myeloperoxidase-negative. These cells are not associated with Auer body formation, the granules having a high frequency of association with T-lymphocyte subpopulations. Cytochemical profiles may reveal residual populations of granulocytes. The presence in the bone marrow of up to 3% of such cells demonstrates that myeloperoxidase reactivity still is considered compatible with acute lymphocytic leukemia.

Burkitt's lymphoma is a malignant childhood tumor found mainly in Central Africa. The Epstein-Barr virus (EBV) genome is identified in approximately 96% of the patients (Harrington et al., 1988), but there is a lack of direct evidence for a causal relationship between EBV and the

disease. It has been suggested that T-cell response is involved.

Cytochemistry in Acute Leukemias

Cytochemical reactions can be beneficial in separating the acute leukemias, particularly the acute lymphocytic forms, from one another and from the M1 type (Figure 13.1). Additionally, these reactions are useful in identifying myeloblastic and monocytic cell lines and in differentiating L1 and L2 types of acute lymphocytic leukemia.

Myeloperoxidase and Sudan Black B. The myeloperoxidase reaction is based on the principle that the enzyme in the leukocyte granules in the presence of hydrogen peroxide oxidizes benzidine or other oxidizable substrates to brightly colored products. Myeloperoxidase activity is present at all stages of neutrophil development and is located in the azurophilic granules. The pattern of positivity in these cells may take the shape of discrete dots or rod-type structures termed *Phi bodies*. More differentiated myeloid cells exhibit an intense reaction product that may obscure the cell nucleus. Eosinophils show an intense reaction, monocytes stain less intensely, and neutrophils have moderate reactivity. On occasion, the reaction can be demonstrated in agranular cells, which might represent peroxidase activity in the perinuclear space, endoplasmic reticulum, and Golgi apparatus.

Sudan black B stains phospholipids and sterols. The stain is positive with both azurophilic and specific granules in neutrophils and eosinophils. Monocytes may be unstained or may contain a few positive staining granules. Lymphocytes and lymphoblasts do not stain with Sudan black B, but occasional myeloblasts exhibit a positive staining reaction.

Both of these stains show similar cytochemical reactions in various cells and are useful in separating the acute lymphocytic from the acute myeloid leukemias. In addition, Auer bodies stain strongly positively by the myeloperoxidase reaction in acute myeloid leukemias. The exact staining mechanism is not fully understood. Occasionally, the number of blasts that stain positively with Sudan black B is greater than the number that stain positively for myeloperoxidase, thereby suggesting that Sudan black B may be more sensitive in detecting these

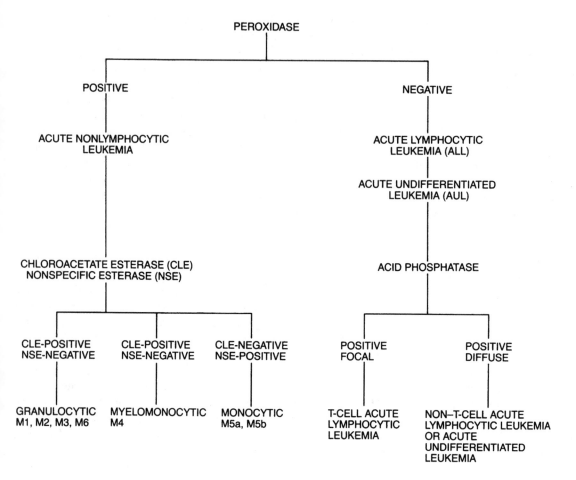

Figure 13.1. Classification of acute leukemia based on the chloroacetate esterase, nonspecific esterase, peroxidase, and acid phosphatase reactions. (Adapted from CY Li. Leukemia identification by immunochemistry. Mayo Med Lab Comm 9:6, 1984.)

cells. This has been supported by the rare finding of Sudan black B–positive, myeloperoxidase-negative acute myeloid leukemia (Hayhoe et al., 1964).

Esterases.   Esterases are a group of lysosomal enzymes capable of hydrolyzing both aliphatic and aromatic esters and are associated with azurophilic granules in the neutrophil. The cytochemical reaction is based on the hydrolysis of a naphthalene ester by leukocyte esterase, which produces a naphthol compound that couples with a diazonium salt to produce a colored product at the site of the enzyme activity. The *chloroacetate esterase reaction* uses naphthol-AS-D-chloroacetate as the substrate and produces positive reactions in neutrophils and immature granulocytes and abnormal normoblasts in

Di Guglielmo syndrome. Weak or negative reactions are found in other cell lines. The staining reaction is similar to the reactions of Sudan black B and myeloperoxidase, except that it appears to be more consistent in monocytes than are the other two stains. Activity develops during granulocytic maturation and usually appears at a later stage than myeloperoxidase activity. Consequently, the enzyme may be lacking in peroxidase-positive myeloblasts and is less helpful in distinguishing type M1 from L1 or L2 leukemias. The principal use for this enzyme is in identifying type M4 leukemia and in differentiating myeloblasts from monocytic cells.

Nonspecific esterases that use α-naphthol acetate as a substrate produce strongly positive reactions in monocytes and frequently negative or weakly positive reactions in neutrophils. Megakaryocytes also stain positively with this reaction. α-Naphthol acetate esterase also produces positive results in basophils, plasma cells, resting T lymphocytes and, occasionally, in normoblasts. The reaction is inhibited by sodium fluoride in monocytes, megakaryocytes, platelets, and plasma cells, but it is not inhibited in neutrophils or lymphocytes (Li et al., 1973). At pH 8.0, this esterase reaction can be used to differentiate subpopulations of T and B lymphocytes, null cells, and monocytes (Higgy et al., 1977). When carried out at pH 7.6, this esterase is seen almost exclusively in monocytes and histiocytes, although occasionally granules may be observed in mature neutrophils and lymphocytes.

Acid Phosphatase.

Seven isoenzymes of acid phosphatase are recognized. The enzyme acts by hydrolyzing naphthol-AS-B1 phosphoric acid, releasing naphthol, which couples with hexazotized pararosaniline, producing a colored precipitate within the cells. A positive reaction occurs in most normal and abnormal leukocytes. Monocytes stain more strongly than do neutrophils and immature granulocytes. The stain is helpful in distinguishing between the T-cell acute lymphocytic leukemias and the other acute lymphoblastic leukemias (Gralnick et al., 1977). Acid phosphatase granules are concentrated in the Golgi region of the T cell, whereas they are more dispersed in other lymphocytes, nucleated red cells, and platelets.

The principal use of the acid phosphatase reaction is in the identification of hairy cells in leukemic reticuloendotheliosis. Most cases of this disorder demonstrate the presence of tartrate-resistant acid phosphatase, although this is not a uniform finding (Katayama and Yang, 1977).

Glycogen (Periodic Acid–Schiff Reaction).

Glycogen is stained by the PAS reaction. Periodic acid splits the carbon bonds of glycogen at the CHOH–CHOH groups to produce aldehydes that react with Schiff reagent to form a magenta product. The reaction is inhibited by amylase. Neutrophils and developing granulocytes at all stages of maturation react with this procedure, the more mature neutrophils reacting most strongly. Earlier cells in the same series show decreasing glycogen content but still stain weakly by the PAS reaction. Lymphocytes and monocytes also are weakly reactive.

Normal red-cell precursors usually are glycogen-negative. In disease states, the stain result often is positive in cells that usually are glycogen-negative. For example, lymphocytes in acute lymphoblastic leukemia, lymphosarcoma, and Hodgkin's disease sometimes stain PAS-positive. Nucleated red cells also occasionally are positive in type M6 leukemia (the Di Guglielmo syndrome) and in thalassemia, as well as in iron-deficiency anemia.

A schematic classification in which the acute leukemias are differentiated using cytochemical stains appears in Table 13.6.

Terminal Deoxynucleotidyl Transferase.

The present FAB classification of acute leukemia distinguishes between cells of myeloid and lymphoid lineage on the basis of cytochemical staining. More recently, the demonstration of terminal deoxynucleotidyl transferase (TdT) has become a diagnostic criterion of lymphoid differentiation. A small percentage of pre–B cells and up to 95% of thymocytes contain the enzyme, in contrast to the lack of TdT in peripheral blood T cells and mature B cells. Expression of TdT activity is seen in most patients with acute lymphoblastic leukemia and lymphoblastic lymphoma and in 20–30% of patients in the blastic phase of chronic myelogenous leukemia (Cuttner et al., 1984). TdT has also been described in cells of individuals with acute myelogenous leukemia (types M4 and M5) (Bertazonni et al., 1982). It is not found in cells of patients with chronic lymphocytic leukemia. Some investigators now believe that TdT activity may signify merely that a cell is at an early maturation stage and probably has limited value in identifying the cell as a member of a particular lineage (Cuttner et al., 1984). It has also been previously reported that blasts simultaneously contain myeloperoxidase and TdT in 29% of patients with acute myeloblastic leukemia and 3% of patients with acute lymphocytic leukemia (Kaplan et al., 1987). TdT first was detected using an enzyme method based on the incorporation of radiolabeled deoxynucleotide monomer into a polynucleotide chain. This procedure has been replaced by immunofluorescent techniques and the use of monoclonal antibodies (Stass et al., 1979; Lanham et al., 1985, 1986). The newer procedure appears to offer several practical and theoretical advantages: Conventional light microscopy can be used; the technique has improved sensitivity over the previous method, allowing long

Table 13.6. Cytochemical Reactions Found in the Acute Leukemias

Leukemia	Peroxidase and Sudan Black B	Chloroacetate Esterase (Specific Esterase)	α-Naphthol Esterase (Nonspecific Esterase)	PAS	Acid Phosphatase	TdT
M1	2+	2+	–	1+	1+	–
M2	2+	2+	–	1+a	1+	–
M3	4+	4+	–	1+	1+	–
M4	2+	1+	3+c	1+b	1+a	–d
M5	1+	e	4+c	1+b	1+a	–d
M6	f	3+	–	4+h	g	–
L1	–	–	3+i	j	k	3+
L2	–	–	3+i	j	k	3+
L3	–	–	–	–	–	3+

PAS = periodic acid–Schiff; TdT = terminal deoxynucleotidyl transferase; – = negative; 1+ = weakly positive; 2+ = moderately positive; 3+ = positive; 4+ = strongly positive.

aDiffuse staining.

bDiffuse or granular.

cFluoride sensitive.

dRare positive.

eGranulocytes positive, monocytes negative.

fIn granulocytes.

gGranulocytes negative to weakly positive (diffuse), erythrocytes strongly positive.

hDiffuse to coarse in early red cells.

iFocal in some cells.

jVariable, negative to positive.

kVariable, negative to positive T-cell acute lymphocytic leukemia.

storage life for smears; and it does not involve auto-fluorescence or quenching.

Adenosine Deaminase. Adenosine deaminase (ADA) is involved in the purine pathway, which catalyzes the conversion of adenosine to inosine and deoxyadenosine to deoxyinosine. It is present in most human tissues, particularly those in which lymphocytes predominate. The enzyme activity is highest in immature T cells and is lowest in B cells. Lymphoblasts demonstrate significantly higher ADA activity than do normal lymphocytes (Smyth et al., 1978). The highest levels are present in T-cell acute lymphocytic leukemia; intermediate levels are seen in null-cell leukemia; and low ADA levels are associated with B-cell disorders, such as acute lymphocytic leukemia, Burkitt's lymphoma, and chronic lymphocytic leukemia (Coleman et al., 1978). ADA has also been reported in acute myelogenous leukemia, although the enzyme level is lower than that seen in acute lymphocytic leukemia (Meier et al., 1976). Owing to the substantial overlapping of results, the diagnostic value of the enzyme is believed to be limited (Hoffbrand and Janossy, 1981). Increased plasma ADA in leukemic patients is thought to reflect an increment of leukemic cells in the bone marrow. It is believed that several determinations of the plasma enzyme may provide a good indicator of the total mass of neoplastic cells present (Morisaki et al., 1985). Decreased ADA (and 5'-nucleotidase) activity has been reported in peripheral blood T cells in Hodgkin's disease (Murray et al., 1986).

Cell Membrane Markers in Acute Lymphoblastic Leukemia

Acute lymphoblastic leukemia can be subdivided into six groups, depending on the blastic reactions to various lymphocytic cell markers. A discussion of each of these groups follows, and classification of the acute lymphoblastic leukemias according to the following criteria is shown in Table 13.7.

E Rosettes. The formation of E rosettes by lymphocytes is the sign most commonly used to identify T lymphocytes. Leukemic cell suspensions are incubated with unsensitized sheep cells. In T-cell leukemia, the sheep cells attach to the surface of the blasts, forming rosettes that can be counted manually. The E rosettes so formed possess the unusual property of remaining stable at 37°C, whereas those formed by normal human peripheral blood T cells undergo dissociation at this temperature.

Surface Immunoglobulins. Surface immunoglobulins (SIgs) are reliable cell surface markers of B-cell lineage. Leukemic cell suspensions react with monospecific fluorescent antisera to the various heavy and light chains of human immunoglobulins. Under the usual test conditions, SIgs appear as distinct, bright, fluorescent dots on the cell membrane. Such surface proteins are found principally on type L3 cells and usually are IgM-κ, thus distinguishing this as a B-cell acute lymphocytic leukemia. Type L3 cells usually do not contain IgD, which frequently is associated with IgM on the cell surface in other B-cell malignancies (Brouet and Seligmann, 1978).

Cytoplasmic Immunoglobulins. Cytoplasmic immunoglobulins can be demonstrated in pre–B-cell acute lymphoblastic leukemia by immunofluorescent methods. The IgM detected can be demonstrated in alcohol-fixed smears with fluorescein-conjugated nonspecific antisera. The resulting fluorescence is very faint. Immunoelectron-microscopic studies have shown that the μ chains are located at the level of free polyribosomes rather than inside endoplasmic reticulum (Preud'homme et al., 1978). Pre–B-cell leukemias are of either the L1 or L2 type.

Immune-Associated Antibodies (Anti-Ia). Ia antigens are glycoproteins that are associated with the HLA-DR locus, and they are reliable markers of early differentiation in granulocytic and erythroid blastic cells and in normal and leukemic B cells. Lack of the antigen is used as a marker of T-cell acute lymphoblastic leukemia.

Acute Lymphoblastic Leukemia Antibodies (Anti-ALL). Anti-ALL reacts with a single glycosylated polypeptide present on the blasts of acute lymphoblastic leukemia of children (common acute lymphocytic leukemia antigen) and shows no reaction with T-cell acute lymphoblastic leukemia, B-cell acute lymphoblastic leukemia, and a proportion of non–T-cell, non–B-cell acute lymphoblastic leukemias known as *null-cell acute lymphoblastic leukemia.*

The antibody is prepared by immunizing rabbits with non–T-cell, non–B-cell acute lymphoblastic

Table 13.7. Classification of Acute Lymphoblastic Leukemia Using Cell Surface Markers and TdT

Leukemia Subtypes	E Rosettes	Surface Immunoglobulins	Cytoplasmic Immunoglobulins	Ia-Like Antigen	Common Acute Lymphocytic Leukemia Antigen	HuThy Antigen	TdT
T cell	+	–	–	–	–	+	+
Common cell	–	–	–	+	+	–	+
Null cell	–	–	–	+	–	–	+
B cell	–	+	–	+	–	–	–
Pre–B cell	–	–	+	+	–	–	+/–

TdT = terminal deoxynucleotidyl transferase; Ia = immune-associated; HuThy = human thymus antigen; + = positive; +/– = weakly positive; – = negative.

Source: Data from FR Davey, DA Nelson. Leukocyte Disorders. In JB Henry (ed), Clinical Diagnosis and Management by Laboratory Methods (17th ed). Philadelphia: Saunders, 1984.

leukemia blasts coated with rabbit antilymphocyte serum, which then is absorbed with normal red cells, leukocytes, and acute myeloid leukemia blast cells.

Anti–Human T-Lymphocyte Antibody (Anti-HuTLA). Anti-HuTLA reacts with some T lymphoblasts that fail to form E rosettes (see earlier section). It is prepared by injecting human thymocytes or T-lymphoid cell lines into rabbits.

Other Cellular Reactions

Leukocyte Alkaline Phosphatase. Leukocyte alkaline phosphatase is detected by hydrolyzing the substrate α-naphthol phosphate, thus liberating free naphthol. This process unites with a diazotized amine such as fast blue or fast violet at an alkaline pH to produce an insoluble colored precipitate. The enzyme is found to be increased in infections, polycythemia, Hodgkin's disease, and myelofibrosis. Decreased enzymatic activity is present in chronic and acute myeloid leukemia, paroxysmal nocturnal hemoglobinuria, aplastic anemia, and some acute viral infections, such as infectious mononucleosis.

Lysozyme (Muramidase). Lysozyme usually is associated with phagocytic cells, the serum level being increased in types M4 and M5 leukemia and in some cases of type M2 leukemia. Demonstration of cellular lysozyme by immunoperoxidase techniques shows activity in mature granulocytes and monocytic cells. The enzyme is detected later in cell maturation than is either nonspecific esterase or acid phosphatase activity. Cellular lysozyme is not helpful in classifying the acute leukemias, although the serum levels are used in monitoring progress of the disease.

Serum lysozyme can be considered a rough test of granulocytic turnover, although its level is increased also in a variety of other disorders, including tuberculosis, sarcoidosis, megaloblastic anemia, and azotemia. There is poor correlation with the total leukocyte count or with preleukemic conditions.

Chromosomal Abnormalities in Acute Leukemia

Since the advent of banding techniques (Rowley, 1973), approximately 60% of cases of acute myelogenous leukemia and a somewhat smaller per-

centage of cases of acute lymphoblastic leukemia have been shown to have nonrandom chromosomal abnormalities. The most common abnormal karyotypes in acute myelogenous leukemia, in order of frequency, are trisomy 8, monosomy 7, t(8q–;21q+), t(15q+;17q–), and 22q– (First International Workshop on Chromosomes in Leukemia, 1981). The cytogenetic notations used to describe this rearrangement are q, which refers to the long arm of the chromosome below the centromere, and p, which refers to the short arm of the chromosome above the centromere. Thus, t(8q–;21q+) refers to the transfer of a small portion of chromosome 8 to the bottom of chromosome 21.

Of interest is the apparent specificity of t(15q+;17q–) for type M3 leukemia. The occurrence of 22q, usually with the translocation t(9q+;22q–), the Ph[1] chromosome, is believed to be an example of chronic myelogenous leukemia presenting in a blastic crisis. It has been suggested that all acute myelogenous leukemic cells may possess a chromosomal defect (Yunis et al., 1981).

The Ph[1] chromosome is found in more than 90% of all cases of chronic myelogenous leukemia. Of these so-called Ph[1]-positive individuals, 90% have the classic 9/22 translocation; the other 10% have a variant form of the abnormality that includes translocation involving the short arm of chromosome 19 (Caimo et al., 1984). The consistent finding in such situations is a shortened chromosome 22 (22q–). The defect is believed to be in the pluripotential stem cell, because the Ph[1] chromosome can be demonstrated in the other cell lines of the bone marrow but is not seen in other tissues such as skin fibroblasts.

Besides this association and that involving types M2 and M3 leukemia, chromosomal aberrations have been identified in type M5 (acute monocytic) leukemia and in type M4 (acute myelomonocytic) leukemia, in which the terminal deletion of the long arm of chromosome 11 has been reported.

The frequency of abnormal karyotypes seen in acute lymphoblastic leukemia approximates 50%. The most common abnormality is the presence of the Ph[1] chromosome identical to that of chronic myelogenous leukemia in approximately 25% of all adult acute lymphoblastic leukemias (type L2) with the 9/22 translocation. These cases, however, actually may represent chronic myelogenous leukemia presenting as acute lymphoblastic leukemia. Other nonrandom abnormalities are trisomy 8, 13, 14, 21, and 6q–, and the translocation t(8q–;14q+), which appears to be a marker for type L3 leukemia and other B-cell proliferative disorders (Hall and Malia, 1984). The t(4;11) and t(9+;20q–) translocations have also been reported (Bjerrum et al., 1985; Di Donato et al., 1986).

T-cell acute lymphocytic leukemia has been reported with the t(11;14) translocation (Barrow, 1989) and the t(5;14) translocation (Baumgarten et al., 1989; Grimaldi and Meeker, 1989). In addition, there have been reports of 18 cases in which chromosome 16 was abnormal. Of these, 13 were type M4 leukemia, 3 type M5, and 2 type M2 leukemia (Bernard et al, 1989).

Chronic Leukemia

Chronic Myeloid Leukemia

Clinical and Laboratory Findings

Chronic myeloid leukemia is a clonal stem-cell disorder of unknown etiology that is associated with a unique acquired chromosomal abnormality in more than 90% of cases. Chronic myeloid leukemia may develop after an individual is exposed to radiation. Other environmental factors have not been implicated (Champlin and Golde, 1985). The major clinical manifestations relate to the unrestricted production of granulocytes in the bone marrow and elsewhere in the reticuloendothelial system. Clinical onset generally is insidious. The usual symptoms are malaise, night sweats, and weight loss. Fever, bone pain, and hemorrhage may also be present, depending on the degree of thrombocytopenia. Anemia and hepatosplenomegaly also may be seen. The disease rarely is diagnosed in persons younger than 20 years and is more common after the age of 30.

The clinical course of the leukemia is frequently divided into three phases. The first is one of asymptomatic granulocytic proliferation. The second is characterized by a persistently elevated leukocyte count. In the third, cellular proliferation is accelerated. During the chronic phase of the disease, myeloid cells mature normally. Extramedullary involvement is uncommon, with the malignant cells generally remaining restricted to hematopoietic tissues, the bone marrow, the spleen, and cords of the liver. The chronic phase of chronic myeloid leukemia is unstable and, at some point, the disease undergoes transformation to a more aggressive form. This may be clinically apparent by an acute or blastic crisis or by a progression of symptoms and resistance to chemotherapy (Karanas and Silver, 1968).

The blastic crisis is characterized by a maturation arrest at the blast or progranulocyte level (Golde et al., 1974). The crisis can be divided into two general forms—lymphoid and myeloid. Lymphoid blastic crises develop in approximately 25% of patients, the cells being phenotypically similar to those seen in the common form of acute lymphocytic leukemia. The cells generally contain TdT and express Ia antigens and common acute lymphocytic leukemia antigen (CALLA) (Catovsky et al., 1978; Marks et al., 1978a). They typically possess immunoglobulin characteristics of pre-B cells.

A myeloid blastic crisis is heterogeneous, the cells appearing morphologically similar to myeloblasts, usually expressing both myeloid antigens and cytoplasmic enzymes (Champlin and Golde, 1985). Chronic myeloid leukemia has also been associated with pure red-cell aplasia, terminating in promyelocytic transformation (Mijovic et al., 1989).

Notable among the laboratory findings is an extreme leukocytosis, with counts as high as 750×10^9/liter. The differential count is characterized by increases in segmented neutrophils, bands, metamyelocytes, and myelocytes. The predominant cell is the neutrophil, but small numbers of promyelocytes are seen occasionally in the peripheral blood. Eosinophils and basophils also are increased, the absolute basophil level being proportional to the total leukocyte count.

A chronic normocytic normochromic anemia may be present. The peripheral blood picture shows varying degrees of anisocytosis, poikilocytosis, polychromasia, basophilic stippling, and reticulocytosis, and the presence of nucleated red cells. Macrocytosis is present in some cases. Platelets are increased in the early stages of the disease, but a thrombocytopenia develops as the leukemia becomes established.

The bone marrow is hypercellular and demonstrates increased myeloid cells at most stages of development, particularly myelocytes. A chromosomal abnormality is seen in approximately 90% of cases and is characterized by the deletion of the long arm of a G22 chromosome to chromosome 9 [t(9q+;22−)], the Ph^1 chromosome (Prieto et al., 1970). A double Ph^1 chromosome, trisomy 8, and an isochromosome 17 are the most common additional abnormalities observed (First International Workshop on Chromosomes in Leukemia, 1978).

These chromosomal abnormalities can be found in red-cell precursors and megakaryocytes but not in lymphoid cells (see comments concerning type L2 leukemia on page 149). Fewer than 10% of all cases appear to be Ph^1-negative, but these usually are associated with a poorer prognosis. Such cases tend to be clinically atypical because of earlier blast cell transformation.

Platelet function is usually abnormal. Aggregation studies demonstrate lack of second-wave adrenalin-induced aggregation as well as impaired collagen platelet aggregation. This is believed to be due to a storage pool deficiency. Platelet aggregation studies also show abnormal thrombin-induced reactions due to a membrane defect involving thrombin receptors (Ganguly et al., 1978).

As a result of the catabolism of large numbers of granulocytes, increased production of uric acid with hyperuricosuria and sometimes hyperuricemia occurs in the untreated disease. Other laboratory findings include a marked reduction of leukocyte alkaline phosphatase levels and increased levels of serum vitamin B_{12}, which is elevated proportionally to the degree of leukocytosis.

Chromosomal Abnormalities in Chronic and Other Neoplasms.

Translocations in chronic myeloid leukemia have been reported at t(9;22), in B-cell lymphoma at t(14;18), and in Burkitt's lymphoma at t(8;22) and t(8;2) (Barrow, 1989).

Morphologic Variants

Eosinophilic Leukemia. *Eosinophilic leukemia* is an extremely rare variant of granulocytic leukemia; both acute and chronic forms have been reported (Zucker-Franklin, 1974). The disease is difficult to distinguish from other hypereosinophilic disorders, but it shows both a marked absolute and a relative eosinophilia, with immature eosinophils in the blood and the bone marrow. The cytochemical picture is characterized by increased glycogen-positive, acid phosphatase, and naphthol-AS-D-chloroacetate esterase reactions. Other findings are a normochromic anemia and thrombocytopenia. Ph^1-negative chronic myeloid leukemia is characterized by a hypercellular marrow with granulocytic hyperplasia, a peripheral granulocytic leukocytosis with left-shift maturation, and a leukocyte count of more than 20×10^3/ml. The morphologic picture is similar to that of Ph^1-positive chronic myeloid leukemia. The FAB classification defines chronic myelomonocytic leukemia as a subtype of myelodysplastic syndrome, in which the absolute number of monocytes in the peripheral blood exceeds 1,000/ml. This form of leukemia is a hybrid disease that shows features of both proliferation and dysplasia (Katarjiam and Kurzrock, 1990). Most neoplastic hypereosinophilias remain controversial and are categorized as chronic myeloid leukemias with eosinophilic components (Chen and Marsh, 1984).

Basophilic Leukemia. *Basophilic leukemia* presents a clinical picture similar to that of chronic myeloid leukemia. The predominant cell is the mature basophil but, in some cases, both eosinophilic and basophilic granules may be present in the same cell. The Ph^1 chromosome may be present or absent and cannot be used as a diagnostic marker. The acute form of the disease, mast cell leukemia, is characterized by the presence of many mast cells (tissue basophils) possessing strong staining reactions for glycogen and naphthol-AS-D-chloroacetate (Parker, 1976).

Chronic Lymphocytic Leukemia

Clinical and Laboratory Findings

Chronic lymphocytic leukemia is the most common leukemia seen in the Western world. It is characterized by a gradual accumulation of well-differentiated lymphocytes in the bone marrow, lymph nodes, reticuloendothelial system, and peripheral blood. Eventually, involvement of other organs and systems, such as skin, lung, liver, and gastrointestinal tract, is found. In the majority of cases, the lymphocytes are abnormal, immunologically inert B cells, although T-cell variants have been described (Marks et al., 1978b). Based on cytology and membrane phenotype, a number of disorders have been defined (Bennett et al., 1989).

Table 13.8. Types of Leukemic B Lymphoid Cells

Cell Type	Size	Chromatin	Nucleolus	Cytoplasm	Other
Small lymphocyte (CLL)	< ×2 RBC	Clumped in coarse blocks	Absent	Scanty; high N/C ratio	Regular nuclear outline
Large lymphocyte (CLL mixed type)	> ×2 RBC	Clumped	May not be seen	Low N/C ratio	Variable size
Prolymphocytic (PLL)	> ×2 RBC	Clumped	One prominent	Low N/C ratio	Variable size
Pleomorphic prolymphocytes	> ×2 RBC	Clumped	Central and prominent	Variable N/C ratio	Variable size
Cleft cells	1–2× RBC	Homogeneous, coarse	Usually absent	Scanty, not visible or narrow rim	One to two shallow or deep clefts

CLL = chronic lymphocytic leukemia; RBC = red blood cell; N/C = nucleus-to-cytoplasm; PLL = prolymphocytic leukemia.

The B-cell disorders include chronic lymphocytic leukemia; chronic lymphocytic leukemia of the mixed type (in which there are more than 10% and fewer than 55% prolymphocytes); prolymphocytic leukemia; hairy-cell leukemia; splenic lymphoma with circulating villous lymphocytes; the leukemic phase of NHLs; lymphoplasmacytic lymphoma with peripheral blood disease; and plasma cell leukemia. T-cell type disorders include T-cell chronic lymphocytic leukemia, which has been differentiated from reactive T-lymphocytosis; T-cell prolymphocytic leukemia; adult T-cell leukemia or lymphoma; and Sézary syndrome (Table 13.8).

Ionizing radiation has not been implicated in chronic lymphocytic leukemia, unlike in chronic myeloid leukemia, and no definite etiologic factors have yet been identified. The occurrence of this form of leukemia is uncommon in individuals younger than 40 years, although B-cell chronic lymphocytic leukemia has been reported in younger patients (Spier et al., 1985).

Clinically, the presenting features are highly variable. In approximately 25% of cases, the individuals appear asymptomatic, but lymphadenopathy, thrombocytopenia, skin infiltration, bone pain, and splenomegaly may be seen. The most striking features in the typical form are lymphadenopathy and hepatosplenomegaly. Fever and bacterial infections are not uncommon, and fungal infections may occur.

The laboratory findings are clear-cut. A moderate to marked leukocytosis, with both an absolute and relative lymphocytosis, is nearly always present. Total leukocyte counts greater than 100 × 10^9/liter are not unusual. Morphologically, the lymphocytes appear identical to the small lymphocytes in normal blood, but variable numbers of cells that appear to be abnormal may be present. Rarely, large cytoplasmic inclusions are observed. A mild to moderate normocytic normochromic anemia is present. The direct antiglobulin test gives positive results in up to 33% of cases, and a mild thrombocytopenia may also be seen. In approximately 5% of patients, there is a monoclonal paraprotein present, and depressed serum globulin levels are commonly seen. The presence of a monoclonal paraprotein is believed to result from maturation failure in immunoglobulin-producing cells (Kay et al., 1979). β_2-microglobulin levels are also elevated in the disorder (DiGiovanni et al., 1989).

Bone marrow examination reveals infiltration by small, morphologically well-differentiated lymphocytes. Most cases of chronic lymphocytic leukemia are disorders of B-cell lymphocytes, on the surfaces of which are found monoclonal immunoglobulins that frequently display both heavy- and light-chain specificities (Pressens et al., 1973). Other B-lymphocyte membrane characteristics include a receptor for C3 and one for aggregated immunoglobulin (Liepman, 1980). These B-cell findings are commonly found; however, T-cell chronic lymphocytic leukemia has been described in which the proliferating cells form E rosettes and undergo lysis when introduced to anti-T antisera (Marks et al., 1978b). Clinically, the disease is characterized by massive splenomegaly without lymphadenopathy and by prominent neutropenia and skin involvement.

Cytochemistry

Unlike the cells of acute lymphoblastic leukemias, the cells of T- and B-cell chronic lymphocytic leukemia are TdT negative (Dunn and Mauer, 1982). Cytochemical methods of differentiation are not helpful.

Cell Markers

Most cases of chronic lymphocytic leukemia are disorders of B lymphocytes with monoclonal SIgs. The proteins most often detected are membrane-bound and of one heavy-chain class and a single light-chain class, usually IgM. Other B-lymphocyte membrane characteristics include a receptor for C3 and one for aggregated immunoglobulin (Table 13.9).

T-cell (CD 2) and B-cell (CD 20) detection has proven useful in the clinical evaluation of immunodeficiency diseases and autoimmune and lymphoproliferative disorders.

Clinical interpretation of lymphocyte T-cell subsets must be made with caution. Relative and absolute values may be abnormal in a wide variety of infectious, inflammatory, autoimmune, and neoplastic disorders. Profound alterations may be seen because of immunosuppressive therapy. A marked decreased ratio of helper-inducer T-cells (CD 4) to suppressor-cytotoxic T-cells (CD 8) resulting primarily from absolute depletion of the T-helper-inducer subset may be seen in AIDS. Markers seen in chronic T-cell leukemia are shown in Table 13.10; those seen in acute and chronic myeloid leukemia are shown in Table 13.11.

Other Hematologic Disorders

Preleukemia

The clinical definition of preleukemia encompasses hematologic syndromes of different severity and outcome linked by a common risk of ending in overt leukemia. *Preleukemia*, then, is a term applied to a disorder in retrospect, after the diagnosis of acute leukemia has been made.

Five principal etiologic groups can be distinguished, as follows: (1) individuals with well-defined hematologic disorders associated with a higher incidence of leukemia, including poly-cythemia vera, idiopathic myelofibrosis, and paroxysmal nocturnal hemoglobinuria; (2) patients with nonhematologic disorders who possess chromosomal abnormalities (the principal example is Down's syndrome); (3) patients having nonhematologic disorders that are not known to develop into leukemia unless they are treated with cytotoxic drugs (examples include carcinoma of the breast or ovary and potential renal transplant patients on immunosuppressive therapy); (4) individuals exposed to known leukemic agents such as benzene or x-rays; and (5) those individuals who have one of several miscellaneous disorders including idiopathic acquired sideroblastic anemia and chronic erythroid myelosis.

Myelodysplastic Syndromes

The myelodysplastic syndromes represent a group of disorders associated with abnormal cell division, maturation, and production. They are characterized by both qualitative and quantitative defects of hematopoietic stem cells, which result in ineffective erythropoiesis. Myelodysplastic syndromes usually are found in individuals older than 50 and are associated with a high risk of progression to acute myeloid leukemia. The classification of myelodysplastic syndromes is shown in Table 13.12. The syndromes exhibit a wide range of morphologic findings in both blood and bone marrow. A normocytic anemia often is seen but, on occasion, a macrocytic picture may be found. There is frequently poor reticulocyte response compared to the degree of anemia, and nucleated red cells often are present. Thrombocytopenia may occur, and giant platelets might be seen. Dysgranulopoiesis is manifested by any of the following: neutropenia, monocytosis, hyposegmentation of granulocytes, reduced myeloperoxidase and alkaline phosphatase activity, and the presence of immature and blast cells.

Erythrocytic autoantibodies are found, usually of the warm-reacting, IgG form, although increased IgM and IgA antibodies have also been observed (Sokol et al., 1989). The bone marrow usually is hypercellular, despite the peripheral blood cytopenia. Megaloblasts, ringed sideroblasts, nuclear fragments, and multinuclearity are features of the erythropoietic picture.

Table 13.9. Markers in Chronic B-Cell Leukemia

Marker	CLL	PLL	Hairy Cell	NHL Follicular	NHL Intermediate	SLVC	Plasma Cell Tumor
SmIg	Weak	4+	4+	4+	3+	4+	–
CIg	–	–/+	–/+	–	–	–/+	2+
M rosettes	2+	–	–/+	–/+	–/+	–	–
CD 5	2+	–/+	–	–	–/+	–	–
CD 19, CD 20, CD 24	2+	2+	2+	2+	2+	2+	–
Anti–class II	2+	2+	2+	2+	2+	2+	–
FMC7/CD 22	–/+	2+	2+	+	+	2+	–
CD 10	–	–/+	–	+	–/+	–	–/+
CD 25	–	–	2+	–	–	–/+	–
CD 38	–	–	–/+	–/+	–	–/+	2+

CLL = chronic lymphocytic leukemia; PLL = prolymphocytic leukemia; NHL = non-Hodgkin's lymphoma; SLVC = splenic lymphoma, villous lymphocytes, hairy-cell variant; – = negative; + = weakly positive; 2+ = positive; 4+ = strongly positive; –/+ = weakly positive or negative.

Source: Reprinted from JM Bennett, et al. Proposals for the classification of chronic (mature) B & T lymphoid leukemia. J Clin Pathol 42:567, 1989.

Table 13.10. Markers in Chronic (Mature) T-Cell Leukemia

Marker	T-CLL	T-PLL	ATLL	Sézary's Syndrome
TdT	–	–	–	–
CD 1a	–	–	–	–
E rosettes	2+	2+	2+	2+
CD 2	2+	2+	2+	2+
CD 3	2+	+	2+	2+
CD 4	–	+	2+	2+
CD 5	–	2+	2+	2+
CD 7	–	2+	–	–
CD 8	2+	+/–	–	–
CD 25	–	–	2+	–
CD 38	–	–	–	–

T-CLL = T-cell lymphocytic leukemia; T-PLL = T-cell prolymphocytic leukemia; ATLL = acute T-cell lymphocytic leukemia; TdT = terminal deoxynucleotidyl transferase; – = negative; + = weakly positive; 2+ = positive; +/– = weakly positive or negative.

Table 13.11. Markers in Acute and Chronic Myeloid Leukemia

Marker	Acute Myeloid	Chronic Myeloid in Blastic Crisis
CD 2	–	–
CD 5	–	–
CD 10	–	–
CD 13	+/–	+/–
CD 19	–	–
CD 33	+/–	+/–

– = negative; +/– = weakly positive or negative.

Table 13.12. Myelodysplastic Syndromes

FAB Term	Other Terms
Refractory anemia (RA)	Chronic erythremic myelosis, refractory megaloblastic anemia
RA with ring sideroblasts	Acquired idiopathic sideroblastic anemia
RA with excess blasts (RAEB)	Smoldering leukemia, subacute leukemia, oligoblastic leukemia
RAEB in transformation	Acute myeloproliferative syndrome, primary acquired panmyelopathy with myeloblastosis
Chronic myelomonocytic leukemia	Subacute melomonocytic leukemia

FAB = French-American-British.

Myeloproliferative Disorders

Myelofibrosis with Myeloid Metaplasia

Idiopathic myelofibrosis is a chronic, progressive clonal disorder characterized by anemia, splenomegaly, extramedullary hematopoiesis, and leukoerythroblastosis. The disease usually occurs in middle age and follows a chronic course. A minority of cases terminate as acute myelogenous leukemia.

The peripheral blood findings are of a normocytic normochromic anemia with marked poikilocytosis and prominent teardrop-shaped cells. Nucleated red cells often are present. The total leukocyte count is variable but, frequently, granulocytic precursors as immature as myeloblasts are seen. The number of basophils often is elevated. A mild thrombocytopenia with giant granulated platelets is found, together with poor platelet function and elevated α-granule secretion. The recognition of acute megakaryocytic leukemia (M7) requires immunologic studies to demonstrate the presence of one or more antigens, such as factor VIII–related antigen, platelet glycoproteins Ib or IIb/IIIa, or Plt 1. One description of

M7 leukemia makes an association with large vacuolated platelets (McClennan and Maddox, 1989).

The bone marrow is difficult to aspirate, and so a biopsy often is the main diagnostic approach. Histologic staining of the bone marrow sections reveals reticulum fibers and patchy fibrosis. The leukocyte alkaline phosphatase stain is variably reactive and is not helpful, but lack of the Ph[1] chromosome is useful in distinguishing this disorder from chronic myelogenous leukemia.

Chloroma

Chloroma is a variant of acute myelogenous leukemia, this disease being characterized by green tumor masses in the bones and soft tissues. The green hue is caused by an elevated level of myeloperoxidase. The disease occurs most often in children and young adults. Its morphologic appearance is similar to that of acute leukemia.

Megakaryocytic Leukemia

Megakaryocytic leukemia is a rare form of acute myeloid leukemia that produces increased megakaryocytes and megakaryoblasts in the bone marrow. The disease is found principally in middle to late life, and clinically it demonstrates a pancytopenia without the presence of hepatosplenomegaly or lymphadenopathy. The bone marrow is hypercellular, with immature cells predominating, particularly megakaryocytes and megakaryoblasts. The megakaryoblasts that are seen possess a large nuclear mass, multiple nucleoli, and multilobed nuclei. These cells stain positively for glycogen and peroxidase and also test positively for α-naphthol esterase activity, which is inhibited in part by sodium fluoride. Megakaryoblasts are negative for α-naphthol butyrate esterase. Blast cells also show surface staining for the IIb/IIIa platelet-specific glycoprotein, suggesting that megakaryocytes may be related to myelonormoblasts.

Polycythemia (Erythrocytosis)

Polycythemia encompasses a number of disorders characterized by increased circulating red cells.

Polycythemia can be classified into several etiologic groups, as shown in Table 13.13. Of those listed, polycythemia vera, secondary polycythemia, and idiopathic erythrocytosis can be classified as true erythremic disorders, having an increased total red-cell mass. Relative polycythemia describes an apparent increase in circulating cells while the absolute number of cells remains within normal limits. The apparent increase is due to a decrease in plasma volume.

Polycythemia Vera

Polycythemia vera, in conjunction with agnogenic myeloid metaplasia and primary thrombocythemia, is considered one of the myeloproliferative diseases characterized by proliferation of bone marrow stem cells. Polycythemia vera is a chronic disorder principally of erythroid hyperproduction. The increased numbers of red cells give rise to increased blood viscosity, impairment of blood flow, local stasis, capillary distortion, and tissue hypoxia. These clinical findings often lead to thrombosis and hemorrhage. The exact cause of the disease is unknown, although several possible mechanisms have been suggested, including the possibility of a neoplastic stem-cell proliferation, the presence of a myeloproliferative factor stimulating normal stem cells, and an increased sensitivity of stem cells to erythropoietin (Prchal and Axelrod, 1974).

Polycythemia vera is a relatively rare disorder found most frequently in middle-aged and elderly men. The patient usually presents with headaches, visual disturbances, weakness, mucous membrane bleeding, hepatosplenomegaly, thrombohemorrhagic complications, and a deep-red skin coloration. Ecchymoses are common, and a wide variety of skin lesions may also be present. The laboratory findings are distinctive. The peripheral blood picture reveals a raised red-cell count, sometimes as high as 15×10^{12}/liter, with a proportional increase in the hemoglobin and hematocrit values. The total leukocyte count also is increased, usually exceeding 12×10^9/liter but potentially being as high as 50×10^9/liter. The differential leukocyte count predominantly shows an increase in mature granulocytes, although occasional metamyelocytes and myelocytes may be seen.

The number of basophils is increased, which parallels an increase in blood histamine levels. The

Table 13.13. Classification of the Polycythemias

Disorder	Cause
Primary polycythemia vera	Myeloproliferative; increased erythropoietin production, decreased blood oxygen saturation (high-altitude), chronic lung disease, heart disease, high-oxygen-affinity hemoglobin, decreased red-cell 2,3-diphosphoglycerate levels
Secondary polycythemia	Inappropriate erythropoietin production, renal tumors, other kidney diseases
Relative polycythemia	Stress polycythemia, dehydration, plasma loss through burns, etc.

Table 13.14. Principal Bone Marrow Features of the Polycythemias

Characteristic	Polycythemia Vera	Secondary Polycythemia	Relative Polycythemia
Bone marrow cellularity	Markedly increased	Increased	Normal
Myeloid-to-erythroid ratio	Normal	Decreased	Normal
Erythroid elements	Increased	Increased	Normal
Granulocytic elements	Increased	Normal	Normal
Megakaryocytic elements	Markedly increased	Normal	Normal
Hemosiderin content	Decreased	Normal to increased	Normal

leukocyte alkaline phosphatase stain always shows an increase but does not correlate directly with the total leukocyte count. Other biochemical findings reflect the increase in granulocytic mass and include elevated levels of serum lysozyme, myeloperoxidase, and lactoferrin. Additional biochemical findings are increases in serum vitamin B_{12} and unsaturated vitamin B_{12}–binding capacity.

Platelets usually are more numerous, and giant forms are seen. The mean platelet size usually is only slightly larger than normal. Platelet α-granule secretion usually is elevated, and platelet in vivo function defects are present in nearly 60% of all cases (Wehmeier and Schnerder, 1989).

The red-cell morphologic appearance is often normocytic and normochromic but, on occasion, a microcytic hypochromic picture is found, probably caused by an iron deficiency secondary to chronic blood loss. Hemorrhage, when present, is frequently the result of platelet dysfunction. Bone marrow fibrosis and marked poikilocytosis, nucleated red cells, and a left shift can also be seen. In this regard, the peripheral blood picture resembles that seen in myelofibrosis. Erythropoietin levels are reduced.

The bone marrow is extremely hypercellular because of the myeloproliferation. There is a lack of fat spaces and increases in red-cell precursors, granulocytic elements, and megakaryocytes. Iron stores are reduced or absent.

The total blood volume is characteristically increased. By definition, the red-cell mass is 36 ml/kg or more in men and 32 ml/kg or more in women with polycythemia vera. Other diagnostic criteria include a normal arterial oxygen saturation and either splenomegaly or two of the following: thrombocytosis of more than 400×10^9/liter, leukocytosis of more than 12×10^9/liter, increased leukocyte alkaline phosphatase, and increased vitamin B_{12} or unsaturated vitamin B_{12}–binding capacity (Berlin, 1975). The Ph^1 chromosome is not present unless there is a rare transformation to chronic myelogenous leukemia.

Polycythemia vera has also been associated with two hemoglobinopathies, hemoglobin J Amiens (Elion et al., 1979), and hemoglobin Villejuif (Wajcman et al., 1989), both being β-chain variants.

Secondary Polycythemia

Secondary polycythemia, unlike polycythemia vera, demonstrates an increased level of erythropoietin either from tissue hypoxia or secondary to the effects of tumors or renal ischemia. Table 13.14 details some of the more common causes leading to this secondary state.

The clinical and laboratory features of the secondary polycythemias of hypoxia resulting from high altitude are principally cyanosis and physiologic emphysema, a normocytic erythrocytosis with an increase in the absolute reticulocyte count, and an increase in iron turnover. In addition, the red-cell mass is increased, but the cellular composition of the bone marrow is not changed significantly. The increased red-cell mass is reflected in increases in hemoglobin and hematocrit values. The leukocyte count, differential leukocyte count, and platelet count are consistently normal. Serum iron levels and iron-binding capacity are usually normal. Erythrocytosis due to pulmonary disease frequently is associated with cyanosis and decreased arterial oxygen saturation. The hematocrit usually is normal, principally because of the concomitant increase in plasma volume. The release of erythropoietin appears to parallel the degree of arterial hypoxia. Secondary polycythemia might also be caused by cardiovascular disease, defective oxygen transport, alveolar hypoventilation, tissue hypoxia, renal impairment and renal tumors, hepatomas, and endocrine disorders.

Congenital heart disease (right-to-left shunt) can cause a marked decrease in oxygen saturation, accompanied by severe cyanosis and a markedly elevated red-cell count. The hematocrit may reach 80%, and the total red-cell mass may exceed 100 ml/kg body weight. Plasma volume is not usually altered.

Secondary polycythemia associated with defective oxygen transport is rare. That due to acquired or congenital methemoglobinemia is caused by an associated leftward shift of the oxygen dissociation curve, but the cause of the disease in patients with methemoglobinemia resulting from the presence of hemoglobin M depends on the specific site of amino acid substitution.

A number of chemicals also are associated with tissue hypoxia and secondary polycythemia. The most common is cobalt, which is an essential component of vitamin B_{12} and reacts by releasing erythropoietin generated by a general tissue hypoxia.

Essential Primary Thrombocythemia

Essential primary thrombocythemia is a myeloproliferative disorder closely related to polycythemia vera. The principal differentiating features of thrombocythemia are the persistently elevated platelet count in the presence of a normal red-cell mass, no splenomegaly, and a megakaryocytic bone marrow hyperplasia. A neutrophilic leukocytosis and microcytic hypochromic anemia are usual peripheral blood findings. The leukocyte alkaline phosphatase level is normal, but there is a typical decrease in platelet aggregation in response to epinephrine and adenosine diphosphate but not to collagen. α-Granule secretion is elevated only moderately (Wehmeier and Schnerder, 1989). The disease must be distinguished from other causes of thrombocytosis, particularly myelofibrosis and polycythemia vera. Patients with myelofibrosis and myeloid metaplasia rarely have elevated hemoglobin levels and usually show characteristic red-cell abnormalities associated with bone marrow fibrosis and splenic hematopoiesis. Poikilocytosis is a common finding. Patients with polycythemia often have a much higher hemoglobin level than that found in thrombocythemia patients, even when there is no bleeding in the latter. Patients with essential thrombocytopenia are at increased risk for large-vessel and microvascular thrombosis. This is because of abnormal platelet numbers and function and because of the presence of decreased levels of protein S (Conlan and Haire, 1989). The Polycythemia Study Group diagnostic criteria for essential thrombocythemia include a platelet count in excess of 600×10^9/liter, a hemoglobin value of less than 13 g/dl or a normal red-cell mass, stainable bone marrow iron, no Ph[1] chromosome, and no bone marrow fibrosis (Murphy et al., 1986).

Nongranulocytic Disorders

Leukemic Reticuloendotheliosis (Hairy-Cell Leukemia)

Leukemic reticuloendotheliosis is a well-delineated entity characterized by splenomegaly associated with pancytopenia, infections, autoimmune disease, and the presence of neoplastic mononuclear cells in the blood and bone marrow. Although there is controversy regarding the cell line of origin of the disorder, most evidence suggests that the disease fits into the spectrum of B-lymphocyte malignancies (Golde et al., 1977).

The peripheral blood picture shows anemia, thrombocytopenia and, frequently, a leukopenia, although a leukocytosis may also be seen (Loukas, 1976). The majority of patients present with leukocyte counts of less than 50×10^9/liter. On the stained blood smear, hairy cells are seen that vary in size from 10 to 20 μ in diameter. There is a distinct nuclear membrane, and the nuclear configuration varies from oval to slightly indented.

The chromatin pattern is stippled. It is coarser than that seen in the lymphoblast but is less mature than that found in mature lymphocytes. One to three small nuclei may be seen in approximately half of the hairy cells, but they may be inconspicuous in the remaining cells. Most of these leukemic cells have a moderate rim of homogeneous or finely mottled, pale, blue-gray cytoplasm, which terminates in irregular, serrated edges with long cytoplasmic villi or pseudopodic extensions. These hairlike projections are seen more easily in phase microscopy than with the conventional light microscope.

The bone marrow is difficult to aspirate but, when obtained, shows increased reticulum fibers with or without myelofibrosis.

The cytochemical reaction of hairy cells shows strong acid phosphatase activity that is resistant to the addition of tartrate. Fluoride-resistant esterase activity with α-naphthol butyrate as the substrate is seen as finely scattered granules, and usually there is elevated neutrophil alkaline phosphatase activity. Glycogen staining (PAS reaction) is often strongly pronounced, with both diffuse and granular patterns seen in the hairy cells.

In a majority of cases, the cells are shown to possess B-cell characteristics by virtue of their ability to synthesize and produce immunoglobulin and to form red-cell rosettes and by the presence of Fc receptors and positive reactions with anti-Ia.

Acid phosphatase tartrate resistance has been described in other lymphoproliferative disorders as well, including lymphosarcoma cell leukemia, prolymphocytic leukemia, and the Sézary syndrome (Katayama and Yang, 1977). The test cannot be considered pathognomonic, as acid phosphatase is not always tartrate-resistant in hairy cells (Hayhoe and Quaglino, 1980). However, the differential diagnosis has been reported using a panel of monoclonal antibodies. Such antibodies include distinctive patterns that establish principal phenotypes distinguished by immunoenzymatic labeling of tissue sections or cell smears (Brunangelo et al., 1985).

Hodgkin's Disease

Hodgkin's disease is considered a malignant lymphoma of unknown cause. It is more common in men, particularly those older than 50 years. Children also are affected but not as commonly. The origin of the diagnostic Reed-Sternberg cells is in dispute, with different investigators presenting evidence that they are forms of T cells or B cells or macrophages. The cells are large, each possessing two or more nuclei that contain a round azurophilic nucleolus.

Clinically, most patients present with lymphadenopathy, principally affecting the cervical nodes. The diagnosis requires biopsy of the affected nodes. The hematologic findings in the peripheral blood are usually only supportive and not diagnostic of the disorder. For purposes of classification, this group of neoplasms is divided into four categories.

The first category, *lymphocyte predominance,* features the proliferation of lymphocytes with minimal fibrosis and few diagnostic Reed-Sternberg cells. This pattern is usually considered to have a good prognosis. The second pattern of *mixed cellularity* displays variable numbers of histiocytes, lymphocytes, eosinophils, and plasma cells. There is a moderate fibrosis, and Reed-Sternberg cells are plentiful. In the third type, *lymphocyte depletion,* the lymph nodes are replaced by an infiltration of connective tissue with few residual islands of normal lymphocytes. Reed-Sternberg cells are abundant and may be present in clusters. A fourth pattern, *nodular sclerosis,* is characterized by bands of fibrous tissue separating the lymphoid area. Large atypical histiocytes are seen, which retract during staining of the node to give the appearance of clear spaces.

The peripheral blood findings are often of a normochromic anemia with variable total leukocyte and differential leukocyte counts. A neutrophilic leukocytosis is present when lymph nodes are involved, and a neutropenia usually is seen if the bone marrow is hyperactive. During the active stage of the disease, the leukocyte alkaline phosphatase level is elevated, but it reverts to normal when the disease is in remission. The most commonly seen peripheral blood picture is a monocytosis accompanied by an eosinophilia. A positive direct anti–human globulin test denoting an autoimmune hemolytic component is found in approximately 5% of patients.

The bone marrow shows a granulocytic hyperplasia with a left shift and a mild monocytosis. Eosinophilia and Reed-Sternberg cells are present in approximately 10% of individuals and are most

Table 13.15. Rye Classification of Hodgkin's Disease

Classification	Description
Lymphocyte predominance	Mature lymphocytes with histiocytes; few Reed-Sternberg cells
Nodular sclerosis	Nodules of lymphoid tissue separated by thick bands of collagen; many Reed-Sternberg variants; necrosis likely
Lymphocyte depletion	Few lymphocytes present; numerous Reed-Sternberg cells; necrosis and fibrosis
Mixed cellularity	Variable numbers of lymphocytes together with reactive histiocytes, neutrophils, eosinophils, and plasma cells; Reed-Sternberg cells
Reed-Sternberg cells	Large binucleate or multinucleate cells having abundant cytoplasm and prominent nucleoli, surrounded by a clear perinuclear halo
Reed-Sternberg variants	Reed-Sternberg variants with similar nuclear features, though occasionally these cells may be smaller and may possess more lobulated nuclei

common in the mixed-cell disease type (see above) (Table 13.15).

Relatively little is known regarding the karyotype pattern of Hodgkin's disease. Hyperploidy is a characteristic feature and is observed in 70% of tumors that have an abnormal karyotype. A gain of chromosomes 1, 2, 5, 12, and 21 is a recurring numeric abnormality; structural rearrangements involving chromosome 1 are often observed (Thangaveln and Le Beau, 1989).

Non-Hodgkin's Lymphoma

The *NHLs* are a heterogeneous group of lymphoproliferative disorders characterized by a neoplastic proliferation of cells. The most common classification used (Rapport, 1966) divides this group of neoplasms into the divisions shown in Figure 13.2.

The laboratory findings are basically unremarkable and generally are not diagnostic. Leukocytosis is uncommon, but there may be a mild neutropenia and thrombocytopenia and occasional variant lymphocytes. Lymphocytes with monoclonal surface IgG are present in approximately 30–40% of cases. Autoantibodies against platelet glycoprotein IIb/IIIa can also be detected (Kubota et al., 1989).

The bone marrow shows lymphoid involvement, particularly in the diffuse lymphocytic well-differentiated forms. Definitive diagnosis is provided by the histologic architecture of lymph node biopsies.

Mycosis Fungoides (Sézary Syndrome)

The leukemic phase of mycosis fungoides (T-cell NHL) is known as *Sézary syndrome* and involves the skin as the primary site of the disease. Clinically, the disorder is characterized by dermatologic changes resembling eczema and a wide variety of dermatitides.

The peripheral blood picture is relatively normal, but occasionally atypical mononuclear cells showing a monocytoid-shaped nucleus are present. Cytochemically, the most characteristic reaction is the PAS stain for glycogen. This reaction is usually negated by diastase digestion but, although a majority of Sézary cells are stained by this technique, it is not a specific marker. Sézary cells are strongly positive for β-glucuronidase activity and for acid phosphatase, the latter reaction being inhibited by tartrate (Faramarz Naeim et al., 1979). A comparison of the cytochemical reactions of these cells and hairy cells to those of normal lymphocytes and monocytes is shown in Table 13.16. More recently, it has been possible to characterize the lymphoid cells in cutaneous infiltrates by the immunochemical staining of frozen sections with monoclonal antibodies (Ralfkiaer et al., 1985; Duncan and Winkelmann, 1978).

Paraproteinemias

Multiple Myeloma

Multiple myeloma is a neoplastic proliferation of plasma cells that occurs mainly in the bone marrow and occasionally in the lymph nodes and spleen. Clinically, the disease is most common in elderly individuals. Patients present with bone pain, anemia, uremia, and often infections, skeletal lesions, and cardiovascular complications. The

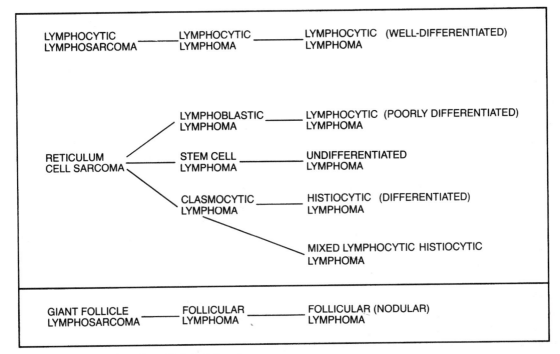

Figure 13.2. Classification of non-Hodgkin's lymphoma.

Table 13.16. Cytochemical Comparison of Sézary and Hairy Cells to Normal Mononuclear Cells

Reaction	Sézary Cells	Hairy Cells	Lymphocytes	Monocytes
Periodic acid–Schiff	Usually positive	Negative	Negative	Negative
β-Glucuronidase	Usually positive	Negative	Usually positive	Usually positive
Acid phosphatase	Usually positive	Positive, uninhibited by tartrate	Usually positive	Usually positive
Peroxidase	Negative	Negative	Negative	Usually positive
Alkaline phosphatase	Negative	Negative	Negative	Negative
Naphthol-AS-D-esterase	Negative	Positive	Negative	Positive

kidney involvement frequently is associated with renal tubular damage due to the precipitation of Bence-Jones protein. The infections found in the disease result from impaired antibody synthesis, reflecting decreases in serum immunoglobulins. Hemorrhage is sometimes present as a result of either a reduction of platelets or their impaired function, which is caused primarily by a coating of myeloma protein on their surface. This increase in abnormal plasma protein produces an increased blood viscosity that can culminate in circulatory impairment and heart failure.

The peripheral blood findings reveal a hypochromic anemia, although frequently the ane-mia is normocytic and normochromic. Rouleaux formation is a common finding, and the erythrocyte sedimentation rate is markedly elevated. Although the total leukocyte count varies, the differential count usually is normal. Plasma cells are not normally a feature of the peripheral blood picture but, if present, they reflect the advanced stage of the disease, in which tissue infiltrates are present. In such situations, the term *plasma cell leukemia* is used.

The bone marrow is hypercellular because of plasma cell infiltration at all stages of maturation. Plasmablasts and proplasmacytes usually are present, as are flame cells, Mott cells, and polyploid

Table 13.17. Protein Abnormalities in Multiple Myeloma

Serum M-Type Protein	Urine Bence-Jones Protein (Light Chains)	Incidence
IgG	κ, λ	52%
IgA	κ, λ	21%
IgD mixed	Variable	2%
None	κ, λ	25%

Source: Data from MJ Inwood, S Thompson. Disorders of Leukocytes and Plasma. In SJ Raphael (ed), Medical Laboratory Technology (4th ed). Philadelphia: Saunders, 1983.

plasma cells. The plasma cells seen in myeloma may be indistinguishable from normal plasma cells but, on occasion, they can be separated from normal cells by their more open nuclear chromatin, large nucleoli, lack of a perinuclear halo, and a less intensely staining cytoplasm. Russell bodies (cytoplasmic mucoprotein inclusions that stain pink by Romanowsky dyes) are seen in many plasma cells. The Mott cell, which also is seen, is a plasma cell containing numerous gray-blue inclusions thought to represent accumulations of immunoglobulins.

Cytochemically, plasma cells seen in myeloma stain strongly for cytoplasmic RNA, reflecting active protein synthesis. This is demonstrated by the pyroninophilia found with the Unna-Pappenheim stain. The PAS reaction for glycogen is negative or weakly reactive, whereas the acid phosphatase reaction is strongly positive, as is the nonspecific esterase reaction.

The principal laboratory feature, other than the obvious bone marrow picture, is the presence of a progressive increase of plasma myeloma protein and the presence in the urine of monoclonal light chains (κ or λ) in addition to the myeloma protein. Serum protein electrophoresis usually shows a definite M protein in the general region of the γ globulin. Immunoelectrophoresis subsequently will identify the specific immunoglobulin, which is IgG in more than half the cases. Table 13.17 summarizes the abnormal proteins found in multiple myeloma.

Subclassification of multiple myeloma by morphologic and immunologic marker characteristics of the tumor cells contributes to the prediction of the therapeutic outcome and prognosis. The plasmablastic type and the subgroup that expresses CALLA are both associated with a poorer survival than other types (Tamura et al., 1989).

Hemorrhagic complications, when not platelet-related, are most commonly associated with the ability of some M-components to interact with various proteins, including coagulation factors V, VII, VIII, prothrombin, and fibrinogen. Some M-components have the capacity to bind to fibrin monomers, resulting in a bulky gelatinous clot with poor fibrin strands and impaired clot retraction. Increased factor VIII activity also is seen sometimes.

Waldenström's Macroglobulinemia

Waldenström's macroglobulinemia is found principally in middle-aged and elderly individuals and is characterized by a lymphocytic and plasma cell proliferation and the presence of at least 1 g/dl of monoclonal IgM protein in the serum. The clinical findings are related to the presence of this abnormal protein, causing hyperviscosity of the blood and both lymphadenopathy and hepatosplenomegaly. Hemorrhagic side effects are seen as a result of macroglobulins adhering to platelets, thereby interfering with adequate platelet function.

The laboratory findings include a normocytic normochromic anemia due to either hemolysis or blood loss (MacKenzie and Fundenberg, 1972), as well as thrombocytopenia and hyperuricemia. A relative lymphocytosis and rouleaux formation also are seen, as is an occasional positive test result on antiglobulin testing.

Bone marrow aspirates are usually difficult to obtain. Lymphocytes are numerous and sometimes possess PAS-positive glycogen inclusions. Serum globulins generally are increased. Immunoelectrophoresis shows the presence of μ-heavy chains and one type of light chain. The Sia water test, based on the insolubility of macroglobulins in aqueous solutions, often gives positive results but is not sensitive and should not be relied on as a diagnostic tool.

Heavy-Chain Disease

Heavy-chain disease is a rare disorder that clinically resembles malignant lymphoma. Patients present with hepatosplenomegaly, lymphadenopathy, fever, severe malabsorption, abdominal pain, weight loss, and infections.

The laboratory findings are of anemia, leukopenia, and thrombocytopenia. Variant lymphocytes and plasma cells are often present in the peripheral blood. The bone marrow picture is one of plasmacytosis, but lymphocytes and increased eosinophils also are present. The diagnostic laboratory tests include protein electrophoresis and immunoelectrophoresis. The former test shows a broad spike in the β-γ region, together with a hypogammaglobulinemia. Immunoelectrophoresis will result in the demonstration of heavy chains or part of a heavy chain. The most common type found is the α chain of IgA, followed in frequency by the γ chain, the μ chain, and the δ chain. One distinguishes heavy-chain disease from Waldenström's macroglobulinemia by recognizing the lack of light chains from the paraprotein. Malabsorption tests often are positive, and infiltrates with *Giardia lamblia* are found. Serum albumin levels are decreased, whereas alkaline phosphatase values often are increased.

Chapter 14

Blood Coagulation (Hemostasis)

Hemostasis is the result of a series of related and overlapping events that culminate in the formation of a fibrin mass encompassing trapped red cells and platelets. The mechanism by which this plug is formed is complex and still is not completely understood. The mechanism consists of at least the following major components: (1) blood vessel wall, (2) blood platelets, (3) plasma clotting factors, (4) clot lysing enzymes, and (5) platelet inhibitors.

In health, a delicate balance exists between hemostasis and dissolution of the clot. When this balance becomes disturbed, either by poor clot formation or by excessive dissolution, hemorrhage can result. Conversely, disproportionate clotting or reduced dissolution results in possible hypercoagulable states. For clarity, it is convenient to review the complicated mechanism involved in clot formation as three separate but overlapping systems, as shown in Figure 14.1. Figure 14.2 provides a review of the total hemostatic mechanism.

General Overview

Blood vessels are lined by endothelial cells that normally are both nonthrombogenic and inhibitory to platelet aggregation because of the production of prostacyclin (inhibitory prostaglandin [PGI_2]). As such, the intact vessel does not promote blood coagulation unless it is ruptured or disturbed in a way that exposes the subendothelium and collagen of the intima of the artery, vein, or capillary. When this takes place, platelets adhere to the materials under-going aggregation and release active chemicals, thereby promoting further aggregation, enhancing vasoconstriction, and accelerating blood coagulation derived from the circulating plasma proteins. These coagulation factors are themselves activated by exposure to the vessel subendothelium and collagen, setting in motion an involved series of step-like reactions that result in the formation of a hemostatic fibrin plug at the site of vessel rupture.

Circulating plasma inhibitors prevent the clotting of circulating blood in the vicinity of the hemostatic plug, and fibrinolytic enzymes activated within the clot slowly begin its dissolution.

Vascular Involvement in Hemostasis

Most of the vascular system is composed of capillaries—both arterioles and venules. The remainder of the vascular tree is made up of the great vessels, which serve principally as conduits of the blood. These vessels consist of large endothelium-lined tubes surrounded by several bands of smooth muscle. They serve to regulate the blood flow to and from the heart and tissues. Capillaries differ from the great vessels in that they are much smaller and are not surrounded by a smooth-muscle layer. These microvessels consist of a single layer of endothelial cells arranged to allow the passage of medium-sized and larger molecules through formed vesicles. Smaller molecules passively diffuse across the endothelium, adjacent to which are supportive layers of basement membrane and collagen.

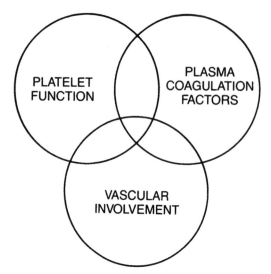

Figure 14.1. Overview of the three principal systems of blood coagulation.

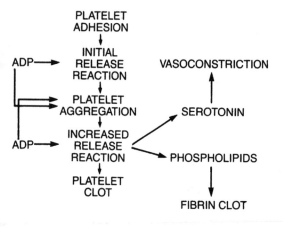

Figure 14.2. Summary of the total hemostatic mechanism involving platelets. (ADP = adenosine diphosphate.)

Blood vessel endothelium is highly active metabolically and allows for a minimum of interaction between the circulatory blood and the cell surfaces. The endothelium contains PGI$_2$ and lacks factors that promote platelet aggregation. PGI$_2$ acts by increasing platelet membrane cyclic AMP (cAMP) levels, thereby decreasing the potential for platelet aggregation. Additionally, the capillary endothelium is rich in a plasminogen activator that, when triggered, produces the stimulation of a fibrinolysin precursor, plasminogen. This sub-

stance then is converted to plasmin or fibrinolysin, the function of which is to lyse any formed fibrin clots in the vessel. Vascular endothelial cells also synthesize factor VIII–related von Willebrand factor (vWF) polymers. These are composed of monomers of 230,000 d covalently linked by disulfide bonds into multimeric structures with a molecular weight of millions of daltons. These polymers are secreted into the circulation or onto collagen-containing subendothelium.

The endothelium thus physically monitors vessel wall integrity, synthesizes and stores hemostatic components, and produces physiologic substances that inhibit platelet adhesion. The principal functions of the endothelium are shown in Table 14.1. An overall view of the interaction of vessel wall, platelets, and plasma factors is shown diagrammatically in Figure 14.3.

Platelets in Hemostasis

Structure

Platelets are disc-shaped particles resembling cytoplasmic fragments of megakaryocytes. The cell does not possess any nucleus, endoplasmic reticulum, or Golgi apparatus. It is surrounded by a fluffy coated peripheral zone termed a *glycocalyx,* which contains plasma proteins and carbohydrate molecules related to coagulation and fibrinolytic and complement systems. Although some of these molecules appear to be adsorbed onto the platelet surface, some are membrane-bound. Most of the circulating plasma coagulation factors, particularly factors I, V, VII, XII, and XIII, have been found to be associated with either the glycocalyx or the platelet membrane.

Below the glycocalyx is the negatively charged platelet membrane, which is a conglomerate of lipid and protein molecules that are in constant motion in relation to one another. This is the *sol-gel zone.* Under the membrane is a series of filaments and microtubules composing the platelet cytoskeleton. This structure maintains the disclike form and the organelle positions in the intact platelet. There is also a secondary system of microfilaments that participate in platelet contraction and secretion, resulting in a morphologic change from a disc to a spiny pseudopodic sphere. Extending through the plasma

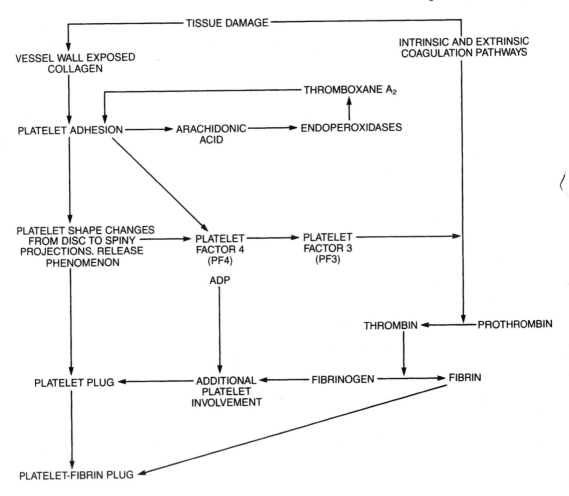

Figure 14.3. The interaction of platelets with endothelial cells and plasma coagulation factors.

membrane into the interior of the platelet is an open-ended canalicular system that allows access to intraplatelet constituents from the granules and cytoplasm to the external environment.

α-Granules and electron-dense bodies are present in the organelle zone. The α-granules are the most abundant and moderately dense. They contain hydrolytic enzymes, fibrinogen, and platelet factor 3. The dense bodies are associated with storable sites for adenosine triphosphate (ATP), calcium catecholamine, serotonin, and prostaglandins. It has also been theorized that platelet factor 4 is stored in these granules (da Prada et al., 1976). Mitochondria, too, are present in the organelle zone and carry out metabolic functions. In the absence of anaerobic glycolysis, they possess

the ability to meet the short-term energy requirements of the cell.

Two additional membrane-connecting structures are found in the platelet, the dense tubular system (DTS) and a surface connecting system. The DTS is composed of smooth endoplasmic reticulum. It has the ability to store calcium and to synthesize prostaglandin for use in platelet function. Figure 14.4 schematically illustrates platelet structure.

Function

Like other hematologic cells, platelets require a source of ATP to be metabolically functional. This is provided by glucose, which is metabolized anaer-

Table 14.1. Principal Hemostatic Functions of Endothelial Cells

Factor	Synthesis	Storage	Release	Binding	Degradation	Physiologic Role
Plasminogen activator	+	+	+	—	—	Fibrinolysis
Factor VIII–related antigen	+	+	+	—	—	Intrinsic pathway
α_2-Macroglobulin	—	—	—	+	—	Inhibitor
Thrombin	—	—	—	+	—	Common pathway
Complement (C3)	—	—	—	+	+	Complement pathway
Basement membrane	+	+	+	—	—	Collagens II and IV,
	—	—	—	—	—	fibronectin cofactors
Prostacyclin (PGI$_2$)	+	—	+	—	—	Inhibitor
Small molecules	—	—	—	+	+	Serotonin

obically by way of the Embden-Meyerhof pathway or aerobically via the Krebs cycle or citric acid pathway or by the pentose-phosphate shunt. Under normal conditions, platelets circulate for approximately 10 days as disc-shaped structures. When endothelial damage occurs, the basement membrane and collagen subendothelial layers become exposed, initiating the conversion of the disc-shaped platelet to a spiny pseudopodic echinocyte. During this transformation, the surface changes from a smooth layer to an adhesive one. Organelles migrate to a central location, and a release phenomenon takes place, which culminates in the release of the contents of both the α-granules and the dense granules into the environment. This takes place by way of the open canalicular system, and it makes available adenosine diphosphate (ADP), serotonin, lysosomal enzymes, platelet factors 3 and 4, and arachidonic acid. The release of ADP causes platelets to aggregate, which is a reversible process (Grette, 1962). The remainder of the released metabolites in this conversion go on to irreversible aggregation, the two-stage process seen in the use of ADP in the platelet aggregation test. Platelet aggregation is shown in Figure 14.5.

Once irreversible aggregation has taken place and the release phenomenon has occurred, platelet factor 3 is made available, and the presence of most clotting factors in the immediate platelet atmosphere leads to thrombin formation. When this takes place, the plasma-platelet clot retracts, the degree being proportional to the number of platelets and to the reaction between ATP and a platelet-contractile protein, thrombosthenin.

This interaction of platelets with plasma coagulation factors is shown in Figure 14.6. The principal platelet procoagulant is platelet factor 3, a phospholipoprotein that interacts with the plasma intrinsic coagulation pathway in two ways. Platelet factor 3, in conjunction with calcium ions, factor VIII, and factor IXa, promotes conversion of factor X to factor Xa. In addition, platelet factor 3 aids in the conversion of prothrombin to thrombin in conjunction with factor V, calcium ions, and factor Xa.

Further platelet-plasma coagulation interaction is evidenced by two feedback mechanisms. First, the platelet release mechanism provides ADP, serotonin, and arachidonic acid, which promote platelet aggregation. Second, this aggregation is enhanced by the presence of thrombin that is generated from prothrombin in the intrinsic pathway.

Many coagulation proteins are found in or on platelets, including factors II, V, VIII, IX, XII, and XIII. In some instances, these factors are found in a slightly different form in platelets in contrast to their form in plasma. The binding of factor IX and factor X to platelets is influenced by factor VIII, which likely acts as a cofactor in the assembly of the factor X activating complex on the platelet surface. Platelet-specific proteins are also present, and platelet factors 1 through 7 have been described.

Other aspects of platelet function involve the maintenance of vascular integrity. The cause of petechial hemorrhages in thrombocytopenic individuals is thought to be related to loss of epithelial cells of the capillaries. Under normal physiologic conditions, platelets are believed to plug the gaps caused by such epithelial loss, so preventing seepage of intact red cells into the surrounding tissues and skin. If the platelet count falls to less than 50×10^9/liter, such hemorrhages occur. This provides the basis for the tourniquet test (Tranzer and Baumgartner, 1967; Huang et al., 1974).

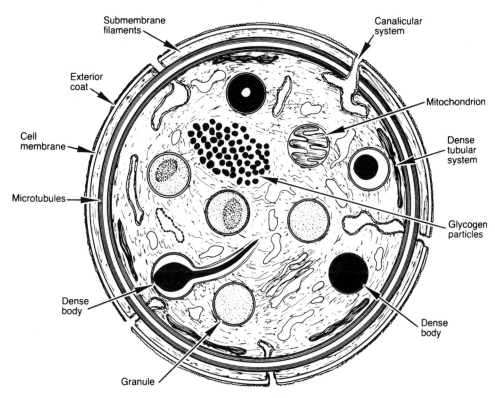

Figure 14.4. Platelet ultrastructure seen by electron microscope. (Courtesy of James White, M.D., Department of Pediatrics, Mayo Clinic.)

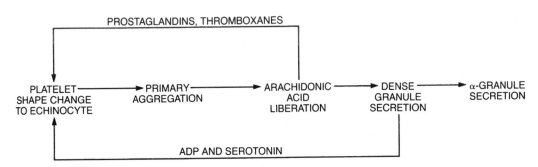

Figure 14.5. Platelet aggregation mechanisms. (ADP = adenosine diphosphate.) (Adapted from H Holmsen. Prostaglandin endoperoxidase-thromboxane synthesis and dense granule secretion as possible feedback loops in the propagation of platelet responses in the basic platelet reaction. Thromb Haemost 38:1030, 1977.)

It is known that, aside from their involvement in these complicated interactions, thrombi found in the arterial and venous circulations depend to some degree on the presence of platelets. Because of the principal differences in flow conditions involving arteries and veins, the composition of the thrombi varies; in the arterial system, the thrombi are mainly platelet-derived, or white, thrombi, whereas in the more static venous circulation, the red thrombi are composed of erythrocytes, platelets, and fibrin.

Platelet adhesion is mediated by many platelet surface receptors. Several of these receptors belong to the integrin family of adhesion receptors present

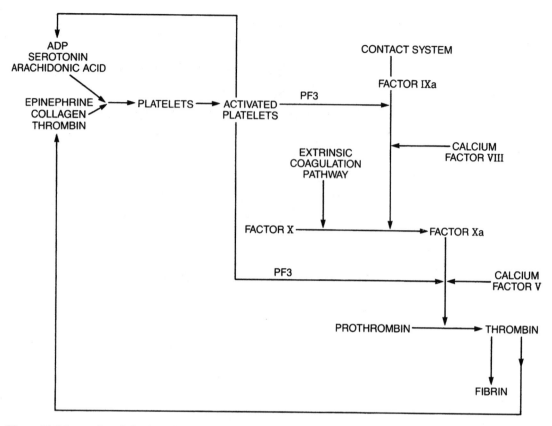

Figure 14.6. Interaction of platelet and plasma coagulation factors. (ADP = adenosine diphosphate; PF3 = platelet factor 3.) (Adapted from D Hutchinson. Platelet Function, Disorders, and Testing. In The Hemophilias. Miami: American Dade, 1983.)

on many different cells. Two subunits are recognized. The beta family contains receptors that mediate the interactions between many types of cells and molecules, such as collagen, fibronectin, and laminin. The β_2 family is present on leukocytes and mediates the interactions in inflammation and immune recognition. The β_3 families (cytoadhesives) include the platelet- and megakaryocyte-specific glycoprotein IIb/IIIa and the vitronectin receptor present on platelets and other cells.

The receptors involved in platelet adhesion are active on resting platelets. Under normal conditions, the intact endothelium covers the adhesive glycoprotein ligands in the subepithelium (vWF, fibronectin, collagen), masking them from the platelet. This limits platelet adhesion to the sites of vascular damage.

Platelet aggregation is mediated by the platelet glycoprotein IIb/IIIa receptor exclusively, which is found only on platelets and megakaryocytes. When

activated, the receptor can bind several different glycoproteins including fibrinogen, vWF, fibronectin, and possibly vitronectin and thrombospondin (Weiss et al., 1989).

Biochemistry

When platelets adhere to the subendothelial lining and exposed collagen, they undergo aggregation and the release of active constituents, which promotes further platelet aggregation, vasoconstriction of blood vessels, and acceleration of blood coagulation (Figure 14.7). The complex platelet cycle begins with prostaglandin formation involving the calcium-dependent hydrolysis of platelet membrane phosphatidylinositol and phosphatidylcholine by phospholipase A_2 to yield arachidonic acid. This fatty acid also is made available from endogenous blood vessel endothelium (Marcus, 1978). Arachidonic acid is acted on by

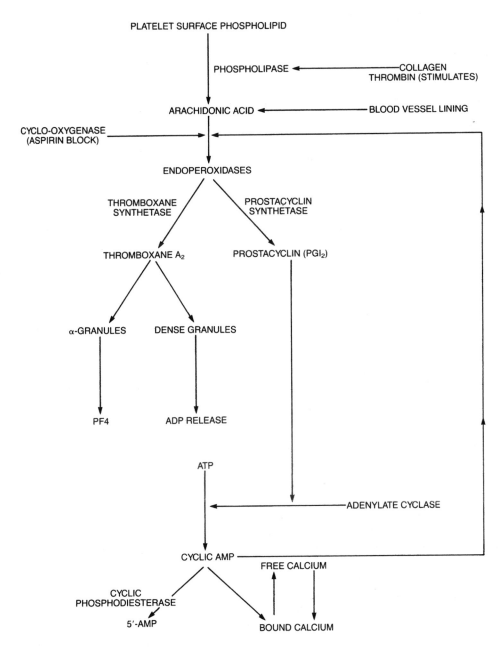

Figure 14.7. Platelet biochemistry and the role of prostaglandins. (PF4 = platelet factor 4; ADP = adenosine diphosphate; ATP = adenosine triphosphate; AMP = adenosine monophosphate.)

cyclo-oxygenase to produce prostaglandin precursors, the endoperoxidases 15-hydroperoxy-9α-11α-peroxidoprosta-5,13-dienoic acid (PGG$_2$) and 15-hydroxy-9-11-peroxidoprosta-5,13-dienoic acid (PGH$_2$) (Hamberg, 1974). These substances are acted on by two enzymes, thromboxane synthetase and PGI$_2$ synthetase. The former enzyme is involved in the production of a potent aggregating agent and vasoconstrictor, thromboxane A$_2$, which additionally promotes the platelet mechanism resulting in the release of both α- and dense granules (Needleman, 1976). Platelet factor 4 is a protein found only in the α-granules. Clinically, its determination is useful in the diagnosis and monitoring of coronary artery dis-

Table 14.2. Factors Affecting Platelet Aggregation

Aggregation-inducing
  Thrombin
  Adrenalin
  Adenosine diphosphate
  Collagen
Aggregation-inhibiting
  Prostaglandin E$_1$
  Caffeine
  Adenosine
  Theophylline

ease. The action of PGI$_2$ synthetase on the endoperoxides results in the formation of PGI$_2$, which acts by stimulating the production of platelet adenylate cyclase.

Two enzymes are known to regulate the concentration of cAMP: adenylate cyclase, which converts ATP to cAMP, and cyclic phosphodiesterase, which converts cAMP to 5'-AMP. Increasing the concentration of cAMP is known to inhibit platelet aggregation. This can be achieved in one of two ways—either by activating adenylate cyclase or by inhibiting cyclic phosphodiesterase activity (Salzman et al., 1977). Table 14.2 illustrates some of the inducers and inhibitors of platelet aggregation that can be shown to relate directly to cAMP concentration.

The stimulation of PGI$_2$ synthesized either de novo from arachidonic acid or in response to stimulation by platelet endoperoxidases (PGG$_2$ or PGH$_2$) via aortic microsomal PGI$_2$ synthetase results in an antiaggregatory response. This is exactly the opposite of the action of thromboxane A$_2$ produced from the same proaggregatory endoperoxidases. Figure 14.8 compares the properties of thromboxane A$_2$ and PGI$_2$ derived from their common precursor, arachidonic acid. It can be seen that PGI$_2$ produced from platelet PGG$_2$ or PGH$_2$ stimulates adenylate cyclase activity, which, in turn, increases cAMP concentrations. This inhibits cyclooxygenase action, with the result of reducing synthesis of proaggregatory thromboxane A$_2$.

The role of calcium in the biochemical platelet pathway is believed to be associated with cAMP, which has been shown to regulate the uptake of calcium ions by isolated platelet membrane vesicles in vitro. An increase in available cytoplasmic calcium is thought to be responsible for activating the platelet contractile process during the release phenomenon (Massini and Käser-Glanzmann, 1978).

Platelet Antigens and Antibodies

Eight human platelet alloantibodies have been described comprising antigens that reside on the major transmembrane glycoprotein. Most clinically significant antibodies are directed against the Pl^{A1} antigen, which depends on a single amino acid polymorphism of the IIa glycoprotein. Rarer alloantibodies are directed against other blood group antigens shown in Table 14.3. Each of these systems has been associated with a specific membrane protein, although many antigens reside on glycoprotein IIIa.

Antibodies to these alloantigens are the major cause of neonatal alloimmune thrombocytopenia.

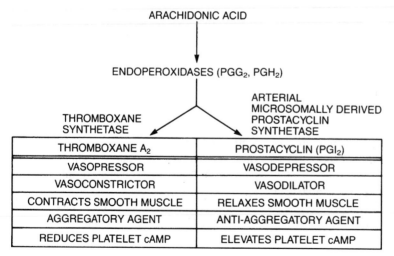

THROMBOXANE A$_2$	PROSTACYCLIN (PGI$_2$)
VASOPRESSOR	VASODEPRESSOR
VASOCONSTRICTOR	VASODILATOR
CONTRACTS SMOOTH MUSCLE	RELAXES SMOOTH MUSCLE
AGGREGATORY AGENT	ANTI-AGGREGATORY AGENT
REDUCES PLATELET cAMP	ELEVATES PLATELET cAMP

Figure 14.8. Differences in the physiologic effects of the generated products of arachidonic acid.

Table 14.3. Human Platelet Antigens

Nomenclature	Antithetical Antigens	Protein	Frequency of Antibody in Neonatal Thrombocytopenia
HPA-1		IIIb	80%
HPA-1a	$Pl^{A1}\ Zw^a$		
HPA-1b	$Pl^{A2}\ Zw^b$		
HPA-2		Ib	—
HPA-2a	Ko^b		
HPA-2b	$Ko^a\ Sib^a$		
HPA-3		IIb	—
HPA-3a	$Bak^a\ Lek^a$		
HPA-3b	Bak^b		
HPA-4		IIIa	—
HPA-4a	$Pen^a\ Yuk^b$		
HPA-4b	$Pen^b\ Yuk^a$		
HPA-5		Ia	15%
HPA-5a	$Br^b\ Zav^b$		
HPA-5b	$Br^a\ Zav^a,\ Hc^a$		
HPA-6		IIIa	—
HPA-6a	$Ca^b\ Tu^b$		
HPA-6b	$Ca^a\ Tu^a$		
HPA-7		IIIa	—
HPA-7a	Mo^b		
HPA-7b	Mo^a		
HPA-8		IIIa	—
HPA-8a	Sr^b		
HPA-8b	Sr^a		

The maternal alloantibody against an antigen inherited from the father causes fetal platelets to be destroyed. This results in the fetus being thrombocytopenic and subject to possible spontaneous bleeding. Post-transfusion purpura, in which a transfusion recipient experiences delayed destruction of his or her own platelets, also is most often caused by anti-Pl^{A1}. The detection of platelet alloantibodies remains difficult, although flow-cytometric techniques now are available and appear to be the most sensitive tool. Enzyme immunoassay methods can also be used.

Plasma Clotting Factors

As already stated, hemostasis is the result of a series of related and overlapping events. If a blood vessel is ruptured, several in vivo changes take place simultaneously. Platelets are attracted to the site of the vessel injury (see preceding discussion), putting into motion a series of involved biochemical reactions that both help to plug the wound physically and as-

sist in the formation of fibrin production. Efficient platelet function alone is not enough to stop the resulting hemorrhage. The original theory of Morowitz postulated a two-stage reaction culminating in the production of fibrin from an intermediate substance, thrombin. More recent theories suggest that coagulation is initiated by two fundamentally different mechanisms—the process of contact activation and the action of tissue factors (Davie and Fujikawa, 1975). These processes involve a series of coagulation factors, which are designated by a Roman numeral, as shown in Table 14.4. Table 14.5 shows other coagulation factors not yet included in the International Committee's classification.

Blood Coagulation Factors

Factor I (Fibrinogen)

Fibrinogen is a glycoprotein dimer produced in the liver, with a molecular weight of 340,000 d. It is a triglobular molecule with three pairs of peptide

Table 14.4. Nomenclature of the Blood Coagulation Factors

International Committee's Factor	Synonyms
I	Fibrinogen
II	Prothrombin
III	Tissue factor, tissue thromboplastin
IV	Calcium
V	Proaccelerin, serum prothrombin conversion accelerator, labile factor, plasma Ac globulin
VII	Proconvertin, stable factor, serum accelerator, stable prothrombin conversion accelerator
VIII	Antihemophilic factor, antihemophilic globin, antihemophilic factor A, platelet cofactor I, thromboplastinogen
IX	Plasma thromboplastin component, Christmas factor, antihemophilic factor B, autoprothrombin II, platelet cofactor 2
X	Stuart factor, Stuart-Prower factor, thrombokinase, autoprothrombin III
XI	Plasma thromboplastin antecedent, antihemophilic factor C
XII	Hageman factor, contact factor
XIII	Fibrin-stabilizing factor, fibrinase, Laki-Lorand factor

Note: Factor VI is not recognized.

Table 14.5. Other Coagulation Factors Not Yet Included in the International Committee's Classification

Principal Name	Synonym
Prekallikrein	Fletcher factor
HMW kininogen	Contact activation factor, Fitzgerald factor, Fleaujeac factor, Williams factor
Protein C	Xa inhibitor

HMW = high-molecular-weight.

chains (α, β, and γ) and interconnecting disulfide bonds. The normal plasma fibrinogen concentration varies between 200 and 400 mg/dl.

Fibrinogen is a natural substrate for the enzyme thrombin. The action of thrombin on fibrinogen results in a cleavage of the α and β chains at their arginyl-glycine bonds. This causes the release of two pairs of peptides—fibrinopeptides A and B—causing the formation of a so-called fibrin monomer, which rapidly polymerizes with other fibrin monomers in an end-to-end and side-to-side fashion, resulting in a fibrin clot. Fibrinogen does not require vitamin K for synthesis and is relatively stable to heat and storage.

Factor II (Prothrombin)

Prothrombin is a liver-synthesized, heat-stable, α_2-globulin that requires vitamin K for its maintenance. Like fibrinogen, it is consumed during the coagulation process. It has a molecular weight of 72,000 d and is present in the plasma at a concentration of approximately 10 mg/dl. Prothrombin, in the presence of ionized calcium, is converted to thrombin by the enzymatic action of products of both the intrinsic and extrinsic coagulation pathways (factors V and Xa, platelet factor 3, and ionized calcium). The half-life of prothrombin is approximately 70–110 hours.

Factor V (Proaccelerin)

Proaccelerin is a liver-synthesized globulin with a molecular weight of approximately 300,000 d. Like prothrombin, it is consumed in the process of blood coagulation, but it differs from prothrombin in that it does not require vitamin K for its production. Factor V is unstable, deteriorating rapidly at room temperature and in oxalated plasma but less rapidly in citrated plasma. The protein also exhibits lability when the pH is increased to 10.5, but it is relatively stable in the pH range of 5–9. Factor V is not removed from the plasma by Seitz filtration or by adsorption with barium sulfate or aluminum hydroxide gel. It possesses a half-life of approximately 16 hours.

Factor VII

Factor VII is a liver-synthesized β-globulin with a molecular weight of 48,000 d. It requires vitamin K for production and is stable in citrated plasma for up to 4 days at 25–37°C and for 2 weeks at 4°C (Miale, 1982). In contrast to its in vitro stability, its in vivo half-life is only 4–7 hours. High levels are present both in stored plasma and in serum, especially when the storage conditions are cool. The action of factor VII consists of the activation of tissue thromboplastins in the extrinsic pathway and the consequential acceleration of thrombin production from prothrombin. This factor is not involved in the intrinsic blood coagulation pathway. Factor VII is removed from plasma or serum by adsorption with barium sulfate, aluminum hydroxide gel, and calcium phosphate.

Factor VIII

Factor VIII is a complex, heat-labile glycoprotein with a molecular weight of 2–20 million d (Miller et al., 1984). It circulates as a two-chain complex consisting of a variable heavy chain (90,000– 210,000 d) and a light chain (80,000 d). It contains high concentrations of sialic acids and other carbohydrates. The molecule is composed of several different fragments (Gralnick and Coller, 1976; Hoyer, 1981). Factor VIII–related antigen (factor VIII:Ag) and the vWF are found in the high-molecular-weight (HMW) region and are believed to be portions of the same molecule, now termed the *von Willebrand protein* (Chavin, 1984). The factor VIII protein is part of a smaller subunit. Dissociation and association of these two fragments can be achieved because they are held together by relatively weak bonds. Factor VIII coagulant antigen is the protein that is deficient or defective in individuals with classic hemophilia. Its function may be measured as factor VIII coagulant activity, which corrects the prolonged clotting time of hemophilic plasma.

The von Willebrand protein is the factor that is deficient or defective in von Willebrand's syndrome, its activity being measured by its ability to agglutinate platelets in the presence of ristocetin or by the adhesion of platelets to collagen. Besides being reduced in von Willebrand's syndrome, this protein has been reported to be present in increased levels in situ in individuals with coronary artery disease (Brody et al., 1986).

Tables 14.6 and 14.7 show the synonyms and relationships for the factor VIII complex, which is believed to be produced mainly by hepatocytes of the liver (White and Shoemaker, 1989), endothelial cells and megakaryocytes (Jaffe, 1977; Piovella and Nalli, 1978) and, in a minor way, by the kidneys (Barrow and Graham, 1974) and spleen (Rizza and Eipe, 1971). Control of factor VIII synthesis is poorly understood. Hormonal influences may be important; it is known that vasopressin and its analogs can increase plasma levels in both normal and hemophilic individuals.

The concentration of factor VIII in plasma is approximately 100–200 ng/ml (Chavin, 1984). It is adsorbed from citrated plasma by aluminum hydroxide and is not present in the serum. Factor VIII coagulant antigen accelerates blood coagulation by its cofactor role in the enzymatic activation of factor X by factor IXa. In the presence of phospholipid and calcium, it markedly enhances this reaction; when factor IXa is not present, this coagulant antigen does not possess any intrinsic capacity to activate factor X. Thrombin activation is essential for factor VIII:C activity, this enzyme acting by cleaving the protein chains of the molecule. The disappearance of factor VIII in hemophilic individuals following transfusion is biphasic. The initial rate is rapid, with a half-life of 3–6 hours, followed by a slower disappearance component, with a half-life of between 8 and 18 hours. Control of factor VIII synthesis is poorly understood. Hormonal influences may be important, and it is known that vasopressin and its analogs can increase plasma levels in both normal and hemophiliac individuals. (Muntean and Leshnick, 1989).

Factor IX

Factor IX, a liver-synthesized β-globulin, requires vitamin K for its production. Factor IX has a mo-

Table 14.6. Synonyms of the Factor VIII Complex

Factor	Importance
Factor VIII antigen	Decreased in classic hemophilia and von Willebrand's syndrome
von Willebrand protein	Normal in classic hemophilia
von Willebrand antigen	Decreased in von Willebrand's syndrome

Source: Data from VJ Marder, PM Mannucci, et al. Standard nomenclature for factor VIII and von Willebrand factor. A recommendation by the International Committee on Thrombosis and Haemostasis. Thromb Haemost 54:871, 1985.

lecular weight of 57,000 d and is usually present in the plasma in the nonactivated form and in the serum as factor IXa. It is completely adsorbed by Seitz filtration from oxalated plasma and by the usual prothrombin adsorbents. The principal function of factor IX is its influence in the rate of conversion of factor X to factor Xa. It is stable at 4°C for several weeks and has a half-life of approximately 20 hours.

Factor X

The proenzyme factor X is a liver-synthesized α-globulin with a molecular weight of 59,000 d. Factor X activation is required to initiate the common pathway of blood coagulation, as it is acted on by the enzymatic end products of both the intrinsic and extrinsic blood coagulation pathways to produce factor Xa. Like factor IX and prothrombin, factor X requires vitamin K for its synthesis. It is adsorbed by barium sulfate and aluminum hydroxide gel and is partially consumed during the coagulation process. It is relatively heat-stable and remains stable at 4°C for up to 2 months. The biological half-life of factor X is approximately 40 hours. It has been found in lymph, which has given rise to the speculation that large extravascular pools exist that act as storage sites (Stutman et al., 1965).

Factor XI

Factor XI is a liver-synthesized β-globulin with a molecular weight of approximately 200,000 d. It normally exists in the circulation in a complex with HMW kininogen. Factor XI is essential for the intrinsic coagulation pathway and constitutes one of the two contact factors of the clotting system. This β-globulin is consumed only partially during clotting, and only small amounts are adsorbed from plasma using the routine inorganic salts. Because of this, factor XI is detected in serum. Plasma levels approximate 7 µg/dl and often are decreased in liver disease. The protein is relatively stable at room temperature and has a half-life of approximately 60 hours.

Factor XII

Factor XII is a single-chain polypeptide migrating as a β- or γ-globulin and having a molecular weight of approximately 80,000 d. The actual site of synthesis of this factor is unknown. Factor XII is not adsorbed from plasma by inorganic salts, but it is adsorbed onto powdered glass and diatomaceous earth such as silica, kaolin, and celite. When factor XII comes into contact with glass, it becomes converted to factor XIIa as part of the contact activation process involving vessel endothelium and the kallikrein and kinin systems (see page 183).

Factor XII is stable and can be stored in oxalated plasma at 4°C for up to 3 months; it also resists heating to 60°C for 30 minutes. Plasma levels of factor XII range from 23 to 47 µg/ml (Ratnoff, 1977). The half-life of factor XII is between 50 and 60 hours.

Factor XIII

Factor XIII is a heat-stable α-globulin, having a high molecular weight of 320,000 d, that acts in the stabilization of the fibrin monomer. Factor XIII is acted on by thrombin in the presence of calcium to produce factor XIIIa. The exact production sites of factor XIII are unknown, although the liver has been implicated in its synthesis.

Table 14.7. Relationships of the Factor VIII Complex

Attribute	Proposed New Abbreviation	Old Terminology
Factor VIII		
Protein	VIII	VIII:C
Antigen	VIII:Ag	VIIIC:Ag
Function	VIII:C	—
von Willebrand factor (vWF)		
Protein	vWF	VIII R:Ag
Antigen	vWF	VIII R:Ag
Function	Ag	VIII R:RCo
		VIII R:vWF

Note: Von Willebrand function abbreviations have been used to indicate ristocetin cofactor activity of vWF. Because neither this test nor any other in vitro test completely reflects vWF activity, no abbreviation is recommended.
Source: Data from VJ Marder, PM Mannucci, et al. Standard nomenclature for factor VIII and von Willebrand factor. A recommendation by the International Committee on Thrombosis and Haemostasis. Thromb Haemost 54:871, 1985.

The biological half-life of this protein is approximately 3–12 days. In cases of factor XIII deficiency, both hemostasis and wound healing are abnormal, which suggests that factor XIII plays a role in scar formation, presumably by modulating collagen synthesis by fibroblasts. Table 14.8 shows the properties of the plasma coagulation factors.

Process of Blood Coagulation

Contact activation triggers a series of reactions involving prekallikrein, HMW kininogen, factors VIII, IX, XI, and XII, and platelet factor 3, which results in the formation of an enzyme that converts circulating factor X to an active state. Such activation may also be accomplished by the initiation of factor VII with tissue factors liberated from ruptured cells. Thus, activation of factor X is carried out by two principal paths—that using mainly circulating plasma coagulation factors (the intrinsic pathway) and that using the tissue factor (the extrinsic pathway).

Intrinsic Pathway of Blood Coagulation

The contact activation of the coagulation mechanism is not completely understood (Hudson, 1983). It is thought that when factor XII is bound to a negatively charged surface, it becomes available for proteolytic activation by other proteases, such as kallikrein.

In the presence of HMW kininogen, prekallikrein is converted to kallikrein, which, in turn, activates factor XII to form factor XIIa. This factor then activates HMW kininogen–bound factor XI to produce factor XIa (Griffin and Cochrane, 1979). Biological surfaces that produce contact activation include unbroken skin, human cartilage, vascular basement membrane, and bacterial lipopolysaccharides. The negatively charged in vitro agents known to promote contact activation of factor XII include the diatomaceous earths such as celite and kaolin, glass, and a tannic acid–related material, ellagic acid.

The interaction between factors XIIa and XI takes place without the aid of free calcium ions and results in the production of factor XIa. This "contact product" acts as a serine protease (Kingdon and Lundblad, 1975), but the mechanism of its production is still unclear. In purified systems, factor XI activation occurs only in the presence of HMW kininogen. It is postulated that this may function to link factor XI to active surfaces (Ratnoff and Saito, 1979; Wiggins et al., 1979).

Activated factor XI (XIa) next acts on a substrate, factor IX, to form a serine protease factor IXa. This reaction requires the presence of calcium ions and takes place in two steps, resulting in the cleavage of factor IX and the subsequent release of a carbohydrate-rich peptide (DiScipio et al., 1977).

Factor IX can also be activated by factor VIIa from the extrinsic pathway (Nemerson and Bach, 1982). After this reaction has taken place, factor IXa, factor VIII, and platelet factor 3 react, leading to the conversion of factor X to factor Xa, an interaction that also requires free calcium ions. This step is ac-

Table 14.8. Properties of the Plasma Coagulation Factors

Factor	Site of Synthesis	Vitamin K–Dependent	Molecular Weight (d) and Chain Structure	Half-Life (hrs)	Minimum Hemostatic Level	Storage Stability	Affected by Coumarin	Mode of Inheritance
Fibrinogen	Liver	No	340,000, α_2, β_2, γ_2	70–120	50–100 mg/dl	Stable	No	Autosomal recessive
Prothrombin	Liver	Yes	72,000, α_2	70–110	40% concentration	Stable	Yes	Autosomal recessive
Factor V	Liver	No	300,000	16	5–10% concentration	Labile	No	Autosomal recessive
Factor VII	Liver	Yes	48,000	4–7	5–10% concentration	Stable	Yes	Autosomal recessive
Factor VIII								
Factor VIIIC	Liver	No	150,000	10–14	30% concentration	Labile	No	Sex-linked recessive
von Willebrand protein	Endothelial cells and megakaryocytes	No	>2,000,000	22–40	—	Labile	No	Autosomal dominant
Factor IX	Liver	Yes	57,000	20	30% concentration	Stable	Yes	Sex-linked recessive
Factor X	Liver	Yes	59,000 (dimer)	40	8–10% concentration	Stable	Yes	Autosomal recessive
Factor XI	Liver	No	200,000 (dimer)	60	20–30% concentration	Stable	No	Autosomal recessive
Factor XII	Unknown	No	80,000	50–60	Not required	Stable	No	Autosomal recessive
Factor XIII	Liver	No	320,000, α_2, β_2	3–12	8–10% concentration	Stable	No	Autosomal recessive
Prekallikrein	Unknown	No	85,000, γ_2	Unknown	Unknown	Unknown	No	Unknown
HMW kininogen	Unknown	No	160,000, α_2	120–144 (5–6 days)	Unknown	Unknown	No	Unknown

HMW = high-molecular-weight.

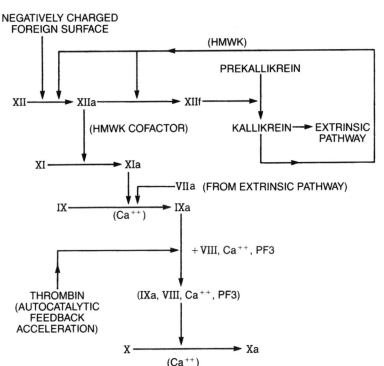

Figure 14.9. Intrinsic coagulation pathway. (HMWK = high-molecular-weight kininogen; PF3 = platelet factor 3.)

celerated by traces of thrombin, generated from the later stages of coagulation in the intrinsic pathway, on factor VIII. Figure 14.9 illustrates the intrinsic coagulation pathway as far as factor X activation.

Extrinsic Pathway of Blood Coagulation

As previously stated, the extrinsic pathway involves the interaction between tissue juices, derived from membrane-bound glycoproteins on subepithelial structures, and factor VII in the presence of calcium ions. The final product is an enzymatic complex capable of activating factor X to factor Xa. The exact mechanism by which this complex acts remains unclear, but it is believed that proteolytic cleavage of factor VII by kallikrein occurs (Saito and Ratnoff, 1975). Other enzymes are known to produce similar actions. They include plasma factor XIIa, factor XIIf, and factor IXa (Nemerson, 1976; Seligsohn and Kasper, 1979). Activation of factor VII by these means is believed to be the mechanism whereby the one-stage prothrombin time is decreased during plasma storage in the cold.

When formed from this activation, factor Xa exhibits an autocatalytic reaction and converts factor VII to factor VIIa. In a similar way, thrombin provides an additional autocatalytic feedback mechanism activating factor VII (Radcliffe and Nemerson, 1976). The extrinsic coagulation pathway is depicted in Figure 14.10.

Joint Pathway of Blood Coagulation

The series of reactions that constitute the joint pathway of blood coagulation begins when factor X is activated by either the intrinsic or the extrinsic pathway to produce factor Xa. From this point, the sequence of reactions is identical for both pathways (Figure 14.11).

Factor Xa next interacts with calcium ions, factor V, platelet factor 3, and ionized calcium, leading to the formation of a *prothrombinase* complex (factors Xa and V, platelet factor 3, and ionized calcium), which catalyzes the prothrombin molecule to the active enzyme thrombin. Once formed, thrombin converts the soluble plasma protein, fibrinogen, into an insoluble material, fibrin. Structurally, fibrinogen is

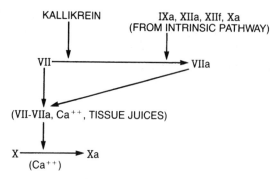

Figure 14.10. Extrinsic coagulation pathway.

a dimer, with each unit consisting of three chains (α, β, and γ) linked by disulfide bonds. Disulfide bridges link the dimers between the two α chains and the two γ chains close to the N terminus, in much the same way that heavy and light chains are colinked in the

immunoglobulin molecules. Figure 14.12 schematically illustrates this primary structure.

The proteolytic conversion of fibrinogen to fibrin by thrombin occurs without the aid of calcium ions and results in the release of four fibrinopeptides per mole of fibrinogen. These split products are designated fibrinopeptides A and B, one being produced from each of the two α and two β chains. The cleavage of these acidic fibrinopeptides promotes fibrin polymerization of the residual molecule, now termed a *fibrin monomer*. Such changes result in the formation of thicker and longer fibrin strands—that is, fibrin units associated both end-to-end and side-to-side (Figure 14.13). These fibrin-soluble aggregates must be stabilized before a firm hemostatic clot can be achieved. Such stabilization involves the formation of hydrogen bonds linking the fibrin monomers.

Fibrin stabilization is achieved through the action of factor XIIIa. This enzyme is formed from its inert

Figure 14.11. The joint pathways of blood coagulation. (PF3 = platelet factor 3.)

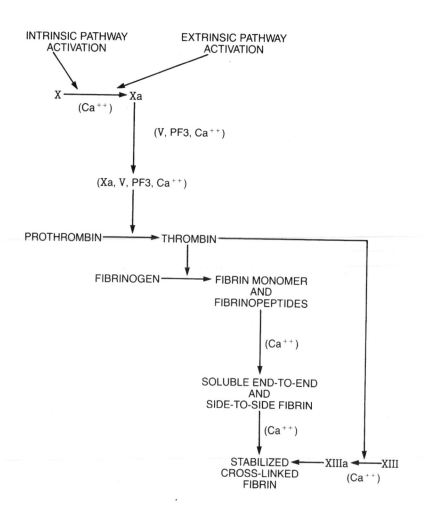

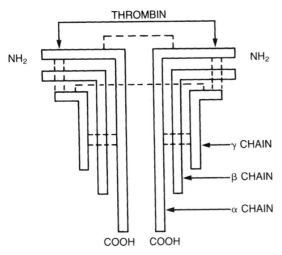

Figure 14.12. Schematic illustration of the fibrinogen molecule. (Dashed lines indicate disulfide bonds.)

precursor, factor XIII, by the action of thrombin. Calcium is not required for this cleavage but, once the cleavage has occurred, calcium is needed to aid in the dissociation of factor XIIIa into an enzymatically active α-chain dimer that contains the active site cysteine and an inactive β-chain dimer. During physiologic fibrin formation in the presence of factor XIIIa, the ε-amino group of lysine from one fibrin monomer forms a peptide bond with a glutamyl residue of an adjacent fibrin monomer, producing a mechanically stronger, stabilized cross-linked fibrin that is more resistant to plasmin action. This reaction occurs rapidly between

the γ chains and more slowly between the α chains of different fibrin monomers. The total number of cross-linkages appears to be approximately six per mole of fibrin, four of which involve the α chain and two of which involve the γ chain.

Thrombin

Thrombin is generated from prothrombin through the concerted action of several factors. Unlike most related serine proteases of the blood coagulation and fibrinolytic pathways, α-thrombin, with high procoagulant and all other thrombin-ascribed activities, has several diverse functions in hemostasis. It is implicated also in wound healing and in various disease processes. Thrombin's principal functions are the activation of plasma proteins (fibrinogen, factors V, VII, and XIII, protein C, protein S, and complement components), and the stimulation of leukocytes and platelets, endothelial cells, and smooth muscle. Although thrombin functions mainly as a serine protease with arginine or lysine-directed specificity, it possesses nonenzymatic activity involving receptor occupancy with monocytes and neutrophils. The regulation of thrombin involves proteinase inhibitors (such as antithrombin III, heparin cofactor II, and α₂-macroglobulin), control of thrombin generation (factors V and VIII), and thrombin partitioning within the clot (Fenton, 1989).

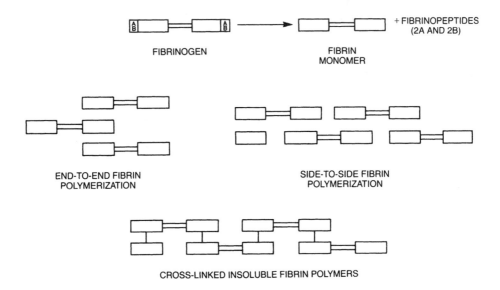

Figure 14.13. The cleavage and stabilization of fibrinogen by thrombin.

Josse Pathway

Although the classic coagulation pathway generally is accepted, there is evidence of an alternate system. Hemophilic plasma does not generate normal amounts of thrombin activity when plasma coagulation is triggered with a diluted thromboplastin solution (Biggs and Nossel, 1961). It is believed that factor VII is essential for the procoagulant activity of diluted thromboplastin (Josse and Prou-Wartelle, 1965). Direct evidence for a possible linkage between both classic pathways was reported (Østerud and Rapaport, 1977) in which a mixture of factor VII and thromboplastin could activate factor IX in a partially purified system. It also was shown that factor VIIa in the presence of thromboplastin can activate both factor IX and factor X (Marlar and Griffin, 1981; Morrison and Jesty, 1984).

The interaction between the intrinsic and the extrinsic pathways of coagulation might explain several different observations. Some patients with a factor VII deficiency have a major bleeding problem, whereas patients with deficiencies in the contact activation system experience little or no bleeding but may suffer thromboembolic episodes (Mr. Hageman). The importance of factors IX and VIII in the thromboplastin-dependent process in these situations in which trace amounts of thromboplastin are present has been postulated. In vivo triggering of thrombin formation by small amounts of thromboplastin, if common, may explain the situation in hemophiliacs, in whom the deficiencies of the intrinsic pathway are uncompensated by the intact extrinsic system (Ma et al., 1989).

Physiologic Limitations of Coagulation

The process of blood coagulation requires the complicated interaction of many enzymes on protein substrates. This cascading mechanism leads to a biological amplification of the process, which, if left unchecked, would culminate in the formation of many thrombi and ultimately would result in death. Physiologic control of this process is divided into three mechanisms: (1) that involving local processes, (2) that involving humoral activity, and (3) that involving cellular action.

Local Control

The local processes of hemostatic control primarily reside in the ability of the circulation to wash away and dilute active coagulants from the injury site. In addition, the fibrin seal covering the injured vessel acts to restrict the active coagulants to the interior of the hemostatic plug.

Humoral Inhibitors

One of the principal methods of controlling the hemostatic mechanism is by the action of physiologic inhibitors. Among these are antithrombin III, α_2-macroglobulin, and plasmin. Table 14.9 shows naturally occurring protease inhibitors.

Antithrombin III is a single-chain glycoprotein synthesized in the liver. It reacts with several proteases, including factors IXa, XIa, XIIa, and VII, but its principal physiologic activity is in its neutralizing effect of factor Xa and thrombin (Barrowcliffe, 1979). Antithrombin III is also the essential cofactor for the action of heparin, a naturally occurring sulfated mucopolysaccharide used as an anticoagulant.

α_2-Macroglobulin is a glycoprotein that forms a complex with various proteolytic enzymes, including thrombin, kallikrein, and plasmin. It differs from antithrombin III in its action on thrombin in that it acts more slowly, but it inhibits plasmin rapidly.

Newer thrombolytic agents, prourokinase and acylated plasminogen streptokinase complex (APSAC), have been developed in the hope that they will act more specifically on fibrin and less on thrombin. Prourokinase is derived from the urine and is a precursor of urokinase. This thrombolytic is capable of significant thrombolysis without causing severe systemic hypofibrinogenemia, hypoplasminogenemia, or depletion of α_2-antitrypsin. APSAC is prepared from pasteurized human plasminogen. Plasmin is discussed below.

Fibrinolysis

Fibrinolysis is a physiologic process of removing unwanted, insoluble deposits by enzymatic cleavage of fibrin to produce soluble fragments. The system involves activation by tissue-related activators of a plasma proenzyme, plasminogen, forming

Table 14.9. Naturally Occurring Protease Inhibitors

Inhibitor	Protease Inhibited	Potentiated by Heparin	Speed of Inhibition
α_1-Antitrypsin	Thrombin, factor XIa, factor Xa, kallikrein, plasmin	—	Slow
Antithrombin III	Factors Xa, XIa, IXa and XIIa, thrombin, kallikrein, plasmin (in the presence of heparin)	—	Slow
α_2-Macroglobulin	Factors XIIa and XIa, thrombin, kallikrein, plasmin	+	Rapid
C' inhibitor	Factors XIIa and XIa, kallikrein, factor XIIf, plasmin	—	Slow
α_2-Antiplasmin	Plasmin	—	Rapid
Protein C	Thrombin	—	Rapid

plasmin, a specific protease that digests stabilized fibrin polymers.

Plasminogen is a β-globulin synthesized by the liver. It exists in serum or plasma in multiple molecular forms, the most important of which has glutamic acid at the NH_2-terminal end. The conversion of plasminogen to plasmin requires splitting an internal arginyl-valine bond, which results in an active enzyme. The outcome is a heavy chain and a light chain combined by a single disulfide bond. The active site of plasmin is on the light chain (Winman, 1977).

Plasminogen undergoes spontaneous activation to plasmin, but the resulting plasmin tends to be unstable. The natural degradation of fibrin involves a pathway similar to that of the intrinsic coagulation pathway. Plasminogen becomes converted to plasmin, which is capable of cleaving fibrinogen, fibrin, factor V, and factor VII. Activation of this conversion is effected by a variety of proteolytic enzymes termed *plasminogen activators* (Figure 14.14). These enzymes are principally concentrated in the lysosomes of most cells, their level being highest in the endothelial cells of the vessels of the microcirculation and lowest in large vessels. Plasminogen activators are found also in small amounts in the plasma, probably having originated from endothelial cells. Urokinase, a polypeptide isolated from urine and synthesized by the kidney, is also a potent activator of plasminogen, as well as streptokinase, thrombin, factor XII, prekallikrein, and kallikrein.

Tissue-type plasminogen activator (t-PA) is the most important plasminogen activator. It is secreted by the endothelial cells and is unique in that it can be released rapidly in large amounts in response to various stimuli. Unlike other coagulation and fibrinolytic factors, t-PA does not circulate as an inactive zymogen but is present in the circulation in an active form, continuously interacting with plasminogen activator inhibitor (PAI) to form an inactive complex.

t-PA is a single-chain glycoprotein with a molecular weight of 65,000 d. Its half-life is between 3 and 5 minutes. It activates its substrate plasminogen to produce plasmin and shows a marked diurnal fluctuation, with levels approximately 25% lower in the afternoon than in the morning. Clinically, t-PA levels are increased slightly with advancing age. High levels have been associated with bleeding tendencies and lower levels with a tendency to develop thrombotic disease.

PAI is a fast-acting inhibitor of t-PA that is present in both plasma and platelets. PAI concentrations in platelets are nearly four times greater than those in the plasma. This inhibitor is a single-chain glycoprotein with a molecular weight of 50,000 d. It is released continuously into the circulation by the endothelial cells and, like t-PA, shows a large interindividual and diurnal fluctuation. Its estimated half-life is approximately 15 minutes. PAI concentrations are increased in thrombi as a result of significant platelet release of the inhibitor. Like t-PA, PAI levels are increased slightly with advancing age, in sepsis, and in pregnancy. High values are associated with a thrombotic tendency. Decreases are seen in the long-term administration of synthetic anabolic steroids and in women taking oral contraceptives (Krutihof et al., 1967).

The action of plasmin on fibrinogen and fibrin produces two principal products: (1) small frag-

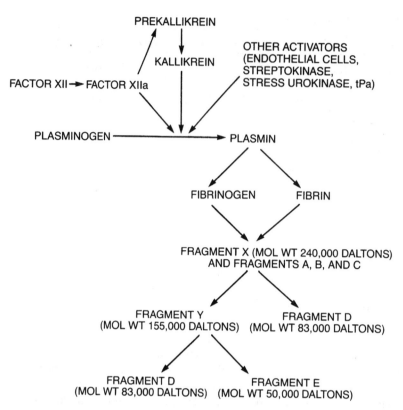

Figure 14.14. The fibrinolytic pathway. (tPa = tissue-type plasminogen activator.)

ments (A, B, and C), which are not clearly defined, and (2) larger HMW fragments, which undergo further cleavage to produce a series of small products, the largest of which is fragment X. This fragment still possesses the clotting property when exposed to thrombin, unlike the other degraded fractions produced. The remainder of the split products—fragments Y, D, and E—are incapable of clotting and actually possess inhibitory effects on clot formation.

Of the fibrin split products produced by this cleavage, only fragments D and E are stable against further plasmin action. Each has been shown to contain an antigenic determinant identical to one of the multiple determinants of the parent fibrinogen molecule. The larger intermediate fragments (X and Y) possess multiple antigenic determinants identical to those of fibrinogen.

Different amidolytic assays for t-PA have been described. One relies on the activation of purified plasminogen to plasmin in the presence of fibrinogen fragments that stimulate the t-PA activity in the test plasma. t-PA activity is measured using a specific chromogenic substrate. Another method uses the capture of t-PA on specific antibodies bound to a solid-phase matrix. Plasminogen is added with a stimulator of t-PA activity, and the plasma produced is measured with chromogenic substrates. Other methods that measure t-PA include enzyme-linked immunosorbent assay and chromogenic substrates specific for t-PA.

The first measurement of increased fibrinolysis was the whole-blood clot lysis test. The procedure is time-consuming and was replaced by the euglobulin lysis time. The latter test uses an acid-precipitated euglobulin fraction of the plasma that contains fibrinogen, plasminogen, plasminogen activator, and plasmin. Shortened clot lysis times indicate accelerated fibrinolysis, whereas prolonged times reflect reduced fibrinolytic activity.

Plasminogen

Abnormal levels of plasminogen have been reported in a variety of diseases and in some physiologic states. Increased levels have been documented in acute bacterial infections, inflammatory conditions, thrombophlebitis, surgery, myocardial infarction, and pregnancy, and after long-term use of oral contraceptives. Reductions in plasminogen have been found in intravascular coagulation and cirrhosis (Lackner and Javid, 1973). Plasma plasminogen levels can be measured by caseinolytic methods (Johnson et al., 1969), fibrin plate methods (Lassen, 1952), chromogen substrate assays (Mattler and Bang, 1977), immunologic methods (Becker, 1969), and fluorescent substrate assays (Pochron et al., 1978).

Cellular Control

Hemostatic control is regulated in part by the removal of active materials by the reticuloendothelial system. The liver has been recognized to clear actively fibrinogen degradation products, prothrombinase, and factors IXa, Xa, and VIIa (Deykin and Cochios, 1968), as well as particulate fibrin and fibrin monomers (Budzynski and Marder, 1977).

Chapter 15

Disorders of Blood Coagulation

Inherited Disorders

Classic Hemophilia (Hemophilia A)

Classic hemophilia is the most common form of a hereditary clotting factor deficiency. It is inherited as an X-linked recessive trait occurring almost exclusively in males. The recessive gene is located on the X chromosome and is closely linked to the chromosome of color blindness (Whittaker et al., 1962) and glucose-6-phosphate dehydrogenase (Boyer and Graham, 1965).

The disorder is the result of a deficiency of a small subunit of the factor VIII molecule termed *factor VIII antigen* (factor VIII:Ag) (see page 181). The frequency of the disease approximates 1:25,000, and it is more commonly found in Germanic peoples than in persons of Asian origin. Female carriers of the trait are generally asymptomatic, being protected by the production of sufficient clotting factor by cells under the control of the normal gene-bearing X chromosomes. Occasionally, symptomatic carriers are found whose levels of factor VIII:Ag are reduced and who exhibit bleeding symptoms similar to those found in mild hemophilia. This is believed to be due in part to the large error of the assay method and to the wide range of factor VIII:Ag in the normal population. The immunoassay methods of measuring factor VIII, which is either normal or increased in the carrier state, appear to improve the carrier detection rate (Ratnoff and Jones, 1977).

Classic hemophilia in females is extremely rare. It can result from the mating of a male hemophiliac with a female carrier, from a chromosomal abnormality that allows homozygous expressions of the trait in a phenotypic female, or from a spontaneous hemophilic gene mutation on the normal gene-bearing X chromosome in the daughter of a hemophiliac or carrier (Mori et al., 1979).

The clinical problems associated with classic hemophilia are related to hemorrhage and its consequences. The first indication that a bleeding disorder is present may be hemorrhage after circumcision or from the umbilical cord. However, there may be a few symptoms during the first few months or even the first year of life. In mild hemophilia, the disorder may not be suspected for years or until prolonged bleeding is encountered following a surgical crisis or major trauma. Hemorrhages can occur both externally and internally, the most common sites being the nose, mouth, eyes, gastrointestinal tract, urinary tract, and joints, and sometimes superficial abrasions. Such bleeding frequently results in large hematomas that cause secondary conditions, especially joint hemorrhages (hemarthrosis). These hematomas often affect the extension and flexion of the joint involved, limiting movement. They are seen most often in the knee and elbow. Hemorrhages into the large muscles, such as the buttocks, can result in considerable blood loss, as can gastrointestinal bleeding. In such situations, a rapidly progressive normocytic anemia results. The major cause of death is intracranial hemorrhage (Aledort, 1976), and the most frequent problem and major cause of disability is hemarthrosis. The usual clinical signs and factor VIII levels are shown in Table 15.1.

Table 15.1. Clinical Severity of Various Levels of Factor VIII Depletion

Degree of Severity	Factor VIII (%)	Clinical Signs
Severe	0–1	Spontaneous joint and soft-tissue bleeding
Moderate	2–10	Rarely, spontaneous bleeding
		Major hemorrhage possible after minor trauma
Minor	10–30	Severe bleeding following surgery
Carrier	30–60	Occasional excessive bleeding with major surgery

Laboratory Findings and Diagnosis

Diagnosis of the disorder should start with a carefully obtained, accurate history. Although this is outside the scope of discussion for this text, it must be emphasized that this is the first and probably most important step in arriving at a diagnosis. The laboratory results in classic hemophilia are often well defined in patients with a severe deficiency. The whole blood clotting time, once recognized as a general screening test, is now acknowledged to be insensitive to factor VIII deficiencies greater than 4% of normal and is considered a nonspecific test for clotting factor deficiencies (Didisheim and Lewis, 1958; Weiss, 1983).

The one-stage prothrombin time (PT) measures coagulation by the extrinsic pathway, as shown in Figure 14.10. This test gives abnormal results in individuals with deficiencies of factors VII, X, or V; prothrombin; or fibrinogen, but it does not detect abnormalities in the intrinsic coagulation pathway. Consequently, factor VIII coagulant (factor VIII:C) deficiencies produce normal one-stage PT tests.

Unlike the one-stage PT, the partial thromboplastin time (PTT) is sensitive to factor deficiencies involving the intrinsic pathway, but it does not detect reductions in factor VII of the extrinsic pathway. As such, this test is an effective and sensitive screening test for classic hemophilia, because it gives abnormal results when the factor VIII level is approximately 25–30% of normal. The abnormality shown by the PTT can be corrected by the admixture of the patient's plasma with approximately 20% fresh adsorbed normal plasma or another reagent that contains factor VIII:C.

Other laboratory test results that are characteristically normal are the platelet count, platelet function tests including bleeding time, and the thrombin time. Prolonged bleeding times in classic hemophilia have been reported in as many as 20% of patients (Buchanon and Holtkamp, 1980; Eyster et al., 1981; Smith et al., 1984). This appears to be particularly emphasized when using the Simplate technique described on page 390, and a distinction should be made between the results obtained using this newer method and those obtained using the older Ivy and Duke procedures. Prolonged bleeding (as determined by the Simplate technique) that is associated with a low factor VIII:C level is not necessarily indicative of von Willebrand's syndrome (Smith et al., 1984). The thromboplastin generation test (TGT) and the prothrombin consumption test (PCT) give abnormal results even in fairly minor cases of hemophilia and are now used only rarely. The more practical and more sensitive PTT is favored. The TGT is useful, however, because it is sensitive to abnormalities of platelet function. In principle, the TGT measures the amount and rate of formation of the prothrombinase complex in the intrinsic pathway. Table 15.2 illustrates the typical laboratory findings in classic hemophilia.

The common screening tests used to separate patients with abnormal findings are usually nonspecific in nature, unless cross-correction studies using factor VIII–deficient plasma and normal plasma are used. Definitive diagnosis requires specific factor assay and exclusion of combined deficiencies or acquired disorders in which factor VIII may be deficient. The assay of factor VIII can be carried out using either a two-stage or a one-stage technique, the former method detecting approximately 20% more factor VIII than the one-stage method (Kirkwood et al., 1977). Such factor VIII:C assays are simple to carry out using lyophilized preparations of concentrated factor VIII or lyophilized citrated plasma. The assay of factor VIII:Ag is based on the use of the immunoradiometric assay or enzyme-linked immunosorbent assay using natural factor VIII and monoclonal antibodies.

Table 15.2. Screening Test Results in Classic Hemophilia

Abnormal Results	Normal Results	Comments
Partial thromboplastin time (PTT)	One-stage prothrombin time (PT)	The PTT is sensitive to factor VIII levels at the 25% range. The one-stage PT measures the extrinsic pathway factors and not those involved in the intrinsic pathway.
Thromboplastin generation test (TGT)	Thrombin time (TT)	The TGT is approximately as sensitive as the PTT but requires the use of serum, barium sulfate–adsorbed plasma, and platelets. The TT measures only fibrinogen levels and is not involved directly in the intrinsic pathway.
Prothrombin consumption test (PCT)	Ivy bleeding time, template bleeding time	The PCT is sensitive to factor VIII levels of approximately 10%. The test is affected by thrombocytopenia and deficient platelet function. The template bleeding time is abnormal 65% of the time in classic hemophilia.*
Plasma recalcification time (PRT)	Platelet count	The PRT has a degree of sensitivity similar to that of the PCT. It can be modified by using platelet-rich or platelet-poor plasma. It now is used rarely.
Coagulation time (CT)	Tourniquet test	The CT is insensitive to factor VIII levels greater than 1%. It is abnormal only in the most severe clinical situations.

*Data from PS Smith, et al. The prolonged bleeding time in hemophilia A: comparison of two measuring technics and clinical associations. Am J Clin Pathol 83:211, 1984.

Methods to detect the carrier state make use of antibodies to purified factor VIII and rely on the fact that classic hemophilia patients have normal amounts of a protein that is antigenically related to factor VIII but possesses no clotting activity (Zimmerman et al., 1971). It has been shown that known carriers of the disease have factor VIII levels similar to those of noncarrier women, but their factor VIII activity levels are only about half that of the antigen levels (Hathaway et al., 1976). Using the ratio of factor VIII activity to factor VIII:Ag, more than 90% of carriers can be detected (Bennett and Ratnoff, 1973). The most sensitive and specific methods for the detection of carrier states appear to be the one-stage factor VIII activity assay and a radioimmunoassay procedure for the quantitation of factor VIII:Ag.

Inhibitors of Factor VIII

The incidence of circulating inhibitors in classic hemophilia is between 3 and 20% of all patients (Weiss, 1975). These inhibitors tend to develop in severely affected young patients, approximately 37% of them presenting before the age of 10 years and more than 60% presenting by 20 years of age (Brinkhous et al., 1972). Besides their spontaneous occurrence, these inhibitors are seen in individuals receiving prolonged treatment of factor VIII–rich cryoprecipitate or concentrates. Additional idiopathic inhibitors are seen during pregnancy.

Inhibitors to factor VIII are specific IgG immunoglobulins that can be neutralized both in vivo and in vitro with factor VIII. The antibody usually contains a single κ light chain, but λ chains also are found. Both alloantibodies and autoantibodies to factor VIII consist of the IgG_4 subclass or mixtures of IgG_4 and other IgG subtypes. The preponderance of the IgG_4 subclass may explain why immune complex disease is not seen and precipitin reactions are not detected.

The kinetics of the interaction of the factor VIII molecule with human anti–factor VIII antibodies is complex. The reaction follows one of two paths. Type I antibodies totally inactivate factor VIII. There is a linear relationship between residual factor VIII activity and antibody concentration. The type I kinetic pattern is seen with antibodies occurring in patients with classic hemophilia.

Most factor VIII antibodies occur in nonhemophilic patients and display a complex reaction known as type II kinetics. Type II antibodies do not completely inactivate factor VIII, and there is a nonlinear relationship between residual factor VIII:C activity and antibody concentration. With type II antibodies, measurable factor VIII:C activity may be present in the patients' plasma even in the presence of detectable inhibitor. Antibodies with type I and type II kinetics are directed against different antigenic sites of the factor VIII complex. Type II antibodies with complex kinetics will display type I kinetics if purified factor VIII, free of von Willebrand factor (vWF), is used. The interaction of type II antibodies with factor VIII is likely sterically hindered by vWF.

The detection of inhibitors usually follows the discovery of the accelerated disappearance of factor VIII after transfusion. In the laboratory, the presence of inhibitors is best recognized by the failure of normal plasma to correct the clotting time of a test plasma. The general screening tests (PTT, TGT, etc.) all show results identical to findings in an uncomplicated hemophilia. The addition of normal plasma to factor VIII–deficient plasma should shorten the PTT to normal but, in the presence of an inhibitor, the factor VIII of the normal plasma will be inactivated so that its corrective effect on the PTT will be reduced. The extent to which the factor VIII of the normal plasma is inactivated depends on the strength of the inhibitor and the conditions of the test system. The action of inhibitors on factor VIII is progressive with time. When an inhibitor is present in high concentration, a large amount of factor VIII can be inactivated rapidly, and the result may be abnormal findings in mixing tests, even without incubation. If the inhibitor level is minimal, sufficient factor VIII may still be active so that the PTT will be corrected to normal: Consequently, the antibody would be missed. By incubating the correction mixture, low levels of inhibitor are allowed to react with the factor VIII, thereby impairing the correction of the clotting test. Factor VIII inhibitors appear to be temperature-dependent, being most active at 35°–40°C (Leitner et al., 1963), and mixing tests for their detection usually are incubated for 1–2 hours.

Procedures for factor VIII assays and factor VIII inhibitor detection are given on page 357.

von Willebrand's Syndrome

The von Willebrand syndrome is the third most common of the hemophilias, found in approximately 10% of all hemophilia patients. The disorder is usually inherited as an autosomal codominant condition, but at least two other variants of the syndrome are recognized: a rare autosomal recessive form (Italian Working Group, 1977) and an X-linked recessive type (Holmberg and Nilsson, 1973).

The syndrome is characterized by a prolonged bleeding time and low levels of factor VIII:C activity, vWF antigen, and an impaired response of platelet aggregation to the antibiotic ristocetin. The exact nature and biochemical makeup of the factor VIII molecule are unclear, but several investigators have proposed that factor VIII is a complex of two molecules: a large fragment (vWF) and a smaller active molecule (factor VIII:C antigen). These are theorized to be linked together by noncovalent bonds (Owen and Wagner, 1972; Van Mourik et al., 1974; Weiss and Sussman, 1974).

According to this theory, the small molecule is produced under the control of an X-linked gene and carries with it both the active site for factor VIII activity and the antigenic site, which reacts with factor VIII inhibitor. The larger molecule is believed to be an aggregate of subunits synthesized under the control of an autosome, and it carries with it a binding site for the smaller active factor VIII:C and one or more sites involved in platelet adhesion and ristocetin-induced platelet aggregation (Weiss, 1983).

In contrast to the low molecular weight of factor VIII (150,000 d), the molecular weight of the von Willebrand protein has been estimated to be in excess of 20 million d (Miller et al., 1984). This protein appears to be constructed of a series of monomers of approximately 2 million d that make up a multimer possessing hemostatic properties (Zimmerman and Ruggeri, 1982). vWF is a glycoprotein synthesized by endothelial cells and megakaryocytes. It is either secreted constitutively or is stored in Weibel Palade bodies or α-granules of the endothelial cells or platelets, respectively. The main role of von Willebrand protein is in platelet adhesion to foreign surfaces, particularly after vessel rupture. Binding sites for heparin, collagen, factor VIII, and the platelet glycoproteins Ib and the IIb-IIIa complex have been identified (Bockenstedt et al., 1986; De Marco et al., 1986; Fujimura et al.,

Table 15.3. Classification of von Willebrand's Syndrome

	Type IA	Type IB	Type IIA	Type IIB	Type IIC	Type IID	Type III
Bleeding time	A	A	A	A	A	A	A
vWF Ag	L	L	N/L	N/L	N	N/LN	L/Ab
vWF Function	L	L	L	N/L	L	L	Ab
Factor VIII:C	L	L	N/L	N/L	N	N	L
Ristocetin-induced platelet aggregation	N/L	N/L	L/Ab	H	L	L	Ab
Genetics	AD	AD	AD	AD	AR	AD	AR

A = abnormal; L = low; N = normal; Ab = absent; AD = autosomal dominant; AR = autosomal recessive; vWF = von Willebrand factor; Ag = antigen.

1986). Platelet vWF is also important in mediating the adhesion of platelets to collagen. vWF is essential in providing a normal platelet thrombus.

von Willebrand's syndrome is not a single disorder but, as the name suggests, a heterogeneous group of diseases that have in common an abnormality in the von Willebrand protein, both quantitatively and qualitatively. The more common autosomal dominant forms generally are classified now on the basis of laboratory tests.

The clinical picture is frequently variable (Zimmerman and Ruggeri, 1983), showing cutaneous and mucosal bleeding in the milder forms. In the more severe form, hemarthroses and bleeding manifestations similar to those in classic hemophilia are seen. Petechial hemorrhages are rare, but epistaxis, gastrointestinal bleeding, and menorrhagia are common.

Laboratory results in patients with von Willebrand's syndrome are known to vary and may be normal on any given occasion (Abildgaard et al., 1980). Another variable is the effect of ABO genes on the vWF; individuals who are group O usually have reduced levels of the factor compared to group A, B, or AB individuals (McCallum et al., 1985; Cox et al., 1987).

Laboratory Findings and Diagnosis

The criteria for definitive diagnosis of von Willebrand's syndrome are unclear. Laboratory tests are used to separate the syndrome into two principal groups (Table 15.3). Type I von Willebrand's syndrome classically presents with decreased levels of von Willebrand protein, ristocetin cofactor, and factor VIII:C. The type II variant is recognized by the lack of the high-molecular-weight (HMW) von Willebrand protein. In type IIa, high concentrations of ristocetin are unable to produce significant platelet aggregation, whereas in type IIb, platelet aggregation is produced with low concentrations (<0.9 mg/ml) of ristocetin. A third type II variant, type IIc, has been documented. In this type, the large vWF multimers are lacking (Ruggeri et al., 1982). The distinguishing characteristic of this disorder is that it is inherited in an autosomal recessive manner. More recently, type IId has been described (Kinoshita et al., 1984). This form of the disorder is characterized by the loss of HMW factor VIII:Ag multimers and the replacement of the normal triplet multimer by a single dense band on agarose electrophoresis. Patients with this variant can exhibit severe bleeding (Hill et al., 1985). The characteristics of the type III variant are shown in Table 15.3. The principle features are the autosomal recessive mode of inheritance combined with an absence of ristocetin-induced platelet aggregation.

An additional disorder showing the selective absence of the HMW multimers of plasma von Willebrand protein has been termed *platelet-type von Willebrand's syndrome* (Miller and Castella, 1982). As in type IIb von Willebrand's syndrome, patients with this form of the disease exhibit an increased platelet aggregation response to low concentrations of ristocetin; in addition, they tend to have borderline thrombocytopenia and marginally abnormal bleeding times, and their platelets exhibit an increased ability to bind circulating vWF. Platelet-type von Willebrand's syndrome also demonstrates increased platelet aggregation between botrocetin-treated platelets (botrocetin is a *Bothrops* venom factor) and vWF. Platelet aggregation is not affected by hexadimethrine bromide in this disorder (Takahashi et al., 1985).

Another von Willebrand variant that has been reported is characterized by increased ristocetin-induced aggregation and plasma vWF containing the full range of multimers (Weiss and Sussman, 1986).

The routine laboratory screening tests can be of value but sometimes are not helpful. The classic picture of a prolonged bleeding time in the absence of aspirin ingestion and of reductions in factor VIII activity are not always seen, and repeated testing may be necessary to establish a diagnosis. This situation may represent the confusing variant picture just discussed. When factor VIII activity is reduced, determination of both the factor VIII:Ag and factor VIII:C levels serves to separate von Willebrand's syndrome from mild classic hemophilia or a hemophilic carrier state. Although abnormal ristocetin-induced platelet aggregation is often found, this test is not specific for the disease, varying quantitatively (as previously stated) in the wide spectrum of the syndrome. The results of this test also are abnormal in the Bernard-Soulier syndrome.

The usual laboratory screening tests often show abnormalities of both the bleeding time and the PTT. This latter test reflects reductions in factor VIII:C. Unfortunately, the PTT data are highly variable and may be normal, reflecting only minor depressions of factor VIII:C. Specific assays are then required to determine the exact concentration of this protein. Factor VIII:Ag is often reduced, reflecting depressions of the von Willebrand protein (see page 181). The ratio of factor VIII:C to factor VIII:Ag is near unity but, in some individuals, normal levels of factor VIII:Ag are seen, as is a low factor VIII:C–factor VIII:Ag ratio.

The PCT results may be abnormal even when the PTT, bleeding time, and factor VIII:C determinations are normal. Platelet adhesion and ristocetin-induced platelet aggregation are more consistently abnormal, but they can occasionally be found to be normal. Table 15.4 illustrates the results of common laboratory screening tests in both classic hemophilia and von Willebrand's syndrome.

Inhibitors of von Willebrand Factor

Inhibitors of vWF are generally IgG antibodies, frequently inactivating factor VIII in the plasma. This inactivation is usually fast rather than a time-dependent reaction, as seen with specific anti–factor VIII antibodies. Factor VIII separated from vWF in high-ionic-strength solutions is not activated by these vWF antibodies.

Acquired vWF antibodies in patients without von Willebrand's syndrome have been associated with autoimmune or lymphoproliferative disorders. These antibodies interfere with ristocetin-induced platelet aggregation in vitro. Patient's with acquired vWF antibodies demonstrate low plasma levels of factor VIII and reduced levels of vWF antigen and vWF activity.

Factor IX Deficiency (Hemophilia B)

Factor IX deficiency is inherited as an X-linked recessive trait, the disorder being nearly five times as rare as classic hemophilia. Patients with this deficiency can be divided into three groups based on the neutralization of factor IX in the patient's blood by anti–factor IX antibody. One group, termed *cross-reacting material, positive* (CRM+), is characterized by full antigenic (but variable) reduced procoagulant activity of factor IX. The second group, *cross-reacting material, negative* (CRM−), shows lack of both antigenic and procoagulant activity, whereas a third group, *cross-reacting material* (CRM^R), is characterized by equally reduced antigenic and procoagulant activity (Roberts and Cederbaum, 1975). The CRM+ factor IX–deficient patients have been further subdivided into those who show prolonged PTs when ox brain thromboplastin is used (hemophilia B$_M$) (Hougie and Twomey, 1967) and those with normal ox brain PTs (hemophilia B$_{CHAPEL HILL}$) (Meyer and Larrieu, 1971; Roberts and Cederbaum, 1975). A fifth variant, hemophilia B$_{LEYDEN}$, has also been reported, in which factor IX concentrations increase and the bleeding tendency improves as the patient ages (Veltkamp et al., 1970).

Factor IX deficiency in females is rare and may be due to X-chromosomal aberrations in a heterozygote or homozygosity for the mutant gene. It is most frequently due to extreme lyonization in a heterozygote—that is, the chance inactivation of the X chromosome carrying the normal gene in a majority of the cells synthesizing factor IX. Most of the reported cases of factor IX deficiency in females have been mild, but moderate factor IX de-

Table 15.4. Laboratory Results in Classic Hemophilia and von Willebrand's Syndrome

Test	Classic Hemophilia	von Willebrand's Syndrome	Comments
Bleeding time	Normal	Normal–abnormal	Sensitivity in von Willebrand's syndrome depends on degree of abnormality in platelet adhesion
Coagulation time	Normal unless disease severe	Normal; very unusual to be abnormal	Very insensitive to factor levels greater than 1% of normal
Platelet count	Normal	Normal	—
Prothrombin time	Normal	Normal	Measures the extrinsic pathway only
Thrombin time	Normal	Normal	Affected only by fibrinogen deficiency or by the presence of high levels of antithrombins
Partial thrombo-plastin time	Prolonged	Normal–prolonged	Sensitive to factor VIII levels greater than 25–30% of normal
Prothrombin consumption test	Abnormal, shortened time	Abnormal, shortened time	Serum prothrombin time is more "normal" (i.e., closer to that of plasma)
Factor VIII: C	Deficient	Low–normal	—
Factor VIII:Ag	Normal	Reduced	—
von Willebrand protein	Normal	Deficient	—
Tourniquet test	Normal	Occasionally abnormal	Parallels platelet adhesion and the bleeding time in von Willebrand's syndrome
Platelet adhesion	Normal	Deficient	—
Platelet aggregation with ADP, collagen, and epinephrine	Normal	Normal	—
Platelet with ristocetin	Normal	Decreased	—

ADP = adenosine diphosphate.

ficiency in a female with a normal karyotype has been reported (Orstavik et al., 1985).

The clinical findings in factor IX deficiency are similar to those seen in classic hemophilia, although there is a tendency for them to be milder.

Laboratory Findings

Laboratory findings in factor IX deficiency characteristically resemble those in classic hemophilia, except that the clotting defect is corrected by aged normal plasma or normal serum but not by barium sulfate–adsorbed normal plasma. The coagulation time often is normal except in the most severe form of the disease, but both the PTT and the TGT are abnormal when the factor IX level decreases to less than 25% of normal. The definitive test is the factor IX assay, which is carried out in a manner similar to the factor VIII assay.

Factor IX Inhibitors

Antibodies to factor IX develop less frequently than in classic hemophilia. They occur in approximately 3% of severely affected deficient patients and are seen more commonly in individuals undergoing long-term therapy with plasma concentrates. Spontaneous factor IX inhibitors in nonhemophilic patients are rare, the antibody usually belonging to the IgG$_4$ subclass of immunoglobulins.

Factor X Deficiency

Factor X deficiency is a rare bleeding disorder that is inherited as an autosomal recessive trait. Both CRM$^+$ and CRM$^-$ variants have been described (Denson et al., 1970), as has as a third variant, factor X$_{FRIULI}$. In this latter disorder, the factor X is antigenically normal but nonfunctional (Girolami et al., 1970).

The bleeding history in factor X deficiency is not clinically distinguishable from that of factor VII deficiency. Neonatal bleeding may be found intestinally or intracranially. Hemarthroses can also be found during later life. Menstruation can be so severe as to be life-threatening but might be normal in some patients. Ecchymoses, hematomas, and epistaxis have all been reported, and severe bleeding can accompany minor surgery (Owen et al., 1975).

The laboratory tests show a normal platelet count, bleeding time, and thrombin time. The PT, PTT, and TGT are prolonged in proportion to the degree of the deficiency. The defect is corrected in vitro by aged normal serum but not by barium sulfate–adsorbed normal plasma. The Stypven time (Russell's viper venom) is usually prolonged, the exception being in factor X_{FRIULI} deficiency, in which normal results are found. Definitive diagnosis requires a specific factor X assay.

Factor XI Deficiency (Hemophilia C)

Factor XI deficiency is a rare autosomal, incompletely recessively inherited bleeding disorder (Rapaport et al., 1961). It is relatively common among Jews. Although usually only homozygous patients show significant bleeding tendencies, heterozygous parents and children of affected individuals often show reduced factor XI levels and exhibit mild hemorrhagic signs (Rimon et al., 1976). The concentration of factor XI in homozygous patients ranges from 5 to 15% of normal, producing mild symptoms that include ecchymoses, hematomas, epistaxis, and menorrhagia. Gastrointestinal hemarthroses and gingival bleeding are uncommon. The severity of the hemorrhages does not appear to be related to the concentration of factor XI. Premature infants have a markedly decreased level of factor XI, though the mechanisms behind this are unknown (Andrew et al., 1981).

The laboratory tests show normal platelet counts, bleeding times, PTs, and thrombin times. The PTT and TGT usually are mildly abnormal, as is the PCT. The PTT and TGT are corrected by both aged normal serum and barium sulfate–adsorbed plasma. The TGT often shows abnormal results only when both the plasma and the serum of the patient are combined. The coagulation time is most often normal and usually is increased only if the defect is severe. The definitive diagnosis is best made with specific factor XI assays.

Factor XII Deficiency

Factor XII deficiency is an inherited autosomal recessive defect, although dominant and codominant variants have been described (Bennett et al., 1972). The clinical effects of the deficiency are minimal. There is usually a lack of bleeding, even during minor surgery, although on occasion patients have complications resulting from thromboembolic disease. Because most individuals with factor XII deficiency are asymptomatic, a diagnosis is usually made during routine presurgical screening.

Factor XII is believed to be involved in the initiation of the intrinsic pathway and the mediation of a variety of other processes such as fibrinolysis, complement activation, inflammation, and chemotaxis.

The laboratory findings show abnormal PTT, TGT, and PCT results. The PTT and TGT are corrected by the addition of aged normal serum and barium sulfate–adsorbed plasma. The whole blood coagulation time is lengthened in severely deficient states and may be as long in glass tubes as it is in siliconized tubes. Bleeding time, platelet count, clot retraction, and PT all are normal. Specific assays for factor XII are diagnostic.

Prothrombin Deficiency

Prothrombin deficiency is an extremely rare autosomal recessive disorder that manifests a mild bleeding tendency with prothrombin levels that are approximately 10% active. Both CRM+ and CRM− variants of the disorder have been reported (Montgomery and Otsuka, 1978).

Clinically, the disorder commonly is diagnosed at or after birth, when bleeding from the umbilical stump or from circumcision is seen. Hematomas, epistaxis, ecchymoses, and hemorrhage from minor wounds are rare, although they are the most common symptoms found in older children and adults

(Weiss, 1983). Gastrointestinal bleeding, hematuria, and menorrhagia are less common.

The laboratory findings show abnormal PTs and PTTs. Coagulation time varies, depending on the severity of the defect. Bleeding time, platelet count, clot retraction, thrombin time, and TGT are normal. Specific assays for prothrombin, such as the two-stage method, are the most reliable tests for establishing the diagnosis.

Factor V Deficiency

Factor V deficiency, a rare autosomal recessive disorder, is characterized by easy bruising, mild to severe bleeding postoperatively, menorrhagia, umbilical hemorrhage, ecchymoses, epistaxis, and minor bleeding after trauma. Recurrent thrombophlebitis has been associated with factor V depletion (Manotti et al., 1989). The frequency of the disease approximates 0.5–1.0 per million population (World Health Organization, 1972).

Laboratory tests show prolonged PT, PTT, TGT, and Stypven times, and the coagulation time is abnormal in severe cases. These tests can be corrected to normal by the addition of barium sulfate-adsorbed plasma but not by the addition of aged serum. The TGT also is corrected by using normal platelets in place of the patient's platelets or platelet substitutes, as they provide a source of normal factor V. The PCT is abnormal and is not corrected by the addition of platelet substitutes. A definitive diagnosis can be made using a specific factor V assay.

Factor VII Deficiency

Factor VII deficiency is a rare autosomal recessive trait having a frequency similar to that of factor V deficiency (World Health Organization, 1972). Both CRM+ and CRM− variants have been reported (Ratnoff, 1972). Clinically, the newborn may bleed from the umbilical stump and following circumcision. Gastrointestinal and intracranial hemorrhages, ecchymoses, hematomas, gingival bleeding, hemarthroses, and bleeding from minor cuts are not uncommon. Menorrhagia is seen in affected females. Surgical and postpartum hemorrhages also are seen.

Most people with a hereditary deficiency of factor VII have bleeding episodes before they reach adulthood. The correlation between clinical bleeding and factor VII activity levels is poor. Studies using rabbit serum containing antibodies to factor VII have shown CRM^R in some patients with a deficiency of factor VII. The use of thromboplastin of different origins (human, ox, rabbit) can produce discrepant results. Patients with factor VII Padua (CRM+) have been found to have reduced factor VII coagulant activity with rabbit brain and rabbit brain-lung thromboplastin but normal factor VII activity using ox brain thromboplastin.

Factor VII deficiency can be divided into congenital and acquired forms. Disorders associated with the acquired form include vitamin K deficiency, malabsorption from the gastrointestinal tract due to antibodies, liver disease, and oral anticoagulant therapy.

The laboratory results show a prolonged PT that can be shortened by the addition of aged normal serum but not by barium sulfate–adsorbed plasma. Because the defect affects only the extrinsic coagulation pathway, the PTT and TGT are normal. Other normal tests include the Stypven time, bleeding time, platelet count, clot retraction, coagulation time, and thrombin time. Specific diagnosis requires factor VII assays.

Fibrinogen Abnormalities

Congenital afibrinogenemia is a rare autosomal recessive disorder. Homozygous individuals have no demonstrable fibrinogen, whereas heterozygous patients show reductions in their fibrinogen level and are termed *hypofibrinogenemic*.

In afibrinogenemia, hemorrhage in the newborn is common. It is seen principally at the umbilical stump and following circumcision and is often severe. Hematuria, gingival bleeding, ecchymoses, and excessive hemorrhage following minor abrasions are common, but major gastrointestinal bleeding, epistaxis, hemarthroses, and menorrhagia are seen less frequently. Wound healing may be defective (Fried and Kaufman, 1980).

Laboratory results are marked by abnormal findings in all tests that use a fibrin clot as their end point. They include the coagulation time, PT, thrombin time, and PTT. The PCT and TGT are normal. The thrombin time becomes abnormal when fibrinogen levels approach 70–100 mg/dl. The bleeding time is abnormal in approximately half of the patients and often is accompanied by mild depressions in the platelet count on the order of 100×10^9/liter. Fibrinogen levels determined by nonclotting assays, such as salting out methods, usually are normal or increased. The clotting time with reptilase is prolonged, sometimes to a greater degree than the thrombin time. Fibrinogen–St. Louis, however, has been associated with decreases in factor VII (Sherman et al., 1972), and fibrinogen–Baltimore IV with delayed fibrin monomer polymerization that remains uncorrected by the addition of calcium (Schmelzer et al., 1989).

Hypofibrinogenemic individuals usually have fibrinogen levels between 20 and 100 mg/dl. If present, bleeding is minor in contrast to that experienced by afibrinogenemic patients. Autosomal dominant and autosomal recessive patterns of inheritance can be seen. The laboratory data are similar to those obtained in afibrinogenemia, but the results are nearly always less severe.

Many qualitative abnormalities of the fibrinogen molecule have been reported. They are usually inherited as incompletely dominant autosomal traits: Homozygotes have only abnormal fibrinogen molecules, whereas heterozygotes have 50% normal and 50% abnormal fibrinogen molecules. These molecular abnormalities result in delayed clot formation due to either abnormal polymerization of fibrin monomers or abnormal cleavage of the fibrinopeptides A and B by thrombin. The bleeding tendency in most of the variants is usually mild, but easy bruising and prolonged bleeding after trauma are characteristic. Clinically, most patients are asymptomatic, although delayed wound healing and a tendency to thrombotic occlusions may be seen.

Congenital Fibrinolysis

Congenital disorders of increased fibrinolysis include increased plasma-plasminogen activator activity and deficiencies of α_2-antiplasmin. Diminished fibrinolytic activity has been associated with a variety of thrombolytic disorders, including plasminogen deficiency, decreased endothe-

lial generation of plasminogen activator activity, and some abnormal fibrinogens. Reduced levels of fibrinolysis have been associated with idiopathic venous thrombosis, oral contraceptive–induced and postoperative venous thrombosis, coronary artery disease, systemic lupus erythematosus (SLE), and thrombotic thrombocytopenic purpura (TTP).

Factor XIII Deficiency

Factor XIII deficiency is a rare autosomal recessive disorder, although families in which only male offspring were affected have been reported (Ratnoff and Steinberg, 1968). CRM$^+$ and CRM$^-$ variants have also been described (Ratnoff, 1972).

Clinical characteristics are often noted first at birth, and fatal hemorrhage from the umbilical cord has been documented (Walls and Losowsky, 1968). Hemorrhage generally is seen from cuts, and ecchymoses, intracranial hemorrhages, and hemarthroses also are common. Prolonged hemorrhage after minor surgery and poor wound healing with prominent scar formation are seen as well.

Laboratory results are mostly normal, including tests sensitive to the intrinsic and extrinsic coagulation pathways. Platelet counts and platelet function tests also are normal. The diagnostic test is the urea solubility test, which is based on the property of 5-M urea or 1% monochloroacetic acid to dissolve the unstabilized fibrin clot. However, this test is normal in the presence of approximately 1% factor XIII, as this small amount is apparently sufficient to induce fibrin cross-linking and to prevent clinical hemorrhage.

Prekallikrein Deficiency (Fletcher Factor)

Prekallikrein deficiency is believed to be inherited as an autosomal recessive trait (Hathaway et al., 1965). The disorder is similar to factor XII deficiency in that it has not been associated with clinical bleeding.

The laboratory results show a moderate lengthening of the PTT when activated by ellagic acid, as well as a lengthening of coagulation times, normal bleeding times, PTs, and thrombin times. The abnormal PTT may be made normal by incubating the plasma for 15 minutes with silicates. Activated PTT tests in which diatomaceous earths are used produce normal times even in moderately deficient plasmas (Abildgaard and Harrison, 1974). Specific prekallikrein assays using chromogenic substrates have been developed (Soulier and Gozin, 1979). Other coagulation tests show a prolonged euglobulin lysis time and abnormally slow contact activation.

High-Molecular-Weight Kininogen Deficiency (Fitzgerald Trait, Williams Trait, Fleaujeac Trait)

HMW kininogen deficiency is an extremely rare disorder that appears to be inherited as an autosomal recessive characteristic (Wuepper et al., 1975). Individuals with this deficiency are asymptomatic.

The laboratory tests include prolonged PTT and coagulation times. The PTT is abnormal when activated by either ellagic acid or diatomaceous earth activators, unlike the reaction seen in prekallikrein deficiency.

Other Inherited Disorders

Passovoy factor deficiency is a mild inherited autosomal dominant bleeding disorder. It is the result of an abnormality in the intrinsic pathway and is manifested by a mildly prolonged activated PTT (APTT).

Acquired Disorders

Vitamin K Deficiencies

The vitamin K–deficiency states include hemorrhagic disease of the newborn, biliary obstruction and other malabsorption disorders, liver disease, oral anticoagulation, and intestinal sterilization.

Hemorrhagic Disease of the Newborn

Hemorrhagic disease of the newborn is the result of a vitamin K deficiency in the infant, resulting in a modest decrease in all the vitamin K–dependent coagulation factors. This causes bleeding with surgical procedures, such as circumcision, and umbilical hemorrhage. The laboratory diagnosis is clear-cut. The PT is always prolonged, as are the PTT and the

coagulation time. Specific assays show deficiencies of prothrombin and factors VII, IX, and X. Factor V and fibrinogen levels are normal.

Liver Disease

Most coagulation factors are produced in the liver, the exception being von Willebrand protein, which is produced in the endothelium. The exact site of production of factor XII, prekallikrein, and HMW kininogen is still unclear, and consequently all coagulation factors (with the exception of factor VIII) may be deficient as a result of inadequate hepatic synthesis. Among these factors is the prothrombin group of vitamin K–related factors (see page 200), which may be deficient because of dietary restrictions or because of malabsorption caused by insufficient production of bile acids. Such a decrease in the wide spectrum of coagulation factors results in potential abnormalities in most laboratory tests, the degree of reduction relating to the severity of the hepatic disease. In addition to such results, fibrinolysins may be increased because of the inability of the liver to remove plasminogen activators, which causes chronic activation of the fibrinolytic pathway.

A number of conditions that cause thrombocytopenia may occur in patients with liver failure. These include splenomegaly, folate deficiency, disseminated intravascular coagulation (DIC) and, occasionally, bone marrow hypoplasia (Counts, 1984).

Oral Anticoagulation

Oral anticoagulants can be divided into two primary groups: the 4-hydroxy coumarins and the 1,3-indanediones. The anticoagulant action of these two groups is the same, but they differ in their absorption rates and the speed of their reaction with the vitamin K–dependent coagulation factors. Oral anticoagulants are absorbed from the intestinal tract, are bound to plasma albumin, and become hydroxylated in the liver. Their physiologic action inhibits normal production of prothrombin and factors VII, IX, and X, and protein C. Such inhibition results in the production of analogs that lack calcium-binding sites, which consequently are nonfunctional but otherwise are identical to normal factors (Stenflo, 1975). The plasma level of these factors falls in a sequence consistent with their in vivo survival times;

Table 15.5. Therapeutic Ranges of Thromboplastins

Thromboplastin	Range (Patient-to-Normal Ratio)
British comparative thromboplastin (UK), human brain	2.0–4.0
Thrombotest (Europe), ox brain–cephalin-adsorbed plasma	2.0–3.5
Rabbit brain-lung	1.5–2.1
Rabbit brain	1.3–1.7

Source: Data from L Poller. Oral Anticoagulant Therapy. In AL Bloom, DP Thomas (eds), Haemostasis and Thrombosis. Edinburgh: Churchill-Livingstone, 1981.

this sequence is factor VII, factor IX, factor X, and prothrombin. Such depressions result in prolonged PTs and, eventually, longer PTT times.

The lack of standardization of the PT test and the wide variations in the nature of the reagents used produce marked differences in tests done in different laboratories. This issue of comparability is compounded by the number of ways that the test results are reported: (1) as a time in seconds, (2) as a percentage activity derived from saline dilution curves, (3) as a prothrombin index, and (4) as a prothrombin ratio. Such poor agreement among PT tests is cause for much confusion and promotes use of different levels of anticoagulant therapy in different locations.

To achieve standardization in PT testing for oral anticoagulant control and thus to ensure reliable oral therapy, the International Committee for Standardization in Haematology and the International Committee on Thrombosis and Haemostasis have agreed on recommendations that are based on the results of international collaborative studies. These recommendations conform with those made by the World Health Organization (WHO), which used reference thromboplastins for testing purposes (World Health Organization, 1983). It has been proposed that manufacturers of thromboplastins used in oral anticoagulant control should indicate the relationship of each batch of material to the WHO International reference preparation by a number that describes the comparative slope (c). This is, at present, referred to as the *international sensitivity index* (ISI). The manufacturers should also provide a table showing the relationship between the conventional terms of expression of results of the test and the *international normalized ratio* (INR). This is calculated by the equation $INR = R_c$, where R is the PT ratio (patient PT:mean normal PT) and c is the comparative slope of the thromboplastin used (Loeliger, 1985; Loeliger et al., 1985). Recommended INR ranges between 2.0 and 3.0 are used to treat the

following disorders: prophylaxis and treatment of venous thrombosis; treatment of pulmonary embolism; prevention of systemic embolism; treatment of acute myocardial infarction; valvular heart disease; atrial fibrillation; and the prophylaxis of valvular heart disease.

INR ranges between 2.5 and 3.5 are recommended to treat recurrent systemic embolism and in patients with mechanical prosthetic valves.

The British comparative thromboplastin, a human brain material, produces longer PTs than the thromboplastin composed of rabbit brain or rabbit brain-lung mixtures that are seen commonly in the United States. The commonly used therapeutic range for the PT ratio in the United States has been 1.5–2.5. If the British ratio, ranging from 2.0 to 4.0, is used as a standard, both the rabbit brain and the rabbit brain-lung reagents at the upper range limit (Table 15.5) result in more aggressive anticoagulant therapy. Consequently, allowing the PT ratio to approach 2.5 may account for the higher frequency of bleeding reported in the United States than in Europe in patients treated with oral anticoagulants.

The American Heart Association recommends that, when using a rabbit brain or brain-lung thromboplastin that produces a control of 12 ± 1 second, anticoagulant therapy should be adjusted to yield a PT ratio of 1.5–2.0 (Wessler, 1984). For example, if the baseline PT is 12.5 seconds, the therapeutic range should be approximately 20–25 seconds. It must be stressed that these times are only approximations, and every laboratory must establish its own range, depending on the test conditions and reagents used (Walsh, 1985). The shortening of the test time when blood is collected in glass will affect this ratio, but this usually plays only a small part in test interpretation if the test is carried out without undue delay. It has also been reported that less intense anticoagulant therapy has been associated

Table 15.6. Common Medications Affecting Oral Anticoagulant Action

Potentiate action
    Anabolic steroids
    Neomycin
    Phenylbutazone
    Dilantin
    Quinidine
    Salicylates
    Quinine
    Tetracycline
    Tolbutamide
Depress action
    Adrenal corticosteroids
    Barbiturates
    Carbamazepine
    Ethchlorvynol
    Glutethimide
    Oral contraceptives

with a lower frequency of recurrent venous thromboembolism and a reduced rate of hemorrhage (Hull et al., 1982).

Many common drugs interfere with the action of oral anticoagulants, acting on mechanisms involving absorption, transportation action, and excretion. Some medications potentiate the action of oral anticoagulants, whereas others are antagonistic to their action. Table 15.6 illustrates some of the medications that interfere with oral anticoagulants.

Heparin Therapy

Heparin is a fast-acting dose-dependent mucopolysaccharide that, when introduced intravenously, has an in vivo half-life of 1–2 hours. Heparin interferes with hemostasis both in vitro and in vivo by inhibiting the action of factors XIII, XIIa, XIa, and IIa, which is accomplished by blocking the conversion of fibrinogen to fibrin and by inhibiting platelet aggregation by thrombin.

The anticoagulant activity of the drug depends on its molecular weight. Low-molecular-weight products obtained from porcine mucosa cause fewer bleeding problems because of limited alterations in platelet function (Triplett, 1982). HMW heparin from bovine lung may produce more hemorrhagic problems unless closely monitored. Three avenues of administration are available: (1) subcutaneous injection, (2) intermittent intravenous infusion, and (3) continuous intravenous infusion. The aim of ther-

apy is to produce an extension of thrombosis with minimal bleeding, which is best obtained at heparin concentrations of 0.2–0.5 units per milliliter of plasma.

The laboratory procedure classically used in monitoring heparin therapy is the Lee and White coagulation time. The test is difficult to reproduce and lacks sensitivity to high heparin doses; however, a modification of the test has been described that can be used at the bedside (Hattersley, 1966). This test, the activated coagulation time (ACT, described on page 345), also is poorly reproducible and is affected by excesses of contact factors liberated at the venipuncture site (Palkuti, 1985). A further modification of this test, the whole blood activated recalcification time test, has also been proposed as a means of monitoring heparin therapy (Reno et al., 1974). This procedure suffers from drawbacks similar to those of the ACT.

The thrombin time has been used as a means of quantitatively monitoring heparin activity, and it possesses the advantage of being able to detect any form of heparin administered. Furthermore, it is not influenced by deficiencies of plasma coagulation factors, such as factor VIII and factor V, as is the coagulation time. The principal disadvantage of the procedure is that it detects only the antithrombin action of heparin and not its action on other coagulation factors. However, when heparin concentrations exceed 0.1 units per milliliter of plasma, thrombin time is the most sensitive procedure available.

The most practical and probably the most commonly used test for the control of heparin therapy is the APTT (Banez et al., 1980). The test is easy to carry out and is relatively simple to control, and it can be readily batch-tested in the laboratory. The therapeutic range commonly used is similar to that used for the PT control of oral anticoagulants—namely, one and a half to two times the control value. This corresponds to a heparin level of 0.3–0.5 units/ml (Hirsh, 1984). Unfortunately, different PTTs vary in their sensitivity to heparin, particularly those activated with diatomaceous earths and, consequently, they may fail to detect therapeutic levels adequately (Brandt and Triplett, 1981). Such reagent variability may contribute to overdosage or underdosage of heparin in the individual patient. It has been found that the average plasma heparin activity required to double the baseline APTT values ranges from 0.11 to 0.27 units/ml for the most sensitive reagents and from 0.19 to 0.67 units/ml for

Table 15.7. Etiology of Disseminated Intravascular Coagulation

Group	Examples
Infectious diseases	Sepsis, gram-negative shock (particularly from *Escherichia coli* and *Pseudomonas*), viral or rickettsial infections, malaria
Obstetric accidents	Premature separation of the placenta, retained dead fetus or placental tissue, septic abortions, amniotic fluid embolism, eclampsia
Intravascular hemolysis	Hemolytic transfusion reactions, acute hemolytic anemia, venomous snake bites
Neoplasms	Acute progranulocytic leukemia, lymphoma, carcinoma of the prostate, ovary, bladder
Autoimmune diseases	Drug reactions, lupus erythematosus, acute glomerulonephritis
Postoperative conditions	Shock, pulmonary surgery
Hematologic disease	Severe sickle cell crises, acute leukemia, paroxysmal nocturnal hemoglobinuria
Miscellaneous	Heat stroke, fat embolism, hyaline membrane disease, burns, congestive cardiac disease, crush injury, tissue necrosis

the least sensitive reagents (Bjornsson and Nash, 1986). Because of this variation, each laboratory should determine its own therapeutic range using its own reagents and instrumentation. However, there is evidence that this traditional approach is of questionable clinical value, as it appears not to correlate well with bleeding levels (Triplett et al., 1978).

One test that does correlate well with clinical efficacy of heparin is the anti–factor Xa assay, but this assay system is not widely available. It has been suggested that subcutaneous or intrapulmonary heparin therapy can be controlled by plasma heparin and antithrombin III levels at approximately 1 hour after the commencement of therapy (Bick and Murano, 1985). If the plasma heparin level is greater than 0.01 unit/ml, it is assumed that adequate heparin is present, and if the antithrombin III level is greater than 60%, it also is assumed that this is sufficient for anti-Xa activity. If both of those criteria are met, no further monitoring is undertaken.

Disseminated Intravascular Coagulation

Etiology

DIC is a syndrome of multiple causes, in which either the intrinsic or extrinsic coagulation pathway is activated to produce intravascular fibrin deposits, leading to a diminution of the coagulation factors required in clot formation. Such reductions of these coagulation factors ultimately leads to hemorrhage when the factor levels drop to less than that required to maintain hemostasis. This process often is accompanied by the activation of fibrinolysins, which intensifies the bleeding tendency.

Table 15.7 shows the etiologic classification of DIC. Most DIC syndromes are acute illnesses and are generalized, but examples of localized reactions include microthrombi and glomerulonephritis. The mechanisms setting off the syndrome often are interrelated and involved and can range from increased platelet adhesion to the liberation of large quantities of *tissue thromboplastin* lipids released from ruptured cells. Such an entry of procoagulant tissue extracts into the circulation, especially from placental tissue, excites the extrinsic pathway to activate factor X to become factor Xa, thereby setting in motion the coagulation sequence. This also occurs in neoplasms, in which breakdown products from tumors act in a similar fashion. In acute leukemia, this activation mechanism results from the release of thromboplastins by leukemic cells, particularly from the granules of the immature cells.

DIC as a consequence of infections often is related to the release of endotoxins from the causative bacteria, which may lead to the activation of factor XII, increased platelet aggregation, and the inhibition of fibrinolysis. Another common triggering event for DIC is intravascular hemolysis. Such lysis can result from hemolytic transfusion reactions or from any intravascular hemolysis regardless of cause. Two basic mechanisms have been suggested in such an event. First, the release of red-cell adenosine diphosphate (ADP) is believed to initiate a platelet release reaction, with the subsequent generation of platelet factor 3 and consequent activation of the whole coagulation system.

Second, the release of larger quantities of red-cell membrane phospholipids during hemolysis may initiate the clotting sequence as well as stimulate the platelet release mechanism (Bick, 1983).

Pathophysiology

Figure 15.1 summarizes the manner in which various diseases can provide mechanisms that initiate DIC, the net result being the generation of thrombin and systemic plasmin. Figure 15.2 shows the pathologic features of DIC once this initiation has taken place. Under normal physiologic conditions, fibrin monomers polymerize into fibrin but, when plasmin is produced rapidly, as in DIC, fibrinogen is degraded, creating fibrin degradation products (FDPs). Increased FDPs form a complex with the fibrin monomer before it can polymerize into fibrin; the outcome of this process is a mixture of FDPs and fibrin monomers called *soluble fibrin monomers*. While this is occurring, other fibrin monomers polymerize, mainly in the microvascular system, and cause blockage of the microcirculation, tissue hypoxia and, ultimately, tissue necrosis. This enhances platelet entrapment and produces a concomitant thrombocytopenia.

Aside from its involvement in the production of degradation products of fibrin and fibrinogen, plasmin is capable of inactivating factors V, VIII, IX, and XI. This occurs as part of the massive DIC syndrome. In fact, it appears that plasmin is largely responsible for the hemorrhages seen in this syndrome. During such a hemorrhagic episode, factor XII often becomes activated to factor XIIa, which then indirectly activates the plasmin system by means of the kallikrein pathway and results in a secondary pathway for the production of FDPs. Plasmin also activates complement, which promotes cell lysis and the release of yet additional phospholipids.

Laboratory Findings

The laboratory results in a patient with DIC are highly variable and depend on the cause and severity of the hemorrhage. In general, the tests shown in Table 15.8 can be found to be abnormal at some point during the progression of the syndrome.

The PTT and PT frequently are increased in DIC for a variety of reasons, including plasmin digestion of factors VIII, IX, and XI, hypofibrinogenemia,

and the presence of FDPs. Occasionally, these tests do not produce prolonged results and are found to be normal or even shortened. The exact reasons for such results are unclear, but they may be due to rapid thrombin action on early degradation products or to the presence of circulating activated clotting factors such as factor Xa (Weiss, 1983).

The thrombin time is primarily increased because of the hypofibrinogenemia. Evidence of fibrinolysis can be obtained from this test by observing the formed clot for 10–15 minutes. The reptilase test is similar to the thrombin time with the exception that this test is useful also in monitoring patients with DIC who are receiving heparin therapy.

In most cases of DIC, thrombocytopenia is present. It is caused by the formation of platelet thrombi in the microcirculation. Recognition of the thrombocytopenia, together with a mild leukocytosis and the presence of schistocytes, can be made on a well-prepared peripheral blood smear.

Schistocytes are the result of a microangiopathic process, in which the red cells become fragmented and distorted as a result of their impact on the formed thrombi. Platelet function studies frequently give abnormal results because of the platelet coating of FDPs and, secondarily, because of the thrombocytopenia present. Consequently, the bleeding time, clot retraction, and tourniquet test results often will be abnormal.

FDPs are elevated significantly. The actual titer is not an indicator of the severity of the disease, as it depends on the interactions that take place between the degree of procoagulant activity and the level of fibrinolytic response, as well as other factors, such as the level of renal failure and the activity of the reticuloendothelial system.

Specific factor assays are of little additional value in obtaining a diagnosis or in establishing the prognosis of the syndrome. Such assays are difficult to carry out with speed and precision and may well produce inconsistent data because of the presence of circulating activated factors such as factor Xa and IXa or thrombin. These materials effectively bypass the factor being assayed and produce erroneous normal or increased outcomes. The protamine sulfate test for paracoagulation detects soluble fibrin monomers even after heparinization and is a good, rapid screening test. Care should be taken in interpreting this test, however, as fibrin monomers can be seen in disorders other than DIC, and the test

208

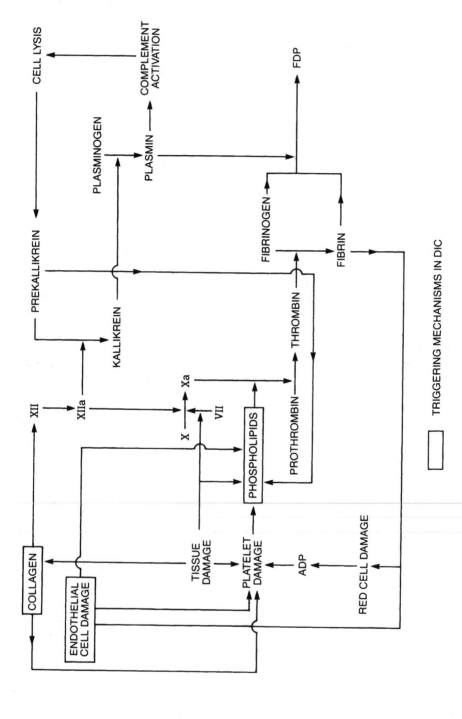

Figure 15.1. The mechanisms of initiation and activation of disseminated intravascular coagulation (DIC). (ADP = adenosine diphosphate; FDP = fibrin degradation products.)

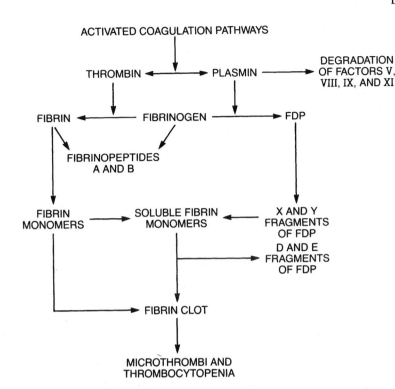

Table 15.8. Laboratory Results Commonly Seen in Disseminated Intravascular Coagulation

Abnormal partial thromboplastin time
Abnormal prothrombin time
Abnormal thrombin time
Abnormal reptilase test
Reduced fibrinogen level
Thrombocytopenia
Presence of fibrin degradation products
Positive protamine sulfate test
Reduced plasminogen levels
Antithrombin III consumption
Reduced factor VIII levels
Reduced factor V levels
Leukocytosis
Peripheral blood schistocytosis

can produce negative reactions in 5–10% of individuals with the syndrome. Like the protamine sulfate paracoagulation test, antithrombin III activity can be used to monitor DIC patients who are receiving heparin and are producing FDPs. Antithrombin III is an α_2-globulin that behaves as an acute-phase reactant and often is consumed by the production of thrombin and other serine proteases (Bick et al., 1976).

The PTT, reptilase test, fibrinogen determination, platelet count, and protamine sulfate test are a good combination for follow-up of DIC patients. These tests together offer the sensitivity and speed necessary for managing DIC and guiding treatment.

Hypercoagulation

Hypercoagulation is the term applied to a poorly defined condition that includes both inherited and acquired disorders associated with an increased risk of thrombosis. Among the hereditary disorders are deficiencies of naturally occurring anticoagulant proteins, and among the acquired disorders is malignancy. One-third of the patients have prolongations of the post–venous occlusion euglobulin lysis time and elevated levels of plasminogen activator inhibitor-1 levels. Two-thirds of the patients have reduced tissue-type plasminogen activator (t-PA), and 12% of these have antiphospholipid antibodies. Hereditary antithrombin III deficiency and hereditary deficiency of naturally occurring anticoagulant factors, protein S, and protein C are present in approximately 2% of such individuals (Doig et al., 1994).

Coagulation Inhibitors

Pathologic inhibitors of the blood coagulation pathways are abnormal endogenous components that may act on any stage of the process. These inhibitors often act on a specific factor and produce a hematologic picture resembling many of the inherited disorders previously discussed.

Factor VIII Antibodies

Factor VIII antibodies are the most common specific inhibitors seen. They are found in approximately 20% of patients with classic hemophilia (Strauss, 1969) and are most common in severely affected individuals. They are detected also in chronic inflammatory disease, in elderly asymptomatic persons, in drug reactions, and during pregnancy. In the patient with classic hemophilia, the use of standard replacement therapy is not effective, and in the nonhemophilic individual, the presence of inhibitors may produce life-threatening hemorrhage.

Most antibodies to factor VIII are IgG immunoglobulins (Shapiro, 1975) and do not appear to fix complement. The clinical symptoms associated with their presence are similar to those seen in classic hemophilia and include massive hemorrhage following minor trauma, diffuse hematomas, and spontaneous epistaxis. The laboratory findings also resemble those found in classic hemophilia. Factor VIII levels usually are so low as to be undetectable. Specific tests for antibodies usually give positive results, but the antibodies can more easily be detected following incubation of the patient's serum with substrate plasma containing factor VIII. Recently, a modified agarose gel procedure has been reported that is more sensitive and easy to perform (Cassidy et al., 1985).

Other antibodies directed against specific coagulation factors include inhibitors of factor IX (Reisner et al., 1977), factor V (Feinstein, 1978), factor XI (Leone et al., 1977), factor XII (Criel et al., 1978), factor XIII (McDevitt and McDonagh, 1972), and vWF (Sarji et al., 1974). Bleeding has been reported after inhibition of thrombofibrinogen

conversion (Marciniak and Greenwood, 1979) and in the presence of antithrombin III in liver disease.

Antithrombin III Deficiency

Antithrombin III is a serine protease that inhibits factors IXa, Xa, XIa, and XIIa. Adequate concentrations of antithrombin III are needed for pharmacologic efficacy of heparin and coumarin. For example, oral anticoagulants are ineffective on their own in preventing recurrent thrombosis unless a concomitant rise in antithrombin III also is present (Rothchild, 1983).

Deficiencies of antithrombin III can be either congenital or acquired. Congenital antithrombin III levels of 40–60% of normal are associated with spontaneous thrombosis—especially in older patients and those with infections, as well as after surgery and during pregnancy. The disease is transmitted as an autosomal dominant characteristic. There is no predictable age at which the antithrombin III deficiency will be manifested, although most cases do not present until the onset of puberty (Shapiro and Anderson, 1977). Causes of acquired deficiency include sepsis, liver disease, nephrosis, DIC, use of oral contraceptives, and eclampsia; acquired deficiency also may occur following the treatment of acute lymphocytic leukemia with L-asparaginase (Schorr and Menaché, 1983; Bick, 1982).

Acquired Fibrinolysis

Acquired disorders associated with increased fibrinolytic activity and bleeding include liver cirrhosis, amyloidosis, acute promyelocytic leukemia, some solid tumors, and snake envenomation syndromes.

Protein C

Protein C is a liver-synthesized protein composed of one heavy chain, the molecular weight of which is 41,000 d, and one light chain, the molecular weight of which is 21,000 d, linked together by disulfide bonds. The heavy chain contains an active serine component, whereas the amino terminal of the light chain contains calcium-binding γ-carboxyglutamic acid residues (La Croix and David, 1985). Also located on the light chain at position 71 is a unique amino acid of unknown function—β-hydroxyaspartic acid (Stenflo, 1984).

Protein C circulates as a zymogen precursor of a vitamin K–dependent protein. It is activated by thrombin, trypsin, and Russell's viper venom (Kisiel et al., 1977). This activation consists of cleaving a 12–amino acid sequence from the heavy chain, thus exposing a serine residue at its active site.

The activation of protein C is enhanced greatly by the presence of an endothelial cell surface cofactor, thrombomodulin, a 74,000-d molecular-weight protein. Thrombomodulin, in the presence of calcium, results in a tightly bound one-to-one complex of thrombin-thrombomodulin, which functions by increasing the activation of protein C 20,000-fold (Esmon and Esmon, 1984). When bound in this complex, thrombin can no longer function as a procoagulant in the cascade pathway, and so it becomes an anticoagulant through its activation role with protein C. This role change does not involve a permanent loss of coagulant ability but appears to be a reversible function.

Once activated, protein C forms a one-to-one complex with a cofactor, protein S. This is a single-chain glycoprotein with a molecular weight of 69,000 d (DiScripio et al., 1977). Like protein C, protein S is a vitamin K–dependent protein with many calcium-binding γ-carboxyglutamic acid residues. Once the protein C–protein S complex has formed, it binds to the surface of the phospholipid vesicle containing its specific substrates. Protein S then acts as a cofactor for protein C (free proteins). A second form of protein S also exists, bound to C4b-binding protein. It inhibits the early steps in the complement pathway and does not appear to be functionally active (Clouse and Comp, 1986).

Only a few cases of dysfunctional protein C have been reported. Of these, only protein C Cadiz has been fully described (Sala et al., 1987). The first variants identified are characterized by reduced amidolytic activity (Barbui et al., 1984). Reduced plasma protein C anticoagulant activities with normal levels of protein C amidolytic activity and protein C antigen have been found.

The ability to detect protein C activity depends on the type of assay used. As with antithrombin III and protein S, antigenic assays measure the total amount of the analyte but do not measure any functional activity. Unlike antithrombin III assays, the chromogenic method measures activity but not all functions of the molecule. The plasma concentration of purified protein C is approximately 4 µg/ml.

The specific substrates for activated protein C are factor V and factor VIII:C. For maximum coagulant activity, factor V and factor VIII:C must undergo proteolysis by thrombin with cofactors Va and VIIIa. Activated protein C causes further inactivation of these substances, inhibiting these cofactor activities in the cascade process. Only the factor VIII:C portion of the factor VIII molecule appears inactivated, the von Willebrand protein being unaffected (Holmberg et al., 1983). Activated protein C also enhances fibrinolysis by increasing circulating plasminogen activator activity (Comp and Esmon, 1981). The activation and formation of the protein C–protein S complex is shown in Figure 15.3.

Protein C deficiency is inherited as an autosomal dominant trait, with the heterozygous state associated with venous thrombosis and the homozygous state manifested by fatal thrombosis in the neonatal period (Griffin et al., 1981; Bertina et al., 1982; Seligsohn et al., 1984). An acquired deficiency state has also been reported in patients with chronic liver disease, in those with DIC, and following surgery (Mannuci and Vigano, 1982; Marlar et al., 1985). Furthermore, reductions of protein C are proportional to the degree of liver impairment and its normalization after acute hepatitis may represent an early marker of recovery. Protein S deficiency has been described in thromboembolic disease (Comp and Esmon, 1984; Schwartz, 1984).

The laboratory findings in protein C deficiency include increases in the APTT, abnormal factor V and factor VIII levels, increased plasminogen levels, and abnormal fibrinolysis. The protein can be quantitated by using rocket electroimmunoassay (Scott et al., 1991; Vasse et al., 1989).

Lupus-Type Antibodies

Lupus-type antibodies are immunoglobulins that inhibit phospholipid-dependent coagulation tests such as the PT, APTT, Russell's viper venom test, and the kaolin clotting time. The antibodies are not directed at any specific coagulation protein but only at the phospholipid epitopes. These inhibitors were believed to be associated directly with SLE but now are known to be found in a wide variety of disorders. They act principally on the inhibition of the conversion of factor X to factor Xa. The laboratory results

Figure 15.3. The activation and complexing of protein C.

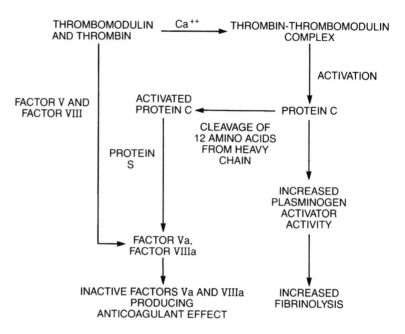

show an abnormal PTT, which is not corrected by the addition of normal plasma. The TGT is normal except when the patient's plasma is used as the substrate. Both the PT and the thrombin time are abnormal. Assays of specific coagulation factors are normal, even in the presence of the inhibitor, if tested by methods other than those using the PTT as a base. However, some PTT reagents are less sensitive to lupus-type antibodies, and these findings appear to be independent of the type of activator used (Brandt and Triplett, 1987). The kaolin clotting time, which is simply the kaolin APTT without platelet lipid substitute of platelet-poor plasma, appears to be more sensitive to the presence of the lupus inhibitor than is the dilute tissue thromboplastin inhibition test (Exner, 1985).

Lupus anticoagulants and cardiolipin antibodies are closely related autoantibodies found in immunologic, neoplastic, and infective disorders, and in asymptomatic individuals. Approximately 30% of patients with these antibodies have arterial or venous thrombosis, thrombocytopenia, and repeated abortions. Clinically, individuals with the lupuslike inhibitor rarely show bleeding tendencies but, if such bleeding does exist, it often is present concomitantly with a mild thrombocytopenia.

A laboratory scheme for the investigation of suspected lupus anticoagulants in serum is shown in Figure 15.4. Alternative commercial methods for the evaluation of lupus anticoagulants are the diluted Russell's viper venom test and the PTT-LA Staclot procedure. The diluted Russell's viper venom test and its confirmation are 80% sensitive, as opposed to the PTT-LA Staclot test, which is only 67% sensitive. However, if both tests are carried out, the combined sensitivity is 97%. False-positive results are not seen (Schjetlein and Wisloff, 1995).

Protein S

Protein S is a polypeptide protein that normally is present in the plasma and in the α-granules of platelets. It functions as a cofactor for the action of protein C. Deficiency of protein S is inherited as an autosomal dominant trait and is associated with life-long thromboembolisms. The protein exists in a free form that is in equilibrium with a nonfunctional form bound to C4b.

Thrombosis is associated with reductions in free or functional protein S. The most common form of the disorder displays reductions in the total protein

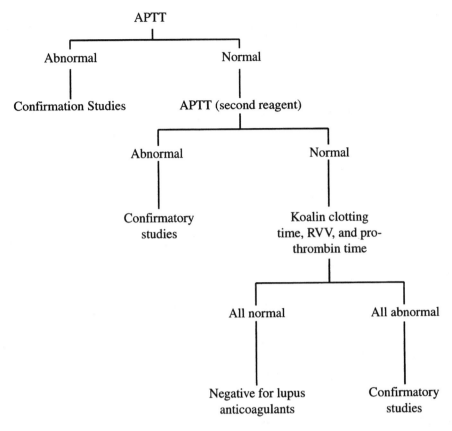

Figure 15.4. Schematic for the investigation of lupus anticoagulants. (APTT = activated partial thromboplastin time; RVV = Russell's viper venom test.)

S antigen and deficiencies of functional protein S. The clinical manifestations of protein S deficiency are identical to those of protein C deficiency.

Hemorrhage Due to Vascular Abnormalities

The etiology of disorders associated with vascular bleeding is shown in Table 15.9.

Autoimmune Purpuras

The autoimmune purpuras include *Henoch-Schön-lein purpura (allergic)* and those purpuras associated with drugs and chemicals. Allergic purpura is most commonly seen in children. Clinically, headaches, fever, and purpura (primarily on the legs and buttocks) are the principal findings. Laboratory data are nonspecific and show a mild neutrophilia or eosinophilia and a positive tourniquet test result. All other tests of blood coagulation, including the bleeding time and platelet count, are normal.

Drug-induced purpura can result from ingestion of a variety of drugs and chemicals. The reaction disappears when the offending agent is removed, and the disorder is not associated with any bleeding tendency or abnormality in any coagulation tests.

Purpura fulminans is characterized by fever, ecchymoses, and skin infarcts and is believed to be brought about by a DIC syndrome (see page 206).

Purpura of Infection

Direct endothelial injury leading to an infection can bring about a DIC syndrome resulting from the release of bacterial toxins or microthrombi. In such situations, a varied set of laboratory results may be produced that are similar to those seen in DIC.

Table 15.9. Etiology of Bleeding from Vascular Abnormalities

Cause	Examples
Autoimmune	Henoch-Schönlein purpura, drug-induced purpura fulminans
Infections	Bacterial, viral, rickettsial, protozoal
Structural	Hereditary hemorrhagic telangiectasia, Ehlers-Danlos syndrome, acquired disorders
Miscellaneous	Paraproteinemias, autoimmune sensitization

Structural Causes of Purpura

Hereditary Hemorrhagic Telangiectasia

Hereditary hemorrhagic telangiectasia is a vascular disorder inherited as an autosomal dominant characteristic in which the vessels are dilated or tortuous, vessel walls are thin, vascular support is abnormal, and the ability of the vessels to undergo normal contraction is diminished. Clinically, the hemorrhages are discrete masses, up to 3 mm in diameter, and are seen most commonly on the face. Symptoms include epistaxis and other mucous membrane bleeding, as well as bleeding from individual telangiectases. Hemorrhage from major vessels or organs is rare. The laboratory findings show a variable anemia and iron deficiency, depending on the severity of the blood loss. Abnormal bleeding times and occasional platelet abnormalities have been reported (Pandolfi and Ehinger, 1978), but no well-defined pattern in coagulation tests is seen.

Ehlers-Danlos Syndrome

The *Ehlers-Danlos syndrome* is a hereditary disorder involving both qualitative and quantitative abnormalities of collagen, which results in abnormal vascular fragility and bleeding related to poor vascular support. Ecchymoses and hematomas are seen commonly. The laboratory test results involving blood coagulation are usually normal.

Acquired Disorders

Acquired disorders of connective tissue include scurvy and senile purpura. *Scurvy* commonly exhibits a positive tourniquet test result and abnormal bleeding time, as well as a mild thrombocytopenia. All other laboratory test results usually are normal.

Senile purpura is a disorder of the aged and involves ecchymoses, particularly on the forearms, hands, and neck. The defect involves impaired dermal support of the microvessels. Like the other purpuras, this condition is associated with an abnormal result on the tourniquet test.

Bleeding Disorders Involving Platelets

Hereditary Disorders of Platelet Function (Qualitative)

Thrombasthenia (Glanzmann's Thrombasthenia)

Thrombasthenia is an autosomal recessive disorder characterized by epistaxis, ecchymoses, gingival hemorrhage, and menorrhagia caused by abnormal platelet aggregation. The platelets exhibit a decrease in surface membrane glycoproteins IIb and IIIa and a normal release mechanism, but they appear to be refractory to the action of ADP, which leads to inadequate platelet plug formation. Deficient levels of glutathione peroxidase and elevated levels of reduced glutathione have been demonstrated.

The laboratory picture includes normal platelet counts and normal platelet morphologic features. Prolonged bleeding times and abnormal clot retraction, prothrombin consumption, platelet adhesion, and platelet aggregation are seen. The platelet aggregation test result is abnormal when challenged by ADP, collagen, thrombin, or epinephrine, but it is normal when exposed to ristocetin. Other laboratory abnormalities include a mild hypofibrinogenemia, abnormal TGT in the serum component, reduced levels of platelet factor 3, and a lack of platelet antigen (HPA-1). Clinical bleeding is severe and usually begins in early life. Spontaneous mucosal and cutaneous bleeding is seen, which is aggravated by trauma. The sever-

Table 15.10. Classification of Platelet Disorders

Type	Group	Example
Qualitative	Hereditary	Thrombasthenia, deficient platelet release, hereditary platelet dysfunction, Bernard-Soulier syndrome
	Acquired	Drug-induced, uremia, disorders of hematopoiesis
Quantitative	Primary	Idiopathic thrombocytopenic purpura
	Secondary	Thrombotic thrombocytopenic purpura, chemical or physical agents, disorders of hematopoiesis, infections

Table 15.11. Platelet Aggregation Results in Inherited Disorders of Platelet Function

		Platelet Aggregation Response			
Defect	ADP	Collagen	Epinephrine	Ristocetin	Thrombin
Defective adhesion to subepithelium					
von Willebrand's syndrome	N	N	N	D[a]	N
Bernard-Soulier syndrome	N	N	N	D	N
Defective platelet release mechanism					
Storage pool disease	D	D	D	—	D[b]
Aspirin-affected disorders	D	D	D[c]	—	N
Deficiency in clot retraction					
Thrombasthenia	D	D	D	—	D

N = normal; D = decreased.
[a]Decrease corrected by factor VIII.
[b]Decreased to a dilute thrombin.
[c]Decreased. Secondary wave blocked.

ity of bleeding often decreases with age. Hemarthroses can occur. Table 15.10 presents the classification of platelet disorders.

Defective Platelet Release

Disorders of defective platelet release are characterized by the platelets' failure to undergo a normal release reaction when stimulated. Consequently, the platelets do not exhibit a secondary aggregation response when challenged by ADP, epinephrine, or ristocetin. Defects in the release mechanism are divided into three principal groups: (1) collagen storage disease, (2) storage pool deficiency, and (3) "aspirinlike" deficiency. Table 15.11 shows platelet aggregation results in inherited disorders of platelet function.

Collagen storage disease type I is believed to be caused by defective nucleotide synthesis secondary to hypoglycemia, the result of a deficiency of glucose-6-phosphatase (Hutton et al., 1976).

Storage pool deficiency is an abnormality resulting from a poor platelet release mechanism that is caused by a deficiency of stored nucleotides. Clinically, bleeding is mild. When associated with albinism and macrophagic ceroid deposits, the disorder is known as the *Hermansky-Pudlak syndrome*. This variant is inherited as an autosomal recessive trait and usually is characterized by a deficiency of dense granules within the platelets.

A second storage pool disease, the *Chédiak-Higashi syndrome*, is also associated with albinism and is inherited as an autosomal recessive characteristic. Patients with this disorder show an increased susceptibility to infections. Giant inclusion bodies are present in the granulocytes and platelets.

A third storage pool disorder, the *Wiskott-Aldrich syndrome*, differs from the other syndromes in that its mode of inheritance is sex-linked. The principal findings include recurrent infections, eczema, and a moderate chronic thrombocytopenia. The laboratory findings show a prolonged bleeding time and no second wave of platelet aggregation when platelets are challenged with ADP, epinephrine, or ristocetin. Aggregation with collagen is impaired or absent. Thrombin aggregation and platelet adhesion are variable; the availability of platelet factor 3 may also be reduced, and the adenosine triphosphate–adenosine diphosphate ratio (ATP:ADP) usually is markedly decreased. The thrombocytopenia in this disease may be due to a shortened platelet survival rate without a compensatory release of young, large platelets. On electron microscopy, these platelets also exhibit decreased numbers of α-granules and dense bodies.

Aspirinlike deficiency is a syndrome in which aspirin blocks prostaglandins and thromboxane formation by interfering with cyclo-oxygenase action (see page 177). This is responsible for the conversion of arachidonic acid to its metabolites (Roth et al., 1975).

In one variant of the syndrome, the *May-Hegglin anomaly*, cyclo-oxygenase is reduced. Both the clinical and laboratory findings in this syndrome are difficult to differentiate from storage pool disorders.

The anomaly is believed to be transmitted in an autosomal dominant manner. These patients have bizarre, giant platelets with basophilic inclusions that are similar in size to Döhle bodies found in the neutrophils. The disease often progresses to other chronic disorders, including leukemia.

Gray Platelet Syndrome

The gray platelet syndrome is a rare autosomal recessive disorder characterized by widely fluctuating platelet counts and the presence of giant platelets lacking α-granules. Thrombocytopenia, hemorrhage, and gray-appearing platelets and megakaryocytes are seen (Raccuglia, 1971).

Bernard-Soulier Syndrome

The *Bernard-Soulier syndrome* is a rare autosomal recessive bleeding disorder that exhibits clinically a moderate to severe bruising pattern, epistaxis, and menorrhagia. The laboratory findings are consistent with a platelet surface membrane defect. The platelet morphologic appearance is striking,

with many large forms seen that occasionally approach the size of lymphocytes (>4 μ). The bleeding time is prolonged, and there is decreased platelet aggregation when ristocetin or purified bovine factor VIII is used. Platelet aggregation is normal with thrombin, ADP, epinephrine, or collagen. Platelet adhesion onto glass usually is reduced, and the PCT also shows abnormalities. The clot retraction and availability of platelet factor 3 both are normal. The inherent defect is believed to be a lack of membrane glycoproteins of type Ib and Is (Solum et al., 1977), which are thought to be essential for normal platelet adhesion during the early stages of primary hemostasis. Glycoproteins Ib and IIb-IIIa complexes are decreased also in myeloproliferative disorders.

Table 15.12 lists other functional abnormalities in qualitative platelet disorders.

Acquired Disorders of Platelet Function

Drug-Induced Disorders

Many drugs have been shown to influence platelet function. The principal agent causing the most disruption of hemostasis is aspirin or aspirin derivatives. Aspirin inhibits the action of platelet cyclo-oxygenase, which is responsible for the conversion of arachidonic acid to endoperoxidases and prostaglandins (see page 176). Small amounts of aspirin are known to affect platelet function for up to 1 week (Weiss and Aledort, 1968).

Platelet aggregation in individuals who have ingested aspirin shows a deficient collagen response and lack of a secondary response with epinephrine as well as low concentrations of ADP. Aspirin-treated platelets fail to release normal ATP, ADP, and platelet factor 4 concentrations. The principal laboratory finding is a prolonged bleeding time and an abnormal aspirin tolerance test. Other drugs affecting platelet function are shown in Table 15.13.

Other Acquired Platelet Dysfunctions

Uremia is associated with defective hemostasis, which is the main abnormality involving a deficient platelet release mechanism. Clinically, ecchymoses and gastrointestinal bleeding are found, and hematomas into serous cavities and large muscle masses

Table 15.12. Other Functional Abnormalities in Qualitative Platelet Disorders

Defect	Platelet Adhesion	Platelet Factor 3 Availability	Clot Retraction	Bleeding Time	Platelet Count	Bleeding Tendency
Defective adhesion						
von Willebrand's syndrome	A	N	N	V	N	V
Bernard-Soulier syndrome	A	N	N	A	N/D	Severe
Defective platelet release mechanism						
Storage pool disease	A	UA	N	A	N/D	V
Aspirin-affected diseases	A	UA	N	A	N/D	Usually mild
Deficiency in clot retraction						
Thrombasthenia	A	A	A	A	N	V

A = abnormal; N = normal; V = variable; N/D = normal or decreased; UA = usually abnormal.

Table 15.13. Drugs that Affect Platelet Function

Drug Class	Action	Examples
Analgesics	Cyclo-oxygenase inhibition	Aspirin and aspirin derivatives, indomethacin, phenylbutazone
Antibiotics	Inhibition of platelet aggregation and release	Carbenicillin
Miscellaneous	Unknown, coats platelet surface, inhibition of platelet ATP-induced aggregation	Heparin, dextran, ethanol, dipyridamole

ATP = adenosine triphosphate.

are not uncommon. Laboratory results show deficient platelet aggregation as well as poor platelet adhesion when platelets are exposed to collagen or epinephrine. The secondary wave in platelet aggregation also is lacking in the face of ADP challenge. Abnormal results are found in the bleeding time, the PCT, and the platelet factor 3 assay.

The bleeding manifestations involving hematopoiesis are varied and nonspecific in nature. Hemorrhage can complicate various paraproteinemias principally because of platelet dysfunction. This involves the macroglobulin coating of platelet surfaces, thereby impairing the release reaction. As a result of such coating, platelet aggregation, platelet adhesion, and platelet factor 3 activity have all been reported to be deficient (Pachter and Johnson, 1959).

Hemorrhage associated with both acute and chronic preleukemia is also well documented (Cowan and Haut, 1972). Acute leukemia often shows abnormal platelet morphologic characteristics, including the presence of giant platelet granules formed by the fusion of several normal-sized granules and abnormal platelet aggregation tests. Chronic granulocytic leukemia often has a bleeding component that is manifested by ecchymoses, epistaxis, and gastrointestinal hemorrhage. This is believed to be the result of a storage pool disease and a deficiency of platelet membrane glycoproteins (Gerrard et al., 1978). The other myeloproliferative diseases associated with platelet dysfunction include hemorrhagic thrombocythemia and myelofibrosis.

Hemorrhagic thrombocythemia is characterized by marked increases in the platelet count and the presence of giant forms in the peripheral blood. Platelet factor 3 activity appears to be reduced, and platelet adhesion is decreased. Myelofibrosis is associated with deficient platelet factor 3 activity (Weiss HJ, 1975), as is polycythemia vera. Cigarette smoking significantly increases in vivo platelet aggregation, and this effect appears to be independent of the nicotine concentrations of the cigarette (Bierenbaum et al., 1978).

Table 15.14. Principal Differences Between Acute and Chronic Idiopathic Thrombocytopenic Purpura

Feature	Acute[a]	Chronic[b]
Preceded by infection	Common	Rare
Onset of bleeding	Abrupt	Insidious
Platelet count	$< 20 \times 10^9$/liter	$< 80 \times 10^9$/liter
Leukocyte changes	Eosinophilia and lymphocytosis	None
Duration of the disease	2–6 wks	Months or years
Remissions	Spontaneous in 80% of cases	Rarely spontaneous

[a]Generally affects children.
[b]Generally affects adults.

Quantitative Disorders of Platelets

Primary Idiopathic Thrombocytopenic Purpura

Two forms of primary idiopathic thrombocytopenia purpura (ITP) are recognized: acute and chronic. Acute ITP usually is seen in children, principally in those children who have experienced a febrile illness such as a viral infection. The disorder is characterized by a marked reduction in the platelet count, a mild eosinophilia, and lymphocytosis. The duration of the disorder is usually 2–6 weeks, and spontaneous recovery is frequently seen.

The chronic form of ITP has an insidious onset and mainly affects adults. Petechial hemorrhages that fuse to form ecchymoses are found commonly. As in the acute form, the laboratory findings reveal a reduced platelet count and a reduction in platelet survival resulting from the formation of specific platelet autoantibodies. The bone marrow shows increases in megakaryocytes and megakaryoblasts. Normal results are found in the PT, PTT, and thrombin time. Table 15.14 differentiates the salient points between the acute and chronic forms of ITP.

Thrombotic Thrombocytopenic Purpura

Thrombotic thrombocytopenic purpura (TTP) is a disorder of unknown etiology and is clinically characterized by fever, hemorrhage, neurologic manifestations, microangiopathic hemolytic anemia, and thrombocytopenia. TTP appears to predominate in young adults and causes platelet aggregates to form in the microvasculature. The laboratory results often show a mild to moderate anemia and the presence of schistocytic red-cell fragments. Occasionally, the

PT is prolonged and the fibrinogen level is decreased. The classic finding, however, is a marked thrombocytopenia that is as low as 10×10^9/liter. The bleeding time, tourniquet test, and clot retraction all are proportionately abnormal. Leukocytosis often is seen, counts being as high as 20×10^9/liter. The bone marrow exhibits an erythroid hyperplasia, reflecting its response to the incurred blood loss and increased numbers of megakaryocytes.

Pseudothrombocytopenia

Pseudothrombocytopenia is an antibody-induced in vitro phenomenon caused by platelet clumping and is usually associated with blood specimens anticoagulated with ethylenediaminetetraacetic acid (EDTA) (Gowland et al., 1969; Shreiner and Bell, 1973; Kjeldsberg and Hershgold, 1974). The spurious nature of the thrombocytopenia is usually supported by a lack of history or physical findings and by a normal bleeding time. Normal counts can be obtained by the use of dry citrate, heparin, or oxalate as anticoagulants (Baele et al., 1978; Fujii et al., 1978; Nilsson and Norberg, 1986).

Pseudothrombocytopenia may be seen in patients with several different types of platelet agglutinins. Cold-reactive antibodies that are active at temperatures of less than 34°C have been reported (Watkins and Shulman, 1970), as have EDTA-dependent agglutinins that are active at room temperature (Shreiner and Bell, 1973). IgG and IgM antibodies that are active in the presence of EDTA at a wide range of temperatures have also been reported (Veehoven et al., 1979; Pegels et al., 1982). Additionally, IgM temperature-independent antibodies have been reported to produce platelet clumping in the presence of all routine anticoagulants (Forscher et al., 1985).

Most of these spurious pseudothrombocytopenias can be resolved by carrying out platelet counts from a capillary puncture directly into a Unopette (Becton-Dickinson, Rutherford, NJ) containing ammonium oxalate and by counting the cells in a hemocytometer. Newer automated instruments H2 also are capable of detecting EDTA-induced platelet clumping. The Coulter counter, with a three-part differential, displays the abnormal platelet population by means of a nonfitted platelet curve, and the H2 illustrates the abnormality in the leukocyte peroxidase X-Y display.

Antibody subpopulations directed against negatively charged phospholipid particles can bind to antigens modified by EDTA on the platelet membrane and may be responsible for pseudothrombocytopenia (Bizzaro and Brandalise, 1995).

Isoimmune Neonatal Thrombocytopenia

Isoimmune neonatal thrombocytopenia is recognized in 1 in 5,000 births. It is analogous to Rh/ABO hemolytic disease of the newborn in that transplacentally acquired maternal antibody is directed against antigens on the fetal platelets. Usually, the HPA-1a (Pl^{A1}) antigen is involved. Firstborn infants are affected in approximately 50% of the reported cases. Without therapy, the mortality is 15% (McIntosh et al., 1973).

Petechiae, ecchymoses, and purpura may appear at birth but more often develop a few hours later when the platelet count usually is less than 30×10^9/liter. The most serious clinical complication is intracranial hemorrhage. The course of the disease is variable, ranging from benign resolution in several weeks to immediate death secondary to hemorrhage. Treatment by attempting the removal of the antibody by exchange transfusion has been attempted (Moncrieff, 1978), but the most successful therapy is transfusion of HPA-1a (Pl^{A1})-negative platelets, which are found in only 2% of the general population (McIntosh et al., 1973), or the transfusion of washed maternal platelets (Keltan et al., 1979; Chandler and Daniel, 1985).

Thrombocytosis

Thrombocytosis occurs as a primary disease of the bone marrow or as a reactive phenomenon in pathologic and physiologic conditions. Increases in platelet numbers can be seen as a reactive process or in association with a myeloproliferation. Spuriously elevated automated platelet counts secondary to in vivo bacteremia have also been reported (Gloster et al., 1985).

Thrombocythemia is characterized by recurrent gastrointestinal bleeding and hemorrhages following surgical procedures and trauma. Thrombosis of veins and arteries may be seen, and pulmonary embolisms and splenomegaly also are found.

The laboratory findings are of a marked increase in the platelet count to as high as 14×10^9/liter. Bizarre platelet morphologic characteristics, including giant forms and abnormalities in shape and granular composition, are also seen. Anemia is uncommon but, if present, it is morphologically normocytic and hypochromic. There is a mild leukocytosis with neutrophilia and a shift to the left. The bone marrow shows a megakaryocytic hyperplasia. Leukocyte alkaline phosphatase, serum vitamin B_{12}, and serum uric acid levels all are increased. Routine coagulation tests usually are normal, but occasionally a low-grade DIC syndrome is present, which may affect the PT, PTT, platelet count, and fibrinogen levels in proportion to the severity of the clotting (see page 206).

Reactive thrombocytosis is an asymptomatic finding that is usually secondary to an inflammatory disorder or an iron deficiency. Platelet counts of up to $1,000 \times 10^9$/liter may be found (Panlilio and Reiss, 1979). Other laboratory results are unhelpful in the evaluation, the increase in platelets being of short duration and usually responding to the treatment of the primary disease.

Familial thrombophilia is a clinical state in which there is a hereditary predisposition to venous thromboembolic disease. Approximately 10–15% of such cases are associated with protein S and protein C deficiency.

Platelet Antibodies

Three classes of platelet antibodies are detectable: (1) autoantibodies (e.g., in idiopathic thrombocytopenic purpura), (2) alloantibodies (e.g., in posttransfusion purpura), and (3) circulating immune complexes (e.g., in drug-induced thrombocytopenia). Table 15.15 provides additional examples of these three platelet antibody classes.

Table 15.15. Platelet Antibodies

Type	Examples
Autoantibodies	Idiopathic thrombocytopenic purpura, neonatal immune thrombocytopenia
Alloantibodies	Post-transfusion purpura, neonatal immune thrombocytopenia
Circulating immune complexes	Drug-induced thrombocytopenia, acquired immunodeficiency syndrome, acute myeloid leukemia, rheumatoid arthritis, systemic lupus erythematosus

Chapter 16
Quality Assurance

The main reasons for assuring laboratory quality are to provide results that can be depended on to aid the physician with the diagnosis, to follow the course of the disease closely, and to monitor the effects of drug therapy. Assuring laboratory quality, though an apparently simple task, is not easy to achieve, as many variables affect the quality of a test result. Laboratory errors can be classified broadly into two main categories: preanalytic and analytic.

Preanalytic Variables Affecting Hematologic Tests

Test Requisition

Each request for a laboratory test must be submitted with a unique number and demographic information, such as the patient's complete name, an identification number, the date, the location, the physician's name, and the time of collection. The test request form should be arranged so that there is ample space in which to document all necessary information.

Patient Identification

This aspect of quality assurance is obvious, but it is often overlooked, especially in a busy laboratory or during a period of stress in which several emergencies arise together. In a hospital setting, the phlebotomist should compare information with the patient's name and identification number on the wristband. If this band is unavailable, the patient should be asked for his or her full name, including the spelling of any unusual names, and his or her date of birth. All too frequently, individuals with the same name are in the same hospital ward or on the same floor, and the use of the date of birth (not age) is an excellent means of avoiding any error. If the patient cannot respond to questions, a member of the immediate family or the charge nurse should be asked to identify the patient positively.

Specimen Collection

Although the principal problems involving the evacuated tubes used for obtaining specimens occur in biochemistry and toxicology, poor hematologic specimen collection can influence a final test result, no matter how well the laboratory carries out the analysis. It is wise to establish a specific quality control procedure for checking evacuated tubes. Parameters to check should include volume draw, stopper removal, and a visual check for the anticoagulant and for the presence of foreign material. The anticoagulated blood should also be checked carefully for the presence of clots.

The actual venipuncture also should be evaluated. Standard procedure, when obtaining a venous specimen, is to apply a tourniquet to make the veins more prominent, thereby facilitating entry and quick drawing of the specimen. To accomplish this, venous flow is occluded and localized stasis may occur, especially if the tourniquet remains in place too long or if it is too tight. This results in a hemo-concentrated specimen with erroneous hematologic values. Because it is difficult to draw blood routinely without the aid of a tourniquet, it is important to limit the time it remains in use and to determine the order of draw for the tests requested.

If multiple tests are required, it is preferable to obtain the hematologic samples first to avoid the effects of stasis and then to collect any remaining samples for tests that require serum for analysis. When multiple tubes are being collected, it is most important to mix the anticoagulated sample immediately, to help minimize the formation of microclots. This is done by gently inverting the tube 5–10 times before additional serum samples are collected.

The effects of hemolysis on hematologic specimens are not well documented. Most laboratories will reject the sample if any sign of hemolysis is present in an anticoagulated specimen, but there is some evidence that the prothrombin time test can be carried out if minimal hemolysis is present, provided that the hemolysis is not the result of a traumatic venipuncture (Engstrom, 1968).

Complete blood cell counts (CBCs) should not be determined on hemolyzed specimens, although hemoglobin determinations can be carried out. Hemolysis may occur during drawing, transporting, or processing a specimen. During specimen collection, blood may hemolyze from a variety of factors, including the expulsion of blood through a small-bore needle, which forms froth, and too-vigorous shaking of the tube when mixing. Technically difficult venipuncture also often results in a hemolyzed blood specimen.

Blood collection from adults should always be carried out using a sharp 20- to 22-gauge needle. Hemolysis occurs more frequently with needles of smaller caliber. It is reasonable to assume that excessive negative pressure from either the syringe or the vacuum tubes not only damages the red cells but may fragment both the leukocytes and platelets. Consequently, the specimen should be routinely examined and rejected if small clots or excessive hemolysis is present. The vacuum tube should be allowed to fill to capacity to assure a correct concentration of anticoagulant. The concentration of ethylenediaminetetraacetic acid (EDTA) should be 1.0–1.5 mg per milliliter of blood. The centrifuged hematocrit may decrease by as much as four hematocrit units, and the total

leukocyte count may be falsely decreased as a result of incomplete filling of the tube when EDTA is excessive (Koepke et al., 1978).

Hemolysis also may occur when blood is collected by skin puncture; it can result from leaving alcohol on the skin as well as from excessive squeezing of the heel or finger. Massaging the site prior to puncture may reduce the cell counts by up to 5%, and squeezing blood through an inadequate wound may elevate the count by as much as 25%. Clotting from liberated tissue juices and local alterations in the marginating leukocytes may account for these discrepancies. Hemolysis of blood collected from newborns and infants is thus more common, and particular attention should be paid to obtaining a free flow of blood from one puncture, without the necessity of making multiple wounds.

For venous specimens, some hematologic parameters will vary sharply in response to changes in the physiologic state of the patient. Apprehensive infants and children may have cyanotic extremities resulting from dilated skin capillaries, which can produce falsely elevated hemoglobin and red-cell count values. Transient leukocytosis may occur, too, in a frightened child in response to the marginal pool's liberation of sequestered cells.

The collection of blood from patients in special situations requires extra care and attention. Obtaining blood from indwelling lines or catheters may be a potential source of test error. It is normal practice to flush these lines with heparin to reduce the risk of thrombosis and, consequently, these lines must be flushed free before any blood is collected and used for testing. It is recommended that at least three times the volume of the line be removed and discarded before a specimen is obtained for analysis (Stockbower, 1982). If intravenous fluids are being administered in an arm, blood should not be collected from that site, to avoid obtaining a hemodiluted specimen. The phlebotomist should obtain blood from the opposite arm or, if that is not possible, from a site below the intravenous infusion. In such a situation, the physician should be notified and, if possible, the intravenous infusion should be stopped for a few minutes prior to venipuncture. A vein other than that used for the intravenous infusion should be selected, and the first 5 ml of blood obtained should be discarded.

The collection and preparation of blood smears requires careful attention. Two types of smears commonly are made: the wedge smear and the coverslip smear. The so-called wedge or push smear has the advantage of being readily prepared by less-skilled workers and is easier to handle than smears made by the coverslip method. Proponents of the coverslip method believe that the cellular morphologic characteristics are better preserved; however, staining and monitoring of coverslip preparations requires special handling that is not easy to integrate into a busy laboratory.

Over the last decade special spinning devices that use standard slides to make monocellular smears have become available. These spinners are used principally in the pattern recognition method of differential leukocyte counting.

Thin blood smears may be made directly from a capillary puncture, from anticoagulated venous blood, or directly from the venipuncture needle. If made from the needle, any delay can affect cytologic detail. Furthermore, endothelial cells caught on the needle tip may contaminate the specimen.

Specimen Processing

Specimen processing in hematologic testing does not present the difficulties encountered in biochemical testing. In general, serum specimens should be centrifuged approximately 30 minutes after collection; this allows adequate time for the blood to clot fully as well as minimizing hemolysis and increasing the serum yield. Anticoagulated specimens for coagulation tests should be centrifuged with the stopper in place and tested as soon as possible after collection (see page 226). Routine hematologic testing for a CBC, sedimentation rates, and reticulocyte counts should be carried out on the freshest blood specimen available. Storage criteria and effects on these tests are discussed on page 224.

Physiologic Variations

Physiologic variations that can give rise to fluctuation in routine hematologic tests include the patient's posture when venipuncture is performed, strenuous exercise, diurnal variation, altitude, cigarette smoking, pregnancy, and the performance of phlebotomy soon after ingestion of food. The effect of patient posture on routine hematologic tests is

well established. Hemoglobin and hematocrit levels, on average, are 5% lower when the individual is recumbent rather than upright (Tombridge, 1968). The change takes place rapidly, usually within 20 minutes, after which time the hemoglobin becomes stabilized at the lower level (Ekelund et al., 1971). In a similar way, the hematocrit is increased 4–6% after prolonged standing (Mollison, 1967). The position of the patient's arm when the venipuncture is carried out also influences the test results. If the arm is held at the atrial level, the hematocrit is 2–4% lower than when the arm is in a vertical position (Eisenberg, 1963).

Strenuous exercise also raises the hemoglobin and hematocrit values and produces a transient leukocytosis. The elevation of hemoglobin is most likely caused by loss of circulating plasma and the re-entry of red cells previously sequestered in marginal capillaries. Increases in the red-cell count of up to 0.5×10^{12}/liter and increases in the hemoglobin of up to 1.5 g/dl can occur (Ekelund et al., 1971). In addition, prolonged exercise can result in a moderate increase in leukocytes of up to 30×10^9/liter, which is mainly due to the release of cells from the marginal pools into the circulatory pool (Dacie and Lewis, 1975). Platelet adhesion and adenosine diphosphate–induced aggregation are accentuated by exercise (Prentice, 1972).

Diurnal variations of the hemoglobin and hematocrit values represent a significant part of the total variation within individuals, with afternoon hemoglobin values being lower than early morning values by approximately 0.3 g/dl. However, hemoglobin differences as great as 1.5 g/dl can occur (Statland et al., 1978). Diurnal variations are also seen in serum iron levels. Maximum values are found in the morning and the lowest values are found in the late evening. Differences of as much as 30% are possible (Hamilton et al., 1950). Differential leukocyte counts, too, show variations within the same day and diurnal trends that are unique for each individual. Exceptions to this finding are eosinophils and basophils, which tend to show a more consistent pattern, with lower afternoon and higher morning values. These values appear to parallel diurnal glucocorticoid changes (Statland et al., 1978).

Increased altitude raises the hemoglobin value and increases the number of circulating red cells. The magnitude of the increase depends on the degree of anoxia. At an altitude of 6,500 feet, the hemoglobin value is approximately 1 g/dl higher than at sea level (Myhre et al., 1970), and a corresponding increase in related test values is also present.

Erythropoiesis is affected by cigarette smoking. Elevated hemoglobin and hematocrit values are found in heavy smokers (Isager and Hagerup, 1971; Smith and Landow, 1978), as are reduced platelet survival and increased platelet ability to aggregate (Hawkins, 1972).

Although pregnancy produces decreases in hemoglobin levels because of increased nutritional demands, it also commonly elevates the leukocyte count as high as 15×10^9/liter. Peak levels occur approximately 8 weeks before parturition, the count returning to normal approximately 1 week after delivery (Cruikshank, 1970).

Leukocytosis and thrombocytosis can be seen following a meal (Priest et al., 1982).

Specimen Stability

In general, anticoagulated specimens for hematologic testing are less stable than all serum samples for serologic and chemical testing. When blood is collected in tripotassium EDTA and is stored undisturbed at room temperature, the hemoglobin, hematocrit, red-cell count, leukocyte count, and red-cell indices are very stable for up to 8 hours, falling within Tonks' "allowable limits of error" (Tonks, 1968). These measurements are stable for up to 24 hours if the specimen is maintained undisturbed at room temperature (Simmons et al., 1978; Simmons, 1982). Blood stored at 4°C produces conflicting data. It has been suggested that EDTA-anticoagulated blood maintains its initial values within 5° for the "hemogram" tests when maintained at 4°C for up to 24 hours (Britten et al., 1969) and that these values remain at an acceptable level when the blood is kept for up to 48 hours in a refrigerator (Lampasso, 1968).

The two problem parameters appear to be the leukocyte count and the mean cell volume (MCV). Leukocytes are stable for 24 hours if stored at ambient temperatures and for up to 48 hours if kept at 4°C. However, individual differences are found, especially if an impedance method of counting is used. After blood has been stored for 8 hours at room temperature, the MCV increases at a progressive rate of 3–4 fl every 24 hours. At 4°C, the MCV is stable for 24 hours and then progressively increases at the same rate as if kept at room temperature (Simmons et al., 1978; Simmons, 1982). However, if the blood is mixed intermittently and is stored at 4°C, the hemoglobin, red-cell count, red-cell indices, leukocyte count, and platelet count are stable for up to 72 hours (Cohle et al., 1981).

Examples of data obtained following undisturbed storage are shown in Table 16.1. One variable that is frequently overlooked is the importance of using the correct concentration of EDTA. For optimal storage conditions, a fully drawn tube (tripotassium EDTA concentration of 1.25–1.75 mg per milliliter of blood) should be used (Sacker, 1975). When using 2-ml pediatric tubes, specimens of less than 0.5 ml produce significant decreases in leukocyte counts and increases in the mean cell hemoglobin concentration (MCHC) because of the hypertonic action of the EDTA, causing cell shrinkage and reduced MCV (Doyle, 1967).

Differential leukocyte counts are stable for an indefinite period provided that the slide is made and fixed within 3 hours of blood collection. Blood smears are best made directly from the venipuncture needle or from a direct skin puncture rather than from EDTA-anticoagulated blood. Slides made from anticoagulated specimens are likely to show morphologic cellular changes even after brief storage. The first changes occur in the neutrophils and other granulocytes, which exhibit swelling and loss of structure in the nuclear lobes. Stretching of the interlobular bridges then occurs, with loss of cytoplasmic granulation. Vacuolation also is seen in the cell cytoplasm. These changes progress to more marked nuclear swelling and nuclear homogeneity, resulting in typical cloverleaf patterns in extreme cases. Ultimately, there is a marked morphologic disintegration of the cell, leaving a bare nucleus (Sacker, 1975). The use of automated cytochemical flow methods to determine the differential leukocyte count reveals that cell stability is acceptable for 36–48 hours (Simmons, personal observations, 1985).

Platelets appear to swell to produce giant forms, which then disintegrate. This causes an artificially high platelet count, as the platelet fragments are sufficiently large to be counted as morphologically normal platelets. Red cells also undergo changes in shape, and both anisocytosis and spherocytosis can

Table 16.1. Examples of Hematologic Test Stability at Different Temperatures and Storage Times*

Parameter	Sample Stored at 21.5°C					Sample Stored at 4°C				
	0	4 hrs	8 hrs	24 hrs	48 hrs	0	4 hrs	8 hrs	24 hrs	48 hrs
Hemoglobin (g/dl)	14.7	14.6	14.7	14.5	14.9	14.7	14.8	14.5	14.6	14.8
RBCs ($\times 10^{12}$/liter)	4.81	4.83	4.87	4.78	4.78	4.81	4.89	4.85	4.85	4.88
WBCs ($\times 10^{9}$/liter)	6.8	6.4	6.6	6.6	6.5	6.8	6.3	6.4	6.6	6.1
MCV (fl)	89.3	89.3	88.0	93.5	98.7	89.3	89.3	90.4	89.0	92.6

RBCs = red blood cells; WBCs = white blood cells; MCV = mean cell volume.

*Tripotassium EDTA anticoagulated blood at a concentration of 1.5 mg/ml EDTA.

Source: Data from A Simmons, JD Wiseman, et al. The stability of hematologic parameters when tested by the Coulter Model S. Proc Int Soc Haematol Meeting Paris, FPS. 371:056, 1978.

Table 16.2. Effects of Storage Conditions on the Prothrombin Time*

Specimen	Fresh Plasma	Plasma Stored at 4°C		Stoppered Vacuum Tube Stored at Room Temperature (24 hrs)
		6 hrs	24 hrs	
1	11.7	11.6	12.7	11.5
2	11.4	11.7	12.7	11.7
3	11.2	11.4	12.3	11.2
4	10.9	10.7	12.4	10.9
5	10.8	10.4	12.0	10.7
6	12.1	11.9	12.7	11.4
Mean	**11.4**	**11.3**	**12.7**	**11.2**
7	19.2	18.9	19.7	19.4
8	18.6	17.2	15.3	18.4
9	25.5	25.8	24.2	27.1
10	25.2	23.7	22.7	26.9
11	26.2	25.1	24.2	26.1
Mean	**22.9**	**22.1**	**21.2**	**23.6**

*All times are in seconds. Each time is the mean of five replicate measurements.
Source: Data from JB Miale, JW Kent. Standardization of the technique for the prothrombin time test. Lab Med 10:612, 1979.

be seen. Macrocytosis occurs on prolonged EDTA contact, leading to cell hemolysis.

Reticulocytes mature in vitro by an aerobic fermentation process. However, the effect of such maturation is minimal when blood is stored at 4°C or at room temperature for up to 48 hours (Lampasso, 1968). Once a blood smear is made and stained, the stability of the reticulocyte preparation is indefinite.

The erythrocyte sedimentation rate remains stable for 4–5 hours when the specimen is stored at room temperature (Lugton, 1987) and for 24 hours when the blood is refrigerated (Gambino et al., 1965). However, it is recommended that the test be set up within 2 hours if blood is left at room temperature or within 6 hours if it is kept at 4°C (International Committee for Standardization in Haematology, 1977). A prestorage normal sedimentation rate is most likely to remain normal after storage, whereas any grossly abnormal test result is likely to diminish in intensity after storage and might still be abnormal or occasionally might revert to the borderline or the normal range. Poststorage changes appear unrelated to the patient's age, gender, clinical state, or other hematologic test results, and it is not possible to predict in advance which samples will show changes.

Coagulation test stability is critical for both diagnosis and the monitoring of anticoagulant ther-

apy. Studies of the stability of blood samples show that, in unopened vacuum-collected tubes, samples do not deteriorate noticeably for at least 6 hours, even when kept at room temperature. Prothrombin time measurements remain constant, but the partial thromboplastin time lengthens 10–15% after 24 hours of storage (Koepke et al., 1975). Others' data support this stability conclusion for prothrombin times (Miale and Kent, 1979; Table 16.2). If prothrombin time tests are collected into buffered sodium citrate, stability appears to be at least 12 hours, even if the samples are unstoppered, when stored at room temperature. Fibrinogen, when stored at room temperature, appears to be stable for up to 6 days (Simmons and Paulo, 1993; Simmons, unpublished observations, 1995).

Special coagulation factor assays should be handled differently from these other test specimens. The venipuncture site must be clean, and there should be a free flow of blood (McPhedran et al., 1974). A two-plastic or siliconized syringe technique is recommended (see page 343) or, if a single-syringe method is used, the first milliliter of blood should be discarded and the sample should be allowed to flow directly into the collecting tubes. Hemolysis, aspiration of air, and prolonged tourniquet application all affect the test results (Beller and Graeff, 1971).

If the patient has a high hematocrit value, there will be a proportionately higher anticoagulant-to-plasma volume. To avoid overdilution and overcitration, the volume of anticoagulant should be reduced to maintain the correct ratio (Koepke et al., 1975). In general, the specimens should be analyzed as soon as possible after venipuncture. Storage is best accomplished by placing the unstoppered specimen on ice or storing it at 4°C. Freezing of the plasma should be avoided, if possible, but if it is frozen, freezing should be done rapidly and the plasma should be kept at –70°C (O'Sullivan, 1979). Factors VII and XI may be activated by freezing (van Royen et al., 1978; Palmer and Gralnick, 1985). The euglobulin lysis time is stable if measured in platelet-poor plasma and stored at –80°C; the euglobulin undissolved precipitates are stable if stored at –20°C (Prisco et al., 1994).

Drug Interference in Hematologic Testing

A large number of drugs are known to affect many hematologic test results (Elking and Kabat, 1968; Sunderman, 1972; Wintrobe, 1981). It is beyond the scope of this text to list all these medications. The following sections discuss the drugs that most commonly influence the final test results.

Hemoglobin, Hematocrit, and Red-Cell Count

More than 60 different drugs or drug groups are known to depress the hemoglobin value. Among these are acetaminophen, aminosalicylic acid, amphotericin B, antimony compounds, antineoplastic agents, arsenicals, chloramphenicol, doxapram, ethosuximide, haloperidol, hydantoin derivatives, hydralazine, hydroxychloroquine sulfate, mefenamic acid, quinacrine, mercurial diuretics, nitrites, novobiocin, oleandomycin, penicillin, primidone, primaquine, pyrazolone derivatives, sulfonamides, thiazide diuretics, thiosemicarbazones, urethan, large doses of vitamin A, and radioactive agents.

Leukocytes

Elevated total leukocyte counts have been reported in some patients after the administration of allopurinol, barbiturates, atropine, diethylcarbamazine, erythromycin, streptomycin, sulfonamides, and the like.

Eosinophilia has been reported after the use of such agents as ampicillin, capreomycin, cephalothin, chlorpropamide, cloxacillin, desipramine, digitalis, epinephrine, hydantoin derivatives, indomethacin, isoniazid, methicillin, methyldopa, methysergide, nalidixic acid, novabiocin, phenothiazines, ristocetin, long-acting sulfonamides, and prolonged use of tetracycline.

Leukopenia has been reported to result from the administration of more than 90 different drugs. Among these are acetaminophen, aminoglutethimide, aminopyrine, antineoplastic agents, bismuth, chloramphenicol, chlordiazepoxide, chloroquine, colistin, desipramine, diazepam, diethylcarbamazine, furosemide, gold compounds, hydantoin derivatives, indanedione derivatives, iodides, iothiouracil, mefenamic acid, quinacrine, meprobamate, methicillin, methsuximide, methyldopa, methysergide, oleandomycin, oxacillin, oxyphenbutazone, phenothiazines, phenylbutazone, primaquine, primidone, procainamide, quinine, ristocetin, sulfonamides, thiosemicarbazones, vancomycin, and prolonged use of vitamin A.

Platelets

Drug-induced thrombocytosis is rare. Thrombocytopenia has been reported to be caused by the action of many drugs, including aminosalicylic acid, amphotericin B, antimony compounds, antineoplastic agents, arsenicals, chloramphenicol, chloroquine, colchicine, ethoxyzolamide, gold salts, iothiouracil, mefenamic acid, methyldopa, oxyphenbutazone, quinidine sulfate, quinine, salicylates, and oral hypoglycemic agents.

Bleeding Time

The bleeding time can be elevated because of the action of dextran, pantothenyl alcohol and its derivatives, streptokinase-streptodornase, and aspirin.

Coagulation Time

Elevated coagulation times can result from the action of anticoagulants or from the excessive use of tetracycline. Decreased times have been reported following the administration of corticosteroids and epinephrine.

Prothrombin Time

Increased prothrombin times can follow the administration of antibiotics, oral anticoagulants, chloral hydrate, hydroxyzine, iothiouracil, methylthiouracil, phenylbutazone, phenyramidol, phosphorus toxicity, propylthiouracil, salicylates, sulfonamides, tolbutamide, vitamin A, and other drugs. Shortened times have been reported from the action of barbiturates, ethchlorvynol, glutethimide, meprobamate, oral contraceptives, and vitamin K.

Sedimentation Rate

Elevated sedimentation rates caused by drug action have incriminated dextran, methysergide, methyldopa, trifluperidol, and vitamin K.

Direct Antiglobulin Test

False-positive results on the direct antiglobulin test can occur from the action of cephalothin, chlorpropamide, melphalan, methyldopa, penicillin, phenacetin, quinidine, quinine, stibophen, and sulfonamides, among other agents.

Statistical Analysis of Data

The sections that follow review briefly some of the statistical tools that can be used by the laboratory staff in assessing test quality. The use of these tools in no way implies that, if the tests are acceptable, they also are accurate, as errors can be introduced in other ways and still go unnoticed. For example, if a large batch of hemoglobin data is submitted and the data from one or two tests are entered incorrectly (i.e., clerical error), the error could go undetected because of the large number of tests involved. The common terminology used in statistical analysis is defined first.

Statistical Terms

Normal distribution is a measure of the dispersion of a group of values around a mean derived from the normal curve, which, in turn, is defined as the distribution curve of a series of analyses obtained from healthy individuals. It has a standard shape

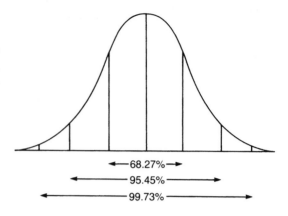

Figure 16.1. Gaussian curve (normal distribution).

that can be found by using an expansion of the binomial theorem $(p + q)^n$ and also is known as a *bell-shaped* or *gaussian curve* (Figure 16.1). The value is calculated from the area under the center of the curve so that the mean value ±1 standard deviation (SD) is 68.27% of the whole area. Likewise, the mean value ±2 SD is 95.45%, and the mean value of the area, ±3 SD, is 99.73% of the curve area.

The *coefficient of variation (CV)* is an alternative method of expressing the SD. The following is the formula to calculate the CV:

$$\frac{SD \times 100}{Mean}$$

The *standard error (SE)* is a measure of the dispersion of the mean of a group of data. The SE is used to compare means and is calculated as follows:

$$\frac{SD}{\sqrt{N}}$$

The *variance (S^2)* is defined as the square of the SD.

Percentile estimates are a method of measuring the dispersion of a series of numbers. If, for example, the ninety-fifth percentile estimates for a series of hemoglobin determinations are 11.0–16.0 g/dl, then 2.5% of all tests carried out had a value of less than 11.0 g/dl, and 2.5% had a value of more than 16.0 g/dl. The percentile estimates are not affected by the shape of the distribution curve but, when the curve is truly bell shaped, the data are identical to the SD calculated conventionally.

Table 16.3. Comparison Between a Standard and a Control

	Standard	Control
Composition	Completely known	Known with a reasonably high degree of reliability
Stability	Very stable	Moderately stable
Physical properties	Completely known	Closely resembles unknown specimens
Reactivity	Well defined	Similar to unknown specimens
Verification	By several different methods or by a reference method	By replicate testing using one method
Information yield	Accuracy and precision	Precision

The *probability (p)* refers to the likelihood that a result equal to or larger than the one obtained would occur only by chance. It is expressed, for example, as 0.05, which denotes that the chance is 5 in 100, or 5%, that these particular data would be found by chance alone.

The *mean* ($\bar{x}$) is the average of a set of data, calculated by dividing the sum of the values by the total number of values.

The *median* is a measurement of the center of distribution of a series of data. It is defined as the value having an equal number of determinations above and below it.

The *student's t test* is used to determine whether the means of two results differ significantly, and it uses the SD in the calculation.

The *F test* determines whether the dispersion of two results around the mean differ significantly: That is, do they differ in their SD?

The *chi-square test* (χ^2) checks for the homogeneity of populations, in which values are reported as positive or negative instead of being reported quantitatively.

Accuracy is the conformity of the test value to the true value.

Precision is the reproducibility of values obtained from replicate testing.

Calibration is the process of relating a measuring instrument to primary physical constants.

Standardization establishes the response of a test method to known standard materials. Standards are usually highly purified materials of known composition.

Control is defined as a known material whose physical and chemical composition more closely resembles the unknown test specimen than the standard. It is used to challenge the test system by checking on the performance of the system against known materials closely related to the unknown. Table 16.3 shows a comparison between a standard and a control.

Control Techniques

Levey-Jennings Charts

In a Levey-Jennings chart, the control results are plotted on the *y* axis (the ordinate) and the data are plotted on the *x* axis (abscissa). On the chart, the expected mean is depicted in the center and the acceptable limits are represented by a broken line. These limits are usually set at either ±2 SD or ±3 SD of the mean (Figure 16.2).

Three principal patterns of data can be obtained by the scanning of Levey-Jennings charts. First, the degree of *scatter or imprecision of the control* can be judged by the dispersion of the data plotted. For example, poor precision or the inability to repeat the results within an acceptable standard are indicated if data randomly extend from +3 SD to –3 SD over a time period.

The second type of pattern observed is a *shift in results*. This pattern occurs when there is an abrupt change, either high or low, of data values. It commonly represents a reagent change or a change in an equipment module such as a colorimetric lamp.

The third pattern that can be observed is a *trend*. This differs from a shift in that it is a slowly developing alteration of data values, either high or low. This progressive drift can result from a variety of factors, including reagent instability or loss of light intensity of a photometric source. If data points are principally on one side of the mean, either high or low, a shift has taken place or a

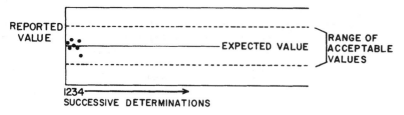

Figure 16.2. Modified Levey-Jennings quality control graph. Control data are graphed as acquired and should fall within the established limits. Values exceeding the limits are indicative of a possible analytic problem or mistake. (Reprinted from JB Henry [ed]. Clinical Diagnosis and Management by Laboratory Methods [17th ed]. Philadelphia: Saunders, 1984. P 83.)

change in the mean value has resulted. Such changes are commonly due to a switch in control lot numbers, or may result from the calculation of incorrect means from a statistically invalid set of data (Figure 16.3).

Cusum Techniques

Systematic errors can be observed using the Levey-Jennings charts, but they can also be illustrated graphically in a more exact way by the use of the cumulative sum method (Woodward and Goldsmith, 1964). The calculation of Cusum for a set of hemoglobin data is shown in Table 16.4. These data can be plotted on a graph with the cusum values on the y axis and time on the x axis.

If there is equal scatter of data above and below the mean or target value, the cusum plot will be a horizontal line but, if a systematic error occurs, the slope of the line will increase, as the error is added daily to the previous cusum data. The larger the error, the steeper the angle of the data plots.

Cusum analysis, in general, provides a better method of observing systematic errors than do the Levey-Jennings plots. This technique is most useful when applied to a computerized quality control program.

Westgard's Multirule

Westgard's multirule approach to the evaluation of quality control data (Westgard et al., 1981) uses

Figure 16.3. Examples of three common changes in quality control data. Dispersion is seen when there is an increased frequency of both high and low outliers. A progressive drift in the reported values from the prior mean value is called a trend. A shift occurs when there is an abrupt change from the established mean value. (Reprinted from JB Henry [ed]. Clinical Diagnosis and Management by Laboratory Methods [17th ed]. Philadelphia: Saunders, 1984. P 83.)

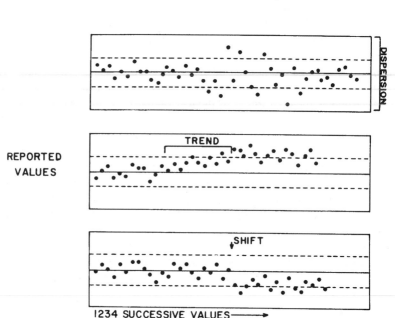

Table 16.4. Examples of Cusum Data for Hemoglobin Determinations

Day	Observed Hemoglobin Value (g/dl)	Control Target (mean, g/dl)	Daily Difference from Mean	Cusum
1	15.1	14.8	+0.3	+0.3
2	14.7	14.8	−0.1	+0.2
3	15.0	14.8	+0.2	+0.4
4	14.8	14.8	0	+0.4
5	14.8	14.8	0	+0.4
6	14.9	14.8	+0.1	+0.5
7	14.7	14.8	−0.1	+0.4
8	14.8	14.8	0	+0.4
9	14.7	14.8	−0.1	+0.3
10	14.7	14.8	−0.1	+0.2

Levey-Jennings charts with several restraining limitations, as follows:

Rule 1. Patient data are rejected for the run if one control exceeds the mean value ±3-SD limits (1:3s rule)

Rule 2. Data are rejected when two consecutive observations exceed the mean ±2-SD limits in the same direction—that is, either both high or both low (2:2s rule).

Rule 3. Data are rejected when one control exceeds the target mean by +2 SD and one control exceeds the mean by −2 SD (4s rule).

Rule 4. Data are rejected when four consecutive control observations exceed the mean by 1 SD, either by four high points (>1 SD) or four low points (<1 SD) (4:1s rule).

Rule 5. Data are rejected when 10 consecutive control points fall on one side of the mean—that is, a shift in data (10 rule).

Westgard's rules can be used when several control levels are run with each batch of tests, such as trilevel controls that are commonly used in routine hematologic testing. In addition to improving the performance characteristics of the quality control program, these rules also provide additional information as to the type of error. Rules 1 (the 1:3s rule) and 3 (the 4s rule) suggest random error in the analysis, whereas rules 2 (the 2:2s rule), 4 (the 4:1s rule), and 5 (the 10 rule) generally suggest systematic errors.

Tests Used to Monitor Quality Control

Standard Deviation

The SD is a statistic used to compare two or more sets of data. The formula used is:

$$SD = \sqrt{\frac{\Sigma(\overline{X} - X)^2}{n - 1}}$$

where $\overline{X}$ is the difference between two sets of results. An example using hemoglobin is shown in Table 16.5.

The SD of ±0.16 g/dl was arrived at by the following processes:

1. The average result ($\overline{X}$) was calculated by adding the sum of the 15 control results and dividing by the number of days run.
2. The result ($\overline{X}$) obtained from rule 1 was subtracted from each day's results, ignoring the ± signs—that is, on day 1, 14.9($\overline{X}$) − 14.7 = 0.2.
3. Each difference value then was squared, and the sum of each squared value totaled—that is, on day 1, 14.9($\overline{X}$) − 14.7 = $(0.2)^2$ = 0.04.
4. The standard formula was used:

$$SD = \sqrt{\frac{\Sigma(\overline{X} - X)^2}{n - 1}}$$

Interpretation of these results shows that 95% of all hemoglobin controls can be expected to fall within the range 14.9 ± 0.32 or 14.6–15.2 g/dl, and

Table 16.5. Example of Calculation of Standard Deviation (SD) Using 15 Consecutive Days of Hemoglobin Control Values

Day	Result	$(\bar{x} - x)$	$(\bar{x} - x)^2$
1	14.7	0.2	0.04
2	14.9	0	0
3	15.2	0.3	0.09
4	14.6	0.3	0.09
5	14.9	0	0
6	15.1	0.2	0.04
7	14.8	0.1	0.01
8	14.8	0.1	0.01
9	14.9	0	0
10	15.0	0.1	0.01
11	14.8	0.1	0.01
12	14.9	0	0
13	14.7	0.2	0.04
14	15.0	0.1	0.01
15	14.9	0	0
	$\bar{x}$ 14.9		SD 0.35*

$$* SD = \sqrt{\frac{0.35}{14}} = \sqrt{0.025} = 0.16$$

99.7% of controls should fall within the range 14.9 ± 0.48 or 14.4–15.4 g/dl.

Duplicate or blind split controls can also be used as an analytic tool to assess quality. When using duplicate specimens, the SD is calculated from the following formula:

$$SD = \sqrt{\frac{\Sigma(\text{differences between duplicates})^2}{2n}}$$

An example of a split-sample SD system using leukocyte counts is shown in Table 16.6. The calculation was carried out by the following processes:

1. The mean of the sets of duplicate results is calculated ($\bar{x}$) from the following formula:

$$\bar{X} = \frac{X_1 + X_2}{2}$$

2. The SD of each set of data is obtained from this formula:

$$\sqrt{\frac{(X_1 - X_2)^2}{2}}$$

That is, the square of the differences between results is divided by 2 (the number of results) and is square-rooted. Using specimen 1 as the example, the mean of the two split samples was 5.0×10^9/liter. The difference between results is 0.4×10^9/liter:

$$SD = \sqrt{\frac{(0.4)^2}{2}} = \sqrt{0.08} = 0.28$$

or $5.2 - 4.8 \times 10^9$/liter.

3. The CV is calculated from the following formula:

$$\frac{SD}{\text{Mean}} \times 100$$

Duplicate or split-sample approaches to quality control allow the technologist to view analytic reproducibility (spread, variability) of the test in two specimens that should give the same result. Split-sample designs are not particularly useful in detecting drift, abrupt changes, or preanalytic changes, but they are helpful in assessing true precision of the test without operator bias. A simple program can be set up by the quality control officer in which duplicate specimens are obtained

Table 16.6. Example of a Calculation of Standard Deviation (SD) Using Sets of Four Split Samples for Leukocyte Counts

Specimen	Result 1 ($\times 10^9$/liter) x_1	Result 2 ($\times 10^9$/liter) x_2	$\bar{x}$	SD	CV (%)
1	4.8	5.2	5.0	0.28	5.7
2	10.4	10.3	10.35	0.07	0.7
3	7.3	7.5	7.4	0.14	1.9
4	5.9	6.2	6.05	0.21	3.5

CV = coefficient of variation.

from both normal and abnormal individuals. If abnormal specimens are difficult to draw in this way, the specimens can be *adjusted* by centrifuging the anticoagulated sample and either removing some of the packed red-cell mass and leukocyte layer or removing plasma. Fictitious names then are given to these split specimens, and they are both afforded accession numbers. Care should be taken not to introduce control specimens sequentially but to introduce them into the test system at different times or even to different laboratory shifts.

The F (Sign) Test

The *F*, or sign, test (Table 16.7) enables a comparison between two series of tests and determines whether there is significant variation between the results. The simplest way to test the null hypothesis that two methods are equivalent, using matching pairs of tests, is to consider only the algebraic sign of the observed differences (d_i). If the null hypothesis is true, whether a pair yields a positive or a negative value depends solely on the difference between the paired subjects and not on the methods.

Therefore, whether or not a particular d_i is positive or negative depends only on random error. As the likelihood that any d will be positive or negative is 0.5, we may consider the signs of the n differences as a random sample of size n from a binomial population where $p = 0.5$.

For example, if a comparison of hemoglobin methods using different automated equipment is under review, application of the *F* test would be as follows:

1. Calculate the difference between the pairs of data $(d = x - y)$.
2. Tabulate the number of pluses, minuses, and zero values.

$$+ = x_1 > y$$
$$- = x_1 < y$$
$$0 = x_1 = y$$

3. Record the smaller of these numbers (+ or –). This is *S*.

4. Using Table 16.8, check for the statistical significance.

Table 16.7. Example of the *F* Test Using Hemoglobin Determinations

Method X	Method Y	$d_i (x_1 - y_1)$
14.2	14.1	+0.1
14.8	14.6	+0.2
7.4	7.6	–0.2
10.3	10.1	+0.2
12.8	12.8	0
13.2	13.1	+0.1
17.0	16.9	+0.1
6.4	6.0	+0.4
15.0	15.1	–0.1
14.9	14.9	0
19.4	19.0	+0.4
9.2	9.0	+0.2
11.4	11.3	+0.1

Table 16.8. Critical Values of *S* for the *F* Test

n	1%	5%	10%	25%
1				
2				
3				0
4				0
5			0	0
6		0	0	1
7		0	0	1
8	0	0	1	1
9	0	1	1	2
10	0	1	1	2
11	0	1	2	3
12	1	2	2	3
13	1	2	3	3

S = sign.
Source: Data from WH Boyer. CRC Handbook of Tables for Probability and Statistics. Boca Raton, FL: CRC Press, 1966.

The following example illustrates application of the *F* test:
1. N = 13
2. $x_1 > y = 9$ = plus
   $x_1 < y = 2$ = minus
   $x_1 = y = 2 = 0$
3. The smallest number attributed to a sign is 2; that is, *S* = 2.
4. From Table 16.8, it can be seen that for n = 13, a value of *S* = 2 is significant at the 5% level. If *S* = 4, the correct conclusion is that there is no statistical significance in the results.

Table 16.9. Percentage Points of the *t* Distribution

df	Area in Two Tails		
	0.10	0.05	0.02
1	6.314	12.706	31.821
2	2.920	4.303	6.965
3	2.353	3.182	4.541
4	2.132	2.776	3.747
5	2.015	2.571	3.365
6	1.943	2.447	3.143
7	1.895	2.365	2.998
8	1.860	2.306	2.891
9	1.833	2.262	2.821
10	1.812	2.228	2.764
11	1.796	2.201	2.718
12	1.782	2.179	2.681

df = degrees of freedom.
Source: Data from ES Pearson, HO Hartley. Biometrika Tables for Statistics (3rd ed). Vol 1. Cambridge, UK: Cambridge University Press, 1966.

The Student's *t* Test

The *t* test is used to compare the means of two or more series of tests. It determines whether the two means are significantly different and should be used only when the *F* test shows no significant difference in variability. This test is a very sensitive analytic tool, particularly if a large number of data are used. In the latter situation, however, false conclusions may be generated, and so the *t* test should be restricted to approximately 30 sets of data.

The test uses paired data, x_1 and y_1, in a way that is similar to the *F* test. Application of the *t* test is as follows:

1. Calculate the difference between the pairs of data ($d_i = x_1 - y_1$).
2. Calculate the SD of the differences and the mean of the differences.
3. Then,

$$\frac{d}{SD/\sqrt{n}} = t(n-1)$$

when n = number of paired sets of data.

Using the hemoglobin data illustrated in the *F* test and applying it to the *t* test, the following is found:

- Number of pairs: 13
- Mean of differences: 0.15
- SD of differences: 0.172

Then,

$$t = \frac{0.15}{1.72} \div \sqrt{13} = \frac{0.15}{1.72} \div 3.6 = \frac{0.15}{0.047} = 3.19$$

Referring to Table 16.9, with n − 1 = 12 df (degrees of freedom), the two-tailed test at the 5% level indicates 2.179 as the appropriate cutoff point. The critical ratio calculated, 3.19, is greater than 2.179; therefore, the *t* value of 3.19 is significant, and it can be concluded that method Y gives results that are different from and higher than those obtained with method A.

Scatter Diagrams

Scatter diagrams are a graphic display of paired data, one variable plotted on the horizontal axis and one variable plotted on the vertical axis. Three principal scatter graphs are identified:

1. Graphs that scatter like "shotgun pellets," denoting uncorrelated sets of data (Figure 16.4A, B).
2. Graphs that produce an upward-sloping ellipse, usually indicating a positive correlation (Figure 16.4C, E).
3. Graphs that exhibit a straight line, denoting either a strong negative correlation (Figure 16.4D) or perfect correlation (Figure 16.4E).

Linear Regression

Linear regression is a mathematic tool that helps to supplement the scatter diagram analyses. It is a method to define the best straight-line relationship between two variables. The so-called best-fit line is that with the smallest sum of the squared distances from each point to the line.

Linear regression is expressed by the equation $y = mx + b$, where y = dependent variable; x = independent variable; m = slope ($\Delta y/\Delta x$), which is a proportionality constant that states that there is a given average change in y for a given change in x; and b = y intercept, which is the point at which the line intersects the y axis where $x = 0$.

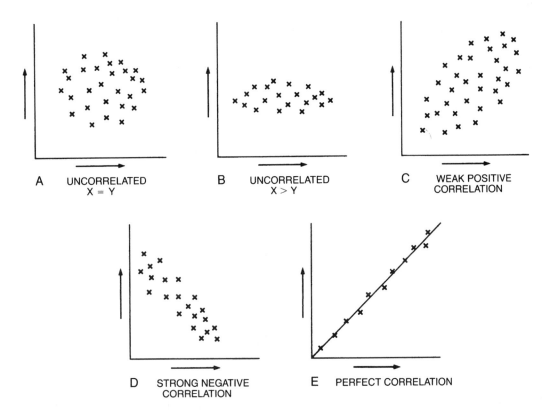

Figure 16.4. Examples of scatter diagrams. A. Uncorrelated data, in which x and y values are equal (round pattern). B. Uncorrelated data, in which x values are greater than y values (elliptic horizontal pattern). C. Weak positive correlation (angled elliptic pattern). D. Strong negative correlation. E. Perfect correlation, in which all the data points fit perfectly along the 45-degree line.

Figure 16.5 illustrates two linear regression graphs. If the line goes through the origin, the y intercept = 0, and the equation simplifies to y = mx. If $\Delta y = \Delta x$, the slope and the equation become y = x. On axes of equal numeric value, the line described by y = x would make an angle of 45 degrees and would pass through the origin (Figure 16.5A).

Figure 16.5B shows a linear regression graph with a positive slope and a positive y intercept. The calculation of linear regression is best carried out by inexpensive pocket calculators and desktop computers, but the following points should be considered when using this analytic tool to compare two sets of data:

1. Beware of outlying points. If most of the points are on one end of the range and only one or two points are at the other end of the range, those outliers carry proportionately more weight and may alter the correlation.

2. The method assumes that the scatter of the data is equal at all levels.
3. The linear regression line should be used only for the range covered by the data. The center of the line is the most reliable.
4. The technique is applicable only if the variables are related linearly.

Linear regression provides the laboratory with two useful tools: a simple method relating one set of data to another and a prediction of future values of the dependent variable.

Youden Plots

When two controls of different values are run, a Youden chart may be plotted (Figure 16.6). The graph is constructed by placing on the vertical axis the mean ±2-SD limits for the abnormal control

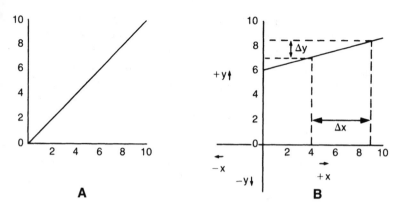

Figure 16.5. Examples of linear regression graphs. A. Perfect agreement. B. Poor agreement; strong positive y intercept, flat curve.

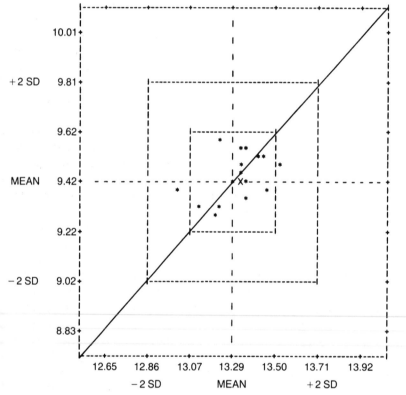

Figure 16.6. Youden plot for hemoglobin.

and on the horizontal axis the same information for the normal control. A square then is drawn to connect the four 2-SD points. A Youden plot is shown in Figure 16.6. The diagonal line from the –2-SD to the +2-SD marks denotes the line of normal distribution and, under normal circumstances, data points will fall on or around this line or will be grouped tightly around the center point. Uneven distribution of points in the corners of the square indicate either high or low shifts of data, and points falling outside the square illustrate that the controls exceeded 2 SD.

Use of Control Samples

The hematology laboratory differs in its approach to quality assurance because of several unique factors that are not present in the chemistry laboratory. First, the controls being analyzed are usually unstable and, even when fixed, possess only a limited shelf life. Second, a large proportion of the results are combinations of both qualitative judgment and quantitative decisions that are unique to the clinical laboratory. Third, until recently, certified calibrated materials had not been available and still are not available for all the equipment in use or for all the tests carried out in the laboratory. Because of these factors, a special effort must be made to modify the quality control approach to ensure adequate controls over the expected range of test results.

Complete Blood Cell Count

Many instruments are currently available that either automatically or semiautomatically determine the CBC, and most of them can be standardized by certified calibrators checked against known manual reference techniques (e.g., Coulter S-Cal). However, it is recommended that these standards be used sparingly at weekly or monthly intervals, or less often, depending on the work volume and the discretion of the technologist. The routine daily control of these instruments, then, presents the laboratory staff with the most cause for concern and takes up the most effort and time.

Commercial and Patient Controls. Commercial controls for a CBC can be obtained from a variety of manufacturers and are usually available at three different levels for all the analytes being measured. It is important to use trilevel samples that cover the expected range of test results because, unlike the control of most chemical tests, CBCs may show nonlinearity over part of the curve and be in control over the remainder.

Besides the standard Levey-Jennings and Youden graphs described on pages 230 and 236, several other methods have been found useful in monitoring control data, particularly for automated cell counters. Many of the newer counters do possess built-in quality control programs, which use either Westgard's rules or Bull's algorithm, and they usually incorporate the use of two different but complementary systems. However, the frequency of running trilevel controls has never been satisfactorily addressed. Many laboratories find it sufficient to run one set every operational shift but, if the laboratory is processing a large volume of tests, it is suggested that multiple sets of controls be run throughout this period.

The testing of commercial controls alone, even at frequent time intervals, adds nothing to the final quality of the test results. Improved quality can come only from the technologist being conscientious and alert to possible analytic problems. All control data should be recorded in such a way as to enable rapid and accurate review. An example of a reporting system is shown in Figure 16.7.

In addition, whenever control data exceed the laboratory's limits, a corrective action report should be generated and signed by the supervisor. Such corrective action should state clearly the problem, the resolution, and the status of the patient data (i.e., whether patient results were released, and, if so, provision of an adequate explanation for this action).

Weighted Moving Averages. The CBC is unique in that it constitutes a test battery that produces interdependent data. As such, the calculated results, the red-cell indices, can be used as a method of ongoing monitoring of test results. This is termed the *weighted moving average* (Bull et al., 1974), or $\overline{x}_B$ *formula*, and is shown in Figure 16.8. One disadvantage of this method is that it controls only the red-cell parameters and not the leukocyte count, the platelet count, or the differential leukocyte count.

Studies on hospitalized patients have shown that the red-cell indices are stable over time (Koepke and Protexter, 1981), and so this can be used as the basis for a quality control system for automated instruments. The formula is mathematically complex but easily implemented with a calculator or computer.

The concept of the weighted moving average is to permit reliable estimates from small samples of the population being tested. It is superior to the traditional moving average because it reacts quickly to changes. The formula both trims the data by giving less weight to the outliers and smooths the data by incorporating information from the previous patient batch in the analysis of the current batch.

The algorithm can detect large shifts effectively, and it has been shown that its power increases with increasing batch numbers. Shifts of

ABNORMAL HIGH CONTROL

DATE _____

SERIAL NO. OF INSTRUMENT _____

TECHNOLOGIST _____ SUPERVISOR _____

CONTROL

MANUFACTURER	LOT NO.	EXP. DATE	ASSAY VALUES							COMMENTS
			WBC	RBC	Hb	Hct	MCV	MCH	MCHC	
ACCEPTABLE RANGE ± 2SD										

LOT NO.	TEST SEQUENCE NO.	DETERMINED VALUES							COMMENTS
		WBC	RBC	Hb	Hct	MCV	MCH	MCHC	

Figure 16.7. Example of control documentation for the Coulter counter. Instructions include the following:

1. Control checks are to be carried out using all three levels of controls at the beginning of each shift and after every 50 patient specimens.
2. The technologist will review the control values, circle the out-of-range values, and document the corrective action as directed in item 3.
3. One or more of the following are to be used in the out-of-range log to document the corrective action taken:
   a. The control result is between the acceptable and action limits (i.e., 2–3 SD). The previous control is within the acceptable limits. Patient's data reported.
   b. The control results exceed the acceptable limit, and the previous control data also are greater than the acceptable limits in the same direction (either both high or both low). Do not report results. Recheck with fresh controls. Repeat patient's specimen as far back as the last acceptable control.
   c. Control exceeds the action range (3 SD). Resolve problem and repeat patient's specimens as far back as the last acceptable control.
   d. One set of controls (low, high, or normal) is consistently out of acceptable range. Open new vial of control; review patient data.
   e. Out-of-range unresolved. Shut down instrument. Rerun on a different instrument all patient specimens as far back as the last acceptable control.
   f. Other (explain in detail).

$$X(B,i) = X(B,i-1) + SGN \left\{ \sum_{j-1}^{N} SGN \left[X(j,i)-X(B,i-1) \right] * \sqrt{|X(j,i)-X(B,i-1)|} * F \right\}$$

$$F = \left\{ \frac{\sum_{j-1}^{N} SGN \left[X(j,i)-X(B,i-1) \right] * \sqrt{|X(j,i)-X(B,i-1)|}}{N^2} \right\}^2$$

WHERE:

$X(B,i)$ = ith $\bar{X}_B$ value
$X(B,i-1)$ = (i-1)th $\bar{X}_B$ value
$X(j,i)$ = the jth value in the ith batch

SGN = the arithmetic sign of number in parentheses
N = number of samples in the batch
$*$ = symbol used to represent multiplication

Figure 16.8. Formula used to calculate the weighted moving average.

Table 16.10. Bull's Weighted Moving Averages

Patient	Mean of Population	MCV (fl)	$(x - \bar{x})$	$\sqrt{(x - \bar{x})}$
1	89	91	2	1.41
2	89	83	6	2.45
3	89	75	14	3.74

MCV = mean cell volume.

less than 2 SD are rarely detected (Cembrowski and Westgard, 1985).

In a manually implemented system, population means are established by analyzing as large a sample as possible—at least 250 blood samples but as many as 1,000 samples, if possible. Once the population means have been established, the weighted moving average analysis can be applied using small samples from the patient population. A 20-patient sample batch is typically used. The red-cell indices are stable to within 1% of the population mean and, using this system in automated analyzers, the test parameters are considered in control when the batch means are within 3% of the expected population means.

When this method is used, changes due to the instrument, the reagent, or sample handling can be detected, as can the direction and amount of this change. An example of this method of analysis is shown in Table 16.10. The square-root function accomplishes the trimming, as it gives proportionally less weight to the results that are further from the population or expected mean. Smoothing of the data is carried out by the use of the previous batch mean as a starting point. As each sample is processed, the means of each of the red-cell indices are subtracted from the corresponding mean of the previous set of samples. The square root of this deviation (the difference between the means) is stored. After 20 samples have been processed, the sum of these square roots is divided by 20, and the result is squared to recover the mean deviation. The individual deviations carry a positive or negative sign, so they can be added to or subtracted from the corresponding previous means. The resulting new mean then is used for the succeeding batch of 20 samples (Coulter Diagnostics, 1981).

Use of Patient Data and Daily Means. The use of daily population means has been proposed as a method of assessing quality assurance (Hoffman and Waid, 1965). Several studies, however, have shown that the method is fairly insensitive to changes in analytic bias (Amador, 1968; Kilgariff and Owen, 1968), whereas others have not demonstrated this insensitivity (Begtrup et al., 1971).

Examples of the use of daily means are presented in Table 16.11. The value of these means and the interpretation of the data are valid only if the initial data are taken from a large number of specimens. The data in Table 16.11 were obtained from 364,800 blood samples collected over a 1-year period. Outliers were excluded by removing all results greater than 3 SD, and the means and ninety-fifth percentile estimates were based on the remaining results.

The percentage spread was calculated from the mean and calculated ranges. Once established, these ranges can act as an excellent secondary source of control for multiphasic hematologic apparatus, either by reviewing data retrospectively or by analyzing data during the run. Batches of at least 20 valid numbers should be used after first removing the outliers. To obtain a database, at least 1,000 specimens should be collected and, if possible, the results transmitted to an on-line computer.

Patient data exceeding either these ranges or the percentage spread from other calculated means are considered a warning sign of a systematic error usually involving calibration of the instrument, reagent problems, or hardware malfunctions.

Use of Patient Specimens as Controls. Aliquots of refrigerated blood samples show no significant change in major hematologic parameters for at least 24 hours. This makes them ideal for run-to-run or shift-to-shift controls. In addition, they can be transferred from major instruments to backup equipment without changes in values. This is in contrast to most

Table 16.11. Analysis of 364,800 Random Ambulatory Patient Specimens of EDTA Blood with Outliers Removed (>3 SD) Using the H6000 Apparatus

Analyte	Mean	± % Spread	Range
Hemoglobin (g/dl)	14.0	2.5	13.7–14.4
Hematocrit (%)	42.2	2.5	41.1–43.3
RBCs ($\times 10^{12}$/liter)	4.82	3.5	4.65–4.99
MCH (pg)	29.3	2.5	28.6–30.0
MCHC (%)	33.1	2.0	32.5–33.8
MCV (fl)	88.0	2.0	86.2–89.8
WBCs ($\times 10^9$/liter)	7.65	8.5	7.00–8.30
Segmented cells (%)	60.0	2.0	58.8–61.2
Eosinophils (%)	2.5	13.5	2.2–2.9
Basophils (%)	0.6	20.0	0.5–0.7
Monocytes (%)	5.8	12.0	5.0–6.5
Lymphocytes (%)	29.7	4.5	28.4–31.1
Large unstained cells (%)	1.0	30.0	0.7–1.3
Platelets ($\times 10^9$/liter)	281.0	7.0	261–301

SD = standard deviation; RBCs = red blood cells; MCH = mean cell hemoglobin; MCHC = mean cell hemoglobin concentration; MCV = mean cell volume; WBCs = white blood cells.
Note: Gender-based differences in hemoglobin, hematocrit, and red-cell count are not separated.

commercial controls, which are subject to instrument method bias. Patient controls can be pooled, provided that the separate samples are the same blood type. If enough specimens are refrigerated immediately at a constant temperature and are stoppered quickly, the pool will provide mean values approaching the patient means, as shown in Table 16.11 for all CBC parameters, including leukocytes and platelet counts.

Use of Red-Cell Indices. A variation of the use of patient data as controls has been proposed (Koepke and Protextor, 1981). The technique depends on the stability of the erythrocyte indices—MCV, mean cell hemoglobin (MCH), and MCHC—within particular population groups. This stability provides a set of standards with known interrelationships among the indices and other cell characteristics, and these indices provide a database for the system.

Distribution of the index data is symmetric and approximately gaussian. The indices for different patient populations show only slight variability, the majority of nonanemic hospitalized individuals having normal indices. Consequently, if the indices are constant within a given population, the means from successive batches of patient samples also remain constant, within ±3% of the standard used. This figure depends not only on the population sampling but

also on the equipment and reagents used. If these data batches are not within the allowable spread, and if there is no significant change in patient population (such as the introduction of pediatric or chemotherapy patients), the technologist can conclude that the instrument has drifted out of control.

The most sensitive indicator for monitoring overall instrument performance is the MCHC (Koepke and Protextor, 1981), probably because it is derived (on Coulter counters) from three directly measured parameters: the hemoglobin, red-cell count, and MCV. MCHC deviations have been associated with more than 80% of malfunctions. The most common abnormality seen is a parallel rise in both MCV and MCH, which indicates protein accumulation in the counting aperture. Routine cleaning procedures will rectify this problem.

Red-cell indices are also similar worldwide and do not appear subject to environmental changes. The mean MCV, MCH, and MCHC has been reported to be 89.5 fl, 30.5 pg, and 34.0 g/dl by one research team (Bull and Hay, 1985) and 88.0 fl, 29.3 pg, and 33.1 g/dl by another (Simmons and Chin, 1987).

Quality Control in Cellular Red-Cell Morphologic Testing. Qualitative tests, unlike quantitative tests, present a difficult problem to control adequately, as the results depend on individual judg-

Table 16.12. Microscopic Quality Control of Leukocyte and Platelet Counts Using a Well-Spread Blood Smear

Average Number of Leukocytes per High-Power Field	Estimated Total Leukocyte Count ($\times 10^9$/liter)	Average No. of Platelets per High-Power Oil-Immersion Field	Estimated Platelet Count ($\times 10^9$/liter)
2–3	4.0–7.0	2–3	50–100
4–6	7.0–10.0	4–6	100–150
7–10	10.0–13.0	7–10	150–250
11–20	13.0–18.0	11–20	250–500

ment and opinion. The best control is to have a group of technologists, trained by the same person in the department, reporting all morphologic conditions. Additionally, the senior technologist should review all abnormal blood smears before releasing the reports.

A standardized scheme for the reporting of red-cell abnormalities should be adopted. Examples of such a scheme are given on page 33. The term *anisocytosis* means little and should be avoided unless a large number of cells do vary in size. More meaningful terms would be *microcytosis* and *macrocytosis*, as these words are more specific and can more easily be translated into a clinical interpretation. Likewise, the term *poikilocytosis* should be reserved for classic teardrop cells. Elongated or fragmented cells are best described as *ovalocytes, schistocytes,* and so on. A well-made blood smear can be used as an adjunct to the quality control of both the leukocyte and the platelet counts. The rules of thumb (discussed later) can be used to assess and control these counts using a freshly made and well-spread smear. Table 16.12 shows the microscopic quality control of leukocyte and platelet counts.

In situations in which there is an excess of 4% nucleated red cells in the blood smear, the leukocyte count should be corrected by the following formula to produce the corrected count:

$$\frac{\text{Total leukocyte count}}{100 + \text{Nucleated red cells}} \times 100$$

Use of Controls in Differential Leukocyte Counting. The two principal methods for determining differential leukocyte counts are by manual or semiautomated subjective review by a technologist, by a pattern-recognition microscopic method, or by an automated flow-through cytochemical method. The control of manual subjective counts cannot be carried out using conventional quality control reagents or procedures. First, the cells are stable in the blood for only a short time, which precludes the reuse of the same sample over a prolonged period. Second, there are no objective standards or control materials available against which to compare results.

One method of controlling manual or pattern-recognition differential leukocyte counts is to make and stain a batch of smears from fresh blood. Both normal and abnormal specimens can be used. Each day, one set of premade methyl alcohol–fixed slides are introduced into the laboratory, and differential counts are carried out. A record should be kept of all results, including the technologist's identification, and these data should be collated and compared to a 500-cell differential count performed by the supervisor and to other technologists' differential counts. Using such a method, it is possible to check leukocyte morphologic features, red-cell morphologic features, and platelet estimates, and to detect any particular weakness in the ability of the staff to recognize individual cells.

The adequate evaluation and control of differential leukocyte counting depends on an adequately prepared and stained blood smear. This is discussed in more detail on page 267, but it should be emphasized that distribution of the cells takes on a nonrandom pattern according to the cells' size and density. Consequently, the larger cells, such as monocytes, neutrophils, and large abnormal cells, tend to be found disproportionately at the lateral and feather edges of the preparation, and the smaller cells, such as lymphocytes, are seen more commonly in the body of the smear. It is advisable to count as many

Table 16.13. Ninety-Five Percent Confidence Limits for Differential Leukocyte Counts

| "Truth" | Number of Cells Counted in the Differential | | | |
	100	200	500	1,000
0	0–4	0–2	0–1	0–1
1	0–6	0–4	0–3	0–2
2	0–8	0–6	0–4	1–4
3	0–9	1–7	1–5	2–5
4	1–10	1–8	2–7	2–6
5	1–12	2–10	3–8	3–7
6	2–13	3–11	4–9	4–8
7	2–14	3–12	4–10	5–9
8	3–16	4–13	5–11	6–10
9	4–17	5–14	6–12	7–11
10	4–18	6–16	7–13	8–13
15	8–24	10–21	12–19	12–18
20	12–30	14–27	16–24	17–23
25	16–35	19–32	21–30	22–28
30	21–40	23–37	26–35	27–33
35	25–46	28–43	30–40	32–39
40	30–51	33–48	35–45	36–44
45	35–56	38–53	40–50	41–49
50	39–61	42–58	45–55	46–54
55	44–65	47–63	50–60	51–59
60	49–70	52–67	55–65	56–64
65	54–75	57–72	60–70	61–68
70	60–70	63–77	65–74	67–73
75	65–74	68–81	70–79	72–78
80	70–88	73–86	76–84	77–83
85	76–92	79–90	81–89	82–88
90	82–96	84–94	87–93	87–92
95	88–99	90–98	92–97	93–97
100	96–100	98–100	99–100	99–100

Source: Data from CL Rumke. Variability of results in differential counts on blood smears. Triangle 4:156, 1960.

cells as possible, because the more cells counted, the more precise the test. On leukopenic blood specimens, it is advisable to make and stain fresh buffy-coat preparations to maximize precision.

Differential precision is a function of the adequacy of the slide and the number of cells counted. Table 16.13 illustrates that if "truth" is 50, a 100-cell differential leukocyte count will fall into the range of 39–61% in 95% of cases. This number is tightened to 42–58% if 200 cells are counted, and narrowed to 46–54% if 1,000 cells are counted. Unfortunately, it is not practical to count more than 100 or 200 cells routinely, and this defines the limits for the precision of the test. It should be noted that there is no available method for determining accuracy, as this denotes "truth" and can be achieved only when the test is compared using a calibrator.

Fully automated differential leukocyte counts carried out by flow-through cytochemical techniques (e.g., H1, H2 Analyzers, Miles Inc., Tarytown, NY) allow large numbers of cells to be counted, the exact number being the function of the total leukocyte count and time. Approximately 10,000 cells are counted, which guarantees excellent precision (Table 16.14). Using patient means data previously described, it is possible to control the differential leukocyte count to less than a 5% spread on all cells except eosinophils, basophils, and monocytes. Large unstained cells usually are present at approximately 1% concentration and do

Table 16.14. Accuracy of Reticulocyte Counts

Desired Accuracy (SE)	No. of Red Cells That Must Be Counted per Percentage of Reticulocytes Present in the Blood					
	1%	2%	5%	10%	25%	50%
5%	40,400	19,600	7,600	3,000	1,600	400
10%	10,100	4,900	1,900	900	400	160
20%	2,525	1,225	475	225	100	25

Note: The chart shows the number of red cells that must be counted at various reticulocyte percentages if an accurate count to within 5, 10, or 20% is to be achieved.
Source: Data from M Seip. Reticulocyte studies: the liberation of red blood corpuscles from the bone marrow into the peripheral blood and the production of erythrocytes elucidated by reticulocyte investigations. Acta Med Scand (Suppl):282, 1953.

not vary as a group beyond 0.7–1.3%. Besides this control mechanism, the cytochemical procedure can be compared with the results of a manual differential count. However, the statistical problem of the number of cells counted complicates the comparison, as it is difficult to compare data adequately when one set of data is based on a 100- or 200-cell test and the other is drawn from a 10,000-cell test. Invariably, such a comparison yields little, and it is doubtful whether it is of any value. Adequate control of the H1 or H2 apparatus is better achieved by photographing or printing the oscilloscope image of the *x-y* threshold displays of the peroxidase channel and of the absorption patterns to ensure a correct setting. In addition, the threshold settings themselves should be monitored on a daily basis to check stability.

Hemocytometer Errors. The random distribution of cells in a hemocytometer conforms to certain absolute theoretical distributions. The SE of such a distribution is given by the formula $SD = \pm\sqrt{m}$, where m is the mean number of cells in the area. This random distribution is termed a *Poisson distribution* and cannot be reduced by improvement of methodology. In practice, $SD = \pm 0.92\sqrt{m}$, but this variation is often neglected in favor of the mathematically simpler form.

If a hemocytometer is filled with standard particles so that the mean particle count is 400, of the counts made on this suspension 95% will be within the range of 360–440 (i.e., 2 SD). In 66% of the total counts made, the number of particles will be in the range of 380–420 (i.e., 1 SD) and, in 99.7% of the counts, the number of particles will be between 340 and 460 (i.e.,

3 SD). This means that if a standard manual dilution is made (1:200) and an improved Neubauer hemocytometer is used, a red-cell count of 4.0×10^{12}/liter will fall between 3.4 and 4.6×10^{12}/liter. This is excluding other errors, such as those in pipetting, counting, the hemocytometer itself, and those attributed to observation. Consequently, manual cell counts, although occasionally still carried out in smaller laboratories, produce such gross errors that their use is limited strictly to cell counts of body fluids that are unsuitable for automated counting equipment.

Reticulocyte Control. Reticulocyte counting requires much attention to detail. The area of the smear that should be chosen for the count is the point at which the cells are undistorted and the staining is good. A common mistake is to make the smear too thin, although the cells should not overlap. Reticulocytes should be counted using a high-power oil-immersion lens and a Miller disc or some other device that restricts the field of the count. The counting procedure should be appropriate to the number of reticulocytes present. Table 16.14 illustrates the mathematic error of the count.

In practice, it is unnecessary to count large numbers of cells, and it is sufficient to survey fields so that at least 100 reticulocytes are counted. The number of red cells in every tenth field should be counted, and the reticulocyte percentage should be calculated from the following formula:

$$\frac{\text{Number of reticulocytes seen}}{\substack{\text{Approximate number of red cells} \\ \text{present in the fields embracing} \\ \text{the reticulocytes}}} \times 100$$

Table 16.15. Analytic Variability of Coagulation Tests

Test	Result Range	Analytic Variation of the Test (CV in the Given Range)	Significant Change in the Test Result (>3 SD)
Prothrombin time	10–12 secs	3%	>1.0 sec
	20–24 secs	5%	>3.0 secs
Activated partial thromboplastin time	26–40 secs	5%	>4.5 secs
	52–80 secs	7%	>14.0 secs
Fibrinogen (clot method)	1.5–4.0 g/liter	6%	>0.4 g/liter

CV = coefficient of variation; SD = standard deviation.
Source: Data from JA Koepke, BS Bull, et al. Hematology. In SL Inborn (ed), Quality Assurance Practice for Health Laboratories. Washington, DC: American Public Health Association, 1978. P 695.

Recently, commercial reticulocyte controls have been made available (Streck Laboratories, Omaha, Nebraska).

Preserved human reticulocytes have also been used as a control (Tsuda and Tatsumi, 1990). If whole blood is collected in acid citrate dextrose anticoagulant and stored at 4°C, the reticulocyte count decreases to 80% of its initial value after 1 week and to 60% after 3 weeks. As this decrease is reproducible and is expedient in vitro, it is believed that this material could be used as a control in the same way as isotopes are used, because of its predictable decay.

Coagulation Tests. Coagulation tests can be controlled in a manner similar to that for routine hematologic testing, using commercially obtained trilevel lyopholyzed plasma. Multiple sets of data can then be analyzed statistically for SD and CV and plotted on Levey-Jennings graphs.

Routine tests, such as the prothrombin time and the partial thromboplastin time, should be tested in duplicate unless the laboratory has shown that the test precision is such that this cross-checking is unnecessary. It has been shown that 99% of duplicate prothrombin times and partial thromboplastin times differ by 0.45 seconds or less and 4.0 seconds or less, respectively (Keshgegian et al., 1986). Regardless of such data, however, it is recommended that patient times in excess of twice the normal control be rerun and that the results be averaged.

The analytic variability of coagulation tests depends on both the equipment and the reagents used. The mean prothrombin time is similar for normal individuals and the control. However, normal patient values for the activated partial thromboplastin time may differ significantly from the control value. Table 16.15 illustrates the analytic variability of the routine tests.

Replicate Controls. A useful means of assessing equipment drift is to run replicate patient samples throughout the run. Depending on the size of the laboratory, replicates can be run as frequently as every tenth specimen or as infrequently as every fortieth. Once the paired data have been recorded, the differences should be examined by standard statistical methods for SD and CV and correlated on a day-to-day basis. Using Coulter equipment, it is useful to run at least one replicate on every rack of specimens.

Rules of Thumb

Certain rules of thumb are well known in the hematology laboratory. These rules, and variations of them, are often used to determine the validity of the red-cell measurements, but they apply only when the patient's red blood cells (RBCs) are normal in size, shape, and hemoglobin content. The rules are as follows:

- Hematocrit = RBC × 9
- Hemoglobin = RBC × 3
- Hematocrit = hemoglobin × 3
- Hematocrit + 6(±3) = first two figures of the red-cell count: that is, 30 + 6(±3) = 33–39

When the hematocrit is 30%, the expected total red-cell count should have a range of 3.3–3.9 × 10^{12}/liter.

Table 16.16. Suggested Limits for Rechecking Hematologic Tests

Test	Decision Level	Action to Be Taken
Hemoglobin	<11.0 and >18 g/liter	Recheck low hemoglobin by second method and examine red cells for unusual morphologic features. Recheck high hemoglobin by a second method to verify results.
Hematocrit	<30 and >54%	Recheck by second method to verify.
Red-cell count	<3.0 and >6.0 × 10^{12}/liter	Recheck by second method to verify.
MCV	<75 and >100 fl	Recheck by second method and examine the blood smear for the presence of either microcytes or macrocytes.
MCHC	<30%	Recheck by second method and examine the blood smear for evidence of hypochromia.
Leukocyte count	<3.0 and >13.0 × 10^{9}/liter	Recheck by second method and examine the blood smear for leukocyte estimation (see page 242).
Differential		Recheck with a second slide by another technologist. If an automated count is carried out, the second or backup procedure should be manual.
Leukocyte count		
Segmental cells	>85%	
Band cells	>10%	
Eosinophils	>10%	
Basophils	>2%	
Monocytes	>10%	
Lymphocytes	>60% (adults)	
Large unstained cells	>2.8%	
(by H1 or H2 analyzer)	(or >5.0% [HI/HII])	
Any immature cells	—	
(manual method)		
Platelets	<100 and >750 × 10^{9}/liter	Recheck by a second method or by examining a well-prepared blood smear (see page 242).

MCV = mean cell volume; MCHC = mean cell hemoglobin concentration.

Additional Control Limits

Despite the statistical evaluation and manipulation of hematologic data, it is sometimes wise to repeat tests that appear perfectly controlled. This decision can be made for a variety of reasons, because no matter how vigilant the technologist may be or how tightly organized the quality control program is, sudden unexplained errors arise that go undetected. Fortunately, hematologic parameters can often be checked by the microscopic review of a well-made blood slide, and this should always be done, particularly when red-cell or hemoglobin parameters are in doubt. Table 16.16 details suggested limits for rechecking, and these should be modified to each particular laboratory regimen. It should be pointed out that various estimations from smears are gross checks only. Rather than acting as a sensitive means of detecting minor errors, blood smear evaluation functions as a method of discovering errors such as mislabeled or interchanged specimens or inadequately mixed samples.

Other quality control adjuncts are used in conditions discussed in the following paragraphs.

Lipemia. Lipemia produces plasma turbidity and elevated hemoglobin, MCH, and MCHC results. To correct this problem, a normal manual cyanmethemoglobin procedure can be carried out using an appropriate volume of patient plasma as the blank so that the spectrophotometer can be adjusted to zero. To calculate the appropriate volume of cyanmethemoglobin diluent to add to 20 μl of patient plasma in preparing the blank, the following formula is used:

$$\frac{N = 5 \text{ ml}}{(1 - \text{Hematocrit})}$$

where N is the volume of cyanmethemoglobin diluent to use.

Leukocytosis. Leukocytosis greater than 30×10^9/liter can produce a significant false elevation of the hemoglobin as a result of turbidity. Leukocytosis exceeding 100×10^9/liter can also result in elevated hematocrits and MCV values, as the leukocytes are counted and sized with the red cells.

Elevated Glucose and Hyperosmolarity. Glucose levels in excess of 400 mg/dl can cause elevated MCV and hematocrit results and decreased MCHC results (Beautyman and Bills, 1982). This artifact can be corrected by incubating a 1:224 dilution of blood at 37°C for 10 minutes.

High-Titered Cold Agglutinins. Elevated MCV results and decreased red-cell counts often are caused by pathologically high cold agglutinin titers. The rise in MCV and decrease in RBC are a result of the sensing of red-cell clumps that pass across the electrical field as one or several large particles, which also produces physiologically impossible elevated MCHC indices (Hattersley, 1971). The problematic test outcomes can be corrected by warming the blood and repeating the count using warmed diluent.

Leukemia. Leukocytes occasionally are fragmented during their passage through the small counting orifice of impedance counters, which produces erroneously low counts if the particles are broken down into such small fragments that they fall beneath the counting threshold. Falsely high counts are found if the particles are sufficiently large to be counted. Manual counts should be carried out if the estimate on the slide disagrees with the counter.

Miscellaneous Problems. Erroneous reductions in the leukocyte count have been noted in uremic patients and individuals receiving immunosuppressive drugs (Luke et al., 1971). Paraproteinemia due to

IgG and IgM also can produce elevations in the leukocyte count (Taft, 1973).

Quality Control of Instruments

Hemoglobinometers

Hemoglobin is the sole hematologic test that can be calibrated by a commercially obtainable primary aqueous standard, available from several commercial companies. These aqueous materials are certified by the College of American Pathologists to be accurate to 2% of the stated value. However, this standard cannot be used in multiphasic equipment and can only be used to calibrate manual spectrophotometers and colorimeters. The practical use of such primary calibrates is found on page 256.

Particle Counters

The plethora of cell counters available makes it impractical to illustrate individual calibration. However, at least two commercial products that can be used as secondary calibrators are now available. Their assigned package values are based on primary accepted methods—cyanmethemoglobin for hemoglobin, centrifuged microhematocrit for hematocrit, and Coulter Model F results for cell counts. With these calibrators, it is possible to adjust the test values of the specific instrument. Once this is done, calibration need not be carried out for awhile, unless test variables change because of reagents or equipment problems. The frequency of the recalibration of multiphasic equipment depends on its usage and the nature of the quality control program in use.

Hemocytometers

Although not widely used for blood counting, hemocytometers still are used in the counting of small numbers of cells in spinal or pleural fluids. Additionally, smaller laboratories may use these counting chambers because of a low work volume and economic considerations. When a manual method is used, it is extremely important to carry out the procedure with absolute diligence to ensure the control of the counts.

Both the hemocytometer and the coverslip should meet the specifications of the National Bureau of

Standards. The chambers are designated so that their depth does not vary more than ±0.01 mm. The coverslip must be plain within 0.002 mm of both sides, optically flat, and 0.4 mm thick. The hemocytometer should be set up so that the coverslip appears flush with the shoulders of the slide and in such a way that the coverslip does not become raised when the diluted fluid is introduced. A common error is to merely lay the coverslip on the raised shoulders of the slide. This introduces errors into the count, as the coverslip is raised off the slide once the chamber is filled. The net result is that the count is carried out on a larger diluted sample than is required, and an erroneously high count is produced. To avoid this pitfall, one should moisten the shoulder of the hemocytometer by gently breathing on the slide. The coverslip then is placed on the raised shoulders by sliding and applying gentle pressure with both thumbs. If the coverslip is placed correctly, it should not fall when the hemocytometer is inverted.

Hematocrit Testing Equipment

Microhematocrit tests are considered the primary standard in the secondary calibration of other instruments. Adequate quality control of the apparatus used in such testing depends on routinely checking the centrifuge speed (10,000–15,000 rpm) and the timer and using certified capillary tubes. The frequency of the speed check varies with the instrument used, but it should not be less than monthly. A strobe-light tachometer should be used, and variations of less than 1,000 rpm should be considered unacceptable. Likewise, timers should be checked with an accurately calibrated stopwatch and should be within 10% of the stated value on the centrifuge. The microhematocrit test should initially be set up using pairs of capillary tubes filled with blood. The tubes should then be spun at increasing time intervals until maximum packing is achieved. This, then, is the correct centrifugal time for the test and centrifuge.

Inaccurately manufactured capillary tubes that have an unequal bore contribute to errors. All hematocrit tubes used should be of high quality and guaranteed uniformity.

Pipettes

Pipettes can be checked by several techniques for accuracy and precision. Automatic pipettes, especially those with disposable tips, should be calibrated for both precision and accuracy before use and intermittently during the life of the instrument. Every 3 months is suggested.

Gravimetry is one method of checking pipettes. Small-volume "to contain" pipettes, which include Sahli hemoglobin pipettes and ultramicropipettes, can be checked by drawing clean, dry mercury into the pipette to the calibration mark, discharging it into a preweighed bottle, and reweighing it. The contained volume is derived from the following formula:

$$\frac{\text{Weight of mercury in pipette}}{\substack{\text{Weight of 1 ml of mercury} \\ \text{at the calibration temperature}}}$$

Pipettes in routine use in hematologic testing should be accurate to within 2% of the stated volume. Alternative methods of calibration can be accomplished by delivery of a dye, such as methylene blue, or a radioactive substance, such as ^{125}I, into a known volume of diluent by both the device to be tested and calibrated volumetric glassware. Serial dilutions may be made. The absorbance or counts per minute of the prepared dilutions may be used to establish both precision and accuracy. The relationship between temperature and density for both mercury and distilled water is shown in Table 16.17.

Verification of automatic pipettes can be carried out using deionized water in a manner similar to that described using mercury. The expected accuracy and precision of these checks are shown in Table 16.18.

Colorimetric methods can be used also. Sahli pipettes can be quality controlled colorimetrically using a hemoglobin reference material. Practically, a normal blood specimen with a hemoglobin value of 12–15 g/dl can be used.

The blood is hemolyzed with a small amount of saponin, and duplicate dilutions of blood are made with the pipettes to be calibrated into 5 ml of standard cyanmethemoglobin reagent. Triplicate dilutions of the same hemolyzed blood are made with a reference pipette, and the percentage transmittance is read spectrophotometrically at 540 nm after first blanking the instrument with cyanmethemoglobin reagent. The allowable limits between the reference and the unknown pipette should not exceed more than 0.5% OT (optical transmission).

Table 16.17. Density Relationships of Water at Various Temperatures

Temperature (°C)	1 ml Mercury (g)	1 ml Distilled Water (g)
20	13.547	0.9972
21	13.545	0.9970
22	13.543	0.9968
23	13.541	0.9966
24	13.539	0.9964
25	13.537	0.9961
26	13.534	0.9959
27	13.532	0.9956

Note: These values do not indicate the true densities and weights of mercury and water but include corrections for various factors, such as the coefficient of expansion of glass.

Table 16.18. Recommended Pipette Quality Control Ranges

Pipette Size	Accuracy Range (ml)	Precision Range (± ml)
25 µl	0.0242–0.0257	0.0010
50 µl	0.0484–0.0514	0.0010
100 µl	0.0968–0.1028	0.0015
200 µl	0.1936–0.2056	0.0030
500 µl	0.4840–0.5140	0.0075

Choice of Hematologic Methods and Reference Ranges

The decision to use a specific apparatus or method in the modern hematology laboratory is not a simple task. With the multitude of apparatuses available and the flood of literature through the mail from the manufacturers, it is often difficult to rely strictly on scientific reasoning to arrive at a decision to purchase. There is no single perfect hematologic analyzer. All have their merits and their shortcomings, and the laboratory director and technologist should be most careful not to be stampeded into a hasty decision. Several points must be carefully considered.

First, the volume of work involved and the projected volume of future work have to be considered. Is a stand-alone apparatus with automatic sampling features required, or will a semiautomatic apparatus suffice? Is hands-on technical time important to the operation? Is there a "stat" capability in the equipment, or is there a delayed start-up time? What is the recommended method of quality control? Are controls freely available, and can other manufacturers' controls and reagents be used?

Are there primary calibrators (standards) available based on acknowledged reference methods? What is the sampling speed of the instruments under consideration, and what is their effective through-put from clean-bench to clean-bench? How much time is expected to be needed for preventive maintenance and for the running of controls and standards?

Consideration should be given to the origin of the specimens, such as oncologic or hemodialysis specimens. Does the equipment produce linear results and, if so, what is its range? Linearity limits should be assessed for all parameters measured, and results should be released only if they fall within these limits. Correlation studies should be set up with other instrumentation to compare results.

The minimum statistical evaluation of new equipment should include the following:

- Precision studies carried out on a statistically valid sampling at all expected levels of results, which should include within-run variabilities and, if possible, day-to-day variability (e.g., hemoglobin)

- Accuracy and correlation studies against known reference methods (cyanmethemoglobin, microhematocrit, and so on)
- Carryover studies, particularly if the instrument uses an automatic pick-up system and probe

The choice of reference, or normal, ranges for hematologic tests should not be made by blindly following the data in the literature. All ranges should be checked by establishing population ranges, or the manufacturer's ranges should at least be verified. Although many laboratories may find it difficult to determine adequately the reference range of a proposed method, a small number of determinations (20–40) should be made in healthy individuals to confirm the published data. If samples are taken from a large number of persons who are disease-free, certain hematologic parameters will describe a near-gaussian distribution.

Given a statistic of the central tendency of the curve, such as the mean, and a statistic of the width or dispersion, such as the SD, a reliable prediction can be made about the population on which the curve is based (see page 228). In any determination of reference ranges, the variations in the base population should be related to age, gender, and the specimen source (i.e., venous, capillary). The laboratory staff should develop its own ranges, particularly if a unique population group is tested.

If large samples are tested, the reference ranges are best determined using a percentile estimate method (nonparametric distribution). However, for this method, at least 120 samples are needed to calculate 90% confidence limits. The central 95% interval of any distribution can be estimated using the ranked sample distribution. If 200 samples are used, the fifth lowest and the fifth highest are estimates of the 2.5 and 97.5 percentiles:

$$i = P_i \times (N + 1)$$
or
$$i = P_i \times (N + 0.2) + 0.4$$

where P_i is the percentile desired, N is the number of samples, and i is the rank of estimate.

Chapter 17

Blood Collection

Two principal methods of obtaining blood samples are by capillary puncture or by venipuncture. The capillary puncture sites most frequently used are the plantar surface of the heel in infants and the finger in older children. Regardless of the method, the first step in obtaining blood is to reassure the patient. It is a relatively easy matter to explain the procedure to adults, but extra care should be taken with children, and some endeavor should be made to win the child's confidence. Identification of the patient should be ascertained by asking the patient's name or by positive identification from a wristband.

Capillary Puncture

The most appropriate site for capillary puncture in infants is the lateral or medial plantar heel surface. In older children, a finger may be used. The site of the puncture should be free of edema and should be warm and dry.

The area is first cleansed with gauze moistened with 70% isopropyl alcohol and allowed to air-dry. A quick, single puncture is made with a sterile, disposable lancet, avoiding excessive squeezing of the area. The first drop of blood is wiped away to avoid excessive tissue juice contamination, and gentle pressure is applied in a milking fashion to obtain a free flow of blood. Excessive squeezing of the heel or finger results in the liberation of tissue juices that contaminate and dilute the collected specimen and promote clot formation. When collection is completed, a dry, sterile pad is applied to the

wound, and pressure is applied to the site until bleeding ceases.

Venipuncture

With the use of venipuncture, blood can be collected from many sites including the antecubital veins of the forearm, the ankle veins, the wrist veins or the veins on the dorsal surface of the hand, the femoral veins, and the scalp or jugular veins in infants. The most common and easiest site from which to obtain venous blood is the forearm. The other sites should be used only by a physician or under a physician's direct supervision, especially in the case of venipuncture of infants and femoral punctures.

Syringe Method from Antecubital Veins

1. The patient is asked to clench his or her fist so that the selected vein is more easily seen and palpable. The area surrounding the site is cleansed with 70% isopropyl alcohol or with 1% povidone iodophor. Beginning at the venipuncture site, the area is cleansed outward in a circular motion, using the circular scrub technique. The area is allowed to dry.

2. A tourniquet is applied around the upper arm, 7–10 cm above the venipuncture site, and a prominent vein is located. If such a vein is not easily seen, the phlebotomist's index finger should be cleansed and the forearm palpated until a vein is felt. Fre-

quently, better veins that are situated deeper in the arm and are less likely to "roll" when punctured are found by this method.

3. If the tourniquet has been applied for more than 1 minute, it should be removed to allow time for normal blood flow to be re-established. The tourniquet is reapplied, and the vein is fixed either by holding it with the finger or by grasping the patient's arm below the elbow and pulling the skin taut.

4. The needle is inserted obliquely into the vein, with the bevel upward. A sensation of resistance will be felt, which is followed by ease of penetration as the vein is entered. The syringe plunger is pulled back slowly until the necessary volume of blood is obtained. The patient is then instructed to open his or her hand, and the tourniquet is released. If several samples of blood are taken, it is best to release the tourniquet before collection of each tube. The tourniquet is never left on the arm for longer than 1 minute or applied so tightly as to cause stasis. This will result in hemoconcentration and falsely elevated cell counts and hemoglobin levels.

5. The needle is removed quickly, and a clean pad is applied over the site in one smooth motion. Moderate pressure is applied to the puncture site.

6. The blood is dispensed into appropriate anticoagulated tubes by removing the needle from the syringe barrel and delivering the specimen directly from the syringe. The stopper is applied, and the blood and anticoagulant are mixed gently by inverting the tube 5–10 times. Avoid shaking the specimen vigorously.

7. The patient's name should be rechecked and the sample labeled with name, location, date, and physician's name.

8. The venipuncture wound is then examined. If it is still bleeding, pressure is applied to the site while the patient's arm is elevated vertically. The patient should not be allowed to bend his or her arm at the elbow. Once bleeding has stopped, a clean sterile dressing is applied to the wound.

Vacuum Tube Method (Vacutainer)

1. Procedures 1, 2, and 3 are carried out as detailed in the syringe procedure.

2. The appropriate Vacutainer (Becton-Dickinson, Rutherford, NJ) tube is then placed in a reusable plastic holder, and a disposable needle is attached by screwing the threaded needle hub to the female end of the holder. The tube is inserted into the holder until the top of its stopper is level with the marked guideline, which causes the tube to recede.

3. The tourniquet is applied and a vein is selected, as previously described. The patient's arm must be in a slightly vertical position. When using this system, venipuncture must not be performed with the patient's arm in a horizontal plane, as a backflow of blood can result. The needle is inserted into the vein as in the syringe technique, and the base of the collection tube is pushed forward, breaking the vacuum seal. Time is allowed for the vacuum tube to fill to exhaustion, and then the procedure continues as is described for the syringe method.

4. If multiple tubes have been requested, the tourniquet is released before collection of each. The tube is removed from the plastic holder while the needle remains in the vein, and other tubes are attached as needed.

Complications of Venipuncture

Prolonged tourniquet application should be avoided if suitable blood samples are to be obtained for hematologic testing. As already stated, tourniquets left in place for more than 1 minute can result in hemoconcentrated specimens that produce falsely elevated cell counts and hemoglobin levels. Excessively tight tourniquets will produce similar effects.

Collapsed veins will be caused occasionally by the use of the vacuum tube method on patients with small veins, especially when performing venipuncture on hand or ankle vessels. In these situations, the syringe technique should be used, as the phlebotomist can more easily control the negative pressure applied to the vessel.

On rare occasions, the vessel wall will be flattened against the needle lumen, occluding the needle and resulting in inadequate specimen collection. The remedy is to disengage the needle gently from the vein wall by slowly withdrawing and rotating it approximately one-half turn, taking care not to remove it completely from the vein. When a vacuum tube is being used, this is more easily accomplished by removing the tube from the tube holder, manipulating the needle, and reinserting a fresh vacuum tube.

Bleeding from the venipuncture site will be seen occasionally, especially following phlebotomy on a patient with hemorrhagic tendencies. Hematomas can be avoided even in such extreme situations by the application of firm and constant pressure to the puncture site for at least 5 minutes. It is essential that the patient's arm not be bent upward, as this opens the wound site, causing further bleeding. Pressure should be applied with the arm held high in a vertical position, and a pressure bandage should be applied after overt bleeding has ceased.

Difficult Venipunctures

If a vein is difficult to puncture, the position of the needle should be changed by slowly and gently moving it either further into the vein or back out. The angle of the needle must not be altered in the vein, as such probing is painful and rarely results in the collection of a satisfactory blood sample. If a vacuum tube is being used, tubes should be changed to eliminate a tube with vacuum loss.

If a second venipuncture is attempted, either a site on the other arm or a site located below the original venipuncture should be chosen. A venipuncture should never be attempted more than twice. If the technologist is in doubt, a physician's assistance should be obtained.

Order of Venipuncture

The recommended order of venipuncture is blood culture tubes first, then tubes without additives, then tubes for coagulation, and, finally, tubes with additives (National Committee for Clinical Laboratory Standards, 1990). Nonadditive tubes should be drawn first to avoid contamination with anticoagulants. Because cross-contamination among different additives has been reported (Jones, 1980), it is recommended that, of the tubes with additives, citrate tubes be drawn first, followed by heparin, and then ethylenediaminetetraacetic acid (EDTA). Finally, any other anticoagulant tubes (oxalate or fluoride) should be drawn (Calam and Cooper, 1982).

Anticoagulants

Whole blood is necessary for most hematologic investigations. The sample must therefore be mixed with an anticoagulant to prevent coagulation. The commonly used anticoagulants are discussed in the following sections.

EDTA, Tripotassium Salt (Versene, Sequestrene)

EDTA removes free calcium ions by chelation. Preparation is accomplished by dissolving 15 g tripotassium EDTA in warm distilled water and making up to 100 ml; then 0.1 ml of this solution is added to a series of tubes. This amount is sufficient to prevent the coagulation of 7 ml of blood.

This anticoagulant has replaced the ammonium and potassium oxalate mixture for routine use. When double oxalates are used, platelet clumping occurs, preventing accurate cell counting. Also, the anticoagulant effect on leukocytes is more severe, making their differentiation more difficult in the differential leukocyte count.

The liquid tripotassium salt is preferred over the disodium salt of EDTA because of its greater solubility. Easier mixing and less frequent clotting result from the use of the liquid anticoagulant.

EDTA-anticoagulated blood can be used for cellular morphologic testing up to 4 hours following collection. The longer the time delay, the greater the chance of cellular aberrations, although acceptable blood smears can occasionally be made as long as 12 hours after collection. Platelet counts can be carried out on blood that is 24 hours old. The changes in cellular morphologic characteristics begin within 30 minutes after contact. Leukocytic changes are variable in that cellular changes vary in intensity and effect in an individual's blood, with progressively increasing numbers of cells. In some individuals, the leukocytes resist change, which gives rise to variation in the extent of anticoagulant alterations, especially with lower concentrations of EDTA.

The first changes in the neutrophils are swelling and loss of structure in the nuclear lobes; stretching of the interlobular bridges then occurs, with loss of cytoplasmic granulation. Vacuolation also takes place in the nucleus or cytoplasm. These changes progress to more marked nuclear swelling, and there then appears to be a crossover of nuclear chromatin, giving rise, in the most extreme form, to the typical cloverleaf pattern. Ultimately, this change progresses to complete morphologic disintegration of the cell, leaving a bare nucleus (Sacker, 1975).

Platelets appear to swell, leaving giant forms that then disintegrate, causing an artificially produced platelet elevation. Red cells are affected principally by shape changes, with increasing anisocytosis, spherocytosis, and macrocytosis. Ultimately, some of these cells become hemolyzed.

EDTA is unsuitable for blood coagulation tests.

Sodium Citrate

Sodium citrate removes free calcium ions by loosely binding them to form a calcium citrate complex. Two different concentrations are used: 3.8 and 3.2%. To prepare the 3.8% concentration, 3.8 g trisodium citrate dihydrate is dissolved in 100 ml distilled water (129 mol/liter). To prepare the 3.2% concentration, 3.2 g trisodium citrate dihydrate is dissolved in 100 ml of distilled water (109 mol/liter).

The 3.8% anticoagulant is suitable for most blood coagulation tests. Nine volumes of blood are added to 1 volume of anticoagulant.

The 3.2% anticoagulant is suitable for Westergren sedimentation rates, in which it is used in a ratio of 4 volumes of blood to 1 volume of anticoagulant. Additionally, this more diluted sodium citrate can be used in place of the usually recommended 3.8% concentration, especially for coagulation testing when the patient's hematocrit is elevated above 60%.

Sodium Citrate–Citric Acid Buffer

The action of sodium citrate–citric acid buffer is identical to that of sodium citrate. It is made up of two stock solutions of citric acid and trisodium citrate dihydrate. The citric acid stock is prepared by dissolving 19.2 g citric acid in 100 ml warm distilled water. For a working solution, 3.7 ml of the citric acid is added to 26.0 ml of the sodium citrate, and the mixture is diluted to approximately 90 ml with distilled water. The mixture then is ad-justed to pH 4.7 and is made up to 100 ml with distilled water.

This buffered sodium citrate can be used in place of the more commonly used 3.8% anticoagulant for coagulation testing. The final pH of the plasma-anticoagulant mixture should be 7.35 ± 0.05 units.

Heparin

Heparin acts as an antithrombin. It is prepared by dissolving 0.4 g powdered heparin in 100 ml distilled water. This preparation is added in 0.25-ml aliquots to collection tubes and is allowed to evaporate to dryness at 37°C.

Heparin is not recommended for cell counting because of its clumping effect on platelets and leukocytes and because blood smears made from it are difficult to stain clearly. Heparin is, however, invaluable for obtaining unhemolyzed and unaltered red cells for osmotic fragility studies and for red-cell enzyme estimations.

Defibrinated Blood

To defibrinate blood, venous blood is delivered directly into an Erlenmeyer flask containing 10–20 small glass beads. The flask is swirled in a rotating motion for 5 minutes or until all of the fibrin has been deposited around the beads. Then the beads are removed and the specimen is centrifuged. Blood defibrinated in this way should not undergo any visible degree of lysis.

Oxalate

Sodium oxalate is now considered obsolete as the anticoagulant for coagulation tests, having been replaced by sodium citrate. The use of the double oxalate mixture composed of potassium and sodium salts has been replaced by the routine use of EDTA.

Chapter 18

Routine Hematologic Procedures

In most hematology laboratories, high-volume routine tests include hemoglobin and hematocrit (Hct) determinations, red-cell and leukocyte counts, differential leukocyte count, reticulocyte count, platelet count, and erythrocyte sedimentation rate (ESR). These procedures constitute a set of screening tests that can be of use in the preliminary hematologic examination of a patient.

Hemoglobin

Hemoglobin is best measured by using the cyanmethemoglobin (hemiglobincyanide, HiCN) method recommended by the International Committee for Standardization in Hematology (1978). Advantages of this technique are that it is standardized and stable standard solutions are available.

Principle

Hemoglobin is oxidized to methemoglobin by potassium ferricyanide. The resulting pigment is then converted to stable cyanmethemoglobin by potassium cyanide. The absorbance of the pigment is measured spectrophotometrically at 540 nm, at which wavelength the pigment produces a broad absorbance peak. The method is calibrated against a standard certified by the American College of Pathologists.

Reagents and Equipment

1. Modified Drabkin's reagent. Potassium ferricyanide (0.2 g), 0.05 g potassium cyanide, and 0.14 g dihydrogen potassium phosphate (anhydrous) are dissolved in distilled water. One milliliter of a nonionic detergent (Triton X-100) is made up to 1 liter with distilled water. The modified Drabkin's reagent should be pale yellow and clear, with a pH of 7.2 ± 0.2 units. At a wavelength of 540 nm, it should give a zero absorbance reading when compared with a water blank.
2. Spectrophotometer.
3. Pipette: 5 ml, graduated.
4. Pipette: 0.02 ml (Sahli).

Specimen

The specimen to be used is whole blood anticoagulated with ethylenediaminetetraacetic acid (EDTA).

Method

1. Capillary or EDTA-anticoagulated blood (0.02 ml) is added to 5 ml of modified Drabkin's reagent. The diluted blood is mixed well by inversion and is allowed to stand at room temperature for at least 3 minutes.

255

2. The spectrophotometer is blanked with reagent, and the transmittance of the resulting cyanmethemoglobin pigment is read spectrophotometrically at a wavelength of 540 nm and compared with the standard graph.

3. Standardization is carried out by preparing a standard curve. The standard purchased commercially is diluted with Drabkin's reagent, as shown in Table 18.1. Transmittance readings for each dilution are measured against a reagent blank and are plotted on semilog graph paper, using the ordinates for absorbance and hemoglobin concentration as the abscissae. The assay value of the standard is present on the vial and commonly is expressed in milligram equivalents. To convert this value to hemoglobin in grams per deciliter, the assay value is multiplied by the dilution of blood used in the test (i.e., 1:251). Consequently, an 80-mg standard is equivalent to 20.08 g/dl (80 × 251). If the spectrophotometer reads optical density rather than percentage of transmittance, the standard values should be plotted on linear graph paper. A straight line passing through zero should be obtained using either method of plotting.

Reference Ranges

Reference ranges for all tests should be determined individually by each laboratory. The following are approximate expected ranges:

Male adult	13.0–18.2 g/dl
Female adult	11.0–16.3 g/dl
Newborn	13.6–19.6 g/dl
Child, 1 month old	9.5–12.5 g/dl
Child, 1 year old	11.0–13.0 g/dl
Child, 10 years old	11.5–14.8 g/dl

Sources of Error

Using this modified Drabkin's solution reduces the time required for the conversion of hemoglobin to cyanmethemoglobin. The detergent functions as an extra lysing agent and also reduces turbidity from protein precipitates. However, some abnormal hemoglobins may still produce some turbidity (Hb S, Hb C), as the cells are more resistant to lysis than is normal. This turbidity can be eliminated by adding 5 ml water to the blood-Drabkin's mixture, mixing well, and allowing the solution to stand for 5–10 minutes. A correction factor of ×2 then is applied to the final result. Turbidity may also result from extreme leukocytosis ($>30 \times 10^9$/liter) or hyperlipemia. All forms of hemoglobin except sulfhemoglobin are measured by this method.

An alternative method using the self-filling, self-measuring dilution pipette (Unopette, available from Becton-Dickinson, Rutherford, NJ) system is available. It produces a 1:250 dilution of blood in cyanmethemoglobin reagent.

Hematocrit (Packed Cell Volume)

Principle

Anticoagulated whole blood is centrifuged, and the total volume of the red-cell mass is expressed as a percentage or decimal fraction. Hematocrit may also be estimated by the product of the mean cell volume (MCV) and red-cell count.

Micromethod

Equipment

1. Capillary tubes (75 ± 0.5 mm × 1.55 ± 0.085 mm internal diameter; wall thickness, 0.20 ± 0.02 mm). Heparinized tubes are used for capillary blood, and plain tubes are used for EDTA-anticoagulated blood.
2. Microhematocrit centrifuge capable of reaching a maximum speed within 30 seconds and of sustaining a relative centrifugal force (RCF) of 10,000–15,000g at the periphery for 5 minutes without exceeding a temperature of 45°C.
3. Hematocrit reader.
4. Plastic vinyl putty.

Specimen

The specimen to be used is EDTA-anticoagulated whole blood or heparinized capillary blood.

Method

1. Two capillary tubes are filled with EDTA-anticoagulated blood to within 5–10 mm of the end of the

Table 18.1. Hemoglobin Standardization*

Tube	1	2	3	4
Standard (ml)	1.5	2.5	4.0	5.0
Reagent (ml)	3.5	2.5	1.0	—
Hemoglobin value (g/liter)	6	10	16	20

*Example using a 20-g/dl standard as the undiluted concentrate.

tubes. They are then sealed with small plastic caps, or the dry ends of the tubes are plugged by placing them in a tray of plastic vinyl putty, ensuring that the seal forms a straight edge across the interior of the tube.

2. The exterior of the tubes are wiped clean of blood and are centrifuged for 5 minutes at 10,000–15,000g. The tubes are removed immediately when the centrifuge has stopped spinning, and the hematocrit is determined using the reader. Duplicate results should agree to within ±1%.

Wintrobe Method

Equipment

1. A Wintrobe tube, which is narrow, hard, and thick-walled, and graduated from 0–100 mm, with an internal diameter of 2.5 mm.
2. Bench-model centrifuge generating at least 2,500g (3,000 rpm with a centrifuge radius of 15 cm).
3. Disposable Pasteur pipettes.

Specimen

The specimen used is EDTA-anticoagulated whole blood.

Method

1. The Wintrobe tube is filled carefully with well-mixed oxygenated blood using a Pasteur pipette. The tube is filled slowly from the bottom, and care is taken not to introduce air bubbles or to allow the blood to foam. This is best accomplished by raising the pipette tip above the meniscus until the blood level reaches the 100-mm mark.
2. The tube should then be balanced and centrifuged at 2,500g for 30 minutes, and the packed red-cell volume should be read directly from the scale on the right side of the tube.

Sources of Error

The microhematocrit values are usually 1–3% lower than those obtained using the Wintrobe method. This difference amounts to approximately 0.01 hematocrit units and is due to the release of trapped plasma between the cells. When testing macrocytic anemias, spherocytic anemias, sickle cell anemia, and hypochromic anemias, this difference becomes slightly larger but still remains fairly small. The mean volume of trapped plasma found in normal individuals using a microhematocrit method is approximately 1.5% and is increased when short-armed centrifuges are used at low speeds (Fairbanks, 1980). There is also an inverse correlation between trapped plasma and the mean cell hemoglobin (MCH) in patients with iron deficiency (Pearson and Guthrie, 1982). The microprocedure is considered the reference method for calibration.

Errors in results occur when the EDTA concentration exceeds 2 mg per milliliter of whole blood. If vacuum tube collection is used, the hematocrit error becomes progressively lower as the concentration of anticoagulant increases, and it reaches 5% when 2 ml of blood are obtained in a 7-ml–draw tube. This error is expanded further to 17% when 0.5 ml of blood is drawn. These differences reflect the hypertonicity of the anticoagulant, but no effect is seen in cyanmethemoglobin values. Other errors of the test involve those of parallax in reading the packed cells in the tube and in excluding the buffy-coat layer of leukocytes and platelets from the actual reading (International Committee for Standardization in Haematology, 1980).

Sampling errors may be introduced by prolonged stasis from the tourniquet, which causes hemoconcentration and falsely high results. Difficult venipunctures may result in sample dilution by interstitial fluid, in clot formation, or in hemolysis due to fine-bore needle trauma. The hematocrit value of deoxygenated blood is approximately 2% lower than fully oxygenated samples, which amounts to approximately 0.01 hematocrit units or 1% packed cells. The effect of posture and muscular activity can also adversely affect the results, causing elevated values in leukocytes, platelets, and erythrocytes.

Besides producing a quantitative relative red-cell result, the hematocrit can provide useful corroborative information. Examination of the relative heights of the buffy coat can support both the platelet count and the total leukocyte count, and a visual inspection of the plasma can correlate with jaundice, bilirubinemia, and a possible hemolytic disorder. When present, overt hemolysis is likely the result of poor venipuncture technique.

Instrument Calibration

The centrifuge should be calibrated regularly with respect to timer accuracy, speed, and maximal packing of cells. Accuracy and precision of the timer is verified using a certified stopwatch, and the centrifugal speed is checked using a calibrated strobe-light tachometer. Constant packing of red cells is checked by a constant volume-time method. Using two fresh EDTA-anticoagulated blood samples, duplicate hematocrit determinations are carried out by centrifuging for 2 minutes and increasing the time by 30-second intervals until the packed cell volume has remained the same for two consecutive time series. The second of these times is the minimum that should be used for the test.

Reference Ranges

	Percent	SI Units
Male adult	36.5–52.0	0.365–0.520
Female adult	33.0–47.0	0.330–0.470
Newborn	40.0–64.4	0.400–0.644
Child, 1 month old	25.6–42.7	0.256–0.427
Child, 1 year old	27.0–45.0	0.270–0.450
Child, 10 years old	33.2–48.4	0.332–0.482

Manual Cell Counting

The use of automated equipment in erythrocyte, leukocyte, and platelet counting is considered in Chapter 23. The fundamentals of manual cell counting are theoretically simple but technically difficult. Blood should be diluted in such a way as to prevent gross changes in the cells being counted while simultaneously destroying unwanted cells. The counting fluid should be free of debris, and the cells in a fixed volume of diluted blood should be totaled accurately. Many types of hemocytometers have been used, but the two most common are the improved Neubauer and the Fuchs-Rosenthal. These are the only hemocytometers currently in routine use in laboratories.

Counting Chambers

The improved Neubauer ruled hemocytometer consists of a thick rectangular glass slide with an H-shaped trough forming two counting areas. It has two raised shoulders supporting an optically flat, thick coverslip at exactly 0.1 mm from the bottom of the chamber. On the reverse side of the slide, a concave indentation is present directly under the ruled area. This prevents scratching of the slide and impairing the count. The total ruled area is divided so that two separate counts can be made. Each area is 3×3 mm, and the depth, if the coverslip is correctly applied, is 0.1 mm. This produces a total counting volume of 0.9 µl. The exact rulings and the dimensions of the squares are shown in Figures 18.1 through 18.3.

The center large square is divided into 25 smaller squares, each being subdivided into 16 smaller units and separated by a triple line. This central area is used for erythrocyte and platelet counts, whereas the four corner 1-mm² areas are used for leukocyte counting.

The Fuchs-Rosenthal chamber is considerably larger than the Neubauer hemocytometer. Its principal use is for performing low cell counts, such as eosinophil counts, spinal fluid counts, and leukopenic blood counts. The ruled area measures 4×4 mm, and the depth is 0.2 mm. The central ruling is divided into 16 smaller squares.

Counting Technique

The hemocytometer should be free of scratches and must be cleaned before use. It should be set up by placing the coverslip on the transverse bars. If the setup is correct, gentle pressure on the bars will pro-

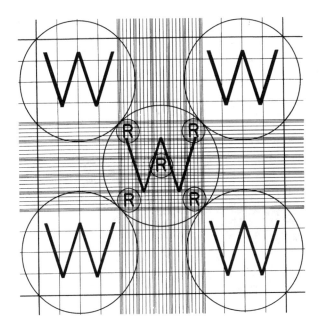

Figure 18.1. Ruled area of the improved Neubauer hemocytometer, showing the four large corner squares usually used in the white cell count (W) and one large center square that can be used in addition. The five smaller squares (R) are used in the red-cell count.

Figure 18.2. Counting red cells and platelets. This figure shows an enlargement of the area marked R in Figure 18.1.

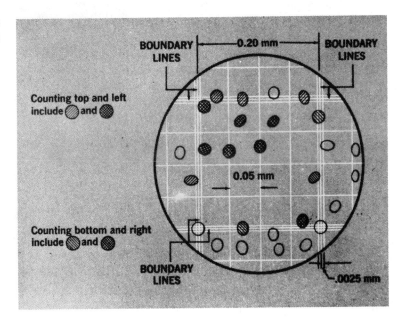

duce concentric refraction spectra (Newton's rings), denoting that the coverslip is in an optically flat plane with the hemocytometer. This is essential if the depth of the counting area is to be uniform. Hemocytometers with frosted glass shoulders do not allow these refraction rings to be observed; in these situations, the raised shoulders should be moist-ened, and the technician should slide the coverslip onto the shoulders with both thumbs. It should be possible to invert the hemocytometer without dislodging the coverslip.

Care must be taken in the filling of a correctly set-up hemocytometer (Figure 18.4). Diluted blood must not overflow into the moats, and the ruled area

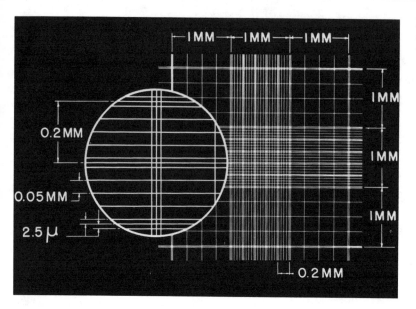

Figure 18.3. Dimensions of the improved Neubauer hemocytometer.

should be filled by allowing one drop of diluted blood to encompass the area. The hemocytometer must not be filled with multiple small drops. Before one attempts to count, the cells must be allowed to settle completely, preferably in a moist atmosphere such as under an inverted Petri dish with a wet pledget of cotton.

Although counting the cells in a fixed, ruled area facilitates a simple calculation, the larger the number of cells counted, the more precise the count. The improved Neubauer hemocytometer is outlined by a triple set of lines, the central line denoting the boundary of the square being reviewed. Cells that touch the top and left boundary lines should be included in the total count, whereas those touching the bottom and right lines should be excluded.

Irrespective of the hemocytometer or technical procedure used, all manual cell counts can be calculated using the following formula, *if* the hemocytometer dimensions and dilution ratios are known (see Figure 18.2):

Total cell count =

Number of cells counted $\times \dfrac{1}{\text{area counted (mm}^2)} \times$

$\dfrac{1}{\text{depth of hemocytometer (mm)}} \times$ dilution ratio

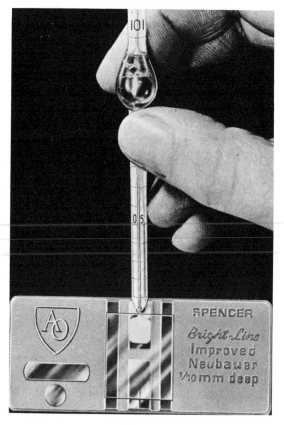

Figure 18.4. The correct method of filling the hemocytometer.

Sources of Error

The errors involved in manual cell counting can be divided into two principal groups: those involving technique and those associated with statistical error. Technical errors involve failure to use accurate pipettes, application of poor technique, incorrect setup and filling of the hemocytometer, and inaccurate counting of cells. All these errors can be minimized by paying attention to detail; however, errors arising from the random distribution of cells in the hemocytometer can be lessened only by counting greater numbers of cells.

The uneven distribution of cells resulting from the momentum that is present as the chamber is charged is known as the *Poisson distribution* and can be calculated from the following formula:

$$SD = \pm\sqrt{M}$$

where *SD* is the standard deviation of the distribution of the cells and *M* is the mean number of cells counted. This inherent error is expressed in more practical terms in the following example.

If 500 cells are counted when determining a manual red-cell count, the SD = $\pm \sqrt{500}$ = $\pm$ 22. Consequently, in 66% of the counts made, the number of cells counted would be 500 $\pm$ 22 (478–522) and, in 95% of the counts, the number of cells would be 500 $\pm$ 44 (456–544). This would result in the following coefficient of variation (CV):

$$\frac{22}{500} \times 100 = 4.4\%$$

An acceptable manual red-cell count range for such a specimen would be 4.56–5.44 $\times 10^{12}$/liter if "truth" is 5.0 $\times 10^{12}$/liter.

By increasing the number of cells, the CV is proportionately reduced. For example, if 1,000 cells are counted, the SD = $\pm \sqrt{1,000}$ $\pm$ 31.6.

$$CV = \frac{31.6}{1,000} \times 100 = 3.16\%$$

If 2,000 cells are counted:

$$SD = \pm\sqrt{2,000} = 44.7$$

and

$$CV = \frac{44.7}{2,000} \times 100 = 2.2\%$$

Use of the Self-Filling, Self-Measuring Dilution Pipette (Unopette)

Principle

The pipette consists of a straight, thin-walled, uniform-bore glass capillary tube, fitted into a plastic holder, and an attached plastic reservoir containing a premeasured volume of diluent. The pipette is closed with a tight-fitting solid plastic plug.

These semiautomated pipetting devices can be obtained in various dilution ratios containing different diluents, depending on the type of count to be carried out. Dilution ratios of 1:100 for leukocyte counts and 1:200 for erythrocyte, platelet, and eosinophil counts are available.

Method

1. The diluent reservoir is opened by forcing the plug into the main chamber with the blunt end of the pipette cap.
2. Blood is drawn carefully into the pipette either from an EDTA-anticoagulated specimen or from a free-flowing capillary puncture. The blood is allowed to fill the pipette without air bubbles being introduced, and the exterior is wiped clean with gauze.
3. The dilution is made by introducing the capillary tube into the reservoir. The reservoir walls are squeezed slightly before inserting the tube so that a slight negative pressure is created when the walls are released. Blood then will be drawn into the diluent from the capillary tube. The tube is rinsed by gently squeezing the reservoir, forcing the fluid into the capillary tube. The pressure is released, allowing the diluent to be drawn back into the reservoir.
4. The diluted blood is mixed, and the dilution pipette is assembled by removing the capillary tube from the reservoir, reversing it, and reattaching it to the reservoir. The reservoir walls are squeezed

gently to force a few drops of diluted blood through the capillary tube, and a previously set up hemocytometer is filled. The procedure of setting up Unopettes is demonstrated in Figure 18.5.

Manual Red-Cell Count

Principle

Whole blood is diluted with an isotonic diluent. The hemocytometer is charged with the diluted specimen, and the number of cells in a fixed ruled area (*volume*) are counted. The final count is expressed as the number of cells in 1 liter of undiluted blood.

Reagents and Equipment

1. Diluting fluids: Dacie's fluid—30% trisodium citrate, 99 ml; formalin, 1 ml, or normal saline–sodium chloride, 0.85 g; distilled water to 100 ml. Hayem's diluting fluid is not recommended, because the erythrocytes tend to agglutinate, particularly in patients with dysproteinemic disorders, including Hodgkin's disease, myeloma, nephritis, and cirrhosis. Dacie's fluid is recommended as a general red-cell diluent.
2. Red-cell pipette. Use either a Thoma bulbed pipette or, for more accurate and precise dilutions, a Sahli hemoglobin pipette (0.02 ml).
3. Improved Neubauer hemocytometer.
4. Microscope.

Specimen

EDTA-anticoagulated whole blood is the preferred specimen. Capillary blood can also be used if it is diluted immediately on collection.

Method

1. A 1:200 dilution of blood is made by one of the following three methods. In the first method, blood is pipetted up to the 0.5 mark of a red-cell Thoma (bulb) pipette, and diluting fluid is added up to the 101 mark, with care taken to avoid introducing air bubbles into the bulb. The pipette is shaken vigorously, and several drops of the diluent are expelled from the stem of the pipette.

The Unopette system, described on page 261, can also be used. These pipettes automatically dilute the specimen in a 1:200 ratio. If this procedure is used, the final results should be calculated accordingly.

Alternatively, a 1:201 dilution of blood can be prepared by adding 0.02 ml of blood to 4 ml of diluting fluid.

2. The hemocytometer is cleaned, and the coverslip is placed firmly over the counting area, as previously described (page 258).

3. The dilution is mixed well and, if the Thoma pipette is used, the first few drops of the diluent from the pipette are expelled. The counting chamber is then filled by capillary attraction. This can best be accomplished by holding the pipette at a 90-degree angle and introducing one sufficiently large drop of diluted blood to fill the counting area completely in one motion.

4. The cells are allowed to settle for 3–5 minutes, and the counting area is then viewed under a low-power microscope lens to check for even distribution.

5. The total cells in five groups of the 16 small squares in the central ruled area are counted. As previously determined, all the cells touching the upper and left lines of each square are included in the count. A variation of more than 25 cells among any of the five areas indicates an uneven distribution and requires that a fresh dilution and new count be made.

Calculation

Total cell count

$$= \text{Number of cells counted} \times \frac{1}{\text{area counted (mm)}} \times$$

$$\frac{1}{\text{depth (mm)}} \times \text{dilution ratio}$$

$$= \text{Number of cells counted} \times \frac{1}{0.2} \times \frac{1}{0.1} \times 200$$

$$= \text{Number of cells counted} \times 1,000$$

Reference Ranges

Male adult	$4.20–6.10 \times 10^{12}/\text{liter}$
Female adult	$3.70–5.50 \times 10^{12}/\text{liter}$

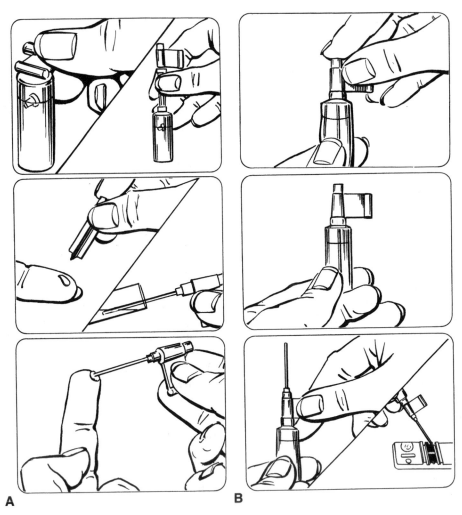

Figure 18.5. The self-filling micropipette. A. The method of removing and filling the capillary pipette. B. The correct method of mixing the blood with the diluent and the filling of the hemocytometer.

Newborn	$4.00–5.60 \times 10^{12}$/liter
Child, 1 month old	$3.20–4.50 \times 10^{12}$/liter
Child, 1 year old	$3.60–5.20 \times 10^{12}$/liter
Child, 10 years old	$4.20–5.20 \times 10^{12}$/liter

Sources of Error

Manual red-cell counts are subject to frequent inherent errors principally caused by random distribution of the cells in the counting area. These errors become magnified if counts are carried out on polycythemic or anemic specimens. In these situations, it is good practice to compensate by varying the initial dilution and adjusting the calculation and final result accordingly. Therefore, a dilution of 1:333 could be made by drawing blood to the 0.3 mark and diluting fluid to the 101 mark on a red-cell pipette for individuals with excessively elevated counts, and dilutions of 1:100 can be made for anemic specimens by drawing blood to the 1 mark and diluting fluid to the 101 level.

In addition to inaccurately calibrated pipettes and hemocytometers, errors can arise from a variety of contaminated diluents, dirty glassware, and poor counting technique. Whenever possible, both sides of the hemocytometer should be filled and the count repeated to reduce the error and improve the precision of the result.

Red-Cell Indices (Absolute Values)

The calculations of the size and hemoglobin content of red cells from the total hemoglobin, hematocrit, and red-cell count were introduced by Wintrobe as a basis for the classification of anemias by morphologic criteria. Because of the errors inherent to manual red-cell counts, these calculated values were used infrequently, but since the advent of hematologic automation techniques, there has been increased use of the data produced. The three most frequently used indices are the MCV, the MCH, and the mean cell hemoglobin concentration (MCHC). The MCV is a calculated index when the individual test parameters are obtained manually, but it is a direct measurement when automated impedance methods are used, such as Coulter and Toa counters. The two methods do not produce identical results, as the MCV produced by impedance automation results in slightly higher values than when the MCV is obtained manually.

Mean Cell Volume

Definition

The MCV is the volume of the average red cell expressed in femtoliters (fl). If the mean red-cell thickness is normal, the MCV bears a linear relationship to the cell diameter.

Factors Required to Calculate MCV

1. Hematocrit.
2. Red-cell count.
3. For the sake of example, assume a hematocrit of 45%. This means there are 0.45 μl of red cells in 1 mm of blood.
4. Also for the sake of example, assume the red-cell count is 5.0×10^{12}/liter. This means these cells occupy a total volume of 0.45 μl. The volume of one red cell (MCV), then, is as follows:

$$\frac{0.45}{5 \times 10^{12}} = \frac{0.09}{10^{12}} = 0.09 \times 10^{-12}/\,liter$$

$$= 90 \times 10^{-15}/\,liter$$

An abbreviated method of calculation is expressed thus:

$$\frac{Hematocrit\ (as\ a\ decimal)}{Red\text{-}cell\ count\ (\times 10^{12}/liter)} \times 1{,}000 = MCV\ (in\ fl)$$

Mean Cell Hemoglobin

Definition

The MCH is the weight of hemoglobin in the average red cell expressed in picograms (pg). If the cell is large, the MCH is raised unless the cell is deficient in iron. If the cell is small and deficient in iron, the MCH is reduced.

Factors Required to Calculate Mean Cell Hemoglobin

1. Hemoglobin.
2. Red-cell count. Let us assume the following calculation example: hemoglobin = 15 g/dl and red-cell count = 5.0×10^{12}/liter.
3. If 1 g = 10^{12} pg and 1 ml = 10^{3} μl, the weight in picograms of hemoglobin in 1 μl of blood is as follows:

$$\frac{Hemoglobin \times 10^{12}}{100 \times 10^{3}\ \mu l} = Hemoglobin \times 10^{7}\,pg/mm$$

Then,

$$\frac{15 \times 10^{7}}{5 \times 10^{6}} = \frac{15 \times 10}{5}\,pg = 30\,pg$$

An abbreviated method of calculation is expressed thus:

$$\frac{Hemoglobin\ (g/dl)}{Red\text{-}cell\ count\ (\times 10^{12}/liter)} \times 10 = MCH\ (in\ pg)$$

Mean Cell Hemoglobin Concentration

Definition

The MCHC is the concentration of hemoglobin per unit volume of red cells expressed as a percentage.

Factors Required to Calculate Mean Cell Hemoglobin Concentration

1. Hemoglobin.
2. Hematocrit. Let us assume a calculation example in which the hemoglobin = 15 g/dl and hematocrit = 0.45 (45%).
3. If the red cells occupy 45% of the total blood volume, and there are 15 g/dl hemoglobin, the hemoglobin concentration is as follows:

$$\frac{\text{Hemoglobin (g/dl)} \times 100}{\text{Hematocrit (\%)}} = \frac{15}{45} \times 100 = 33.3\%$$

Reference Ranges

MCV	75–100 fl
MCH	27.0–35.0 pg
MCHC	31.0–37.0%

Sources of Error

The accuracy of the red-cell indices depends on the accuracy of the primary tests used to calculate them. The data should always be checked by a visual observation of a well-made, stained peripheral blood smear. Elevations of the calculated indices can result from either rouleaux formation or autoagglutination.

Clinical considerations include elevated MCV data found in macrocytic blood pictures (including megaloblastic anemias, liver disease, and the bone marrow response to hemorrhage) and cases in which the reticulocyte count is elevated. Reductions in MCV are found most commonly in iron-deficiency anemia and thalassemia.

The MCH is of less value than either the MCV or the MCHC, but it is a useful check of these two values. Reductions in MCH correlate with microcytic blood pictures and with normocytic hypochromic anemia. Elevations in MCH are found in macrocytic normochromic anemia but, if the macrocytes are also hypochromic, the MCH will be either normal or depressed, depending on the degree of hypochromia.

The MCHC is a useful index for iron deficiency and correlates with the degree of hypochromia. Elevated values are found only when the red cell is

not a biconcave disc—that is, in spherocytosis. Hyperchromic red cells other than spherocytes are physiologically impossible as the cell would, by definition, be supersaturated with hemoglobin and would hemolyze.

Manual Leukocyte Count

Principle

Whole blood is diluted with a fluid that hemolyzes the red cells, leaving all nucleated cells. The number of nucleated cells is counted in a fixed volume of fluid in the hemocytometer, and the final result is expressed as the number of cells in 1 liter of undiluted blood, after first correcting for the presence of nucleated red cells, if appropriate.

Reagents and Equipment

1. Diluting fluids: 2% aqueous acetic acid tinged with gentian violet or 1% hydrochloric acid.
2. Leukocyte pipette: Either a Thoma bulbed pipette or, for more accurate results, a Sahli hemoglobin pipette (0.02 ml).
3. Improved Neubauer hemocytometer.
4. Microscope.

Specimen

EDTA-anticoagulated whole blood is the preferred specimen. Capillary blood can also be used if diluted immediately on collection.

Method

1. A 1:20 dilution of blood is made by any of the following methods: Blood may be pipetted up to the 0.5 mark of a leukocyte Thoma (bulb) pipette, and diluting fluid is added up to the 11 mark. Care must be taken to avoid introducing air bubbles into the bulb. The pipette is shaken vigorously, and several drops of the diluent are expelled from the stem of the pipette.

The Unopette system, described on page 261, can also be used. These pipettes automatically dilute the specimen in a ratio of 1:20 using 25 μl blood to 4.98 ml diluting fluid. If this procedure is used, the final result should be calculated accordingly.

Alternatively, a 1:21 dilution can be prepared by adding 0.02 ml blood to 0.4 ml diluting fluid.

2. The hemocytometer is cleaned, and the cover-slip is placed firmly over the counting area, as previously described (page 258).

3. The dilution is mixed well. If the Thoma pipette is used, the first few drops of diluent are expelled from the pipette, and then the counting chamber is filled by capillary attraction by holding the pipette at a 90-degree angle and introducing one sufficiently large drop of diluted blood to completely fill the counting area in one motion.

4. The cells are allowed to settle for 3–5 minutes, and the counting area is viewed under a low-power microscope lens to check for even distribution.

5. The total cells in each of the four large corner squares in the counting chamber are counted using the same procedure as described in the section on manual red-cell counting. A variation of more than 10 cells among any of the four areas counted indicates poor distribution and requires that the procedure be repeated.

Calculation

Total cell count = Number of cells counted ×

$$\frac{1}{\text{area counted (mm}^2)} \times \frac{1}{\text{depth (mm)}} \times \text{dilution}$$

$$= \text{Number of cells counted} \times \frac{1}{4} \times \frac{0}{0.1} \times 20$$

$$= \text{Number of cells counted} \times 50$$

Note: If the 1:21 dilution is made, the final concentration is the number of cells counted × 52.5.

Reference Ranges

Adult	$3.9–10.9 \times 10^9$/liter
Newborn	$10.0–25.0 \times 10^9$/liter
Child, 1 month old	$7.0–15.0 \times 10^9$/liter
Child, 1 year old	$6.0–15.0 \times 10^9$/liter
Child, 10 years old	$4.5–12.0 \times 10^9$/liter

Discussion and Sources of Error

A number of studies have shown lower leukocyte counts in blacks than in whites (Brown et al., 1966; Caramihai et al., 1975; Rana et al., 1985). The National Health and Nutrition Examination Survey (Fulwood et al., 1982) showed that, in all age groups, blacks had lower mean leukocyte counts than did whites. The differences ranged from 0.6 to 1.3×10^9/liter among male subjects and from 0.2 to 1.4×10^9/liter among female subjects. However, such ethnic differences have not been found consistently (Orfanakis et al., 1970), and recent data show similar ranges for males and slightly wider and higher ranges for females (Rana et al., 1985). The diluting fluid used in the leukocyte count hemolyzes all non-nucleated red cells but, in many bone marrow–responsive anemias, immature erythrocytes may be prematurely released into the circulation in an attempt to compensate for reductions in the oxygen-carrying capacity of the blood. In such an occurrence, these nucleated cells will be counted as total leukocytes and may give an unacceptably high bias to the final result if present in sufficiently large numbers.

Therefore, any time there are more than 4 nucleated red cells present per 100 leukocytes in the differential leukocyte count, a corrected total count should be made using the following formula:

Corrected leukocyte count =

$$\frac{\text{Uncorrected}}{100 + \text{the number of nucleated red cells/100 leukocytes}}$$

If the uncorrected count were 7.0×10^9/liter and there were 10 metarubricytes present for every 100 leukocytes, the corrected count would be

$$\frac{7 \times 10^9}{1.10} = 6.36 \times 10^9 / \text{liter}$$

Manual leukocyte counts are subject to technical problems similar to those encountered in red-cell counts: The glassware should be clean and accurately calibrated, and the diluting fluid should be free of contaminants. For more accurate results, as large a number of cells as possible should be counted, which can be achieved by setting up the hemocytometer in duplicate, using both sides of the chamber.

In many myeloproliferative and lymphoproliferative disorders, the total leukocyte count may be extremely elevated. If the count exceeds 30.0×10^9/liter, it is best to repeat the count using a larger dilution of blood—either 1:100 or 1:200, depending on the degree of the leukocytosis. Conversely, in leukopenic conditions, a more accurate count will be made by using a smaller dilution ratio, such as 1:10 or 1:5.

Differential Leukocyte Counts

Preparation of Blood Smears

Wedge (Slide) Method

The wedge, or slide, method is depicted in Figure 18.6.

1. A drop of blood, approximately 2 mm in diameter, is placed at one end of a clean, grease-free slide.
2. A smooth glass spreader slide is then placed at an angle of 40 degrees, touching the drop of blood. As the blood spreads along the edge of the spreader slide, it is pushed evenly and with moderate speed away from the drop.
3. The blood smear is allowed to air-dry completely before staining.

Coverslip Method

The coverslip method is illustrated in Figure 18.7.

1. Two grease-free coverslips are held carefully by their edges, one in each hand. A small drop of blood is touched to one of the coverslips and is superimposed immediately on the other in a diagonal fashion.
2. The two coverslips then are drawn smoothly apart in a horizontal plane, and the resulting smears are allowed to air-dry, as described previously. The advantage of the coverslip method is that there is a more even distribution of cells, which allows for a more accurate count. However, the handling of coverslip preparations is more difficult—in staining, in labeling, and in storage—so that it is not often carried out.

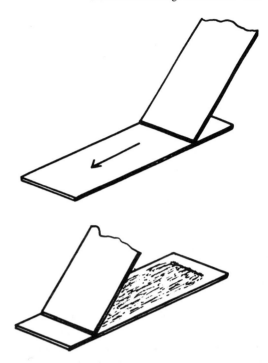

Figure 18.6. The wedge method of blood smear preparation.

Spinner Method

Blood smears that combine the advantages of ease of handling of the wedge method and the uniform distribution of cells of the coverslip preparation can be made with a special type of centrifuge that accepts glass slides. Approximately 0.2 ml EDTA-anticoagulated blood is placed on the center of the slide, and the cover is closed. This activates the centrifuge motor, which spins the slide at approximately 5,000 rpm for a few seconds. The exact centrifuge time can be adjusted for personal preference by an external rheostat knob.

The resulting monolayer blood smear is uniformly thick and enables both leukocyte and red-cell morphologic features to be easily examined. Cellular distribution is even and scattered randomly, but the red cells often appear to have an eccentric central pallor resembling that of spheroidocytes (Rogers, 1973).

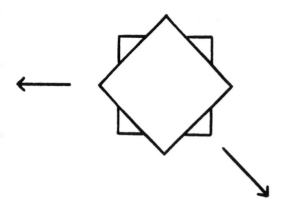

Figure 18.7. The coverslip method of blood smear preparation.

Counting Methods

One of the problems associated with producing accurate and precise manual differential leukocyte counts is in the uneven distribution of the cells even when the best techniques are followed. Two principal counting methods, the longitudinal and the battlement methods, have been used in an attempt to minimize these distribution problems.

Longitudinal Method.   In the longitudinal method, the cells are counted in three strips running from the head to the tail of the smear. The procedure successfully minimizes distribution problems but suffers because leukocyte morphologic features are difficult to determine at the thicker end of the smear. Consequently, it is recommended that the procedure be modified by counting the leukocytes only to the point at which red cells do not overlap.

Battlement Method.   For the battlement method, leukocytes are counted in two microscopic fields near the edge of the smear, then in four to six fields toward the center, in two fields parallel to the edge, and in four to six fields toward the edge. This process is repeated until a sufficient number of cells are counted.

Sources of Error

The differential leukocyte count can be carried out only on well-made, stained blood smears. Al-though experience and technique are vital to adequate preparation, the following are useful criteria and helpful suggestions for the preparation of such smears:

- Blood smears should be of a reasonable thickness. On microscopic examination, the red cells in the center area of the smear should be present without overlapping.
- The smear should possess a smooth appearance when viewed macroscopically.
- There should be a smooth graduated "tail" at the end of the smear.
- A margin of approximately 2–3 mm on each side of the smear should be present. This is made by using a spreader slide with the corners clipped at 45 degrees so that the spreading area is less than the width of the slide being spread.
- The patient's name and date or other identifiable data should be written in pencil on the thick end of the smear.

A number of technical problems are associated with the preparation of adequate blood smears. First, a smooth spreader should be used. The spreader slide edge should be ground lightly to produce a smooth bevel. If a rough-edged spreader is used, many of the leukocytes become aggregated at the edges and in the tail. Moreover, neutrophils and monocytes predominate at the margins and tail, and lymphocytes tend to be seen in greater numbers in the middle of the smear.

In addition, slides should be clean and free of grease and finger marks. Only a moderate-sized drop of blood should be used, approximately 2 mm in diameter. If too large a drop is used, the smear will be unacceptably thick or, if too small a drop is used, the smear is usually thin and shows distorted morphologic characteristics.

The angle of the spreader slide as it touches the blood and as it is used should be approximately 40 degrees. If the angle is greater than this, a thin smear is produced, whereas if it is less, a thicker smear will result.

The motion used in pushing the spreader slide should be smooth. Erratically pushed spreaders produce "chatters" (i.e., uneven layers of cells) and poor cellular distribution. The speed with which the slide is made helps to determine the smear thickness. The quicker the smear is made, the thicker it will be.

The best smears are made from blood taken directly from the needle of the syringe or vacuum collection device or from a capillary puncture. If EDTA-anticoagulated blood is used, the smear should be made as soon after collection as possible, preferably within 4 hours, to produce acceptable morphologic features.

The Differential Leukocyte Report

Two principal methods of reporting leukocyte differentials exist: by percentage and by absolute numbers. The most common procedure is to count 100 cells and categorize the cells seen into their various types. Although this is the easiest method of carrying out the test, it can lead occasionally to erroneous interpretation unless care is taken to review the complete blood cell count. For example, a differential count showing 10% eosinophils would, in most situations, be considered abnormal. The eosinophilia interpretation may cause additional and expensive testing and produce incorrect diagnostic conclusions. In this example, an eosinophilia would exist if the total leukocyte count was 7.0×10^9/liter, producing an absolute eosinophil count of 0.70×10^9/liter, but a report of 10% eosinophils would be within the reference range if the total leukocyte count were 4.0×10^9/liter. This would result in an absolute count of 0.28×10^9/liter. Similarly, care should be taken in interpreting other results. The absolute differential count is calculated from the following formula:

$$\frac{\text{Total leukocyte count} \times \text{percentage differential}}{100}$$

For example:

$$\frac{7.0(\times 10^9)}{100} \times 10 = 0.7 \times 10^9 / \text{liter}$$

Reference Ranges

Manual Method

	Percent	Absolute Numbers ($\times 10^9$/liter)
Adults		
Neutrophils	50–75	2.5–7.5
Bands	2–6	0.1–0.6
Eosinophils	1–5	0.05–0.4
Basophils	0–2	0–0.2
Monocytes	2–9	0.1–0.9
Lymphocytes	20–44	1.0–4.0
Infants (birth)		
Neutrophils	21–81	2.1–20.3
Eosinophils	0–5	0–1.3
Basophils	0–1	0–0.3
Monocytes	0–6	0–1.5
Lymphocytes	8–38	0.8–9.4
Children (8–14 years)		
Neutrophils	33–54	1.5–6.5
Eosinophils	0–5	0–0.6
Basophils	0–2	0–0.2
Monocytes	0–7	0–0.8
Lymphocytes	33–54	1.5–6.5

Cytochemical Method (H1, H2 Analyzer; Miles, Inc., Tarrytown, NY)

	Percent	Absolute Numbers ($\times 10^9$/liter)
Adults		
Neutrophils	47.6–74.6	2.1–7.8
Eosinophils	0.3–5.5	0.04–0.39
Basophils	0.1–1.5	0.010–0.136
Monocytes	1.4–11.6	0.13–0.86
Lymphocytes	15.9–38.6	1.25–3.38
Large unstained cells	<2.8	1.0–2.5

Discussion

The principal limitation of the differential leukocyte count is the inherent error in counting randomly distributed cells influenced by the physical character-

Table 18.2. Normal Differential Leukocyte Counts in Infants and Children

Age	Percentage of Total Leukocytes					
	Segmented	Bands	Eosinophils*	Basophils*	Lymphocytes	Monocytes*
Birth	32–62	10–18	2.2	0.6	26–36	5.8
4 wks	15–35	6–12	2.8	0.5	41–71	6.5
4 yrs	23–45	5–11	2.8	0.6	35–65	5.0
10 yrs	31–61	5–11	2.4	0.5	28–48	4.3
16 yrs	34–69	5–11	2.6	0.5	25–45	5.1

*Data for eosinophils, basophils, and monocytes represent mean numbers.
Source: Data from JB Miale. Laboratory Medicine: Hematology (6th ed). St Louis: Mosby, 1982.

istics of the smear. The various counting methods previously discussed do not remove this source of error completely even in the best-made wedge blood smears. The use of the battlement pattern sometimes produces excessively high neutrophil counts derived from their marginal distribution. The disadvantage of the longitudinal method is that in the thicker part of the smear, the leukocytes appear smaller and more condensed, making their identification more difficult. Both of these two major disadvantages are removed, at least theoretically, by using the spinning technique. However, the improvement over wedge-made smears appears fairly insignificant (Koepke, 1977).

The most acceptable method used to reduce the inherent error of the differential count is to count a larger number of cells. It is impractical to routinely count more than 200 cells in a differential count; the only practical approach is to use an automated method, whereby up to 10,000 cells are counted, sized, and identified rapidly. Several different systems are currently in use but, irrespective of the theoretical approach of each one, the inherent error is reduced in relationship to the number of cells counted.

The second main problem in manual differential counting is in cell identification and subjective morphologic assessment of the red-cell and platelet populations. Several techniques for quality control of the test have been suggested (page 241) but, at best, these are still only mildly helpful.

The differential count, besides determining the relative number of each type of leukocyte present, also provides valuable information as to red-cell and platelet status. During the count, morphologic abnormalities in any of the three cell lines should

be noted, and an estimate of the total leukocyte and platelet count should be made as part of the quality control of the complete blood count (see page 241).

The normal range for the test is established by puberty. Thereafter, there are no significant differences in the values related either to age or gender. In infancy and childhood, the values show a mild-to-moderate lymphocytosis. During the period from 1 month through 4 years of age, the percentage of lymphocytes is greater than 50% of the total cells, peaking at 8–10 months of age at more than 60%. An approximation of the reference range for children is shown in Table 18.2.

Stains

Romanowsky Stains

The most commonly used Romanowsky-type stains are Wright's, Giemsa, May-Grünwald, and Jenner's. These compound stains are mixtures of two or more dyes that interact to produce a new compound possessing new staining properties. The differences among stains are mainly in the proportion of the reagents used and in the methods of preparation. The crux of producing a satisfactory stain is the oxidation of the methylene blue, which, when added to eosin derivatives, produces a neutral stain. Methylene blue and its oxidation products are basic dyes that stain acidic cell components, whereas acidic eosin stains basic cell structures. The thiazine dyes produced by the interaction and chemical treatment of the stain are responsible for the subtle shades of staining seen when using these types of stains. Consequently, the characteristic appearance of Romanowsky-stained blood reveals pink-red cells, purple-black chromatin, blue leukocytic cytoplasm, black basophilic granules, pink-orange eosinophilic granules, lilac neutrophilic granules, and pale blue nucleoli.

Most Romanowsky stains are of little value if water is present because neutral dyes have precipitated from solution, or if acetone is an impurity of the alcohol. The staining action probably depends on partial dissociation of the components after dilution of the stain with buffered water. The intensity of the staining varies with the extent of stain dilution and with both the staining time and the nature and quality of the dyes.

Wright's Stain

Wright's stain is a polychromatic stain producing multicolored staining reactions from a single application. Wright's stain, like other Romanowsky stains, is a complex mixture of oxidized methylene blue and various eosin azures. It is best obtained commercially as a dry powder, although various modifications can be obtained in a ready-to-use state.

Preparation

1. Pure Wright's stain (0.2 g) is added to 100 ml anhydrous acetone-free methyl alcohol. The mixture is shaken to suspend and dissolve the stain and is placed on an electric plate at 60°C until the stain has dissolved completely.
2. The stain solution then is allowed to cool and is filtered through dry, coarse filter paper to remove any large particles.
3. The filtered stain is aged or oxidized by placing it in a 37°C incubator for approximately 30–45 days, shaking the reagent daily to resuspend and dissolve any particulate material that may be present.
4. The stain is refiltered before use.

Method

1. The air-dried blood smear is placed on a level staining rack with the smear side up and is then fixed by adding 1 volume of undiluted stain to the smear with a Pasteur pipette or a dropping bottle.
2. Two to three volumes of buffered distilled water (pH 6.4) are then added to the stain, with care taken not to wash off the stain. The diluted stain is mixed either by gently blowing air on the slide or by repeatedly sucking the dilution up and down in a Pasteur pipette. If the correct dilution has been made, a metallic scum will be present on the surface of the diluted stain after mixing.
3. The blood smear is allowed to stain for 5–10 minutes, the exact amount of time being determined by experimentation.
4. The stain is removed from the smear with a stream of buffered water, and the water is allowed to differentiate the smear for 1 minute or so or until the edges of the smear become faintly pink.
5. The water is drained from the slide. The underside of the slide is wiped with damp gauze to remove any concentrated stain and is allowed to air-dry. The slide must not be blotted dry.

Giemsa Stain

Preparation

1. Powdered Giemsa stain (1.0 g) is dissolved in 66 ml glycerol by placing the mixture on an electric plate at 60°C for 2 hours.
2. The stain is allowed to cool to room temperature, and an equal volume of pure anhydrous acetone-free methyl alcohol is added. The solution is mixed and allowed to stand for nearly 30 days in direct sunlight, or it is incubated at 37°C for 30–45 days to ripen. The stain is mixed daily to redissolve any precipitated stain.
3. The stain is filtered before use.

Method

1. The blood smear is fixed by placing it in a Coplin jar of anhydrous acetone-free methyl alcohol for 1–2 minutes.
2. The concentrated Giemsa stain is diluted by adding 1 volume of stain to 9 volumes of buffered distilled water (pH 6.8).
3. The fixed blood smear is placed either on a level staining rack or in a second Coplin jar. The 1:10 diluted Giemsa stain is added and allowed to stand for 5–10 minutes. The stain is washed off with a stream of distilled water and differentiated, as in the Wright's staining procedure, for 1–2 minutes.
4. The water is removed, the underside of the slide is wiped free of stain, and allowed to air-dry.

Wright-Giemsa Stain

The Wright-Giemsa stain is a modification of both the Wright and the Giemsa stains. The addition of Giemsa stain produces subjectively more delicate staining characteristics to blood cells, and it is preferred by many workers for routine use.

Preparation

1. Pure Wright's stain (9.0 g) is added with 1.0 g of Giemsa powder to 2,910 ml anhydrous acetone-free methyl alcohol. The mixture is made up to 3 liters by the addition of glycerin.
2. The stain is mixed by shaking and is allowed to age at 37°C for 30–45 days, care being taken to mix the stain daily.
3. The stain is filtered before use.

Method

1. The air-dried blood smear is placed on a level staining rack with the smear side up and is fixed by flooding with anhydrous acetone-free methyl alcohol for 1–2 minutes or by immersing in a Coplin jar filled with freshly poured methyl alcohol.

2. The methyl alcohol is drained from the slide, which then is flooded with the Wright-Giemsa stain and allowed to stand for 4 minutes.

3. An equal volume of buffered distilled water (pH 6.4) is added to the stain, taking care to avoid washing the stain off the smear. The diluted stain is mixed either by gently blowing air on the slide or by repeatedly sucking the dilution up and down in a Pasteur pipette. If the correct dilution has been made, a metallic scum will be present on the surface of the stain after mixing.

4. The blood smear is allowed to stain for 7 minutes.

5. The stain is rinsed from the slide with a stream of buffered water, the underside of the slide is wiped with damp gauze to remove any concentrated stain, and the smear is allowed to air-dry.

May-Grünwald-Giemsa and Jenner-Giemsa Stains

Preparation. The *May-Grünwald stain* (0.25 g, stock) is dissolved in 100 ml pure anhydrous acetone-free methyl alcohol by heating it to 60°C on an electric plate. The mixture then is allowed to cool to room temperature and is filtered through dry, coarse filter paper into a dry bottle and stored stoppered in a cool place.

Jenner's stain (stock) is prepared exactly as is the May-Grünwald stain.

To prepare the working solutions of these stains, stock May-Grünwald or Jenner's stain (100 ml) is diluted with 150 ml buffered distilled water (pH 6.8), or 100 ml stock Giemsa stain (prepared as already described) is diluted with 400 ml buffered distilled water (pH 6.8).

Method

1. The air-dried blood smear is placed on a level staining rack with the smear side up and is fixed by flooding with anhydrous acetone-free methyl alcohol for 1–2 minutes or by immersing in a Coplin jar filled with freshly poured methyl alcohol.

2. The methyl alcohol is drained from the slide, which then is flooded with the working solution of either the May-Grünwald or the Jenner's stain and allowed to stain for 3 minutes.

3. The stain is removed with a stream of buffered water, and the working Giemsa stain is added and allowed to stand for 15 minutes or longer. The Giemsa stain is washed off with buffered water, and the smear is allowed to differentiate in the water for 1–2 minutes or until the edge of the smear is a faint pink.

4. The water is removed, the underside of the slide is wiped free of stain, and the smear is allowed to air-dry.

Composition of the Buffers Used to Dilute the Romanowsky Stains

The buffers used to dilute the Romanowsky stains are potassium dihydrogen phosphate, anhydrous (0.067 M), and dibasic sodium phosphate, anhydrous (0.067 M). The salt form of either buffer (9.08 g potassium dihydrogen phosphate or 9.47 g dibasic sodium phosphate) is dissolved in 1 liter distilled water. The dilutions listed in Table 18.3 can be used as a guide to preparing buffered solutions of varying pH levels.

Table 18.3. Composition of Buffer Solutions

pH	Potassium Dihydrogen Phosphate (ml)	Dibasic Sodium Phosphate (ml)
5.2	98.2	1.8
6.4	73.0	27.0
6.8	50.8	49.2
7.2	28.0	72.0

Sources of Error

A well-stained blood smear will show pink-red cells and well-differentiated, stained leukocytes. Poorly stained smears result from a variety of conditions, which include staining of thick smears, incorrect pH of water, inappropriate staining times, air-drying of smears in a humid atmosphere, and the presence of precipitated stain.

Thick blood smears, even if correctly stained, often appear darkly stained and are unacceptable for examination. If the pH of the buffer is too acidic, the red cells appear pinker and the leukocytes stain lightly or with an overall pink hue. If the pH of the buffer is too basic, the red cells appear purple-blue, and the leukocytes stain uniformly blue or shades of blue-black. In either situation, the smear should be remade and restained.

On occasion, air bubbles are present in many of the red cells, giving the superficial appearance of punched-out holes or even of a marked atypical hypochromic cell. This is caused principally by either allowing a thick smear to dry slowly or by air-drying smears in a humid atmosphere. Usually, this problem can be corrected by remaking a thinner blood smear and blowing warm air over its surface or by waving it vigorously.

The staining times detailed in the procedures are merely guides. Each batch of stain or each lot of dried stain will produce its own individual staining characteristics, and the staining times will vary accordingly and should be individually tested. The times suggested have been for blood smears. However, when staining bone marrow preparations, staining times should be increased. Again, the exact times should be determined individually.

Stain precipitate on either blood or bone marrow preparations is caused by inadequate removal of the stain by washing with buffered water or by allowing the stain to dry on the slide. If it is desirable to restain the smear, the precipitate may sometimes be removed by destaining the smear, which is accomplished by immersing the smear in a Coplin jar of methyl alcohol until the stain is removed.

Reticulocyte Count

Principle

Reticulocytes are young red cells that contain within the cell membrane a proportion of ribonucleoprotein derived from the more immature nucleated red-cell precursors. The more immature the reticulocyte, the greater the ribosome content of the cell. This ribonucleoprotein is gradually lost as the reticulocyte matures. The number of reticulocytes is then used as an index of bone marrow activity and red-cell production. Recognition of reticulocytes in unfixed preparations is based on the ability of the ribosomal material of the cell to be stained with certain nontoxic dyes, the so-called supravital technique.

Anticoagulated blood is mixed with a supravital dye and, after staining, blood smears are made and the reticulocyte count is estimated by visual inspection. The smear may be counterstained, but this is an individual choice and is not necessary for the identification of the cells. The results are expressed as a percentage of the total number of red cells or as a corrected count relative to the hematocrit.

Reagents and Equipment

1. Staining fluid. New methylene blue (1.0 g) is dissolved in 80 ml normal saline and 20 ml 3% sodium citrate. Brilliant cresyl blue can be substituted for new methylene blue.
2. Microscope with eyepiece stock or equipped with a Miller disc.
3. Pasteur pipette.

Specimen

EDTA-anticoagulated blood is the preferred specimen. Capillary blood also may be used. Blood should be less than 24 hours old.

Method

1. Approximately equal volumes of blood and freshly filtered stain are mixed in a tube and are allowed to stand at room temperature or at 37°C for 15–30 minutes.

2. The cells are resuspended, and several blood smears are made using a Pasteur pipette to deposit a small aliquot of stained cells on a slide. The smears are made using the same technique as that used in making smears for differential leukocyte counts.

3. The stained smears are allowed to air-dry and are then examined under the high-power oil-immersion lens of the microscope. Mature red cells stain a gray-blue, and reticulocytes are identified by the presence of a deep blue filamentous web or isolated granules within the cell. Any cell that contains two or more particles of blue-stained material is classified as a reticulocyte (National Committee for Clinical Laboratory Standards, 1993).

4. An area of the slide in which the red cells are not overlapping is scanned, and 1,000 cells are counted. The total number of reticulocytes seen is divided by 10 to express the result as a percentage.

Calculation

If 22 reticulocytes were seen when counting 1,000 red cells, the reticulocyte count expressed as a percentage is as follows:

$$\frac{22 \times 100}{1,000} = 2.2\%$$

An alternative procedure is to survey sufficient microscopic fields so that at least 100 reticulocytes are counted. The number of red cells present in every tenth field is counted. The reticulocyte result then is expressed by this formula:

$$\frac{\text{Number of reticulocytes counted}}{\substack{\text{Approximate number of red cells} \\ \text{present in the fields embracing} \\ \text{the reticulocytes}}} \times 100$$

For example, if 100 reticulocytes are present in 200 fields, and 3,000 red cells also are present in 20 fields, the 100 reticulocytes are present with 30,000 red cells, which yields the following percentage of reticulocytes:

$$\frac{100}{30,000} \times 100 = 0.33\%$$

A third method of enumerating the reticulocyte count is to use a Miller disc. This optical aid is inserted into the eyepiece of the microscope and allows for a more accurate count. The disc ruling consists of a center square containing a secondary square ruled area that is one-ninth the area of the larger square. Reticulocytes are counted in the total larger area and red cells in the small square. The count is expressed as this formula:

$$\frac{\text{Number of reticulocytes in large square}}{\text{Number of red cells in small square} \times 9} \times 100$$

If 25 reticulocytes were counted in the large square and 111 red cells were counted in the smaller area, the reticulocyte count would be calculated thus:

$$\frac{25}{999} \times 100 = 2.5\%$$

Reticulocyte counts can also be reported as absolute numbers in a manner similar to absolute differential leukocyte counts. The following formula is used:

$$\frac{\% \text{ Reticulocytes} \times \text{red - cell count } (\times 10^{12}/\text{liter})}{100}$$

$$= \text{Reticulocytes} \times 10^9/\text{liter}$$

Reference Ranges

Adults   0.5–1.5% (25–75 × 10⁹/liter)
Infants   2.0–6.0%

Sources of Error

The reticulocyte count, like other quantitative tests, should be controlled using blood of known composition. Recently, a commercial control has been made available that produces stable values of approximately 3.5% (Streck Laboratories Inc., Omaha, NE).

As stated previously, a reticulocyte is an immature red cell and is not demonstrated in Romanowsky-stained blood smears but is readily seen if stained supravitally by either new methylene blue or brilliant cresyl blue. During the counting process, other types of red-cell inclusions may be seen and erroneously counted as reticulocytes. These include Howell-Jolly bodies, Pappenheimer bodies, Heinz bodies, Hb H inclusions, and basophilic stippling. Fortunately, it is relatively easy to separate most of these inclusions, but the presence of Hb H can present the technologist with identification difficulties. Hb H inclusions are often found in relatively large numbers in Hb H disease, and they appear as uniform, rounded inclusions randomly scattered within the cell (page 39).

The technical and biological factors affecting the reticulocyte count are numerous. The concentration and purity of the stain as well as differences in the staining characteristics can be reflected in the final result. Low staining concentrations can result in staining that is too pale, whereas stains that are too concentrated often lead to stain precipitation and interpretive errors. Impure stains may contain contaminating metallic salts, which can falsely elevate the result (Peebles et al., 1981).

The anticoagulation of blood samples has been shown to affect the final test result. Sodium citrate decreases the reticulocyte count (Cudak, 1982), but defibrinated blood is stable if it is kept at refrigerated temperatures for up to 3 weeks (Pepper, 1922). EDTA is the anticoagulant of choice and does not affect the final result for 24 hours, irrespective of the storage temperature (Koepke, 1979).

Temperature and pH can also have an effect on the number of reticulocytes counted. Warming the stain and giving it an acidic pH can produce a fine reticular granulation, making it easier to miss the reticulocytes.

The expression of reticulocyte counts as a straight percentage of the red cells is not necessarily a true indicator of bone marrow response and, consequently, a corrected value may be used to overcome this problem (Crosby, 1981). The method involves setting up a ratio between the patient's hemoglobin, red-cell count, or hematocrit and the normal value for each of these parameters. Such a choice of corrections is as follows:

Corrected count =

$$\frac{\text{Patient's red cell count}}{5.0} \times \text{raw reticulocyte count}$$

or

$$\frac{\text{Patient's hematocrit}}{0.45} \times \text{raw reticulocyte count}$$

or

$$\frac{\text{Patient's hemoglobin}}{15} \times \text{raw reticulocyte count}$$

Although these correction criteria are useful in assessing bone marrow output, the formula assumes that the release of bone marrow reticulocytes is occurring normally. Ferrokinetic data should be used to obtain a true index of bone marrow red-cell reduction, and account must be taken of the reduced reticulocyte transit time in the marrow, as this time is influenced and reduced by the degree of anemia. The reticulocyte production index (RPI) should be used in such situations (Hillman and Finch, 1967). Using this approach, it is seen that as it changes, the patient's hematocrit influences the rate at which reticulocytes are released from the bone marrow. As the hematocrit drops, the bone marrow releases more immature reticulocytes, which take longer to develop into mature cells. Using the RPI, a true corrected reticulocyte result is expressed as shown in Table 18.4.

The reticulocyte count is also limited by the statistics of counting relatively small numbers of these cells. It has been shown that the technical error associated with the test is approximately 30%; in addition, the Poisson distribution error could add another 40% error to the result. This then reduces the test to a semiquantitative estimation (Peebles et al., 1981). The statistical error of the count can be expressed as follows:

$$R \pm 2 \times \sqrt{R \frac{(100 - R)}{N}}$$

where R is the reticulocyte count in percentage and N the number of red cells counted.

Discussion

Reticulocytes can be counted using an argon laser–based flow cytometer. Whole blood samples

Table 18.4. Reticulocyte Production Index (RPI)

RPI	Patient Hematocrit (%)
1.0	45
1.5	35
2.0	25
2.5	15

are stained directly with a fluorescent dye (auramine O) and are passed through a laser beam. A 100-µl blood sample is used, which allows use of the same tube for blood and reticulocyte counts and the analysis of capillary and finger-stick samples. Compared with the standard microscopic techniques, the automated method possesses excellent correlation ($r = 0.98$), and improved precision (CV, 4.1%). Preanalytic storage of specimens at 4°C for up to 48 hours does not affect the result (Lofsness et al., 1994). The presence of red cells containing DNA inclusions, such as malarial parasites or Howell-Jolly bodies, produces erroneously high results.

Erythrocyte Sedimentation Rate

If anticoagulated blood is allowed to stand for some time, the erythrocytes gradually sink and the plasma becomes displaced upward. The rate of this action is constant in health and is known as the *erythrocyte sedimentation rate*. Increased rates occur when the cells become aggregated or form rouleaux. The rate is directly proportional to the size of the aggregate.

The ESR is affected principally by three factors: (1) the number, size, and density of the red cells, (2) the plasma composition, and (3) miscellaneous technical factors.

Red cells possess a net negative charge derived from cell membrane sialic acid moieties. When cells are suspended in normal plasma, rouleaux formation is minimal and the sedimentation of the cells is slow. However, if changes in the proportion and levels of various proteins occur, particularly asymmetric macromolecules, the negative charge or ς-potential is reduced, and the rate of rouleaux formation increases. This causes an acceleration in the ESR. Cells that do not readily form rouleaux are unable to exhibit increased sedimentation unless there is a severe anemia. Consequently, red cells that show alterations in their biconcavity, such as spherocytes and sickle cells, usually do not exhibit increased rates and frequently produce normal and even reduced ESRs even in the presence of moderate anemia.

As previously stated, changes in plasma composition are the principal cause of rouleaux formation. These alterations often result from inflammatory processes caused by hydrophobic protein fractions such as fibrinogen and α_1- and α_2-globulins, which reduce the ς-potential of the red cells. Besides these abnormalities, sedimentation of red cells also depends on plasma viscosity, and this most closely correlates with the presence of acute-phase reactants, total protein, albumin, and γ-globulin (Crook et al., 1980).

Technical factors are divided into three groups: (1) those due to mechanical influences, (2) those due to temperature variations, and (3) those due to physical vibrations. The laboratory conditions under which the ESR test is carried out have a direct effect on the result. It is most important that the sedimentation tube be perpendicular and placed in a rack equipped with a bubble level. Deviations as small as 3% from the absolute vertical can increase the result by 30%. Wide in vitro temperature changes also can promote falsely elevated results owing to a reduction in plasma viscosity, but this is unlikely unless the test is set up in direct sunlight. In general, however, minor temperature variations such as those found in most laboratories do not affect the result.

The effect of vibration is believed to increase the test result falsely by cell agitation, but this has not been substantiated even when the ESR test is set up on the same bench as a centrifuge (Hazelton, 1968).

Westergren's Standardized Method for the Erythrocyte-Sedimentation-Rate Test

Principle

Westergren's standardized ESR test measures the rate of settling of red cells in diluted plasma (International Committee for Standardization in Haematology, 1977; National Committee for Clinical Laboratory Studies, 1978). The reported value is obtained by the measured drop in the red-cell meniscus after 1 hour. The result is reported as the number of millimeters the red-cell meniscus falls in 1 hour.

Reagents and Equipment

1. Anticoagulant: Trisodium citrate dihydrate (0.109 mol/liter), 32.08 g/dl. Tripotassium EDTA may be used as an alternative anticoagulant at a concentration of 1.4–1.6 mg per milliliter of blood. An exact dilution of 4 volumes of blood to 1 volume of 9 g/dl sodium chloride or 32.08 g/dl trisodium citrate dihydrate must subsequently be made before testing.
2. Pipette. The Westergren pipette must be made of thick-walled glass or plastic that is straight and free from visible defects. The ends must be smooth and flat and at right angles to the long axis. The pipette must have the following dimensions: overall length, 300.5 ± 0.5 mm; external diameter, 5.5 ± 0.5 mm; tube bore, 2.55 ± 0.15 mm; and uniformity of bore, ± 0.05 mm. The pipette must be inscribed with a graduated scale numbered from 0 at the top to 200 mm at the bottom, in increments of 10 or less. For use, the tube must be clean and dry.
3. Rack. The tube rack should hold the tubes in a vertical position to within ±1 degree and should be constructed so that no leakage of diluted blood can occur from the tube when it is in place.

Specimen

The specimen should consist of citrated whole blood in a ratio of 4 volumes blood to 1 volume trisodium citrate dihydrate (32.08 g/dl). Alternatively, venous blood collected in EDTA can be used, provided that it is diluted as described previously.

Method

1. Blood is obtained by clean venipuncture and dispensed into the anticoagulant. When possible, collection should be completed within 30 seconds without allowing stasis to occur.

2. Before the diluted specimen is transferred to a Westergren tube, it is mixed thoroughly by gentle inversion, and the tube then is filled to the 0 mark using a rubber bulb or mechanical suction device.

3. The tube is placed in the rack in a strictly vertical position (±1 degree) under room-temperature conditions. The tube must not be exposed to direct sunlight, and the rack must be free of vibrations. The distance the red-cell meniscus falls in 1 hour is recorded. Care should be taken to exclude any buffy coat from the reading.

Reference Ranges

According to Westergren (1920), the following reference ranges apply:

Men   0- to 10-mm fall in 1 hour
Women   0- to 20-mm fall in 1 hour

Wintrobe Method

Principle

The principle of the Wintrobe method (Wintrobe, 1936) is similar to that of the Westergren method.

Reagents and Equipment

1. Wintrobe tube, which is a thick-walled tube, 120 mm long, with an internal diameter of 2.5 mm. The tube is closed at one end and is graduated from 0 to 100 mm.
2. Sedimentation rack with bubble level and adjustable leveling feet.
3. Long-stemmed Pasteur pipette.

Specimen

EDTA-anticoagulated blood is the preferred specimen.

Method

1. The Wintrobe tube is filled carefully with well-mixed blood using the Pasteur pipette. The tube is filled slowly from the bottom, with care taken not to introduce air bubbles or to allow the blood to foam. This is best accomplished by raising the pipette tip above the meniscus until the blood level reaches the 100-mm mark.

2. Once filled, the tube is placed in a vertical position in the rack for exactly 1 hour. The distance the red-cell meniscus falls in that time then is recorded.

Reference Ranges

Men   0- to 7-mm fall in 1 hour
Women   0- to 15-mm fall in 1 hour

Zetafuge Method

Principle

The Zetafuge is a device that implements a new approach to ESRs. Anticoagulated blood is pipetted into micropipettes, which are then placed in a slow-speed centrifuge. The gravitational force applied causes the red cells to migrate across the diameter of the tube toward the outer wall, accelerating rouleaux formation. After the centrifugal force has been applied for 45 seconds, the Zetafuge stops, the sample tube is rotated 180 degrees, and the apparatus restarts. During the second cycle, centrifugal force removes the red-cell rouleaux from what is now the inner wall of the capillary tube and partially disperses the rouleaux, moving them across the diameter of the tube and allowing them to form on the opposite wall. Each time the rouleaux traverse the tube diameter, they gently form sediment toward the bottom of the tube as a result of the gravitational force applied. After four 45-second cycles, the Zetafuge percentage is determined by a comparison of the Zetacrit percentage to that of the microhematocrit.

Reagents and Equipment

1. Plain capillary tubes 75 mm long with an internal diameter of 2.0 mm and an external diameter of 2.3 mm.
2. Zetafuge (Coulter Electronics, Hialeah, FL).
3. Clay.

Specimen

The specimen used is EDTA-anticoagulated blood.

Method

The Zetafuge method has been described previously by Bull and Brailsford (1972).

1. Approximately 100 μl anticoagulated blood are drawn into a capillary tube, and one end is plugged with clay to a depth of 5 mm.
2. The tube then is centrifuged for 3 minutes, and the degree of compaction achieved by the red cells is measured immediately.

Calculation

The Zetacrit is read using conventional microhematocrit readers, and the zeta sedimentation rate (ZSR) is calculated from the following formula:

$$ZSR = \frac{\text{True hematocrit (\%)}}{\text{Zetacrit (\%)}} \times 100$$

Reference Range

The reference range for all adults is 40–51%.

Interpretation

Doubtful elevation	51–54%
Mildly elevated	55–59%
Moderately elevated	60–64%
Markedly elevated	>65%

The Zetafuge is now unavailable, but the principle of an alternative ESR method is unique and is of value in assessing tissue destruction.

Microsedimentation Rate

Principle

EDTA–sodium citrate–anticoagulated blood is allowed to form sediment into plastic disposable micro-Westergren tubes (Barrett and Hill, 1980).

Reagents and Equipment

1. Microsedimentation tubes (commercially available as Dispette tubes, Becton-Dickinson, Rutherford, NJ) and stand.
2. Reservoir cap (Dispette).
3. Trisodium citrate, 31.3 g of the salt dissolved in 1 liter distilled water.

Specimen

The specimen used is EDTA-anticoagulated whole blood. Capillary samples are collected into 1.8% wt/vol dipotassium EDTA.

Method

1. EDTA-anticoagulated blood (0.2 ml) is added to 0.05 ml trisodium citrate in a funneled reservoir cap and mixed. Care should be taken to avoid air bubbles.
2. A plastic disposable microsedimentation rate tube is inserted. It should be 230 mm long with an internal bore of 1 mm into the cap. This creates positive pressure and results in blood entering the tube. The height of the column is adjusted to zero by manipulating the tube within the cap.
3. The tube is allowed to stand in a vertical position, and the sedimentation rate of the red cells is read in a conventional way by observing the markings on the tube.

Reference Ranges

Men	0- to 10-mm fall in 1 hour
Women	0- to 20-mm fall in 1 hour

Sources of Error

Besides the general sources of error and precautions in carrying out the ESR test, several other technical variables exist. These include the errors associated with the introduction of air bubbles and those found when hemolyzed specimens are used. Heparin should never be used, as it alters red-cell membrane ς-potential.

Red-cell sedimentation takes place in three principal stages. The cells start to cling together, beginning rouleaux formation during the first 5 minutes. Once rouleaux have formed and maximum aggregation has occurred, the falling rate remains constant and then slows down because of packing at the bottom half of the tube.

The effect of anemia on the ESR is well documented. Several different correction schemes have been proposed for the Wintrobe method. However, none is truly satisfactory, and such anemia corrections are not recommended. The effect on the re-

sult caused by delays in testing is discussed on page 226.

The ESR is a nonspecific test that is frequently increased in inflammatory disorders, principally because of the role of plasma proteins and their effect on rouleaux formation. There is agreement that acute-phase reactants become elevated in a variety of disorders and that their presence induces elevations in the ESR (Ritzmann and Daniels, 1975). Those most frequently cited are fibrinogen, C-reactive protein, α-acid-glycoprotein, α_1-antitrypsin, ceruloplasmin, and haptoglobin. In chronic diseases, the ESR elevation is probably caused by fibrinogen or by monoclonal or polyclonal increases of IgG, IgA, and IgM, alone or in combination (Talstad and Haugen, 1979). Despite this, there are significant differences in the clinical utility of the test. Most authorities consider the ESR a general screening procedure, but others have found it insensitive to some inflammatory disorders, such as gout, neoplasms, and thyroid disease in young adults (Froom et al., 1984).

It has been shown (Zacharski and Kyle, 1967) that fewer than 0.4% of patients have abnormal test results if the history, physical examination, and routine laboratory screening tests do not supply a clear diagnosis and, although unexplained elevations are found, there will be one and one-half times as many false-positive as true-positive results. Because no studies indicate the number of patients with disease who have normal results, the false-negative rate is unknown. The sensitivity of the test is believed to be less than 50%, with more than half the patients with active disease producing normal results (Galen, 1981).

The Westergren procedure, adopted as the international reference method, does not have well-established reference ranges. Several surveys suggest that the upper limit of normal in a person younger than 50 years may be as high as 15–20 mm in men and between 25 and 33 mm in women (Böttiger and Svedberg, 1967; Rafnsson et al., 1979).

Statistical analysis of large numbers of healthy adults has shown that the Westergren method produces considerably skewed results relative to patient age and that a gaussian distribution cannot be used to construct these ranges. Consequently, it has been proposed that the following formula be used (Miller et al., 1984):

$$Men = \frac{Age\ in\ years}{2} \ mm\ fall\ in\ 1\ hour$$

$$Women = \frac{(Age\ in\ years + 10)}{2} \ mm\ fall\ in\ 1\ hour$$

Contrary to general opinion, the Westergren method is less sensitive than the Wintrobe procedure to minimal elevations of asymmetric molecules. It is nonlinear in its response at these low levels but, in contrast, the rapid onset of the packing phase renders the Wintrobe method insensitive to marked elevations of these molecules, an area in which the Westergren test is the more sensitive (Bull and Brecher, 1974).

Neither the Westergren nor the Wintrobe procedure is adapted easily to micromodifications, although several capillary methods have been proposed (Hackett et al., 1983) and are commercially available (Barrett and Hill, 1980). The ZSR, like the other general tests, responds to an increase in the plasma content of asymmetric molecules that commonly accompany inflammatory disease. Unlike these methods, the ZSR is insensitive to hematocrit fluctuations, but it possesses the advantages of speed and of using small volumes of blood.

Manual Platelet Counts

Principle

Anticoagulated blood is diluted with a diluent that hemolyzes the red cells, leaving platelets and nucleated cells. The hemocytometer is charged with the diluted specimen, and the platelets are counted in a fixed ruled area. The final count is expressed as the number of cells in 1 liter of undiluted blood.

Reagents and Equipment

1. Diluting fluids. Using Brecher-Cronkite fluid (1% aqueous ammonium oxalate), the diluent is filtered and stored at 4°C. This fluid should be used if the count is to be carried out by phase microscopy. Alternatively, Dacie's fluid (stock: sodium citrate dihydrate, 5.0 g; formalin, 1 ml;

distilled water to 100 ml) can be used. One milliliter of 0.2% brilliant cresyl blue is added to 19 ml of the stock diluting fluid just before use and then is filtered. Another option is Rees-Ecker fluid (sodium citrate dihydrate, 3.8 g; brilliant cresyl blue, 0.1 g; formalin, 0.2 ml; distilled water to 100 ml).

2. Improved Neubauer hemocytometer. If a phase microscope is used in the procedure, it must be a special flat-bottomed phase hemocytometer, as routine hemocytometers are concave on the underside of the counting area.

3. Red-cell pipette. Either a Thoma bulbed pipette or a Sahli hemoglobin pipette (0.02 ml) can be used.

4. Phase-contrast or light microscope.

Specimen

EDTA-anticoagulated whole blood is the preferred specimen. Capillary blood can also be used if it is diluted immediately on collection.

Method

1. A 1:200 dilution of blood is made by one of the following methods: Diluting fluid is pipetted up to the 0.5 mark on a red-cell Thoma bulbed pipette, and the blood is drawn up carefully so that the level of the diluting fluids is at the 1 mark and that of the blood is at the 0.5 mark. The external surface of the pipette is wiped free of blood, and the dilution is completed by pipetting diluting fluid to the 101 mark, taking care to avoid the introduction of air bubbles.

An alternative is the Unopette system, described on page 261. These pipettes automatically dilute the specimen 1:100—20 ml blood to 1.98 ml diluting fluid. If this procedure is used, the count should be carried out using a phase microscope, and the final result should be calculated accordingly. Another method, a 1:101 dilution of blood, can be prepared by adding 0.02 ml blood to 4 ml diluting fluid.

2. The hemocytometer is cleaned, and the coverslip is placed firmly over the counting area, as previously described (page 258).

3. The dilution is mixed well. If the Thoma pipette is used, the first few drops of diluent are expelled from the pipette, and then both sides of the counting chamber are filled by capillary attraction.

This can best be accomplished by holding the pipette at a 90-degree angle and introducing one sufficiently large drop of diluted blood to completely fill the counting area in one motion.

4. The platelets are allowed to settle in a moist atmosphere for 3–5 minutes, and the counting area then is viewed under a low-power microscope lens to check for even distribution. A suitable moist environment can be produced by placing the slide and a damp pledget of cotton under a Petri dish.

5. The total number of platelets in the large center square (1 × 1 mm) on both sides of the counting chamber are counted. Platelets will be recognized more readily if the focus of the light microscope is altered carefully with the fine adjustment and if the illumination is reduced by closing the iris diaphragm. Using a high, dry objective, platelets will appear as highly refractile particles. If phase microscopy is used, the platelets appear as round or oval bodies with a light purple sheen. When focusing up and down, the platelets may be seen to have one or more fine processes. Dirt and debris are distinguishable because of their high refractility.

Calculation

Total platelet count

= Number of platelets counted ×
$$\frac{1}{\text{area counted (mm}^2)} \times \frac{1}{\text{depth (mm)}} \times \text{dilution ratio}$$
= Number of platelets counted $\times \dfrac{1}{2} \times \dfrac{1}{0.1} \times 200$

= Number of platelets × 1,000

Reference Range

The reference range is 150–450 × 10^9/liter.

Sources of Error

The choice of diluting fluid depends on the type of microscope used in the count. In general, ammonium oxalate diluents are most efficient when phase microscopy is used, but the choice of either conventional light or phase microscopes does not alter the procedure or the final result. The advantage of the phase technique is in the easier recognition of the platelets, which helps in distinguishing them from contamination and dirt particles. However, little difference between the techniques is found if attention is paid to cleaning the pipettes and hemocytometer scrupulously and filtering the diluting fluid just before use.

Platelet counts carried out directly from capillary blood obtained from the heel (in infants), finger, or earlobe are less satisfactory than those obtained from venous specimens. If capillary specimens are taken, the Unopette system should be used to minimize dilution errors. If these microspecimens are used, extra attention has to be given to the collection procedure, as outlined on page 251. It is essential that a free flow of blood be obtained without undue pressure and that the first few drops of blood be wiped away and not used in the dilution. Whenever possible, duplicate sets of Unopettes should be used and the results averaged to minimize the technical error of collection.

Platelets are technically more difficult to count than either red cells or leukocytes. This is because of their small size and confusion with extraneous dirt in the hemocytometer and because of their propensity to form agglutinates, especially if the specimen collection is poorly performed. Because of the many technical errors involved in the procedure, all manual platelet counts should be checked with a microscopic review of a well-made, stained blood smear, using the approximate quality control criteria, as shown on page 242. The presence of platelet clumps in the counting chamber invalidates the procedure, and a fresh specimen, collected in sodium citrate, should be obtained. Because the standard citrate collection tube combines one part of citrate solution with nine parts of blood, platelet counts done on such specimens would be slightly decreased because of the dilution. The raw platelet count should then be corrected by multiplying by 10/9 (1.11) to arrive at the correct result.

Chapter 19

Tests Useful in the Evaluation of Hemolysis

General Tests

Osmotic Fragility

Principle

The osmotic fragility test (Dacie and Lewis, 1975) determines the resistance of red cells to hemolysis at room temperature in varying concentrations of hypotonic saline solutions.

Reagents and Equipment

1. Stock solution: 10% buffered sodium chloride (pH 7.4); sodium chloride, 90 g; disodium hydrogen phosphate dihydrate, 17.115 g; sodium dihydrogen phosphate dihydrate, 2.43 g; distilled water to 1 liter.
2. Pipettes: 1 ml, graduated in 0.011-ml divisions; 10 ml, graduated in 0.1-ml divisions; 0.1-ml micropipette; 10-ml volumetric pipette.
3. Volumetric flask: 100 ml.
4. Spectrophotometer.
5. Centrifuge.
6. Linear graph paper.

Specimen

Heparinized venous or defibrinated blood should be used. Specimens anticoagulated with ethylene-diaminetetraacetic acid (EDTA) or sodium citrate cannot be used.

Method

1. A working saline solution is made by diluting 10 ml of the stock solution to 100 ml with distilled water. Serial dilutions of the working saline are made as shown in Table 19.1.
2. Each tube is mixed well to ensure uniformity, and 0.1 ml of blood is added to each dilution.
3. The tubes are mixed again by inversion and are allowed to stand at room temperature for 2 hours. They are then remixed and centrifuged for 5 minutes at 2,000 revolutions per minute (rpm).
4. The supernatants are read spectrophotometrically at 540 nm, using the 0.85% saline dilution as a blank (tube no. 18) and the distilled water tube (tube no. 1) as the 100% lysis standard.
5. The degree of hemolysis of each tube supernatant then is calculated from the formula

$$\frac{\text{Optical density of the test dilution}}{\text{Optical density of the standard (tube no. 1)}} \times 100$$

and the percentage of hemolysis against each saline concentration is plotted on linear graph paper. A typical normal fragility curve is shown in Figure 19.1.

Reference Ranges

Table 19.2 gives reference ranges for the osmotic fragility test.

Table 19.1. Serial Dilutions of Working Saline Used in the Osmotic Fragility Test

Tube	1% Working Saline (ml)	Distilled Water (ml)	% Final Saline Dilution
1	—	10.0	0
2	2.0	8.0	0.20
3	2.5	7.5	0.25
4	3.0	7.0	0.30
5	3.5	6.5	0.35
6	3.75	6.25	0.375
7	4.0	6.0	0.40
8	4.25	5.75	0.425
9	4.5	5.5	0.45
10	4.75	5.25	0.475
11	5.0	5.0	0.50
12	5.5	4.5	0.55
13	6.0	4.0	0.60
14	6.5	3.5	0.65
15	7.0	3.0	0.70
16	7.5	2.5	0.75
17	8.0	2.0	0.80
18	8.5	1.5	0.85

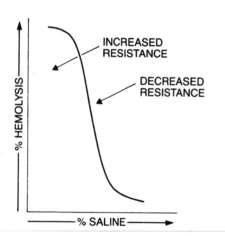

INCREASED	DECREASED
RESISTANCE	
LIVER DISEASE	HEREDITARY
SPLENOMEGALY	SPHEROCYTOSIS
THALASSEMIA	ABO HEMOLYTIC
IRON-DEFICIENCY	DISEASE
ANEMIA	
HEMOLYTIC DISEASE	
OF THE NEWBORN	

Figure 19.1. A characteristic osmotic fragility curve and findings in various disorders.

Table 19.2. Reference Ranges for the Osmotic Fragility Test

% Saline	% Hemolysis
0.2	97–100
0.3	90–97
0.35	50–95
0.4	5–45
0.45	0–6
0.5	0
0.55	0
0.6	0
0.65	0
0.7	0

Control

A normal fresh-blood control specimen should be run in parallel with the test to ensure reagent adequacy.

Sources of Error

The osmotic fragility test should be carried out within 2 hours of sample collection or within 6 hours if the blood is kept at 4°C. Many technical and physiologic variables influence the accuracy of the test. Technically, errors in the saline dilutions and pipetting of blood obviously affect the test results adversely and, for this reason, the Unopette system (Becton-Dickinson, Rutherford, NJ) offers significant advantages. It has been shown that the Unopette reagents are stable for at least 2 years at room temperature (Ray and Noteboom, 1970), and the method produces comparable results and reference ranges for both the routine procedure and for the incubated variation. In addition, pipetting errors are eliminated and the test is less time-consuming to set up.

Physiologically, the osmotic fragility test is influenced by both the pH and the relative proportions of blood and saline. A ratio of 1 volume of blood to 99 volumes of saline is such that the added plasma has little effect on the tonicity of the mixture. If the ratio of the mixture is decreased to 1:20, the plasma volume substantially increases the effective tonicity of the lysing solution. However, if weak suspensions of blood in saline are used, it is necessary to control the pH of the hypotonic solution. A shift of 0.1 pH units is equivalent to an alteration of tonicity of 0.01% saline.

The incubated osmotic fragility test is more sensitive to mild alterations of red-cell fragility than is the routine procedure. When red cells are placed in a hypertonic solution, they lose fluid until an equilibrium is established; they then become crenated. In hypotonic solutions, the cells take up fluid and swell until either an equilibrium is attained or the cell ruptures. In some types of hemolytic anemia, the resistance of the red cells to hypotonic solutions is reduced, whereas in others it is increased.

Clinical Correlation

Characteristic reductions in cell resistance or increased fragility are present in hereditary spherocytosis and in some of the acquired hemolytic anemias. The opposite is found—that is, increased resistance or decreased fragility—in most of the hemoglobinopathies, thalassemia, iron-deficiency anemia, liver disease and, occasionally, in myelosclerosis, leukemia, lymphosarcoma, and postsplenectomized individuals. Such findings indicate the presence of unusually flattened cells in which the ratio of volume to surface area is decreased.

Increased red-cell fragility is related to cell shape. The more spheric the cell, the greater is its fragility relative to saline concentrations. Normal hemolysis is preceded by a phase in which the red cell assumes a spheric form and, consequently, in a spherocyte less water intake (compared to cells of other shapes) will incite rupture from the increased volume–surface area ratio.

When normal cells are incubated under sterile conditions, metabolic changes occur, including loss of red-cell cholesterol (Murphy, 1962), accumulation of sodium, and loss of potassium. These cation exchanges are determined by the membrane properties of the cell and the ability of the cation pump to continue to function despite the gradual reduction of available glucose as an energy source. These factors are discussed on page 8. Osmotic fragility tests are therefore useful and sensitive indicators of the ability of the red cell to resist both membrane and enzymatic stress.

Unopette Method for Osmotic Fragility

Principle

The principle underlying the Unopette method for testing osmotic fragility (Ray and Noteboom, 1970) is the same as that outlined for the osmotic fragility test.

Reagents and Equipment

1. Unopette fragility kit, which consists of premeasured volumes of buffered sodium chloride solution of 10 concentrations, packaged in plastic containers, and self-filling, self-measuring microvolume capillary tubes.
2. Spectrophotometer.
3. Centrifuge.
4. Linear graph paper.

Specimen

Heparinized venous blood is used. EDTA- or sodium citrate–anticoagulated specimens cannot be used.

Method

1. Heparinized blood (20 µl) is added to each of 10 Unopette reservoirs, each containing 3.98 ml of buffered (pH 7.4) sodium chloride solution, which is osmotically equivalent to sodium chloride in the following concentrations: 0%, 0.30%, 0.35%, 0.40%, 0.45%, 0.50%, 0.55%, 0.60%, 0.65%, and 0.85%.

2. The diluted blood is allowed to stand at room temperature for 20–30 minutes and then is transferred to tubes and centrifuged for 5 minutes at 2,000 rpm.

3. The supernatant is examined as described in step 4 of the section on the routine osmotic fragility test, and the degree of hemolysis is plotted as previously illustrated.

Reference Ranges

Reference ranges are listed in Table 19.2.

Sources of Error and Clinical Correlation

The sources of error and clinical correlation for this variation of the osmotic fragility test are discussed in the preceding section.

Incubated Osmotic Fragility

Principle

The principle for the incubated osmotic fragility test (Dacie and Lewis, 1975) is the same as for the routine osmotic fragility test.

Reagents and Equipment

This test uses the same reagents and equipment as does the routine osmotic fragility test.

Specimen

Sterile defibrinated blood is the specimen of choice, but sterile heparinized blood can also be used.

Method

Sterile defibrinated or heparinized blood is incubated at 37°C for 24 hours. The method is as outlined in the sections on the routine osmotic fragility and Unopette procedures.

Reference Ranges

Table 19.3 shows the reference ranges for blood incubated at 37°C for 24 hours at a pH of 7.4.

Table 19.3. Reference Ranges for the Incubated Osmotic Fragility Test

% Saline	% Hemolysis
0.2	95–100
0.3	85–100
0.35	75–100
0.4	65–100
0.45	55–100
0.5	40–100
0.55	15–70
0.6	0–40
0.65	0–10
0.7	0–5

Sources of Error and Clinical Correlation

The sources of error and clinical correlation for this variation of the osmotic fragility test are discussed in the section on osmotic fragility.

Haptoglobin

Principle

Haptoglobins are glycoproteins that migrate electrophoretically in the α_2-globulin region. Several methods exist for their quantitation, including immunodiffusion, electrophoresis, gel filtration, and nephelometric and spectrophotometric techniques. Of these, the radial immunodiffusion method is reliable and simple and produces useful data. The technique is based on the principle of single-gel diffusion, in which there is movement of one reactant through an inert medium containing a reacting substance. Antisera are incorporated in an agarose plate, and the test specimen containing the antigen is placed in a well in the agarose. The antigen then diffuses into the antibody, resulting in a white precipitin zone around the antigen well, the diameter of the ring being proportional to the concentration of the antigen.

Three basic methods for reading the diffusion exist. Two of these are the end-point method and a timed-diffusion method. It is known that the precipitin ring diameter stops increasing at the point at which diffusible antigen has been reduced and antigen-antibody complexes have attained equivalence. At this point of equivalence, there is a linear relationship between the antigen concentration for equal volumes of test solutions and the squares of their corresponding ring diameters. These measurements, although independent of time and diffusion rates, are affected by marked fluctuations in temperatures. In the second method, the diffusion rates are read before equivalence is reached. The third method, which provides improved accuracy and precision, uses a nephelometric procedure and offers the additional advantage of fast turnaround (i.e., rapidly obtained results) to the physician.

Reagents and Equipment

1. Diffusion plates (Endoplates, Kallestad Laboratories Inc., Chaska, MN): Each plate contains up to 7.6 ml of a pH 7.2 buffered saline–agarose–antiserum mixture and up to 1.6 ml of monospecific equine or goat antiserum to human haptoglobin. The plates should be stored at 4°C.
2. Standard reference serum: A trilevel reference serum is used (available from the manufacturer of the diffusion plates), containing approximately 370 mg/dl, 150 mg/dl, and 40 mg/dl.
3. Micropipette: 5 μl.
4. Linear graph paper.
5. Normal control serum.
6. Measuring device capable of measuring precipitin ring diameters in 0.1-mm increments.

Specimen

Venous blood is allowed to clot for at least 15 minutes and then is centrifuged at approximately 900 rpm to obtain at least 0.5 ml of unhemolyzed, cell-free serum. If separated, the serum is stable for up to 5 days at 4°C or for longer periods if it is kept frozen. Hemolyzed specimens are unacceptable.

Method

1. The diffusion plate and reference sera are removed from the refrigerator and are allowed to reach room temperature. The plate is kept in the reclosable plastic bag until it is to be used.
2. If moisture is on the plate, it is left uncovered at room temperature until the moisture evaporates.

3. The trilevel reference sera, the control, and the patient's serum (5-μl volumes) are dispensed into five wells. The plate is covered and repacked into the reclosable plastic bag, and it is left at room temperature on a level surface for 48 hours.
4. At the completion of the incubation period, the diameters of the precipitation rings that have developed are measured.
5. The concentrations of each reference serum are plotted on the ordinate axis against the square of their precipitin ring diameters on the abscissa axis. The best-fit straight line is drawn through the adjacent points, and the concentrations of the control and test samples are determined from the intersection of the square of the sample's ring diameter and the reference curve (Figure 19.2).

Reference Range

The reference range is 60–270 mg/dl.

Sources of Error

The end-point procedure described can be modified to produce a faster result by reading of the precipitin ring diameters after 18 hours of incubation at room temperature. If this is done, all reference sera and control samples should be read to the nearest 0.1 mm at the same time and the results plotted in the same way as previously described, but using semilogarithmic graph paper, as shown in Figure 19.3.

If the precipitin ring is greater than the highest reference, the specimen should be diluted in normal saline and the test rerun. The resulting concentration then is multiplied by the appropriate dilution factor. If the test result is less than the lowest reference, the result should be expressed as being less than the value for the lowest reference serum.

A number of technical problems can affect the test. Care should be taken in filling the wells of the agarose plates. The pipette tip should enter the well in a vertical position, and the sides of the well should not be touched during this procedure.

In addition, the incubation temperature should be 21–25°C. If the end-point method is used, the plates should be left undisturbed for at least 48 hours after the addition of the antigen. When using the timed-diffusion method, the plates should be read at between 17.5 and 18.5 hours. Shorter diffusion times result in

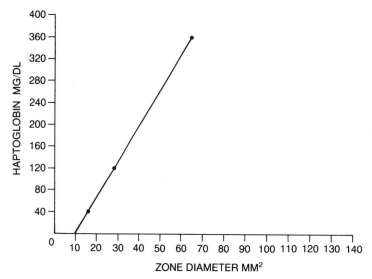

Figure 19.2. An example of a calibration graph using the haptoglobin end-point diffusion method.

decreased test sensitivity, and longer times or significant increases in temperature greater than 25°C will cause the graph to be nonlinear. If the room temperature varies, the plates should be incubated at a constant temperature.

Clinical Correlation

Variations in the haptoglobin level occur in several pathologic conditions. Haptoglobin is an acute-phase protein, elevation of which is a characteristic, though nonspecific, finding in infections and inflammatory conditions. There is a significant positive correlation between increased haptoglobin levels and red-cell sedimentation rates. Haptoglobin concentration rises slowly with the onset of infection and, as the condition is contained, the level returns slowly to normal.

Haptoglobin quantitation is useful in assessing the degree of a hemolytic crisis. In the majority of diseases with normal liver function, depletion of the haptoglobin level is most likely due to increased haptoglobin consumption. The level will decrease approximately 100 mg/dl for every 10 ml of red cells lysed, and even a small amount of lysis may cause significant reductions in the serum level. A fall in serum haptoglobin to less than 30 mg/dl or a drop in the serum level of 50–70 mg/dl from the original value is considered indicative of a hemolytic crisis. The haptoglobin concentration is inversely related to the degree of hemolysis as well as to the length of the hemolytic episode. Because the normal reference range is so wide, a single observation of a reduced level is of questionable value in assessing the clinical condition.

A haptoglobinemia is usually indicative of increased red-cell destruction; however, there is a genetic condition (Hp 0-0) in which there is little or no demonstrable serum haptoglobin.

Plasma Hemoglobin

Principle

Toluidine blue O and hydrogen peroxide, in the presence of hemoglobin, produce a green-blue complex, the intensity of which is compared against a hemoglobin standard.

Reagents and Equipment

1. One Hematest tablet (Ames Co, Elkhart, IN), crushed and dissolved in 8 ml warm distilled water, using a magnetic stirrer and vigorous action. The reagent is filtered into a clean bottle and stored at 4°C.
2. Standard: The whole-blood hemoglobin of a fresh blood sample is determined in duplicate, and the specimen is diluted with an equal volume of distilled water to reduce the value to 50%

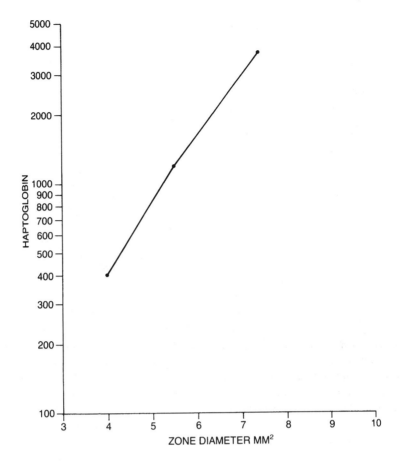

Figure 19.3. An example of a calibration graph for using the haptoglobin timed-diffusion method.

of normal. This stock dilution (0.1 ml) is added to 100 ml distilled water to produce a working standard. For example, for whole-blood hemoglobin assayed at 14 g/dl, the working plasma hemoglobin standard is 70 mg/liter.

3. Acid-washed glassware: 0.02-ml micropipettes, 5-ml graduated pipettes, 12- × 75-mm tubes.
4. Hydrogen peroxide 1%: One volume 3% hydrogen peroxide is added to two volumes deionized or distilled water. This is prepared fresh when the test is run.
5. Spectrophotometer.
6. Centrifuge.

Specimen

Heparinized blood is the specimen of choice. The venipuncture is performed using a syringe and an 18-gauge needle. The syringe is removed from the needle, and blood is allowed to flow directly from the needle into a heparinized tube.

Method

1. The heparinized blood is centrifuged at 2,000 rpm for 15 minutes to obtain an adequate plasma sample.
2. One milliliter of aqueous Hematest reagent is added into each of four tubes (blank, standard, control, and test).
3. Distilled water (0.02 ml) is added to the blank tube, 0.02 ml of the working standard is added to the standard tube, 0.02 ml of a normal heparinized plasma is added to the control tube, and 0.02 ml of unknown plasma is added to the test tube.
4. One milliliter of freshly made 1% hydrogen peroxide is added to all tubes, and the contents are mixed and allowed to stand for exactly 10 minutes

at room temperature. The optical density is read at 600 nm against the blank tube.

Calculation

Plasma hemoglobin =

$$\frac{\text{Optical density of test}}{\text{Optical density of standard}} \times \text{standard value (mg/dl)}$$

Reference Range

The reference range is 10–70 mg/liter.

Discussion

If the optical density of the test is greater than 0.7, the test should be repeated using a diluted test sample. Because the developing color is unstable, the test must be read exactly 10 minutes after the hydrogen peroxide is added to the reaction tube, and all the readings should be completed within a 2-minute time span.

A macroscopic examination of the centrifuged heparinized whole blood can be used as an additional quality check and guide to the plasma hemoglobin level. If the plasma is pink to eye examination, the plasma hemoglobin is in excess of 250 mg/liter. This procedure is suitable for specimens with plasma hemoglobin concentrations that are too low (<1,500 mg/liter) to be measured by conventional cyanmethemoglobin methods.

Clinical Correlation

Plasma hemoglobin levels are elevated in hemolytic anemias, in which hemolysis is sufficiently severe for the available haptoglobin to be fully bound. The highest levels are found when hemolysis is predominantly intravascular. This marked hemoglobinemia may be found with or without hemoglobinuria, particularly in microangiopathic anemias, paroxysmal nocturnal hemoglobinuria (PNH), paroxysmal cold hemoglobinuria (PCH), and cold hemagglutinin disease.

In warm autoimmune hemolytic anemia, hemoglobinopathies, and severe thalassemia, the plasma hemoglobin may be mildly raised but, in hereditary spherocytosis, it is an uncommon finding as the he-

molysis is principally extravascular, occurring in the spleen. The presence of elevated plasma hemoglobin levels should be taken as a reliable sign of intravascular hemolysis only if it is certain that the elevated hemoglobin level has not been caused by either faulty venipuncture technique or mistreatment of the blood after phlebotomy.

Urine hemoglobin levels may be quantitated using the same methodology as described in the section on plasma hemoglobin. Special care should be taken before proceeding with the test to centrifuge the urine to remove any organized deposit. When the urinalysis result is positive for heme pigment, the presence of myoglobin may be distinguished from that of hemoglobin by the addition of approximately 2.8 g ammonium sulfate to 5 ml urine. The specimen is centrifuged, and the supernatant is observed. If a heme-positive pigment remains in the solution after this treatment, myoglobin is present. If the pigment is precipitated, hemoglobin is present.

Although the use of the diphenyls—such as benzidine, toluidine blue O, and dianisidine—once were believed to be potentially harmful, the restrictions on their use have been removed (Federal Register, 1976). However, as an alternative chromogen, 3-methyl-2-benzothiazolinone hydrazone has been proposed (Elson et al., 1978). This couples with N,N-dimethylaniline to form a water-soluble indamine dye, which, under suitable reaction conditions, produces a color that is proportional to the hemoglobin concentration.

Plasma hemoglobin levels can also be quantitated using spectrophotometry. If the latter method is used, the test can be carried out even in the presence of bilirubin, myoglobin, or marked turbidity (Solani et al., 1986).

Hemosiderin

Principle

Ferric iron reacts with a potassium ferrocyanide solution to form ferric ferrocyanide, which produces a Prussian blue color (Perl's reaction).

Reagents and Equipment

1. Hydrochloric acid 20%.

2. Potassium ferrocyanide 10%, stored in a dark bottle: The solution is stable for approximately 3 weeks. Just before use, the staining solution is prepared by mixing equal volumes of hydrochloric acid and potassium ferrocyanide and filtering the solution into a Coplin jar, ready for use.
3. Safranin O, 0.5% aqueous solution.
4. Methanol.
5. Centrifuge.
6. Slides.
7. Coplin jars.
8. Microscope.

Specimen

Freshly voided urine is used.

Method

1. The urine is centrifuged at 1,500 rpm for 15 minutes. The supernatant is decanted, and the centrifuged deposit is transferred to a slide. It is spread out to occupy an area of approximately 1–2 cm and is allowed to air-dry.
2. The dried deposit is fixed by immersing in a Coplin jar containing methanol for 10–20 minutes.
3. To stain the specimen, the fixed deposit is placed for 30 minutes in a Coplin jar containing freshly prepared staining mixture. The slide is rinsed with distilled water and is counterstained using 0.5% safranin for 5 minutes.
4. The slide is rinsed with distilled water, air-dried, and examined microscopically for the presence of hemosiderin.

Reference Range

No hemosiderin should be detected.

Sources of Error

The glassware used for the collection and test should be new and scrupulously clean or acid-washed in order to avoid a false-positive reaction. Intracellular blue particles should be identified before a positive test result is reported. The finding of only extracellular blue material is frequently artifactual, and consequently caution should be used in interpreting such results.

Clinical Correlation

Hemosiderinuria is a diagnostic sign of chronic intravascular hemolysis, because the urine often is found to have iron-containing granules in the absence of hemoglobinuria. Hemosiderin is usually not present in the early stages of a hemolytic crisis but may persist for several weeks after such an episode.

Qualitative Porphobilinogen Determination

Principle

Porphobilinogen reacts with Ehrlich's reagent in acid solution to produce a red color that is not extractable with amyl alcohol containing 25% benzyl alcohol (Rimington, 1971). Urobilinogen forms a similar pigment but differs from porphobilinogen in that it is completely extractable by the organic solvent mixture.

Reagents and Equipment

1. Ehrlich's reagent: *p*-Dimethylaminobenzaldehyde (0.7 g) is dissolved in 150 ml concentrated hydrochloric acid and is brought carefully up to 250 ml with distilled water.
2. Saturated aqueous sodium acetate.
3. Amyl alcohol–benzyl alcohol mixture: Three volumes of pure amyl alcohol are added to one volume of pure benzyl alcohol.
4. Pipettes: 1 ml and 5 ml, graduated.
5. Centrifuge.

Specimen

Freshly voided urine is used for this test.

Method

1. Urine (1 ml) is mixed with 1 ml Ehrlich's reagent and is allowed to stand for 2–3 minutes at room temperature. Saturated aqueous sodium acetate (2 ml) is added, and the solution is mixed.
2. Two milliliters of the amyl alcohol–benzyl alcohol reagent is added to the urine-Ehrlich's mixture. The tube is capped, and the solution is mixed gently by inversion for 1–2 minutes.
3. The tube is centrifuged at 2,000 rpm for 5 minutes, and the supernatant is examined.

Interpretation

A pink color in the lower layer of the supernatant indicates the presence of porphobilinogen, whereas a red color in the upper layer denotes the presence of urobilinogen.

Qualitative Coproporphyrin Determination

Principle

Examination of urine under ultraviolet light will show a pink to red fluorescence when either coproporphyrin or uroporphyrin is present (Benson and Chisholm, 1960). Uroporphyrin can be distinguished from coproporphyrin by the different solubilities of the two substances in acidic solution.

Reagents and Equipment

1. Wood's light (ultraviolet).
2. Glacial acetic acid.
3. Hydrochloric acid 5%.
4. Ether.
5. Volumetric flask: 25 ml.
6. Separatory funnel: 100 ml.
7. Pipettes: 10 ml, graduated.

Specimen

The test specimen is freshly voided urine.

Method

1. Glacial acetic acid (10 ml) is added to 25 ml freshly voided urine in a separatory funnel. Ether (50 ml) carefully is added to the mixture, and the funnel is shaken vigorously for 2–3 minutes, ensuring that the stopper is loosened at intervals to release ether vapors.
2. The solvents are allowed to separate, and the urine is drawn off. The separation is repeated on the same urine sample with 50 ml of fresh ether, in the same manner as described, taking care to release the stopper at frequent intervals to release ether vapors.
3. The urine is separated, and the two ether extracts are combined. These extracts are examined under ultraviolet light.

4. Ten milliliters of 5% hydrochloric acid are added to the ether extract. The solution is mixed well, the acid is drawn off, and the specimen is examined under ultraviolet light.

Results

A strong red fluorescence in the ether extract before the acid wash indicates the presence of uroporphyrin. If the fluorescence persists after the acid wash, the presence of coproporphyrin is indicated.

Clinical Correlation

Coproporphyrin normally is excreted in the urine in small amounts, but the level is increased whenever erythropoiesis is hyperactive, particularly in the bone marrow response to hemolytic anemias, polycythemia, and pernicious anemia. Coproporphyrin levels are also elevated in lead poisoning and in liver disease, but they are reduced in renal disorders.

Qualitative Urobilinogen Determination

Principle

Urobilinogen, along with other aldehyde-reacting substances present in urine, reacts with Ehrlich's reagent to produce a red color, the intensity of which is proportional to the urobilinogen present (Watson and Schwartz, 1941).

Reagents and Equipment

1. Ehrlich's reagent: p-Dimethylaminobenzaldehyde (0.7 g) is added to 150 ml concentrated hydrochloric acid. This mixture is added slowly to 100 ml deionized water. The reagent should be stored in a dark bottle and is stable for 3–6 months at room temperature.
2. Saturated aqueous sodium acetate.
3. Chloroform.
4. Butanol.

Specimen

The specimen should be freshly voided urine that has been cooled to room temperature before testing.

Table 19.4. Interpretation of the Qualitative Analysis of the Urobilinogen-Porphobilinogen Test

	Urobilinogen	Porphobilinogen	Other Ehrlich's Compounds	Urobilinogen and Other Compounds
Urine acetate layer	—	Color	Faint color	Faint color
Chloroform layer	Color	—	—	Color
Butanol layer	Color	Faint color	Faint color	Color

Method

1. Equal volumes of freshly voided urine and Ehrlich's reagent are combined and are mixed well by repeated inversion.

2. A volume of sodium acetate equal to the total volume of the mixture is added immediately, and the mixing procedure is repeated. Positive test results show colored reactions in the supernatant that range from light pink to cherry red. Peach- and orange-colored reactions are not considered positive. If the test result is positive after the addition of the sodium acetate, the procedure continues as follows.

3. The colored supernatant is divided into two equal parts. Chloroform, 2 ml, is added to one, and the solution is mixed vigorously. The layers are allowed to separate, and one takes note of whether the color is extracted into the lower chloroform layer. Urobilinogen will be extracted into the chloroform layer, whereas color resulting from porphobilinogen will not be extracted and will remain in the upper aqueous layer.

4. If the pink color is not extracted by the chloroform, 2 ml butanol is added to the other portion of the supernatant (described in step 1). This mixture is shaken vigorously, and the layers are allowed to separate. The solution is observed to determine whether the color is extracted completely into the upper butanol layer. If color remains in the urine-acetate layer, extraction takes place again with more butanol. Color from urobilinogen and other Ehrlich's-reactive compounds will be extracted into the butanol, but porphobilinogen-produced color will remain in the lower aqueous layer.

Results

Table 19.4 shows the interpretation of the qualitative results of the urobilinogen-porphobilinogen test.

Sources of Error

This test is not specific for urobilinogen. The finding of other Ehrlich's compounds is due to interfering substances such as procaine, 5-hydroxy-indoleacetic acid, and sulfonamides that react with Ehrlich's reagent and methyldopa to produce reactions identical to porphobilinogen. An increase in urinary urobilinogen occurs in hemolytic anemia because of the increased production of unconjugated and conjugated bilirubin. The conjugated form is converted to urobilinogen in the colon. Increases in urinary urobilinogen levels are found also in liver disease because the hepatic cells do not remove the pigment from the enterohepatic circulation.

Reductions in urinary urobilinogen are found in obstructive jaundice, as conjugated bilirubin does not reach the colon for conversion, and when *Escherichia coli* function is altered by the use of a broad-spectrum antibiotic.

Tests for Detection of Abnormal Hemoglobin Pigments

Hemoglobin pigments are most easily detected and identified by their unique spectroscopic patterns. The common pigments show the following absorption bands:

Carboxyhemoglobin: 572 nm and 535 nm. These bands are similar to those seen with oxyhemoglobin.
Oxyhemoglobin: 578 nm and 540 nm.
Reduced hemoglobin: 540 nm and 570 nm, with a maximum peak at 556 nm.
Sulfhemoglobin: 618 nm, 578 nm, and 540 nm.
Methemoglobin: 630 nm, 578 nm, 540 nm, and 500 nm.

Table 19.5. Differentiation Between Methemoglobin and Sulfhemoglobin

Pigment	Absorption Bands (nm)	Principle Band (nm)	Band Characteristics When Added to		
			Sodium Dithionite	Alkaline Sodium Dithionite	Hydrogen Peroxide
Methemoglobin	630, 578, 540, 500	630	Disappears	Disappears	—
Sulfhemoglobin	618, 578, 540	618	Remains	Disappears	Disappears

Methemalbumin: 624 nm, 540 nm, and 500 nm.
Myoglobin: 581 nm and 542 nm.

Qualitative Methemoglobin and Sulfhemoglobin Determination

Principle

Heparinized or EDTA-anticoagulated blood is hemolyzed and examined spectroscopically for definitive absorption bands in the red region of the spectrum.

Reagents and Equipment

1. Recording spectrophotometer.
2. Sodium dithionite.
3. Sodium hydroxide 10%.
4. Pipettes: 1 ml and 10 ml, graduated; 0.1-ml micropipette.

Specimen

The specimen used is EDTA-anticoagulated or heparinized blood.

Method

1. Whole blood (1 ml) is added to 9 ml distilled water. It is mixed and centrifuged at 2,000 rpm for 2–3 minutes.
2. The supernatant hemolysate is examined for characteristic absorption peaks in a recording spectrophotometer at a wavelength of 600–650 nm.

Results

Differentiation between methemoglobin and sulfhemoglobin can be accomplished by the following procedure: Methemoglobin is recognized if there is an absorption band at 630 nm that disappears on the addition of 5 mg of sodium dithionite. Sulfhemoglobin is evidenced by an absorption band at 618 nm that disappears on the addition of a mixture of 5 mg sodium dithionite and 2 ml 10% sodium hydroxide. Alternatively, the band disappears on the addition of freshly made 3% hydrogen peroxide. The differentiation of these pigments is shown in Table 19.5.

Methemalbumin Screening Test

Principle

Plasma from heparinized or EDTA-anticoagulated blood is spectroscopically examined for absorption bands at 624 nm.

Reagents and Equipment

1. Recording spectrophotometer.
2. No reagents required.

Method

EDTA-anticoagulated or heparinized whole blood is centrifuged, and the plasma is removed for spectroscopic examination, as described previously.

Result

A specific absorption pattern for methemalbumin is found at 624 nm. This pattern disappears after the addition of 5 mg of sodium dithionite. The test result should be confirmed by performing a Schumm's test.

Schumm's Test

Principle

Yellow ammonium sulfide is added to the plasma-containing methemalbumin to produce ammonium hemochromogen, which is identified by a spectroscopic band at 558 nm.

Reagents and Equipment

1. Diethyl ether.
2. Yellow ammonium sulfide.
3. Recording spectrophotometer.
4. Pipettes: 1 ml, graduated.

Specimen

Heparinized plasma is the specimen used.

Method

Ether is layered carefully over 2 ml fresh heparinized plasma, and 0.2 ml yellow ammonium sulfide is added. The solution is mixed and placed in the recording spectrophotometer. The absorption bands are recorded.

Results

If methemalbumin is present in the plasma, absorption bands of ammonium hemochromogen are present at 558 nm.

Controls

Control samples should be made up and used whenever blood or plasma is examined spectroscopically for abnormal hemoglobin pigments. The control samples can be made in the laboratory by the method to be described and can be examined spectrophotometrically to ensure that the instrument is satisfactory for their detection.

Reagents

1. Potassium ferricyanide, 10% aqueous.
2. Phenylhydrazine hydrochloride, 0.1% aqueous.
3. Water saturated with hydrogen sulfide.

Method for Sulfhemoglobin

1. Heparinized blood (0.1 ml) is mixed with 9.9 ml distilled water, and 0.1 ml of a 0.1% aqueous solution of phenylhydrazine hydrochloride then is added.
2. To this mixture, one drop of water saturated with hydrogen sulfide is added, and the solution is read spectrophotometrically. A strong band at 618 nm will be present if the test is positive.

Method for Methemoglobin

1. Heparinized blood (1 ml) is mixed with 4 ml distilled water, and 5 ml 10% potassium ferricyanide then is added.
2. The absorption bands are read spectrophotometrically. A strong band at 630 nm will be present if the test is positive.

Quantitative Methemoglobin Determination

Principle

Methemoglobin has a maximal absorption peak at 630 nm. When cyanide is added, this band disappears, and the resulting change in optical density is directly proportional to the concentration of methemoglobin present. The total hemoglobin concentration of the sample is measured after complete conversion to cyanmethemoglobin by the addition of ferricyanide-cyanide reagent. The conversion will measure hemoglobin and methemoglobin but not sulfhemoglobin.

Reagents and Equipment

1. Disodium hydrogen phosphate, 0.067 M: The salt form of disodium hydrogen phosphate, 1.78 g, is dissolved in 100 ml distilled water.
2. Potassium dihydrogen phosphate, 0.067 M: The salt form of potassium dihydrogen phosphate, 0.91 g, is dissolved in 100 ml distilled water.
3. Phosphate buffer, 0.067 M (pH 6.6): 125 ml 0.067-M disodium hydrogen phosphate are added to 375 ml of 0.067-M potassium dihydrogen phosphate. The mixture is adjusted to pH 6.6 with either the disodium salt, if too acidic, or with the potassium salt, if too alkaline.

4. Phosphate buffer, 0.067 M: 250 ml 0.067-M phosphate buffer are added to 750 ml distilled water.
5. Sodium cyanide, 10% aqueous.
6. Acetic acid 12%.
7. Potassium ferricyanide, 20% aqueous.
8. Pipettes: 10 ml, graduated; 0.12-ml and Pasteur micropipettes.
9. Spectrophotometer.

Specimen

The specimen of choice is either EDTA-anticoagulated or heparinized fresh whole blood.

Method

1. Fresh anticoagulated blood (0.2 ml) is added to 10 ml phosphate buffer (0.067 M). The dilution is mixed by inversion several times and is allowed to stand at room temperature for 5 minutes.
2. The optical density of this solution is read spectrophotometrically at 630 nm. This is optical density no. 1.
3. Equal volumes of 10% sodium cyanide and 12% acetic acid are added carefully, using a bulbed Pasteur pipette. The technologist performing this procedure should wear rubber gloves and use a safety cabinet. One drop of this mixture is added to the hemolysate solution, the tube is stoppered and inverted several times, and the mixture is allowed to stand 2–3 minutes at room temperature.
4. The optical density of this solution is recorded spectrophotometrically at 630 nm. This is optical density no. 2.
5. One drop of 20% potassium ferricyanide is added to 8 ml phosphate buffer (0.067 M), and then 2 ml of the freshly made hemolysate described in step 1 is added. This mixture is allowed to stand at room temperature for 2–3 minutes, and one drop of the sodium cyanide–acetic acid mixture is added, the same precautions being taken as are detailed in step 3. The tube is stoppered, and the solution is mixed by inversion and allowed to remain at room temperature for 2–3 minutes.
6. The optical density of this solution is read spectrophotometrically at 540 nm against a blank containing 10 ml distilled water and one drop each of sodium cyanide and potassium ferricyanide. This is optical density no. 3.

Calculation

$$\frac{\text{Optical density no. 1} - \text{Optical density no. 2}}{\text{Optical density no. 3}} \times 100$$
$$= \% \text{ Methemoglobin}$$

Reference Range

The reference range is 0–2%.

Sources of Error

The sodium cyanide–acetic acid mixture should be prepared just before use, the preparer taking extreme caution in its handling. A pipette aid or rubber bulb is used to transfer the reagent, and rubber gloves are used to avoid skin contact. It is best to carry out the handling of sodium cyanide in an exhaust hood whenever possible.

Myoglobin can be differentiated from hemoglobin in the urine by dissolving 2.8 g ammonium sulfate in 5 ml urine and centrifuging. Myoglobin will not be precipitated, and the supernatant will be pigmented. The specimen can be spectrophotometrically examined for absorption bands at 582 nm and 542 nm. Hemoglobin will be present in the precipitate, and the supernatant will be normal in color.

Tests for Red-Cell Membrane Disorders

Acid Hemolysis

Principle

Red cells become hemolyzed when exposed to acidified normal or autologous serum (pH 6.5–7.0; Ham and Castle, 1940).

Reagents and Equipment

1. Hydrochloric acid 0.2 N.
2. Normal saline 0.85%.
3. Water bath.
4. Centrifuge.
5. Normal defibrinated blood of the same ABO group as the patient. (For preparation, see later.)
6. Pipettes: 10 ml and 9 ml, graduated; 0.05-ml and Pasteur micropipettes.
7. Tubes: 12 × 75 mm.

Table 19.6. Acid Hemolysin Methodology

	Tube 1	Tube 2	Tube 3	Tube 4	Tube 5	Tube 6
Cells (0.05 ml)	P	P	P	P	N	N
Serum (0.05 ml)	P	—	N	—	P	—
Acidified serum (0.05 ml)	—	P	—	N	—	P

P = patient derived; N = normal derived.

Specimen

Defibrinated blood is used for this test. Approximately 20–25 ml of patient's blood is added to an Erlenmeyer flask containing 20–25 glass beads (3–4 mm in diameter). The flask is rotated continuously for 10–15 minutes and then is centrifuged at 2,000 rpm for 5 minutes.

Method

1. Five percent suspensions of both normal and patient red cells obtained after defibrination are prepared by adding 0.5 ml packed cells to 9.5 ml saline.
2. Acidified patient serum and normal serum are prepared by adding 0.05 ml of 0.2-N hydrochloric acid to 0.95 ml serum.
3. Samples of the 5% red-cell suspensions (0.5 ml) are introduced into 12- × 75-mm tubes and are centrifuged at 2,000 rpm for 2–3 minutes. The saline-serum supernatant is removed completely with a Pasteur pipette.
4. Six tubes are set up, as shown in Table 19.6, and the solutions are mixed by shaking. The tubes are incubated at 37°C for 1 hour and centrifuged at 2,000 rpm for 5 minutes. The supernatants are examined for hemolysis.

Result

A positive test result is indicated by hemolysis in the tubes containing the patient's cells with acidified serum (tubes 2 and 4). The remaining tubes are unaffected.

Sources of Error

Patient's serum is best obtained by the defibrination method described. If the blood is allowed to clot at 37°C, it may be hemolyzed in patients with PNH. A positive test result for acid hemolysins usually is diagnostic of PNH, but positive results may also be found in congenital spherocytosis, in hereditary erythroblastic multinuclearity with a positive acidified serum (HEMPAS) lysis, and in rare immune-mediated hemolytic anemias.

To confirm and separate PNH from these other disorders, the test should be repeated after first inactivating acidified serum at 56°C for 30 minutes. Such heating destroys serum complement components necessary for hemolysis in PNH and, consequently, the acid hemolysin test result will be negative in PNH but will remain positive in congenital spherocytosis. PNH cells are not sensitive to acidified serum per se; the addition of the acid adjusts the serum pH to the optimum for activity of the hemolytic system. The factor in normal serum that is responsible for the hemolysis of PNH red cells is complement, principally the C3 component.

Differentiation of HEMPAS red cells can be made by the fact that these cells are not hemolyzed by their own serum and will be hemolyzed only by approximately 30% of normal sera. Further differentiation can be made using the sucrose lysis test.

Hemolysis of PNH red cells is commonly incomplete and may be as little as 5% or less. A possible cause of a false-negative test result is the presence of iron-deficiency anemia. The test result becomes positive when the anemia is corrected.

Sugar Water Test

Principle

PNH red cells hemolyze when incubated with compatible normal serum in a sucrose solution of low ionic strength. The test depends on the absorption of complement components even in the absence of an antibody. PNH cells undergo lysis in these conditions by virtue of their increased sensitivity to complement (Hartmann et al., 1970).

Reagents and Equipment

1. Phosphate buffer, 0.005 M (pH 6.1): Sodium dihydrogen phosphate (690 mg) is dissolved in 1 liter of distilled water. 135 mg dibasic sodium phosphate are dissolved in 1 liter of distilled water. To make a working buffer, 90 ml of the disodium hydrogen phosphate is added to 910 ml sodium dihydrogen phosphate. This can be stored indefinitely at 4°C.
2. Sodium hydroxide, 0.75 N: 3 g sodium hydroxide are dissolved in 100 ml distilled water.
3. Hydrochloric acid, 0.75 N: 6.25 ml 12-N (concentrated) hydrochloric acid are added to 100 ml of distilled water.
4. Isotonic sucrose solution: Sucrose (924 mg) is dissolved in 8 ml of the phosphate buffer (pH 6.1) described in step 1. The pH is adjusted to 6.1 with either 0.75-N sodium hydroxide or 0.75-N hydrochloric acid to make up a total volume of 10 ml with buffer.
5. Normal saline 0.85%.
6. Pipettes: 1 ml, graduated; 0.05-ml micropipette.
7. Incubator.
8. Centrifuge.

Specimen

Clotted whole blood from the patient and ABO-compatible whole blood from a normal donor are needed to perform this test.

Method

1. Serum is separated from the clotted blood of both the test specimen and the normal specimen. A 50% suspension of cells from the clots of each sample is prepared in 0.85% saline. The test serum is saved.

2. To each of two tubes, 0.85 ml of a sucrose solution and 0.05 ml nonacidified autologous serum are added.

3. To one of the tubes, 0.1 ml of a 50% suspension of patient cells is added, and to the other tube, 0.1 ml of a 50% suspension of normal control cells is added.

4. Both tubes are mixed and incubated at 37°C for 30 minutes. They are centrifuged at 2,000 rpm for 1–2 minutes and are macroscopically examined for hemolysis.

Results

Marked hemolysis is found in the tube containing cells from patients with PNH but is not found in the control tubes.

Sources of Error

The sucrose lysis test is based on the adsorption of complement by red cells from serum at low ionic concentrations. PNH cells are more sensitive to complement attachment and consequently undergo hemolysis more easily than do normal red cells. Red cells from patients with some myeloproliferative disorders occasionally show mild hemolysis (Catovsky et al., 1971; Rosse, 1973) but, in such cases, the acid hemolysin test result usually is negative. Red cells from patients with HEMPAS typically show no lysis in this test. Hence, this and the acid hemolysin test can be used to differentiate these two disorders (Table 19.7).

Blood collected in EDTA or heparin is unsuitable for the test, although defibrinated whole blood or citrated blood may be used.

Tests for Enzymopathies

Autohemolysis Test

Principle

When normal sterile defibrinated blood is incubated at 37°C for 48 hours, little or no hemolysis takes place. In certain hemolytic disorders, the increase in hemolysis can be reduced by the addition of either glucose or adenosine triphosphate (ATP). This then forms the basis for separating some of the hemolytic anemias (Selwyn and Dacie, 1954).

Reagents and Equipment

1. Sterile 125-ml Erlenmeyer flask containing 25 glass beads (diameter 4.0 mm).
2. Sterile 5-ml capped tubes.
3. Sterile glucose 50%, diluted 1:5 with sterile water just before use (10%).
4. ATP, disodium salt 0.4 M: ATP (2.5180 g) is added to 5 ml distilled water, is adjusted to pH 7.0 with sodium hydroxide, and is made up to 10 ml with

Table 19.7. Differentiation Between PNH and HEMPAS-Derived Cells

	PNH Cells	HEMPAS Cells
Acid hemolysins (Ham's test)	Positive	Positive
Sucrose lysis test	Positive	Negative

PNH = paroxysmal nocturnal hemoglobinuria; HEMPAS = hereditary erythroblastic multinuclearity with positive acidified serum.

distilled water. ATP is frozen in 1-ml aliquots. This reagent is stable for an indefinite time.

5. Sterile pipettes: Sahli 0.02-ml hemoglobin pipettes; 0.2-ml micropipettes.
6. Water bath.
7. Cyanmethemoglobin diluent (Drabkin's solution).
8. Sterile tuberculin syringes and needles.
9. Spectrophotometer.

Specimen

Approximately 25 ml venous blood is added to a sterile Erlenmeyer flask containing 25 glass beads. The specimen is defibrinated by gently swirling the flask for 5–10 minutes or until the noise of the beads can no longer be heard. A normal control specimen should be obtained and treated in the same way as the test specimen.

Method

All steps in the procedure should be completed using sterile techniques to avoid bacterial glycolysis.

1. Into each of six sterile tubes, 2 ml defibrinated blood is added.
2. Into two of these tubes, 0.1 ml 10% glucose is added, using the sterile tuberculin syringe. The solution is mixed well by inversion.
3. Into two other tubes, 0.1 ml 0.4-M ATP is added, using the same procedure described in step 2.
4. The remaining two tubes, containing 2 ml defibrinated blood, are left undisturbed.
5. All six tubes are incubated for 48 hours in a 37°C water bath.
6. Two milliliters of preincubated stock defibrinated blood are centrifuged in a clean (though not necessarily sterile) tube. The serum is separated and stored frozen.
7. The sterile incubated tubes are removed, and each is inspected for signs of contamination (usually indicated by a dark brown color or white bacterial growth). Tubes are discarded if contaminated. Each tube is inverted gently to mix thoroughly. Hematocrits and hemoglobin determinations are set up immediately on all vials.

8. The hematocrit is determined using the microhematocrit procedure (page 256).

9. The hemoglobin is determined by adding 0.2 ml blood to 5 ml cyanmethemoglobin reagent (Drabkin's) and allowing this to stand at room temperature for 10 minutes, after which time the optical density is determined spectrophotometrically at 540 nm, as described on page 255 (optical density of blood = p).

10. The remaining blood in each tube is centrifuged, and 0.2 ml of the serum is placed into 5 ml Drabkin's reagent. The optical density is recorded as described on page 256 (optical density of serum = p).

11. Preincubated serum (0.2 ml) (from step 6 in this section) is placed in 5 ml Drabkin's reagent, and the optical density is read as described previously (optical density of serum = a).

12. The percentage of hemolysis is calculated from the following:

$$\left[\frac{\text{Optical density of serum p} - \text{optical density of serum a}}{\text{(Optical density of whole blood p)} \times 10}\right] \times 100 - \text{hematocrit (\%)} = \% \text{ Hemolysis}$$

where p is the postincubation specimen and a is the specimen before ("ante") incubation.

13. All duplicate results are averaged.

Reference Ranges

Table 19.8 gives the reference ranges for autohemolysis.

Table 19.8. Reference Ranges for the Autohemolysis Test (% Lysis)

Disorder	Initial	Incubated	10% Glucose	0.4 M ATP
Type I autohemolysis	0–0.94	3.0–5.0	0–2.2	0.5–2.3
Type II autohemolysis	—	12.0–16.0	12.0–16.0	0.5–2.3
Type III autohemolysis (hereditary spherocytosis and triosephosphate isomerase deficiency)	—	12.0–15.0	3.0–5.0	3.0–5.0
Normal	0–0.94	0.2–2.7	0–2.2	0.5–2.3

ATP = adenosine triphosphate.

Sources of Error

Little hemolysis occurs in normal blood when it is incubated under sterile conditions after 48 hours, and the hemolysis that is produced is reduced markedly in the presence of added glucose. The hemolysis so formed is a function of the red-cell membrane and the metabolic ability of the cell to continue to produce energy. In red-cell membrane disorders, such as hereditary spherocytosis, the rate of glycolysis is increased, which leads to hemolysis unless extra glucose or energy in the form of ATP is added.

Clinical Correlation

Three principal patterns of autohemolysis are seen. Type I is characterized by a mild degree of hemolysis that is reduced by the addition of glucose and ATP. These findings have been observed in glucose-6-phosphate dehydrogenase (G6PD) deficiency and other disorders of the pentose-phosphate pathway, including hexokinase deficiency and nonspherocytic hemolytic anemia.

In type II patterns, there is a marked increase in autohemolysis that is uncorrected by the addition of glucose but is corrected by the addition of ATP. This is seen principally in pyruvate kinase deficiency and in acquired spherocytic hemolytic anemia.

The type III pattern is characterized by a marked increase in hemolysis, which is corrected in part by the addition of either glucose or ATP and has been referred to previously. This pattern is found in triosephosphate isomerase deficiency as well as in hereditary spherocytosis.

Glucose-6-Phosphate Dehydrogenase Screening Test: Ascorbate-Cyanide Method

Principle

When sodium cyanide and sodium ascorbate are added to blood, catalase is inhibited by the cyanide. This allows hydrogen peroxide to be produced from the coupled oxidation of ascorbate and hemoglobin. G6PD-deficient red cells are oxidized quickly by the hydrogen peroxide, producing a brown methemoglobin pigment (Jacobs and Jandl, 1966).

Reagents and Equipment

1. Ascorbate: 10 mg of sodium ascorbate and 5 mg glucose are added to a series of 13- × 100-mm tubes. This reagent may be stoppered and stored indefinitely at –20°C.
2. Isosmotic phosphate buffer, 0.067 M (pH 7.4): Potassium dihydrogen phosphate (anhydrous), 0.91 g, is dissolved in 100 ml distilled water or 0.95 g disodium hydrogen phosphate (anhydrous) is dissolved in 100 ml distilled water. A working buffer is made by adding 19.6 ml of the potassium dihydrogen phosphate to 80.4 ml of the disodium hydrogen phosphate.
3. Cyanide solution: 500 mg sodium cyanide are dissolved in 50 ml distilled water and added to 20 ml of the isosmotic phosphate buffer (pH 7.4). The reagent is neutralized to pH 7.0 using hydrochloric acid. It is diluted to 100 ml with distilled water. The reagent is stable indefinitely at room temperature.
4. Pasteur pipette.

Specimen

EDTA-anticoagulated or heparinized patient blood and normal control blood are used.

Method

1. The anticoagulated blood is aerated to a bright red color either by passing oxygen or air through it or by gently swirling the specimen in an Erlenmeyer flask.

2. Two milliliters of the aerated specimen are added to a tube containing the ascorbate reagent, and two drops of the sodium cyanide solution are added. The solution is incubated at 37°C unstoppered for 4 hours. During this incubation period, the solution is remixed by use of a Pasteur pipette to blow air into the mixture.

3. The color of the suspension is noted after each mixing.

Results

G6PD-deficient red cells become brown within 1–2 hours, whereas normal blood darkens slowly over several hours and should remain red for at least 2 hours. Blood from heterozygotes with intermediate levels of enzyme activity also becomes brown within 2 hours.

Sources of Error

This G6PD screening test is not specific for G6PD deficiency. Other enzymes of the hexose monophosphate shunt produce abnormal results, as does glutathione deficiency.

Fluorescence Spot Method for G6PD Deficiency

Principle

G6PD catalyzes the oxidation of glucose-6-phosphate (G6P) in the glucose metabolic pathways. It then reduces nicotinamide adenine dinucleotide phosphate (NADP) to the reduced form of NADP (NADPH) by transferring two electrons from G6P. The NADPH becomes fluorescent when exposed to long-wave ultraviolet light. When whole blood is mixed with G6PD screening reagent, this reduction reaction takes place if G6PD is present, and the samples become fluorescent under ultraviolet light (Beutler, 1966).

Reagents and Equipment

1. G6P, 0.01 M: 305 mg of G6P are dissolved in 100 ml distilled water.
2. NADP, 0.0075 M: 60 mg of NADP disodium salt are dissolved in 10 ml distilled water.
3. Saponin: 1 g is dissolved by shaking in distilled water.
4. TRIS–hydrochloric acid buffer, 0.75 M (pH 7.8): TRIS(hydroxymethyl)aminomethane, 90.8 g, is dissolved in 250 ml water and acidified by adding 33 ml 1-N hydrochloric acid. The reagent is made up with distilled water to 1 liter.
5. Oxidized glutathione (GSSG), 0.008 M: GSSG, 49 g, is dissolved in 10 ml distilled water.
6. Working reagent: Combined are 1 ml G6P, 1 ml NADP, 2 ml saponin, 3 ml buffer (pH 7.8), 1 ml GSSG, and 2 ml distilled water. This working reagent is stable for 2 years if stored frozen and for 2 months if stored at 4°C.
7. Filter paper.
8. Pipettes: 0.01-ml and 0.1-ml micropipettes; Pasteur pipettes.
9. Ultraviolet light source.

Specimen

Fresh EDTA-anticoagulated or heparinized blood is used, and the specimen is tested as soon as possible, as hemolysis resulting from poor storage invalidates the results.

Method

1. Whole blood (0.01 ml) is added to 0.1 ml working reagent and is incubated at room temperature. Aliquot drops of the mixture are added to filter paper after 5-, 10-, and 30-minute intervals.

2. The spots are allowed to dry thoroughly for 10–15 minutes and then are examined under longwave ultraviolet light in a darkened area.

Results

Normal blood becomes fluorescent; G6PD-deficient samples show little or no fluorescence.

Sources of Error

Fluorescence is produced by NADPH, which is formed by the action of G6PD on the substrate NADP. This test is useful as a screening procedure but is limited in its usefulness by its sensitivity to deficiencies of G6PD, with only levels of less than 20% being detected. Blood from heterozygotes usually appears normal by this procedure.

A normal control sample should be treated in the same way as the patient blood and should show strong fluorescence. If qualitative procedures show the presence of a potential G6PD deficiency, a quantitative test should be carried out to confirm the finding.

Quantitation of G6PD

Principle

G6PD catalyzes the reaction that takes place when G6P is converted to 6-phosphogluconic acid (6PG). The rate at which NADPH is produced is measured spectrophotometrically (Lohr and Waller, 1963).

$$\text{G6P} + \text{NADP} \xrightleftharpoons{\text{G6PD}} \text{6PG} + \text{NADPH}$$

Reagents and Equipment

1. Triethanolamine buffer, 0.5 M (pH 7.5): Triethanolamine hydrochloride, 0.93 g, is added to 0.2 g disodium EDTA in 50 ml distilled water. The pH is adjusted to 7.5 with 0.1-N sodium hydroxide, and the total volume is made up to 100 ml with distilled water.
2. NADP, 0.01 M: Triphosphopyridine, 25 mg, is added to 1 ml 1% sodium bicarbonate solution. The reagent is stable for 3 months if kept frozen and for 2–3 weeks if stored stoppered at 4°C.
3. G6P: 130 mg are dissolved in 10 ml distilled water. This reagent is stable for 3 months if kept frozen and for 2–3 weeks if stored stoppered at 4°C.
4. Digitonin, saturated: Digitonin, 1 g, is dissolved in 100 ml distilled water by shaking the mixture vigorously. It then is filtered.
5. Normal saline.
6. Spectrophotometer, ultraviolet range with constant-temperature cuvette.
7. Centrifuge.
8. Pipettes: 1 ml and 5 ml, graduated; 0.05-ml micropipettes.
9. Refrigerator.
10. Stopwatch.

Specimen

The specimen consists of EDTA-anticoagulated blood.

Method

1. Approximately 0.5 ml blood is washed two to three times with normal saline, and the washed packed cells are resuspended in approximately 1 ml saline so that the red-cell suspension approximates 2×10^{12}/liter. A red-cell count is carried out on the suspension to confirm the correct dilution.
2. The following reagents are combined: 1 ml red-cell suspension, 1 ml distilled water, 0.7 ml buffer, and 0.3 ml digitonin. The mixture is allowed to stand for 15 minutes at 4°C. It then is centrifuged, and the insoluble precipitated material is discarded.
3. The following are pipetted successively into the spectrophotometer cuvette: 2.85 ml buffer, 0.05 ml red-cell hemolysate (from step 2), and 0.05 ml NADP.
4. A blank is set up by putting into a second cuvette 2.90 ml buffer and 0.05 ml red-cell hemolysate.
5. The contents of both cuvettes are mixed with a glass rod that is flattened at one end. The cuvettes are kept at 25°C for 5 minutes. Reagent G6P (0.05 ml) then is added to each cuvette.
6. The test cuvette is read against the blank at 340 nm. (Spectrophotometric requirements are a 1-cm light path and 25°C constant-temperature cuvette.) The optical density increase should not be more than 0.030 per minute. If the increase is greater, the test is repeated using a sample that has been diluted accordingly.
7. An optical density of approximately 0.020 is the test end point. A stopwatch is started and the optical density is read at 2-minute intervals for 10 minutes. The mean optical density change per minute is calculated.

8. The red-cell count is determined by a standard method.

Calculation

The ΔE_{340}/minute $\times$ 60,000 = G6PD units/ml red-cell suspension:

$$\text{G6PD activity (in U/10}^9 \text{ red cells)} = \frac{\frac{\text{U/ml red cells}}{\text{Red cell count}}}{} \times 10^9$$

Reference Range

The reference range is 6.5–7.9 units/10^9 cells.

Sources of Error

The optimal pH of the G6PD reaction is 8.3, but between pH 7.4 and 8.6 there is little change in the enzyme activity. The test measurements are made at pH 7.5 because this is nearest to physiologic conditions and allows for comparison with other enzyme activities that usually are measured near this pH.

Phosphate buffers should not be used in this procedure because of their inhibitory action on the test. Blood specimens possessing high reticulocyte counts also should not be tested, as this can result in falsely elevated G6PD levels because of the high concentrations of the enzyme in younger red cells.

The metabolism of glucose is essential for the survival of the red cell. It takes place in two pathways—the Embden-Meyerhof and the pentose-phosphate pathways (page 19). G6PD is active in the latter pathway, which accounts for nearly 20% of the energy supplied to the red cell. The action of G6PD is:

$$\text{G6PD} + \text{NADP} \rightleftharpoons \text{6 phosphate gluconolactone} + \text{NADPH}$$

The NADPH formed is used by glutathione reductase to maintain glutathione in a reduced state. This seems to be essential for red-cell maintenance and for the integrity of the globin part of the hemoglobin molecule. Consequently, the pentose-phosphate pathway, although playing a minor role in supplying red-cell energy, is essential for safe-guarding red-cell integrity by maintaining sufficient intracellular reduced glutathione.

G6PD deficiency is believed not to be caused by lack of a gene product but rather by the replacement of the normal enzyme with an enzyme containing an altered molecule. There appear to be at least six enzyme mutants, the two most common resulting in severe deficiencies in Mediterranean people (Greek, Italian, Sardinian), Asians, and Kurdish Jews, and the remainder resulting in more moderate deficiencies found in African and American blacks. These two principal forms of G6PD deficiency can be separated electrophoretically using commercial equipment and either cellulose acetate or acrylamide gel as a supporting media (Vupio et al., 1973).

Fluorescent Spot Method for Pyruvate Kinase Deficiency

Principle

A phosphate group (phosphoenolpyruvate [PEP]) is transferred to adenosine diphosphate (ADP), forming pyruvate and ADP in the presence of red-cell pyruvate kinase (PK). Lactate dehydrogenase (LDH) in the red-cell hemolysate catalyzes the reduction of pyruvate to lactate, with the resulting oxidation of the reduced form (DPNH) to disphosphopyridine (DPN). DPNH becomes fluorescent when exposed to long-wave ultraviolet light, in contrast to DPN, which does not fluoresce (Beutler, 1966).

Reagents and Equipment

1. PEP, trisodium salt, 0.067 M: PEP, 0.6980 g, is dissolved in 8.5 ml distilled water and is adjusted with 0.25-N sodium hydroxide to pH 7.8 and diluted to 10 ml with distilled water. It is stored frozen in 0.5-ml aliquots. The reagent is stable for 1 month.
2. ADP, 0.03 M: ADP, 0.1508 g, is dissolved in 8.5 ml distilled water and is adjusted with 0.25-N sodium hydroxide to pH 7.8 and diluted to 10 ml with distilled water. It is stored frozen in 5-ml aliquots. This reagent is stable for 1 month.
3. The reduced form of nicotinamide adenine dinucleotide (NADH), 0.015 M: NADH, 0.1063 g,

is dissolved in 10 ml distilled water. This reagent should be freshly prepared and kept on ice during use.

4. Magnesium sulfate ($MgSO_4 \cdot 7H_2O$): This salt, 1.9720 g, is dissolved in 100 ml distilled water and is stored frozen in 5-ml aliquots.

5. Potassium phosphate buffer, 0.25 M (pH 7.4): Potassium dihydrogen phosphate, 3.403 g, is dissolved in 85 ml distilled water and is adjusted to pH 7.4 and diluted to 100 ml. It is stored frozen in 5-ml aliquots. This reagent is stable for 1 month.

6. Working reagents: The stock reagents are thawed, and 0.03 ml PEP, 0.1 ml ADP, 0.1 ml NADH, 0.1 ml magnesium sulfate, 0.05 ml buffer, and 0.62 ml distilled water are added (total volume made up to 1 ml). Alternatively, a commercially prepared working reagent can be obtained from Sigma Chemical Company, St. Louis, MO. The working solution is stable for 7 hours at room temperature.

7. Normal saline.

8. Ultraviolet light.

9. Filter paper.

10. Pipettes: 1 ml, graduated; 0.05-ml, 0.1-ml, and Pasteur micropipettes.

11. Centrifuge.

12. Water bath, 37°C.

Specimen

EDTA-anticoagulated or heparinized blood is used. Both patient blood and normal control blood should be obtained. Blood is stable for 5 days if kept at room temperature.

Method

1. Approximately 2 ml anticoagulated blood is washed with large volumes of normal saline, and the supernatant plasma-saline layer is removed carefully without disturbing the packed red-cell layer.

2. One volume of packed red cells is pipetted carefully from the bottom of the centrifuged cells into four volumes of normal saline, with care taken to wipe off the outside of the pipette to ensure that it is free of contaminating white cells and platelets. The pipette is rinsed several times with the saline.

3. The cell suspension (2 ml; as prepared in step 2) is added to 0.20 ml of the working reagent. One

drop is placed on filter paper immediately and allowed to dry for 10–15 minutes. The remainder of the cells and working reagent is incubated in a 37°C water bath for 30 minutes, and one drop is removed and placed on the filter paper as before. It is allowed to dry for 10–15 minutes.

4. The spots are examined under long-wave ultraviolet light in a darkened area.

Results

There should be strong fluorescence from the first applied spot (0 time), but the spot applied after 30 minutes' incubation should show no fluorescence. Red cells deficient in PK show fluorescence in both spots.

Quantitation of Pyruvate Kinase

Principle

PEP is converted by PK to pyruvate in the presence of ADP. The pyruvate then is converted to lactate by LDH in the presence of NADH. The decrease in absorbance of NADH due to its oxidation to NAD^+ is a direct measurement of the concentration of pyruvate kinase (Valentine et al., 1961).

$$ADP + PEP \underset{PK}{\rightleftharpoons} ATP + pyruvate$$

$$Pyruvate + NADH + H^+ \underset{LDH}{\rightleftharpoons} lactate + NAD^+$$

Reagents and Equipment

1. Triethanolamine buffer, 0.025 M (pH 7.4): Triethanolamine hydrochloride, 4.62 g, is dissolved, along with 16.79 g potassium chloride and 5.92 g $MgSO_4 \cdot 7H_2O$, in approximately 900 ml distilled water. The pH then is adjusted to 7.4 with either hydrochloric acid or potassium hydroxide, and the volume is made up to 1 liter with distilled water. Five-milliliter aliquots are stored frozen.

2. ADP, 0.013 M: ADP, 0.645 g, is dissolved in 10 ml distilled water. It is kept on ice during use.

3. NADH, 0.005 M: NADH, 0.035 g, is dissolved in 10 ml distilled water. The reagent should be prepared fresh and kept on ice during use.

Table 19.9. Test Procedure for the Quantitation of Pyruvate Kinase

Reagents	Test (ml)	Blank (ml)	Control (ml)
Triethanolamine	1.00	1.00	1.00
Distilled water	1.48	1.58	1.48
NADH	0.10	—	0.10
ADP	0.10	0.10	0.10
LDH	0.02	0.02	0.02
PEP	0.20	0.20	0.20

NADH = the reduced form of nicotinamide adenine dinucleotide; ADP = adenosine diphosphate; LDH = lactate dehydrogenase; PEP = phosphoenolpyruvate.

4. LDH, 60 units/ml (Boehringer Corp., Indianapolis, IN), should be used in the suspension provided.
5. PEP: In 1 ml distilled water, 0.0073 g PEP is dissolved. The reagent should be prepared fresh and kept on ice during use.
6. Dextran 6%.
7. Spectrophotometer, ultraviolet range (1-cm optical path).
8. Normal saline.
9. Pipettes: 5 ml and 1 ml, graduated; and Pasteur.
10. Stopwatch.

Specimen

The specimen is fresh EDTA-anticoagulated or heparinized blood. Blood stored at 4°C for 24 hours can be used provided that a control sample stored under the same conditions is assayed.

The blood is hemolyzed by adding 1 ml 6% dextran to 3.5 ml anticoagulated blood. It is mixed by inversion and is allowed to stand at room temperature for 30 minutes. The red cell–free plasma is removed with a Pasteur pipette, 1 ml dextran is added, and the mixture is brought up to the original volume of 4.5 ml with normal saline. Mixing is accomplished by inverting the suspension, and the procedure is repeated six times to ensure that the red-cell suspension is free of leukocytes.

Immediately before use, 0.1 ml of the leukocyte-free red-cell mass is added to 4.0 ml ice-cold distilled water, and that hemolysate is frozen until tested.

Method

1. The reagents are placed into three silica cuvettes, as shown in Table 19.9.

2. The cuvettes are warmed at 37°C for 2–3 minutes, and then the test cuvette is placed in the spectrophotometer. Test hemolysate (0.1 ml) is added, and the optical density of the reaction is recorded at 340 nm at 30-second intervals for 5 minutes.

3. The procedure is repeated after 0.1 ml hemolysate is added to the blank cuvette. These optical densities are recorded at 30-second intervals for 5 minutes.

4. The procedure is repeated, but 0.1 ml normal saline is added to the control cuvette. This step checks for absorbance from the oxidation of NADH in the absence of hemolysate.

Calculation

PK activity

$$= \frac{\Delta_A / \text{minute} \times 10^3}{6.22 \times \text{volume of red cells /cuvette } (\mu l)}$$

$$= \frac{\Delta_A / \text{minute} \times 10^3}{6.22 \times \frac{0.1}{4.1} \times \text{packed cell volume of cell suspension}}$$

Reference Range

The reference range is 1.2–2.2 IUs per milliliter of red cells.

Sources of Error

The PK unit is expressed as the micromoles of NADH oxidized in 1 ml of red cells per minute at 37°C. Care should be taken when screening or quantitating PK to avoid the introduction of any buffy-coat layer when preparing the red-cell he-molysate. Leukocytes must be removed completely from the sample, because normally they contain nearly 300 times as much PK as do red cells. In type 2 hemolytic anemia, the red cells are deficient in PK, and the leukocytes have normal levels of PK.

Clinical Correlation

PK deficiency is the most common red-cell enzyme disorder involving the Embden-Meyerhof pathway. The abnormality results in a mild-to-moderate hemolytic anemia that often is tolerated well by individuals because of the high levels of 2,3-diphosphoglycerate (2,3-DPG) found as a result of the block in glycolysis. Consequently, with some PK variants, the assay of 2,3-DPG can be helpful in further identifying a suspected enzymopathy. The International Committee for Standardization in Haematology (1979) has published recommended procedures for the characterization of such variants.

Glutathione Assay

Principle

Glutathione reacts with 5,5'-dithiobis-(2-nitrobenzoic acid) (DTNB) to produce a stable yellow complex, the intensity of which is proportional to the glutathione concentration (Beutler et al., 1963).

Reagents and Equipment

1. Precipitating solution: Glacial metaphosphoric acid, 1.67 g, is dissolved, along with 0.2 g dipotassium EDTA and 30 g sodium chloride, in 100 ml distilled water. The solution is stable for 3 weeks when stored at 4°C.
2. Phosphate reagent (disodium hydrogen phosphate [$Na_2HPO_4 12H_2O$]), 0.3 M: The salt, 107.5 g, is dissolved in 1 liter of distilled water. This reagent is stable indefinitely if stored at 4°C. If crystals are formed during storage, they can be dissolved by warming. Discard the reagent if molds are present.
3. DTNB reagent: DTNB, 0.04 g, is dissolved in 10 ml 1% sodium citrate. The reagent is stable for at least 3 months if stored at 4°C.

4. Stock glutathione standard: Metaphosphoric acid, 0.002 g, and 0.0625 g glutathione (Sigma Chemical Company, St. Louis, MO) are dissolved in 100 ml saturated aqueous sodium chloride. The solution is buffered by adding 4 ml of the phosphate reagent to 2-ml aliquots of stock standard. One milliliter of the DTNB reagent is added to each aliquot, and these are stored frozen at –20°C.
5. Filter paper.
6. Pipettes: 2 ml and 5 ml, graduated; 0.2-ml micropipettes.

Specimen

Heparinized or EDTA-anticoagulated whole blood is the specimen of choice. A normal control is obtained and treated exactly as is the test specimen.

Method

1. The hematocrits of both the test and control specimens are determined using a standard method (page 255).
2. Blood (0.2 ml) is added to 1.8 ml distilled water. This is mixed and allowed to hemolyze. Three milliliters of the precipitating solution then are added.
3. The mixture is allowed to stand for 5 minutes and is filtered. Four tubes are set up, as shown in Table 19.10.
4. The tubes are mixed by inversion, and their optical densities are read in a spectrophotometer at a wavelength of 412 nm.

Calculation

$$\frac{\text{Optical density of (test} - \text{blank)}}{\text{Optical density of (standard} - \text{blank)}} \times \frac{62.5}{\text{hematocrit} \times 10}$$
$$= \text{Red-cell glutathione (mg/l)}$$

Reference Range

The reference range is 600–900 mg per liter of red cells.

Table 19.10. Procedure Used for the Assay of Glutathione

Reagent	Test	Control	Standard	Blank
Test filtrate (ml)	2.0	—	—	—
Control filtrate (ml)	—	2.0	—	—
1:25 Dilution of stock standard (ml)	—	—	2.0	—
Phosphate reagent (ml)	8.0	8.0	8.0	8.0
DTNB (ml)	1.0	1.0	1.0	1.0
Precipitating solution 3 vol:2 vol water (ml)	—	—	—	2.0

DTNB = 5.5'-dithiobis-(2-nitrobenzoic acid).

Sources of Error

This procedure is insensitive to temperature variations. Therefore, a standard calibration is not needed for each batch of tests once the procedure has been established and the spectrophotometer accurately calibrated. Glutathione is relatively stable, and so the specimen can be stored at 4°C for 2–3 weeks.

Clinical Correlation

Glutathione is a tripeptide of glycine, glutamic acid, and cysteine. In the blood, it is found exclusively intracellularly and is reduced in individuals who are sensitive to the hemolytic action of oxidizing drugs, particularly acetylphenylhydrazine.

Glutathione Stability Test

Principle

When normal red cells are incubated with acetylphenylhydrazine, there is little effect on the glutathione content but, in G6PD-deficient cells, the glutathione content is markedly reduced (Beutler et al., 1963).

Reagents and Equipment

1. Acetylphenylhydrazine: 0.1 g of acetylphenylhydrazine is dissolved in 1 ml acetone, and 0.05-ml aliquots are dispensed into tubes. The reagent is allowed to evaporate to dryness in an incubator. The tubes are stoppered and then stored in the dark until used.
2. Water bath, 37°C.
3. As in the glutathione assay (page 306).

Specimen

Freshly collected heparinized or EDTA-anticoagulated blood is used. A normal control sample should be run simultaneously with the test.

Method

1. Patient blood and control blood (1 ml each) are added to tubes containing 5 mg acetylphenylhydrazine. The specimens are mixed and incubated at 37°C for 2 hours. The tubes should be remixed by gentle inversion during the incubation.
2. The glutathione level of each tube is determined by the method described on page 306.

Results

In normal blood, the glutathione level is reduced by less than 20% after incubation with acetylphenylhydrazine. In G6PD-deficient cells, the glutathione reduction is greater than 50% in the heterozygous patient and may be absent in hemizygous men.

Fluorescent Spot Test for Glutathione Reductase Screening

Principle

When glutathione reductase is present in the test blood, oxidized glutathione is reduced to glutathione, and NADPH is oxidized to NADP. This reaction can be detected by the presence of fluorescence when examined under ultraviolet light (Beutler, 1966).

Reagents and Equipment

1. Phosphate buffer, 0.067 M (pH 7.4): Sodium dihydrogen phosphate ($NaH_2PO_42H_2O$), 2.34 g, is dissolved in 100 ml distilled water (0.067 M). Disodium hydrogen phosphate, 2.13 g, is dissolved in 100 ml distilled water (0.067 M). A working solution is made by adding 18.0 ml 0.067-M sodium dihydrogen phosphate to 82.0 ml 0.067-M disodium hydrogen phosphate.
2. GSSG, 0.033 M: GSSG, 0.404 g, is dissolved in 2 ml distilled water.
3. NADPH, 0.015 M: NADPH, 0.45 g, is dissolved in 10 ml distilled water.
4. Saponin, 1% aqueous.
5. Reaction mixture: The following are added together: 0.1 ml glutathione (0.033 M), 0.1 ml NADPH (0.015 M), 0.06 ml phosphate buffer (pH 7.4), and 0.2 ml 1% saponin. This reagent is stable for 10 days when stored frozen.
6. Filter paper.
7. Pipettes: 1 ml, graduated; 0.1-ml and Pasteur micropipettes.
8. Ultraviolet light.
9. Water bath, 37°C.

Specimen

Heparinized or EDTA-anticoagulated blood is used. A normal control sample should be tested with the patient blood. Blood as old as 6 weeks is satisfactory if kept at 4°C.

Method

1. A 1:10 dilution of blood to reaction mixture is made by adding 0.02 ml blood to 0.2 ml reagent. This is incubated at 37°C for 1 hour.
2. A spot of the blood-reaction mixture is placed immediately on the filter paper and at 15-minute intervals during the incubation for up to 1 hour.
3. The spots are allowed to dry and are examined under long-wave ultraviolet light.

Results

The first spot should become fluorescent and, if glutathione reductase activity is high, the fluorescence will disappear within the first 30 minutes.

Decreased glutathione reductase activity may produce fluorescence for up to 1 hour.

Clinical Correlation

Glutathione reductase deficiency has been implicated as the cause of chronic hemolytic anemia (Waller, 1968; Chang et al., 1978). However, it now is recognized that, in most cases, the deficiency is due to suboptimal riboflavin intake and that partial deficiency of the enzyme has no known hematologic effect. In fact, a complete deficiency of glutathione reductase is extremely rare, having been documented in only one family (Loos et al., 1976; Beutler, 1979).

Heinz Bodies

Principle

Heinz bodies are not detected in Romanowsky-stained smears. They are seen when supravital staining techniques are used under light microscopy and by examining unstained preparations under phase microscopy. Heinz bodies are produced by an oxidant stress of drugs or chemicals, by an instability of hemoglobin molecules, or by defects in the red-cell glycolytic pathways.

Reagents and Equipment

1. Methyl violet 0.5%, in normal saline, filtered before use.
2. Pasteur pipettes.
3. Microscope.

Specimen

EDTA-anticoagulated or heparinized whole blood is used.

Method

1. Equal volumes of anticoagulated blood and stain are mixed and are allowed to stain for 10–15 minutes at room temperature.
2. A small drop of the stained cells is placed on a slide, a coverslip is applied, and the specimen is examined under the high-power oil-immersion lens.

Result

Heinz bodies will be seen as refractile red-cell inclusions, 1–3 μ in diameter, found most frequently at the red-cell periphery.

Clinical Correlation

These inclusions represent denatured hemoglobin and are found in certain hemoglobinopathies, in deficiencies of G6PD and other enzymopathies, in the presence of oxidant drugs, and in some splenectomized individuals. The common drugs associated with their presence include analgesics (e.g., acetylsalicylic acid, acetophenetidin), antimalarials (e.g., primaquine, quinine, chloroquine), nitrofurans (e.g., nitrofurantoin, nitrofurazone), sulfonamides (e.g., sulfisoxazole, sulfnilamide), and a miscellaneous group that includes chloramphenicol, dilantin, fava beans, naphthalene, phenylhydrazine, quinidine, streptomycin, and water-soluble vitamin K.

Heinz bodies are seen also in patients with polycythemia who are treated with phenylhydrazine. If drug-induced hemolysis is suspected, the test should be carried out as soon as possible, as the cells in which the hemoglobin has been denatured disappear from the circulation within hours to days after the toxic event.

An alternative method of staining using brilliant green has been recommended, and it appears to possess greater specificity for the inclusion (Schwab and Lewis, 1969). Relatively little of the stain is taken up by the remainder of the red cells, which makes it possible to enhance the prominence of the particles by using neutral red as a counterstain.

Solubility Test for Hemoglobin S

Principle

Hemoglobin S (Hb S) in the deoxygenated state has reduced solubility and, when fully oxygenated, forms a precipitate when placed in a high-molarity phosphate buffer solution. The precipitate is the result of the formation, by the deoxygenated hemoglobin molecule, of tactoids that refract and deflect light, producing a turbid solution (Nalbandian et al., 1971; Wright and Brosious, 1977).

Reagents and Equipment

1. Phosphate buffer-lysing reagent: To approximately 900 ml distilled water in a 1-liter volumetric flask, 215 g anhydrous dipotassium hydrogen phosphate and 169 g anhydrous potassium dihydrogen phosphate are added. This is mixed to dissolve and warmed, if necessary, to hasten solution. Sodium hydrosulfite (dithionite, 5 g) is added and mixed until dissolved. Saponin (1 g) is added and diluted to 1 liter with distilled water. This reagent is stable for 1 month at 4°C.
2. Pipettes: 0.02-ml and 0.05-ml micropipettes.
3. Tubes: 12 × 75 mm.
4. Volumetric flask: 1 liter.
5. Test tube rack, prepared as follows: A heavy sheet of white paper, on which horizontal black lines have been drawn approximately 6 mm apart with heavy black ink, is attached to the back of the rack. The rows in the rack are covered so that the only open holes are positioned 2.5 cm in front of the white paper.

Specimen

The specimen is EDTA-anticoagulated blood.

Method

1. Well-mixed blood (0.02 ml) is pipetted into 2 ml reagent. This is mixed and left at room temperature for 5 minutes.
2. The horizontal lines are viewed through the hemolyzed specimens.
3. Control specimens consisting of known normal and sickled blood should be run with the test.

Interpretation

A positive test result, indicating the presumptive presence of Hb S, will be represented by turbidity sufficient to prevent visibility of the lines behind the tube. Normal specimens will show only a faint haziness; many will be completely transparent.

Sources of Error

Other hemoglobins besides Hb S produce positive solubility tests. They include Hb C Harlem, Hb S Travis, Hb C Ziguinchor, and Hb Bart's. Marked

Table 19.11. Percentage of Reduced Hemoglobin in Phosphate Buffer Solutions of Different Concentrations

Hemoglobin Type	1.10 M (%)	2.49 M (%)	2.87 M (%)
AA	100	90–95	13–20
AD	100	90–95	13–20
AS	100	25–35	5–20
SS	100	3–10	2–4

AA = normal; AD = heteozygote AD; AS = sickle cell trait; SS = sickle cell anemia.

polycythemia, hyperlipidemia, and dysglobinemia also may produce false results, although the use of washed cells eliminates the errors caused by plasma proteins and lipids. False-negative test results can be caused by the use of outdated reagents, recent transfusions of normal blood, and tests carried out on anemic patients (Hb <7g/dl) and on newborns' and infants' blood.

Modified Solubility Test for Hemoglobin S

Principle

This modification of the standard ferrosolubility test (Jonxis and Huisman, 1968) differentiates between the homozygote and heterozygote states by using a standard spectrophotometer to assess lysis more accurately at different concentrations.

Reagents and Equipment

1. Phosphate buffer, 2.87 M (pH 6.5): Anhydrous dipotassium hydrogen phosphate, 289.2 g, and 164.7 g anhydrous potassium dihydrogen phosphate are dissolved in 800 ml distilled water and diluted to 1 liter.
2. Phosphate buffer, 2.49 M: The 2.87-M buffer, 86.7 ml, is diluted to 100 ml with distilled water.
3. Phosphate buffer, 1.10 M: The 2.87-M buffer, 3.83 ml, is diluted to 100 ml with distilled water.
4. Sodium hyposulfite (dithionite).
5. Spectrophotometer.
6. Filter paper: Whatman no. 1.

Specimen

EDTA-anticoagulated blood is used for this test.

Method

1. Approximately 50 mg sodium hyposulfite is added to 4.5-ml volumes of each of the phosphate buffers.
2. EDTA-anticoagulated blood (0.5 ml) is added to 9.5 ml distilled water and is mixed and allowed to remain at room temperature for 5–10 minutes to hemolyze completely.
3. One-half milliliter of this hemolysate is added to each of the phosphate buffers, and they are mixed and left overnight at room temperature. The solutions are filtered and read at 540 nm.

Results

Table 19.11 shows the percentage of reduced hemoglobin in phosphate buffer solutions of different concentrations.

Discussion

This procedure is useful in confirming the presence of Hb S following electrophoresis. Like the standard solubility test, other sickling hemoglobins will produce false-positive test results, and so the same precautions apply.

Sickle Cell Preparation (Sodium Metabisulfite Method)

Principle

When whole blood is mixed with a reducing agent, deoxygenation takes place, causing the Hb S molecule to assume a tactoid form and produce morphologic sickle cells.

Reagents and Equipment

1. Sodium metabisulfite, 2% aqueous, which should be prepared fresh. The reagent is stable for 8 hours.
2. Microscope.
3. Slides.
4. Pasteur pipettes.
5. Syringe (5 ml) and 19-gauge needle.
6. Petroleum jelly.

Specimen

The specimen is EDTA-anticoagulated blood.

Method

1. A small drop of blood is placed on a clean slide, and two drops of 2% sodium metabisulfite reagent are added. The solution is mixed with an applicator stick and covered with a coverslip. This is allowed to stand for 30 minutes.
2. Using the high-dry microscope objective, the preparation is examined for the presence of sickle cells or holly leaf–shaped red cells. If sickling is not observed, the coverslip is rimmed carefully with petroleum jelly using the syringe and needle.
3. The preparation is allowed to stand at room temperature overnight and is re-examined for the presence of sickle cells.

Discussion

Sodium metabisulfite and sodium bisulfite can be used interchangeably to promote a deoxygenated atmosphere. Using this screening procedure, the number of sickled cells is not proportional to the Hb S level, and the method cannot be used to differentiate the heterozygous from the homozygous state.

Demonstration of Hemoglobin H and Other Unstable Hemoglobins (Brilliant Cresyl Blue Test) for Inclusions

Principle

Unstable hemoglobins are easily denatured intracellularly. The resulting denatured hemoglobin is detected as stained bodies enhanced by the presence of a redox dye—brilliant cresyl blue (Papayannopoulou and Stamatoyannopoulos, 1974).

Reagents and Equipment

1. Sodium citrate, 3% aqueous.
2. Normal saline.
3. Brilliant cresyl blue.
4. Filter paper: Whatman no. 42.
5. Microscope.
6. Test tube: 10×75 mm.
7. Water bath.
8. Pasteur pipette.
9. Working reagent: 20 ml of 3% sodium citrate is added to 80 ml of normal saline, and 1 g brilliant cresyl blue is dissolved in this solution. The stain is mixed and filtered just before use. The reagent is stable for 2 months when stored at room temperature.

Specimen

Fresh EDTA-anticoagulated blood is used.

Method

1. Four drops of fresh blood are added to two drops of filtered working reagent, and the mixture is incubated in a 37°C water bath for 2 hours.
2. Smears are made after 20 minutes, 1 hour, and 2 hours, and are examined under an oil-immersion objective.
3. The tube is removed from the water bath and is allowed to incubate overnight at room temperature. An aliquot is removed, and a smear is prepared and examined in the same way.

Results

Unstable hemoglobin (e.g., Hb H) inclusions appear as multiple green-blue bodies arranged in a pitted sequence like the pattern on the surface of a golf ball. These bodies might be confused with reticulocytes but can be differentiated by their presence in most cells examined and by their green color, in contrast to the dark blue filamentous material seen in reticulocytes.

This test also detects inclusion bodies found in splenectomized patients. Such inclusions are usually large spheric single bodies found only after prolonged overnight incubation.

Sources of Error

A normal control sample should be tested simultaneously with the patient sample, and the control sample should not show any inclusion bodies even after overnight incubation. A positive test result for unstable hemoglobins should always be confirmed by other tests, including the isopropanol precipitation test, the heat denaturation test, and hemoglobin electrophoresis.

Isopropanol Precipitation Test for Unstable Hemoglobins

Principle

Three main factors affect the stability of hemoglobin: bonding within the globin subunit, bonding of the globin to heme, and bonding between hemoglobin chains. Decreased stability of the hemoglobin molecule may result from any of these alterations. This is reflected by the exposure of the hemoglobin molecule to either heat or isopropanol precipitation (Carrell and Kay, 1972).

Reagents and Equipment

1. Water bath, 37°C.
2. pH meter.
3. Centrifuge.
4. Normal saline.
5. Carbon tetrachloride or toluene.
6. Isopropyl alcohol.
7. Hydrochloric acid.
8. Potassium cyanide, 2% aqueous (prepared with rubber gloves in an exhaust hood).
9. TRIS buffer (2-amino-2-hydroxymethyl-1,3-propandiol).
10. Pipettes: 1 ml and 5 ml, graduated; 0.2-ml micropipette.
11. TRIS buffer 17% isopropanol, 0.1 M (pH 7.4): TRIS primary standard, 12.11 g, is added to 170 ml isopropyl alcohol and is diluted to 1 liter with distilled water. It is adjusted to pH 7.4 by adding concentrated hydrochloric acid. This reagent is stable at room temperature for 2 months if kept stoppered.

Specimen

EDTA-anticoagulated blood of the patient and a normal control should be used. Hemolysates of both test and control blood specimens are prepared by washing an aliquot of red cells in copious volumes of normal saline. This procedure is repeated at least twice. After the last wash, an equal volume of distilled water and one-half volume of carbon tetrachloride or toluene are added. The mixture is stoppered and shaken vigorously for 5 minutes. It is centrifuged at 2,500 rpm for 10 minutes. The hemolysate is removed, and one volume of 2% potassium cyanide is added to five volumes of the hemolysate. It is prepared fresh just before testing.

Method

1. Buffer (2 ml) is added to each of two tubes and is allowed to warm to 37°C for 10 minutes in a water bath.
2. Test and control hemolysates (0.2 ml each), prepared as previously described, are then added to each tube. They are stoppered, mixed by inversion, and incubated at 37°C for 30 minutes.
3. Both tubes are examined for the presence of a precipitate after 5 and 30 minutes of incubation.

Results

After 5 minutes of incubation, a normal specimen will remain clear. However, if the specimen contains an unstable hemoglobin, it will show a faint precipitate that becomes flocculent within 20 minutes.

Sources of Error

False-positive results may occur with hemolysates containing large amounts of fetal hemoglobin (Hb F) and with blood specimens containing methemoglobin. The most frequently encountered unstable hemoglobins are Hb E, Hb H, Hb Köln and Hb Hasharon. All other unstable hemoglobins are extremely rare. Old hemolysates and samples that have been stored at room temperature for more than 48 hours will give false-positive results because of methemoglobin formation. False-negative results may occur if cyanide is added to the hemolysate.

Heat Denaturation Test for Unstable Hemoglobins

Principle

The principle underlying the heat denaturation test for unstable hemoglobins is the same as that for the isopropanol precipitation test (Jonxis and Huisman, 1968). If unstable hemoglobin is heated at 50°C for 2 hours, it will precipitate. By comparing the optical density of the supernatant before and after heating, unstable hemoglobin can be quantitated.

Reagents and Equipment

1. Hydrochloric acid, 0.1 N.
2. Sodium bicarbonate.
3. Potassium cyanide.
4. Potassium ferricyanide.
5. Toluene.
6. Normal saline.
7. TRIS buffer.
8. Volumetric flask: 1 liter.
9. Pipettes: 5 ml, graduated; 0.1-ml and Pasteur micropipettes.
10. Centrifuge.
11. Spectrophotometer.
12. Water bath, 50°C.
13. TRIS buffer, 0.1 M (pH 7.4): TRIS, 12.1 g, is dissolved in 25 ml 0.1-N hydrochloric acid and diluted to 1 liter with distilled water.
14. Cyanmethemoglobin reagent: Sodium bicarbonate, 1.0 g, along with 0.5 g potassium cyanide and 0.2 g potassium ferricyanide, is dissolved in 1 liter of distilled water.

Specimen

Fresh anticoagulated blood is used.

Method

1. Three milliliters of freshly collected blood are washed in a large volume of saline. The washing is repeated twice, and the saline is decanted. The packed red cells are lysed by adding five volumes of distilled water and one volume of toluene. This is mixed well and centrifuged at 2,500 rpm for 15 minutes.

2. The clear supernatant is removed with a Pasteur pipette, and 3 ml hemolysate is added to an equal vol-

ume of TRIS buffer. Two-milliliter volumes of this mixture are pipetted and added to each of two tubes.

3. One tube is placed in the refrigerator at 4°C, and the other tube is placed in the water bath at 50°C. The tubes are allowed to remain for 2 hours, and then both are centrifuged at 2,500 rpm for 10 minutes.

4. The supernatant (0.1 ml) is removed from each of the tubes and is added to 5-ml volumes of the cyanmethemoglobin reagent. The tubes are allowed to stand 10 minutes at room temperature and are centrifuged at 3,000 rpm for 30–45 minutes.

5. The supernatants are removed carefully from each tube, and their optical densities are read spectrophotometrically at 540 nm. The instrument is blanked using 0.1 ml buffer added to 5 ml of the cyanmethemoglobin reagent.

Calculation

$$\text{Optical density of tube at 4°C} - \left(\frac{\text{optical density of tube at 50°C}}{\text{optical density of tube at 4°C}} \right) \times 100$$

$$= \text{Precipitated hemoglobin (\%)}$$

Reference Range

Less than 5% of normal hemoglobin precipitates at 50°C.

Sources of Error

Blood should be less than 72 hours old to be suitable for testing. The presence of an unstable hemoglobin should always be confirmed by other tests, including the isopropanol precipitation test, the examination of red-cell morphologic features, hemoglobin electrophoresis, and tests for red-cell inclusion bodies. It is important to monitor the water bath temperature carefully, as false-positive test results may be found if the temperature exceeds 50°C.

Alkali Denaturation Test for Fetal Hemoglobin—Middle Range

Principle

A hemolysate is prepared and converted to cyanmethemoglobin, which then is exposed to a strong alkaline solution. Normal hemoglobin becomes denatured after this exposure, but Hb F is resistant and is not destroyed. After a specific time, denaturation is stopped by the addition of ammonium sulfate, which lowers the pH and precipitates the denatured hemoglobin (Singer et al., 1951).

Reagents and Equipment

1. Potassium hydroxide, 0.465 M (pH 12.7): Potassium hydroxide, 0.465 g, is dissolved in 100 ml distilled water.
2. Ammonium sulfate, 50% saturated: Approximately 500 g of the salt is added to 500 ml cold distilled water. It is mixed well and allowed to stand at room temperature for 20–30 minutes. One volume of the supernatant-saturated solution is removed and diluted with an equal volume of distilled water. Two milliliters of 10-N hydrochloric acid are added. The pH should be 2.8–3.0.
3. Normal saline.
4. Saponin.
5. Chloroform.
6. Spectrophotometer.
7. Stopwatch.
8. Water bath, 20°C.
9. Thermometer.
10. Pipettes: 5 ml, graduated; 0.02-ml and 0.1-ml micropipettes.
11. Filter paper: Whatman no. 14.
12. Centrifuge.
13. Tubes: 13 × 100 mm.

Specimen

EDTA-anticoagulated blood is used.

Method

1. A red-cell hemolysate is prepared as follows: 3–5 ml of anticoagulated blood are washed in double their volume of normal saline. The cell washing is repeated twice. Approximately 1 mg saponin is added. The solution is mixed and left for 10–15 minutes. An amount of chloroform equal to half the volume of packed red cells is added. The tube is stoppered and placed on a rotating mixer for 5 minutes. It is examined macroscopically for hemolysis. If not complete, lysis is accelerated by freezing

and quickly thawing the specimen. The specimen is centrifuged at 2,500 rpm for 15 minutes to remove stroma. It is kept until the following tubes are set up. The hemolysate is stable for at least 7 days at 4°C.

2. Potassium hydroxide (1.6-ml volumes of 0.465 M) is placed into two tubes (test and control). These are allowed to attain room temperature or are placed in a 20°C water bath.

3. Five milliliters of distilled water are placed into each of two tubes. Then 0.02 ml of patient hemolysate is added to one tube and an equal amount of control hemolysate is added to the other.

4. The optical densities of these tubes are read spectrophotometrically at 540 nm, using distilled water as a blank. This is the total hemoglobin reading.

5. Patient and control hemolysates (0.1 ml each) are added to the potassium hydroxide tube described previously. After *exactly* 60 seconds, 3.4 ml of the 50% saturated ammonium sulfate is added to the mixture, and the tubes are mixed well. They are left undisturbed for 30 minutes and then are filtered through double-thickness filter paper. The optical density is read spectrophotometrically at 540 nm. This is the Hb F reading.

Calculation

$$\frac{\text{Optical density of fetal hemoglobin}}{\text{Optical density of total hemoglobin}} \times$$
$$0.203 \times 100 = \text{Hb F } (\%)$$

Reference Range

The reference range is 0–2%.

Sources of Error

The alkali denaturation test is useful in quantitating Hb F and other resistant hemoglobins, such as Hb Bart's, if present in concentrations in the middle range (15–40%). It is not sufficiently sensitive to detect small amounts of resistant hemoglobin found in many cases of thalassemia minor but may be of use in detecting hereditary persistence of Hb F (HPFH). To detect low levels of Hb F accurately, the Betke method can be used. This method is sensitive for Hb F levels between 1 and 15%.

Decreased test sensitivity can result from making up a hemolysate containing less than 10 g/dl hemoglobin, and falsely decreased Hb F values may occur if the pH of the ammonium sulfate is less than 2.7. Fresh half-saturated ammonium sulfate reagent should be made when values of Hb F appear to be falsely elevated.

Clinical Correlation

Increased levels of Hb F are found in neonates (55–85%). They usually decline to adult normal levels by the age of 2 years. Hb F is increased also in sickle cell anemia, thalassemia, aplastic anemia, acute leukemia, and HPFH. The levels found, however, do not exceed 4% of the total hemoglobin.

Alkali Denaturation Test for Fetal Hemoglobin— Low Range

Principle

The alkali denaturation test for Hb F in the low range (Betke et al., 1959) is founded on a principle similar to that described for the Singer middle-range procedure (page 314).

Reagents and Equipment

1. Cyanmethemoglobin reagent: Potassium ferricyanide, 0.2 g, and 0.2 g potassium cyanide are dissolved in distilled water and diluted to 1 liter. This reagent should be stored in a dark bottle at room temperature and is stable for 2 months under these conditions.
2. Sodium hydroxide, 1.2 N: Stock 2.5-N sodium hydroxide, 1 ml, is diluted with 1 ml distilled water. It is stored in a plastic bottle at room temperature.
3. Ammonium sulfate, saturated aqueous: 500 g of the salt are added to 800 ml distilled water. The mixture is warmed and then diluted to 1 liter.
4. Pipettes: 1 ml, 2 ml, 5 ml, and 10 ml, graduated.
5. Stopwatch.
6. Filter paper: Whatman no. 1.
7. Volumetric flasks: 25 ml.
8. Spectrophotometer.
9. Balance.
10. Tubes: 17 × 100 mm.

Specimen

The specimen should be EDTA-anticoagulated blood.

Method

1. A red-cell hemolysate is prepared as described in the previous section on middle-range testing (page 314) and is diluted with cyanmethemoglobin reagent to make a 4.5- to 6.0-mg/ml solution. This is done by adding 0.2–0.5 ml hemolysate to 8 ml cyanmethemoglobin reagent.
2. Sodium hydroxide (0.2 ml of 1.2-N solution) is pipetted into 2.8 ml of the diluted hemolysate in a tube. It is mixed, and the stopwatch is started immediately.
3. After exactly 2 minutes, 2 ml saturated ammonium sulfate is added. The solution is mixed by inversion and is allowed to stand at room temperature for 5 minutes.
4. The mixture is filtered through a double layer of filter paper, and the filtrate is collected. This is the fetal filtrate, which should be clear. The optical density of the filtrate then is read spectrophotometrically at 540 nm against a blank composed of 2.8 ml cyanmethemoglobin reagent, 0.2 ml 1.2-N sodium hydroxide, and 2 ml saturated ammonium sulfate.
5. Cyanmethemoglobin hemolysate (2.8 ml), described previously, is added to a volumetric flask and diluted to 25 ml with distilled water. The optical density of this solution is read as before against the same blank as described in step 4. This is the total filtrate.

Calculation

$$\frac{\text{Optical density of fetal tube}}{(\text{Optical density of total tube} \times 5)} \times 100 = \text{Hb F}\,(\%)$$

Reference Range

The reference range is 0–2%.

Sources of Error

Known normal and abnormal control samples should be run simultaneously with this test. Abnormal control specimens can be made by mixing ABO-compatible adult and cord blood together in various proportions and establishing acceptable limits by replicate testing.

Detection of Intracellular Fetal Hemoglobin Modified

Principle

Hb A is eluted from the red cells by an acid phosphate buffer. Hb F resists elution and can be seen intracellularly after counterstaining (Kleihauer et al., 1957).

Reagents and Equipment

1. Fixative, 80% ethyl alcohol.
2. Phosphate buffer (pH 3.2): Disodium hydrogen phosphate (0.2 M), 14.2 g, is dissolved and diluted to 500 ml with distilled water. Citric acid (0.1 M), 10.5 g, is dissolved and diluted to 500 ml with distilled water. A working solution is made before use by adding 13.3 ml 0.2-M disodium hydrogen phosphate to 36.7 ml 0.1-M citric acid. The buffer is checked before use and is adjusted accordingly to pH 3.2. The buffer is stable for 6 months when stored at 4°C.
3. Eosin, 0.5% aqueous solution, which is stable for 6 months when stored at 4°C.
4. Coplin jar.
5. Normal saline.

Specimen

The specimen consists of EDTA-anticoagulated blood. Positive and negative control specimens should be set up routinely and run with the test. Two positive control samples should be used, one consisting of cord blood and the other containing one volume of cord blood and nine volumes of an ABO-compatible adult blood. A negative control sample of adult blood should also be used.

Method

1. One volume of whole blood is diluted with one volume of normal saline. The mixture is placed in a clean stoppered tube and is mixed. A thin blood smear is prepared according to the method described on page 267.

2. The smear is allowed to air-dry and then is placed in a Coplin jar containing 80% ethyl alcohol to fix for 5 minutes. All smears should be fixed within 1 hour of preparation.

3. The acid buffer is warmed to 37°C in another Coplin jar, and the fixed smears are immersed for 10 minutes. The slide is agitated continuously. If the preparation is successful, the buffer becomes slightly tinged with hemoglobin whether or not fetal cells are present.

4. The smears are washed in distilled water for 10–20 seconds and are stained with eosin for 5 minutes.

5. The smears are rewashed under running tap water for 1 minute, are allowed to air-dry, and are examined microscopically using a ×40 objective.

Interpretation

Cells containing Hb F are stained proportionately to the concentration present. Normal cells appear as pale gray-pink "ghosts" in the background.

Sources of Error

Reticulocytes may resist elution and can appear as Hb F–containing cells. Hb F may be present in normal adult blood in small quantities (0–1%) and, consequently, occasional stained cells may be seen. Usually, they have intermediate staining properties, lacking the highly refractile and deeply stained appearance of the characteristic fetal cell.

Technical problems associated with the test are primarily in the buffer pH and in the environmental testing temperature. Buffer pH should be closely checked because, if it is increased, more adult hemoglobin is retained in the cells, producing false-positive results. Temperatures greater than 25°C during slide fixation inhibit adult hemoglobin elution and also promote false-positive results.

Detection of Hemoglobin A_2 by Column Chromatography

Principle

In certain buffer systems, the interaction of charged groups on the ion exchange resin with charged groups on the hemoglobin molecules causes the separation of different hemoglobin fractions. Hb A_2 can be separated using TRIS–hydrochloric acid buffer (Efremov, 1974).

Reagents and Equipment

1. Potassium cyanide, 2% aqueous.
2. Hydrochloric acid, 10 N.
3. Stock buffer (TRIS, 1 M): TRIS primary standard, 121.1 g, is dissolved in 1 liter of distilled water.
4. Working buffers (pH 8.5, 8.3, and 7.0): Potassium cyanide, 0.6 g, is added to 300 ml of the stock buffer. The solution is divided into three equal parts, and these are adjusted to pH 8.5, 8.3, and 7.0, respectively, by adding concentrated hydrochloric acid. Each buffer is diluted to 2 liters with distilled water, and the solutions are stored at room temperature.
5. Anion exchanger—diethylaminoethylcellulose (DE-52): The DE-52 is washed several times with large volumes of the working buffer (pH 8.5), prepared as previously described. The supernatant is poured off after the last wash, and the pH is checked. The DE-52 is stored as a slurry in a covered container with the supernatant volume of buffer equal to approximately 0.7 times that of the settled anion exchanger. The solution is stored at room temperature.
6. Columns: Disposable Pasteur pipettes are set up in a vertical position on stands, and small cotton plugs are placed loosely in the narrow end of the tube. The column and cotton plug are moistened with pH 8.5 buffer, and the column is filled with DE-52 to a height of 5 cm. The tube is sealed until ready to use.
7. Spectrophotometer.
8. Pipettes: 1 ml and 5 ml, graduated; Pasteur.
9. Volumetric flasks: 10 ml, 25 ml, 100 ml, 1 liter, 2 liter.
10. Tubes: 12×75 mm.
11. Normal saline.
12. Centrifuge.
13. Toluene.

Specimen

EDTA-anticoagulated blood is the specimen used. Hemolysate preparation consists of 1 ml EDTA-anticoagulated whole blood added to 15 ml normal saline. It is mixed by inversion and centrifuged at 2,500 rpm for 10 minutes. Approximately 0.2–0.3 ml of packed red cells are removed with a Pasteur pipette, with care taken to bypass the buffy coat. The cells are washed three times with normal saline. Six to 10 volumes of distilled water and one-half volume of toluene are added to the packed cells and are mixed well by constant inversion of the tube. The cells are allowed to hemolyze for 5–10 minutes, and the hemolysate is centrifuged to separate the red-cell stroma. The supernatant is transferred to a clean tube and is stoppered and stored at 4°C until one is ready to use it. The hemolysate (one volume) is diluted with six volumes of distilled water and one volume of 2% potassium cyanide.

Method

1. Excess buffer is removed from the top of the column, and the diluted hemolysate is added slowly to the column.
2. The buffer, pH 8.3, is applied to the top of the column and, when the Hb A_2 has begun to move away from the remaining hemoglobin at the top, the effluent dripping from the bottom is collected in a 10-ml volumetric flask.
3. After the Hb A_2 has eluted, the pH 7.0 buffer is added to the top of the column, and the effluent that contains the remaining hemoglobin is collected in a 25-ml volumetric flask.
4. The optical densities of the eluted hemoglobins are read spectrophotometrically at 415 nm.

Calculation

$$\frac{\text{Optical density of Hb } A_2}{\left[\begin{array}{c}\text{Optical density} \\ \text{of Hb } A_2\end{array} + \left[2.5 \times \begin{array}{c}\text{optical density} \\ \text{of remaining hemoglobin}\end{array}\right]\right]}$$
$$\times 100 = \text{Hb } A_2 \ (\%)$$

Reference Range

In normal individuals, the reference range is 1.7–3.5% Hb A_2. In individuals with β-thalassemia trait, the reference range is higher at 3.9–6.5% Hb A_2.

Sources of Error

When the DE-52 column is being packed, one can avoid creating bubbles in the packed resin by moistening the cotton plug and the column with buffer. The diluted sample must be placed slowly on the resin. If it is squirted down the column, poor separation will take place.

This method also is useful for quantitating Hb A_2 and Hb S in hemolysates that contain Hb S, using a 15-cm column and the modifications that follow: Hb A_2 is eluted with pH 8.35 buffer and is collected in a 10-ml flask, starting when the hemoglobin has reached the lower part of the column. The Hb S zone is eluted with pH 8.2 buffer, and the residual hemoglobin is eluted with pH 7.0 buffer. The volumes of the later two eluates are adjusted to 25 ml with appropriate buffer. If this modification is used (Miale, 1982), the procedure requires 5 hours to complete. The eluates are read spectrophotometrically, as previously described.

Clinical Correlation

Hb A_2 levels are increased in thalassemia trait, Hb Zurich, Hb Tacoma, and pernicious anemia. Using column chromatography, Hb C, Hb E, and Hb O cannot be distinguished from Hb A_2.

Determination of Bart's Hemoglobin by Column Chromatography

Principle

The principle underlying the determination of Hb Bart's by column chromatography is similar to that of Hb A_2 separation by column chromatography (Henson et al., 1980). A hemolysate of whole cord blood is absorbed onto a preconditioned CM-52 cellulose column bed. Hb Bart's is eluted selectively from the column under specific conditions of pH and chloride ion concentration.

Reagents and Equipment

1. Chromatographic columns.
2. Eluting reagents: Hb Bart's other hemoglobins.
3. Sample preparation reagent: All three reagents are available from Isolab, Akron, OH.

4. Spectrophotometer.
5. Normal saline.
6. Carbon tetrachloride.
7. Tubes: 12 × 75 mm.
8. Pipettes: 1 ml, graduated; 0.2-ml micropipettes.
9. Centrifuge.

Specimen

The specimen is either EDTA-anticoagulated or heparinized cord blood. It is stable for up to 2 weeks when stored at 4°C. The specimen must not be frozen or stored as a hemolysate.

Method

1. All reagents and columns should be allowed to reach room temperature.

2. A hemolysate is prepared by washing the test cells three times with normal saline and lysing with an equal volume of water plus two-tenths volume of carbon tetrachloride. Twenty minutes are allowed for complete lysis to occur, and cell stroma is removed by centrifugation at 2,000 rpm for 10–15 minutes. Hemolysate (0.2 ml) is added to 0.6 ml of sample preparation reagent and is mixed by inversion.

3. Fresh columns are set up by removing the column's top cap and then the bottom closure. The top disc is pushed down until it just contacts the top of the chromatographic bed. The remaining buffer is aspirated to remove resin particles from the top disc.

4. The prepared hemolysate (0.4 ml) is added to the top of the column. The column is allowed to drain until the liquid level reaches the top disc.

5. The test sample is rinsed from the sides of the column with approximately 0.2 ml of the Hb Bart's elution reagent, and the liquid is allowed to flow until the level reaches the top disc. The solution that has eluted from the column is discarded.

6. A clean tube is placed under the column, and 4 ml of the elution reagent is added to the column. It is allowed to drain until the liquid level reaches the top disc. This should take less than 30 minutes. The eluate contains Hb Bart's.

7. The column is placed over a second clean tube, and 4 ml of the "other" hemoglobin elution reagent is added to the column until the liquid

reaches the top disc. The second tube contains the remaining hemoglobin in the test sample.

8. Each of the two eluates is mixed and read spectrophotometrically at 415 nm, according to the following procedure: After first zeroing the spectrophotometer with water, the optical density of the Hb Bart's fraction is read and recorded. One milliliter of the other hemoglobin fraction is diluted to 20 ml with distilled water and is read as described.

Calculation

$$\frac{\text{Optical density of Hb Bart's fraction}}{\left[\text{Optical density of Hb Bart's fraction} + \left(20 \times \begin{array}{l}\text{optical density}\\\text{of other hemoglobin fraction}\end{array}\right)\right]}$$

$$\times 100 = \text{Hb Bart's } (\%)$$

If the optical density of the Hb Bart's fraction exceeds one, 1 ml of the fraction is diluted to 5 ml with distilled water, and the optical density is read again. The formula to calculate the percentage of Hb Bart's then is as follows:

$$\frac{\text{Optical density of Hb Bart's fraction}}{\begin{array}{l}\text{Optical density of Hb Bart's fraction} + \\ (4 \times \text{optical density of the} \\ \text{other hemoglobin fraction})\end{array}} \times 100$$

Reference Range

The reference range is 0–1% for cord blood.

Sources of Error

This chromatographic separation should not be used on adult blood. Common hemoglobinopathies such as Hb S and Hb C do not interfere with the test, although it is possible that hemoglobin variants possessing electrophoretic mobilities faster than Hb A, such as Hb J or Hb N, may interfere by chromatographing with Hb Bart's. The test is useful in the identification of α-thalassemia, as the percentage of Hb Bart's present is a direct reflection of the extent of the disease.

Clinical Correlation

In homozygous α_1-thalassemia, all α-chain genes are nonfunctional. This is the most severe manifestation of the disorder and is always fatal. Hb Bart's is present as 80% or more of the total hemoglobin. The mildest form, heterozygous α_2-thalassemia, with only one gene inactivated, usually shows Hb Bart's levels of 0.8–3%. This mild abnormality is asymptomatic and can easily escape detection. Heterozygous α_1-thalassemia and homozygous α_2-thalassemia have the same Hb Bart's level, as well as similar clinical pictures that may be confused with iron-deficiency anemia and other microcytic hypochromic pictures (Adams and Steinberg, 1977).

The incidence of the various forms of α-thalassemia varies among different populations. The frequency of the α_2-thalassemia disorders (both heterozygous and homozygous) is approximately 30% in American blacks and is found less frequently in Mediterranean and Asian peoples (Dozy et al., 1979).

Hemoglobin C Inclusions

Principle

Hb C crystallizes in vitro when the level is greater than 44% and under conditions that favor partial drying and hemolysis of the red cells.

Reagents and Equipment

1. Sodium citrate, 3% aqueous solution.
2. Petroleum jelly.
3. Microscope.
4. Slides and coverslips.

Specimen

Citrated whole blood is used.

Method

1. An aliquot of the red cells is washed three times in 3% sodium citrate and then is resuspended in five volumes of the citrate. The cell suspension may be stored at 4°C for a day.

2. The suspension is mixed, and one drop is placed on a slide together with one drop of sodium citrate. A coverslip is made of the preparation, and it is partially sealed with petroleum jelly.

3. The specimen is examined microscopically under the high-dry objective daily for a week.

Interpretation

Hb C crystals, when present, can be identified as dark intracellular crystals of diamond, hexagonal, or tetragonal shape.

Hemoglobin Electrophoresis on Cellulose Acetate (pH 8.5)

Principle

Electrophoresis is the movement of charged particles in an electrical field. At a pH of 8.4–8.6, hemoglobin is negatively charged and migrates toward the anode, with cellulose acetate as its support medium. During this migration, various hemoglobins separate because of differences in charge resulting from structural variations of the molecule.

Reagents and Equipment

1. Chamber, which consists of the buffer reservoir separated by bridges on which the supporting media are placed.
2. Power supply, which should have adequate grounding to prevent electrical shock and should be able to generate variable voltages up to 450 V.
3. Cellulose acetate medium.
4. Applicator that allows approximately 0.5–0.6 μl of sample to be applied to the cellulose acetate. All of these first four items can be obtained from commercial manufacturers.
5. TRIS buffer (pH 8.4): TRIS, 10.2 g, along with 0.68 g EDTA and 3.2 g boric acid, is placed in deionized water and diluted to 1 liter. It should be prepared fresh daily. The pH is checked before use.
6. Ponceau S stain, 0.5%: 0.5 g of the stain and 5.0 g trichloroacetic acid are dissolved in distilled water and diluted to a final volume of 100 ml.
7. Destaining and clearing reagents: Any of the following reagents can be used for destaining and clearing—5% aqueous acetic acid, 95–100% methyl alcohol, 20% acetic acid in absolute methyl alcohol.
8. Normal saline.
9. Pipettes: Pasteur.
10. Abnormal hemoglobin control specimens.

Specimen

The specimen used is EDTA-anticoagulated blood. A hemolysate is prepared by centrifuging the anticoagulated blood at 2,500 rpm for 5 minutes. The plasma is removed with a Pasteur pipette, and the packed red cells are washed three times with large volumes of normal saline. The red cells are lysed after the final washing by adding an equal volume of distilled water and one-fourth volume of toluene. One drop of 3% potassium cyanide is added. The solution is mixed by inversion and is centrifuged to remove any red-cell stromal material that may be precipitated. The hemolysate then is transferred to a clean tube and stored in the refrigerator.

Method

Individual manufacturers usually suggest modifications of the procedure. If the instructions given in this section differ from those published by the manufacturer, the method printed for the specific product should be followed.

1. The buffer is poured into the electrophoresis chamber, and the wicks are soaked and positioned.
2. The cellulose acetate plate is presoaked in buffer for 20–30 minutes, and then excess moisture is removed by placing the plate between layers of absorbent paper.
3. The hemolysate samples are applied to the cellulose acetate side of the plate approximately 3 cm from the cathode, and at least two abnormal control specimens are set up for each plate.
4. The plate is placed in the chamber and is covered with a microscope slide.
5. Four hundred fifty volts are applied for 20 minutes, after which the power is turned off and the cellulose acetate plate is removed.
6. The specimen is stained by immersing in ponceau S for 3 minutes. The plate is washed with three consecutive washes of 5% acetic acid and is fixed in absolute methyl alcohol for 5 minutes.

7. It is cleared in 20% acetic acid in absolute methyl alcohol for 10 minutes and is dried in a warm oven at 65°C for 10 minutes.

8. The cellulose acetate plate is scanned with a scanning densitometer that produces a graphic interpretation of the hemoglobin migration.

Interpretation

The relative mobilities of the unknown sample are compared with known control samples applied on the same cellulose acetate plate. Such comparisons should be made both visually and by scanning densitometry. Controls containing at least two different hemoglobin variants should be used on each plate (e.g., Hb S and Hb C). Except for Hb Bart's and Hb H, the more commonly encountered hemoglobins that migrate faster (i.e., move more anodally) than Hb A include Hb N Baltimore and Hb J Baltimore, both of which are β-chain abnormalities and are clinically benign.

Sources of Error

Factors that influence electrophoresis include the ionic strength of the buffer, the pH, the voltage applied to the unit, the running time, and the type of supporting media. In general, ionic strengths of 0.01–0.10 M are used, and pH ranges of 8.4–8.6 are considered optimal for these media. The lower the ionic strength and the higher the voltage, the faster is the migration. However, if the voltage is too high, greater heat is produced, which ultimately denatures the hemoglobin.

Sources of error include the contamination of sample wells, applicators, blotter, or cellulose medium plates with dirt, blood, or other proteins; cloudy or deteriorated hemolysate that is old, contains red-cell stroma, or is bacteriologically contaminated; improper presoaking of the strips in buffer, causing trapped air or peeling; improper blotting of the strips, causing drying out or excess buffer retention; delay in applying samples to blotted strips, in applying current, or in removing and staining strips after electrophoresis; and improper sample application and placement of samples on the medium. (They should be placed cathodic to the midpoint to allow the proteins to migrate to the anode.) These errors are applicable also to agar gel electrophoresis.

Cellulose acetate electrophoresis is principally a screening test for abnormal hemoglobins, as it cannot separate Hb S from Hb D, Hb Lepore, or Hb G, nor can it separate Hb E from Hb A_2 (Figure 19.4). Any hemoglobin migrating in these positions should be retested using citrate agar electrophoresis.

Table 19.12 shows abnormal hemoglobins migrating closely or with Hb S on cellulose acetate electrophoresis at pH 8.4.

Hemoglobin Electrophoresis on Agar Gel (pH 6.15): Method 1

Principle

The basic principle underlying hemoglobin electrophoresis on agar gel is similar to that for hemoglobin electrophoresis on cellulose acetate (page 320; Schneider et al., 1981). Agar gel in an acidic buffer can be used to separate abnormal hemoglobins that migrate together on alkaline cellulose acetate hemoglobin electrophoresis.

Reagents and Equipment

1. Chamber, power supply, wicks, and applicator, as used for cellulose acetate electrophoresis (page 320).

2. Stock buffer, 0.5 M (pH 6.0): Stock buffer is made by dissolving 147 g sodium citrate dihydrate and 4.3 g citric acid in deionized water. It is diluted to 1 liter.

3. Working buffer: One volume of stock buffer is diluted to 10 volumes with deionized water, and the pH is adjusted to 6.0 by the addition of citric acid (30 g/dl).

4. Agar plates (Difco Bacto), 8.75 × 10 mm: Glass plates are precoated by dipping in a hot solution of 0.1% agar. They are allowed to drain and placed in an incubator at 37°C for 2–3 hours. One gram of agar is dissolved in 100 ml working citrate buffer (pH 6.0). This is heated until completely dissolved and is allowed to cool to approximately 60°C. The pretreated plates are placed on a level surface, and approximately 4 ml of the cooled agar is poured evenly on the slides. The mixture is allowed to gel and is stored by wrapping in plastic and placing in a tight box containing moistened wool.

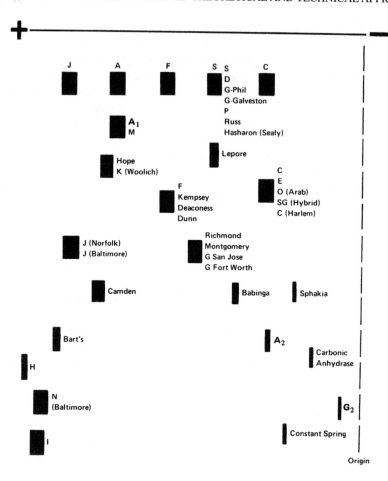

Figure 19.4. Relative mobilities of hemoglobins on cellulose acetate electrophoresis (TEB) at pH 8.4 (TEB = TRIS EDTA boric acid). (Reprinted from RM Winslow [ed]. Laboratory Methods for Detecting Hemoglobinopathies. Atlanta: Centers for Disease Control, 1984;143.)

5. Stain (amido black 10B): 10 g of the dye are dissolved in 100 ml glacial acetic acid and is diluted with distilled water to 1 liter.
6. Clearing agent: This is composed of five volumes of absolute methyl alcohol, five volumes of distilled water, and one volume of glacial acetic acid.
7. Abnormal hemoglobin control specimens.

Specimen

The specimen used is EDTA-anticoagulated blood. The hemolysate is prepared as in the alkaline cellulose acetate electrophoresis method described on page 320. It can be stored at 4°C for up to 1 week.

Method

1. Working buffer is poured into the electrophoresis tank and is cooled by placing in the re-

frigerator for 15–20 minutes. The filter paper wicks are draped on the tank shoulders.
2. The hemolysate is applied lightly to the agar plate surface with the applicator, with care taken not to break the surface of the agar. The hemolysate is placed approximately 3 cm from the anodal end of the plate. For reference, at least two abnormal control samples are set up on each plate.
3. The impregnated agar plate is placed agar-side down on the wicks and is covered with the lid; then nearly 70 V are applied for 1 hour. The electrophoresis time depends on the agar thickness, the current used, the concentration of the specimen, and the number of gel samples run concurrently. If the chamber lid becomes warm to the touch, the voltage is reduced and the specimen is rechecked.
4. The current is turned off, and the plates are placed in the amido black 10B stain for 15 minutes. They are removed, lightly rinsed in distilled water,

Table 19.12. Abnormal Hemoglobins Migrating Close to or with Hemoglobin S on Cellulose Acetate Electrophoresis at pH 8.4

Bibba
Memphis
Russ
D Los Angeles
D Ibadan
Flatbush
Zürich
Köln
G Philadelphia
G Coushatta
G Galveston
G San Jose
Lepore
L Ferrara
Shiminoseki
P
Stanleyville II
Richmond
Sabine
Ft. Worth
Hasharon

placed agar-side down on filter paper, and dried in an oven at 65°C for 1–2 hours.

5. The plates are washed in tap water and are transferred to the clearing solution until cleared. They then are returned to the oven and allowed to dry.

Hemoglobin Electrophoresis on Agar Gel (pH 6.15): Method 2

Reagents and Equipment

Reagents and equipment for this method are exactly the same as those for the previous method with the following exception: Commercially obtained cellulose acetate plates are impregnated with citrate agar by lowering a rack of plates into a container of 0.05-M citrate buffer (pH 6.0) for 30 minutes. The rack is removed and is allowed to drain. The plates are lowered into a solution of 1% melted citrate agar at 60–70°C and are allowed to stand for 30 minutes. They are removed and the agar is allowed to gel and drain. It is stored, wrapped well in plastic bags, at 4°C.

Method

1. The hemolysate is applied and the chamber is set up as previously described on page 322.
2. It is electrophoresed at 90 V for 30–45 minutes and is stained and dried as described on page 322.

Interpretation

The relative mobilities of the unknown sample are compared with known control samples applied on the same plate.

Sources of Error

Citrate agar electrophoresis cannot serve as a primary screening method for detecting hemoglobinopathies, as many of the abnormal hemoglobins migrate like Hb A and Hb F. However, the method is particularly useful in confirming the presence of Hb A, Hb F, Hb S, and Hb C. Under the test conditions described, the abnormal hemoglobins migrate as shown in Table 19.12. The procedure is particularly useful in the differentiation of Hb S from Hb D or Hb G, and Hb C and Hb E, from Hb O Arab, or Hb C Harlem

The alternative procedure using cellulose acetate–impregnated citrate agar plates is a more sensitive technique and is particularly useful in the separation of Hb Bart's and Hb Korle Bu (Figure 19.5). However, such extreme sensitivity is not required for most of the routine variants found, such as Hb F, Hb S, Hb O, and Hb C.

The control samples used in citrate agar electrophoresis should include both anodal and cathodic moving hemoglobins. Hb S and Hb C can be used easily as the anodally moving control, and Hb F can be used as the cathodically migrating hemoglobin.

Hemoglobin Electrophoresis on Starch Block (pH 7.4)

Principle

To effect hemoglobin electrophoresis on starch block (pH 7.4), red cells are lysed, and the hemoglobin is separated by using a starch gel support (modified from Smithies, 1955). The gel is in contact with a

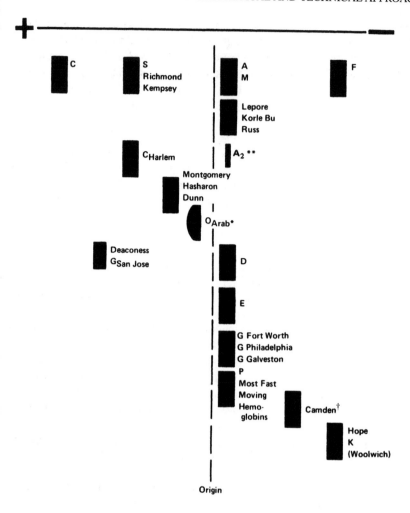

Figure 19.5. Relative mobilities of some hemoglobins on citrate agar electrophoresis at pH 6.0–6.2. (* = indicates variable between A and S; ** = depending on sample concentration; † = degradation, if present, may be observed between A and F.) (Reprinted from RM Winslow [ed]. Laboratory Methods for Detecting Hemoglobinopathies. Atlanta: Centers for Disease Control, 1984;145.)

barbital buffer through which a constant voltage is passed. The isolated fractions are then separated and quantitated spectrophotometrically at 540 nm.

Reagents and Equipment

1. Potato starch (available from Fisher Scientific, Pittsburgh, PA).
2. Phosphate buffer (pH 7.4): Disodium hydrogen phosphate, 26.7 g, is dissolved in 1 liter distilled water (1 M), and 13.65 g potassium dihydrogen phosphate is dissolved in 1 liter of distilled water (1 M). Disodium hydrogen phosphate, 112 ml (1 M), is added to 496 ml 1-M potassium dihydrogen phosphate and diluted to 8 liters with distilled water. The pH is checked and adjusted to 7.4.
3. Barbital buffer pH 8.6: Sodium barbital, 82.4 g, and 14 g barbital are dissolved in 1 liter of warm distilled water and diluted to 8 liters. The pH is checked and adjusted to 8.6.
4. Power pack.
5. Casserole dishes: Four glass baking dishes, each approximately 24 × 10 × 5 cm.
6. Wire coils: Nichrome wire, diameter 0.25 mm; two coils approximately 90 cm long and 7.5 cm in diameter.
7. Cellulose sponge cloths (two): each 20 × 12.5 cm.
8. Spatula.
9. Sodium cyanide, 2% aqueous.
10. Acetic acid 10%.
11. Toluene.
12. Normal saline.
13. Potassium ferricyanide, 5% aqueous.
14. Tuberculin syringe and 22-gauge needle.
15. Glass funnel: 2 liter.

16. Filter paper: Whatman no. 3.
17. Glass or plastic sheet: 45 × 25 cm.
18. Pipettes: 0.5-ml and 0.05-ml micropipettes.
19. Known control samples (treated as described for the test).

Specimen

EDTA-anticoagulated or heparinized blood is used.

Preparation of Hemolysate

1. Five milliliters of anticoagulated blood are centrifuged at 2,000 rpm for 5 minutes. The plasma is discarded, and the red cells are washed three times with copious volumes of normal saline.
2. Distilled water (1.4 ml) is added to 1 ml of packed cells. This is shaken well to mix, and 0.4 ml toluene is added to the laked red cells. The tube is stoppered and shaken vigorously for 5 minutes. It is centrifuged at 3,000 rpm for 15–20 minutes.
3. The toluene layer is removed by absorbing with filter paper, and the hemolysate is removed with a Pasteur pipette, with care taken not to disturb or include any red-cell stroma. The specimen is stored frozen.

Preparation of the Starch Plate

1. A sheet of heavy glass or plastic is washed thoroughly with soap and water and then is rinsed in distilled water and dried. Strips of adhesive masking tape are placed along the plate so that they extend to approximately 5 cm around the corners. The tape should be placed so that it is 8–12 mm above the plate. Blotter pads are placed against the open ends of the plate and are held in place temporarily with a heavy object. The plate now is ready for the application of the starch.
2. Approximately 500 g purified potato starch is dispensed into a 1-liter beaker. Sufficient barbital buffer is added until a uniform paste is formed. The paste is filtered through several thicknesses of Whatman no. 3 filter paper using a fritted glass funnel attached to a vacuum line or pump.
3. The washed starch is mixed with 400 ml barbital buffer and is allowed to settle for several minutes. The foam and excess buffer are removed with a pipette.

4. The starch paste is poured onto the prepared plate. The consistency should be similar to that of freshly prepared plaster. All air bubbles are removed, and the block is allowed to dry on an even surface at room temperature.

Method

1. The prepared hemolysate is converted to cyanmethemoglobin pigment by adding 0.05 ml 5% potassium ferricyanide to 0.3 ml hemolysate. The mixture is allowed to stand for 5–10 minutes.
2. A mixture composed of 11 volumes 2% sodium cyanide and 3 volumes 10% acetic acid (0.05 ml of this mixture) is added to the hemolysate-ferricyanide mixture and is allowed to stand for 5–10 minutes.
3. Slits are cut in the starch block using the spatula blade. Each slit should be approximately 10 mm long and spaced at 2.5-cm intervals down the width of the plate. If the starch fuses the slits after they are cut, the block is allowed to dry for a longer period and the slits are reopened with the spatula blade. The block is ready for use when the spatula blade can be inserted into the starch and the slit remains discrete.
4. Approximately 0.02 ml hemolysate is applied to the starch slit with a tuberculin syringe and 22-gauge needle or a plain capillary tube. The hemolysate should spread evenly through the slit. If the starch block is too wet, the slits will fuse, and if it is too dry, the hemolysate will not spread evenly. To aid in the spreading of the hemolysate, a few drops of buffer may be placed around the application.
5. After the sample has been applied, the tape is removed from around the plate, and the slits are closed by simultaneously moving the spatula gently in the slits and applying a drop of phosphate buffer. The starch will flow together when sufficiently wet.
6. Three thicknesses of Whatman no. 3 filter paper are cut into 10 × 20–cm strips and are soaked in the barbital buffer. Two and one-half centimeters of the long side of the filter paper are placed over the ends of the starch block and are folded down the other end so that it is ready to be placed in the barbital buffer dishes of the equipment.
7. The four dishes are placed in the refrigerator. The two center dishes are half-filled with phosphate buffer, and the outside dishes are half-filled with barbital buffer.

8. The nickel-chromium wire coiled electrodes are placed in the phosphate buffer dishes, and the paired buffer dishes (one barbital and one phosphate) are joined by immersing the cellulose sponge cloths in each dish.

9. The starch plate level is set on the dishes so that three thicknesses of filter paper are immersed in the barbital buffer.

10. The wire coils are connected to the power pack through the rubber gasket of the refrigerator door so that the negative pole is connected to the coil on the side of the plate nearest the hemolysate application. The positive electrode is connected to the remaining coil.

11. The refrigerator door is closed, and electrophoresis is begun and maintained for 18 hours at 500 milliamperes (mA) and 410 V at 4%.

12. The power is turned off, the starch plate is removed, and the *underside* of the starch block is examined. It is possible to invert the plate without disturbing either the starch or the hemoglobin migration.

13. Quantitative estimations can be made of each hemoglobin band by cutting the starch, removing the band, and eluting the hemoglobin by washing the starch four times with an equal volume of distilled water. All washings are pooled and read spectrophotometrically at 540 nm.

Results

Qualitative results are obtained by comparing the migration rates against known control samples. For a permanent record of the electrophoresis, a record is made by photographing the *underside* of the plate within 30 minutes of discontinuing electrophoresis, because discrete hemoglobin bands tend to diffuse into the surrounding starch.

Sources of Error

To obtain optimal resolution, the hemolysate initially applied to the starch should have a hemoglobin concentration of 3–4 g/dl but, if small amounts of a minor hemoglobin are present, the hemolysate concentration should be made to be between 10–12 g/dl. Figure 19.6 illustrates the relative mobilities of some abnormal hemoglobins on starch-block electrophoresis at pH 7.4. The starch-block electrophoresis technique

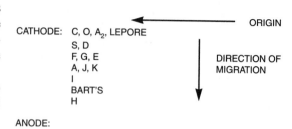

CATHODE: C, O, A_2, LEPORE
S, D
F, G, E
A, J, K
I
BART'S
H

ANODE:

ORIGIN

DIRECTION OF MIGRATION

Figure 19.6. Relative mobilities of some hemoglobins on starch-block electrophoresis at pH 7.4.

can be modified by using a variety of different buffers varying in pH from 6.5 to 9.0. The buffer system described is useful in detecting small quantities of Hb Bart's and Hb H and separates the fast-moving hemoglobins, such as Hb H from Hb I.

Hemoglobin Isoelectric Focusing

Principle

Hemoglobin is applied to a 1-mm precast agarose gel containing Ampholytes (Isolab, Akron, OH) at pH 6.8. These are low-molecular-weight amphoteric molecules having varying isoelectric points. The Ampholytes migrate to their isoelectric points along the gel, the result of which is the formation of a stable pH gradient.

The hemoglobin variants also migrate through the gel until they reach the area where their individual isoelectric points equal the corresponding pH on the gel. At this point, the charge on the variant will be zero, and the migration will stop. The electrical field will counteract diffusion, and the hemoglobin variant will form a sharply defined band. This band is then stained with O-dianisidine, which becomes oxidized by the heme in the presence of hydrogen peroxide to form an insoluble precipitate. The precipitate is formed proportional to the amount of hemoglobin present.

Reagents and Equipment

A Resolve Hemoglobin Neonatal Screening Kit (available from Isolab, catalog no. FR-9400) is used as follows:

1. Agarose isoelectric focus gels containing Resolve Ampholytes, 2.5% wt/vol, pH 6.8 (gel size 203 × 240 × 1 mm): Store at 2–8°C.
2. Anode solution (no. 1): acetic acid (0.5 mol/liter, pH 2.5), stored at 15–30°C.
3. Cathode solution (no. 2): ethanolamine (0.5 mol/liter) and potassium cyanide (0.1% wt/vol), stored at 15–30°C.
4. Hemoglobin eluting solution (no. 3): potassium cyanide (0.05% wt/vol), sodium azide (0.01% wt/vol), and 1% Triton X-100, stored at 15–30°C.
5. Blotting paper.
6. Sample application templates.
7. Isoelectric focus electrode wicks.
8. Trichloroacetic acid 10% (Isolab catalog no. 1981995101).
9. Isoelectric focusing unit (LKB Pharmacia, Summitt, NJ).
10. Pipette: 0–10 μl.
11. Scanning densitometer.
12. Sample application guide.
13. Hole punch.
14. Panogel blotters (Princeton Separates, Princeton, NJ, catalog no. DR47617).
15. Semiautomatic pipettes: 200 μl–5 ml.
16. Oven: 55–60°C.

Specimen

The specimen used is EDTA-anticoagulated blood, which can be stored at 4°C for 3 weeks. Pediatric samples can be collected on filter paper and stored at room temperature.

Whole blood, 25 μl, is added to 200 μl hemoglobin elution solution (bottle no. 3), mixed, and allowed to stand for 10 minutes. If the filter-paper collection method is used, punch out two 7-mm circles and place into 200 μl elution solution. Allow to stand for 10 minutes.

Method

1. The cooling plate and power supply are prepared. The cooling plate should be at 15°C before electrophoresis.
2. The gel is removed from the package and placed on the sample application guide. It must be blotted gently.

3. Two wicks are placed on a clean Panogel blotter, and each is saturated with 5 ml anode solution (no. 1). The excess is blotted gently on the blotter pad, and the wicks are placed along the centerline of the gel. If they overlap the gel, the wicks must be trimmed.

4. Any of the anode solution is cleaned from the equipment, and another precut wick is placed on a separate Panogel blotter and saturated with cathode solution (no. 2). Any excess fluid is blotted from the blotter pad, and the wick is positioned along the centerline of the gel. If it overlaps the gel, the wick must be trimmed.

5. Two sample templates are positioned along both sides of the center cathode wick. These are smoothed down to ensure that there are no bubbles that might cause the sample to leak into adjacent wells.

6. Hemoglobin solution, 3 μl (5 μl if the pediatric collection system is used), is added to each sample well by way of a microdispenser. The samples are allowed to dry into the gel for 5–10 minutes. The templates are removed before isoelectric focusing is carried out. These are rinsed in deionized water.

7. Water, 5 ml, is spread onto the cooling plate, and the gel then is transferred onto this plate. Air bubbles must be prevented from forming between the plate and the gel. Excess water is blotted from around the gel.

8. The three electrodes (anode, cathode, anode) are adjusted so that they make even contact along the center of all the wicks when the lid is in the "run" position.

9. The leads are connected to the power supply, and the power is turned on to 40 watts. Electrophoresis is carried out for 1.5 hours or until forward migration ceases and tight thin bands are formed.

10. The gel is submerged immediately in 10% trichloroacetic acid for 10 minutes.

11. The trichloroacetic acid is poured off, and the gel is soaked in 1–2 liters of deionized water for 20 minutes. Two more rinses are conducted using fresh water.

12. The water is poured off, and the gel is allowed to dry in an oven at 55–60°C for 30–45 minutes. Then the gel is scanned in the densitometer at 540 nm.

Interpretation

Hemoglobins migrate from the anode to the cathode as follows:

Anode H
Bart's
N Baltimore, I Texas, Hopkins II
J
Campertown
Strasbourg
F
A1c
A, Hammersmith, Brigham, Bethesda
Milwaukee, Köln
Saki
M Saskatoon
G Georgia
M Boston
G San Jose
Mobile
G Coushatta, P Galveston, Philadelphia
D Ouled, Baylor
D Punjab
Korle Bu
Montgomery
S
G Galveston, G Norfolk
Hasharon
D Iran, Zuridi
Methemoglobin
E, C Harlem, O Arab
A_2
C
C Ziguinchor
Constant Spring

If Hb N Baltimore is suspected, electrophoresis should be done on cellulose acetate to differentiate Hb N Baltimore from Hb I Texas. In addition, Hb N usually shows a 1:1 ratio with Hb A, whereas Hb I shows a 3:1 ratio with Hb A. If Hb E is suspected, electrophoresis on citrate agar is recommended to separate Hb E from Hb C Harlem and Hb O Arab.

Identification of Abnormal Hemoglobins

Cellulose Acetate Electrophoresis

Hb A_2, Hb C, Hb O, and Hb E cannot be differentiated on the basis of electrophoretic mobility on cellulose acetate. Likewise, Hb D, Hb G, and Hb Lepore cannot be distinguished from Hb S. Hb F is poorly resolved from Hb A, and Hb H and Hb

I are indistinguishable from each other. However, Hb A_2 rarely constitutes more than 10% of the total hemoglobin and, consequently, if a very slow-moving band constitutes more than 20% of the total hemoglobin, it may be presumed to be Hb C, Hb O, or Hb E. Hb C and Hb O are virtually limited to peoples of Central African ancestry, whereas Hb E is found commonly in Southeast Asian populations.

Hb Lepore may be separated from Hb S, Hb D, or Hb G by the fact that it commonly represents 25–45% of the total hemoglobin. In a similar way, Hb H constitutes approximately 10–15% of the total hemoglobin, whereas Hb I usually is 25% or so.

Thus, by measuring the proportions of these hemoglobin bands densitometrically and by knowing the ethnic origin of the patient, the probable nature of the abnormal hemoglobin may be determined. However, additional confirmatory tests often are necessary before a definitive result is established. Such tests should include hemoglobin solubility (to confirm the presence of Hb S) and a thermostability test (to establish the presence of an unstable hemoglobin). The quantitative relationship of hemoglobins in sickling disorders is shown in Table 19.13.

Other hemoglobins that migrate in the same positions as Hb A on cellulose acetate electrophoresis include Hb Seattle and Hb Porto Alegre. Hemoglobins migrating similarly to Hb S include Hb Zürich and Hb Stanleyville. Hemoglobins migrating between S and C include Hb O, Hb Ube 1, and Hb Köln. Findings in the common hemoglobinopathies are listed in Table 19.14.

Agar Gel Electrophoresis

Agar gel electrophoresis is valuable in differentiating Hb C from Hb E, and Hb O or Hb S from Hb D and Hb G. Hb A_2 cannot be quantitated accurately by this procedure, so in order to rule out β-thalassemia minor, any Hb A_2 level that is greater than 3.5% should be confirmed by column chromatography. Values greater than 8% indicate the presence of additional hemoglobin variants such as Hb C, Hb E, Hb O, Hb D, or Hb G.

Hemoglobins that migrate in the same position as Hb A on citrate agar electrophoresis include Hb J

Table 19.13. Quantitative Relationships of Hemoglobins in Sickling Disorders

Hemoglobinopathy	% Hb S	% Hb Non-S
Sickle cell trait	25–40	60–75 Hb A
Sickle cell anemia	80–95	5–20 Hb F
Sβ⁰-thalassemia	80–95	5–25 Hb F
		Slight increase in Hb A₂
Sβ⁺-thalassemia	75–90	10–25 Hb A and F
		Slight increase in Hb A₂
HPFH	70–80	20–30 Hb F
		Decrease in Hb A₂

HPFH = hereditary persistence of fetal hemoglobin.
Source: Data from RG Schneider et al. Proposed Guidelines for Citrate Agar Electrophoresis for Confirming Identification of Mutant Hemoglobins. Vol 1 (no. 15). Villanova: National Committee for Clinical Laboratory Standards, 1981.

Table 19.14. Results Found in the Common Hemoglobinopathies

Disorders	Hemoglobin	Hemoglobin A₂	Hemoglobin F
Hb S trait (AS)	55% Hb A; 40% Hb S	Normal	Normal
Sickle cell anemia (SS)	95% Hb S	Normal	<15%
Heterozygote C disease (AC)	55% Hb A; 40% Hb C	Normal	Normal
Heterozygote E disease (AE)	60% Hb A; 35% Hb E	Normal	Normal
S/C disease	48% Hb S; 48% Hb C	Normal	Normal
Heterozygote β-thalassemia	90% Hb A	4–8%	<5%
Homozygote β-thalassemia	40–80% Hb A	4–8%	10–50%
Homozygote β°-thalassemia	No Hb A	4–8%	90%
α₁-Thalassemia	Normal	Normal	Normal
α₂-Thalassemia	Trace Hb H	Normal	Normal
α₃-Thalassemia	5–30% Hb H	Normal	Normal
α₄-Thalassemia	100% Hb Bart's	0	0
S β⁺-thalassemia	55% Hb S; 30% Hb A	4–8%	<5%
S β°-thalassemia	90% Hb S	4–8%	<5%
S α-thalassemia	65% Hb A; 30% Hb S	Normal	Normal

Oxford, Hb I, Hb Winnepeg, Hb Inster, and Hb Bromssais.

Other Methods

Globin-chain electrophoresis (pH 8.6 and 6.0) allows for the identification of several variants, especially HbE, Hb O, Hb D, and Hb G. Isoelectric focusing on polycrylamine gel in the pH range of 6–8 allows resolution of at least 70 hemoglobin variants. Genetic probes (DNA and RNA) have been used also to identify substitutions in structural hemoglobinopathies as well as gene deletion and transcriptional translation mutations in thalassemia.

revision 3

Globin-Chain Electrophoresis at Alkaline pH

Principle

Cellulose acetate electrophoresis is used to separate polypeptide chains of hemoglobin that have been dissociated with 6-M urea. In the presence of mercaptoethanol, heme is removed from globin. The globin migrates toward the cathode, and the heme moves toward the anode (Schneider, 1974; Schneider et al., 1981).

Reagents and Equipment

1. Power supply, chambers, applicator, and cellulose acetate strips as for cellulose acetate hemoglobin electrophoresis.
2. Urea.
3. 2-Mercaptoethanol.
4. Trichloroacetic acid, 5% aqueous.
5. Stock buffer (pH 8.6–8.7): Acid barbital, 11.2 g, is dissolved in 1 liter of boiling deionized water, and 82.4 g sodium barbital is added. The mixture is diluted to 4 liters with deionized water.
6. Working buffer (pH 8.9): Urea, 36 g, is dissolved in approximately 70 ml of the stock buffer. The volume is adjusted to 100 ml with additional buffer. It is prepared fresh just before use.
7. Stain: Ponceau S, 0.5 g, is dissolved in 100 ml 5% aqueous trichloroacetic acid.
8. Destaining reagent: acetic acid 5%.
9. Pipettes: 1 ml and 5 ml, graduated.
10. Filter paper.

Specimen

EDTA-anticoagulated blood is used. A hemolysate is prepared as described on page 320. Control samples containing at least two different abnormal hemoglobins are treated in the same way.

Method

1. Equal volumes of working buffer, 2-mercaptoethanol, and hemolysate are combined in a small tube, are mixed, and are covered and left at room temperature for 0.5–1 hour but not longer than 4 hours.

2. One and one-half milliliters of 2-mercaptoethanol are added to the working buffer. The cellulose acetate strips are soaked in this reagent for an hour or so.

3. Fifty milliliters of the buffer are poured into each side of the chamber, and the strips are blotted and draped across the supports of the electrophoresis chamber.

4. Hemolysate buffer (step 1), 2–5 μl, is applied to the center of the strip, and electrophoresis is performed for 1 hour at approximately 200 V.

5. The strips are removed and stained by placing them in 0.5% ponceau S for 5 minutes.

6. The strips are rinsed with 5% acetic acid until the background is void of color, and then the strips are allowed to air-dry.

Results

Almost immediately after the current is applied, several heme-containing bands will be seen moving rapidly toward the anode. They disappear into the buffer in approximately 15 minutes. All of the globin chains migrate toward the cathode. Figure 19.7 illustrates some of the hemoglobin variants.

Globin-Chain Electrophoresis at Acid pH

Principle

The principle underlying globin-chain electrophoresis at acid pH is the same as that in globin-chain electrophoresis at alkaline pH (Schneider, 1974; Schneider et al., 1981).

Reagents and Equipment

1. Power supply, chamber, applicator, and cellulose acetate strips as for cellulose acetate hemoglobin electrophoresis.
2. Urea.
3. 2-Mercaptoethanol.
4. Citric acid, 30% aqueous.
5. Trichloroacetic acid, 5% aqueous.
6. Stock buffer (pH 8.4): TRIS, 10.2 g, along with 0.6 g EDTA and 3.2 g boric acid, is dissolved in deionized water and diluted to 1 liter.

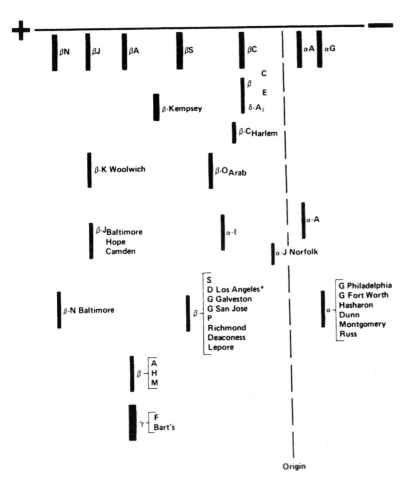

Figure 19.7. Relative mobilities of globin chains on cellulose acetate (TEB-urea buffer) at pH 8.8–9.5. (* = may move slightly off S anodally; TEB = TRIS EDTA boric acid.) (Reprinted from RM Winslow [ed]. Laboratory Methods for Detecting Hemoglobinopathies. Atlanta: Centers for Disease Control, 1984;63.)

7. Working buffer (pH 6.0–6.2): Urea, 36 g, is dissolved in approximately 70 ml of the stock buffer. The pH is adjusted to 6.0–6.2 with 30% citric acid, and the total volume is diluted to 100 ml with deionized water. The working buffer is prepared just before use.

8. Stain: Ponceau S, 0.5 g, is dissolved in 100 ml 5% trichloroacetic acid.

9. Destaining reagent: 5% acetic acid.

10. Pipettes: 1 ml and 5 ml, graduated.

11. Filter paper.

Specimen

The specimen used is EDTA-anticoagulated blood. A hemolysate is prepared as described on page 320.

Control samples containing at least two different abnormal hemoglobins are treated in the same way.

Method

1. Equal volumes of working buffer, 2-mercaptoethanol, and hemolysate are combined in a small tube, are mixed and covered, and are left at room temperature for 0.5–1.0 hour but not longer than 4 hours.

2. One and one-half milliliters of 2-mercaptoethanol are added to the working buffer. The cellulose acetate strips are soaked in this reagent for an hour or so.

3. Fifty milliliters of the buffer are poured into each side of the chamber, and the strips are blotted

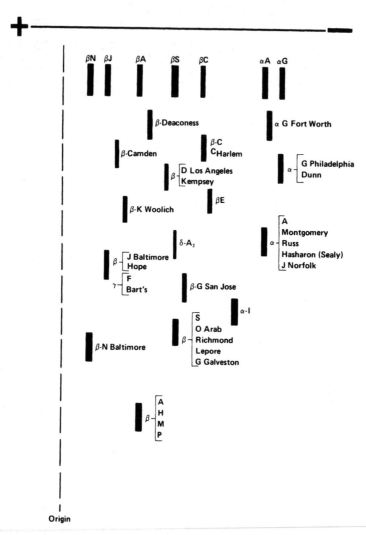

Figure 19.8. Relative mobilities of globin chains on cellulose acetate (TEB-urea buffer) at pH 6.0–6.2. (TEB = TRIS EDTA boric acid.) (Reprinted from RM Winslow [ed]. Laboratory Methods for Detecting Hemoglobinopathies. Atlanta: Centers for Disease Control, 1984;148.)

and draped across the supports of the electrophoresis chamber.

4. Hemolysate-buffer (step 1), 2–5 μl, is applied approximately 1 cm from the anodal end of the strip, and electrophoresis is performed for 2 hours at 250 V.

5. The strips are removed and stained by placing them in 0.5% ponceau S for 5 minutes.

6. The strips are rinsed in 5% acetic acid until the background is void of color, and then they are allowed to air-dry.

Results

The migration bands are compared with the control samples as in other electrophoretic procedures. Figure 19.8 illustrates the positions of some of the hemoglobin variants.

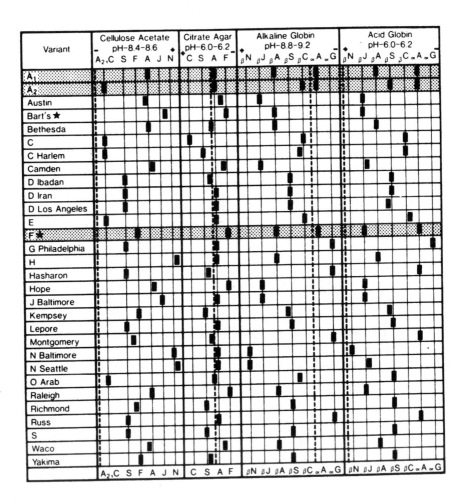

Figure 19.9. Electrophoretic patterns of some hemoglobin variants. Shaded areas indicate normal hemoglobin patterns; broken lines indicate origins; asterisk indicates that γF moves in $_β$J position on acid globins and in $_β$A position on alkaline globins. (Reprinted from RM Winslow [ed]. Laboratory Methods for Detecting Hemoglobinopathies. Atlanta: Centers for Disease Control, 1984;150.)

Sources of Error

The characterization of abnormal hemoglobins using standard cellulose acetate and citrate agar electrophoresis depends on the resolving power of these systems, which tends to be rather poor. Consequently, electrophoresis of the globin chains on cellulose acetate at acid and alkaline pH allows a better separation of the mutant chains because of the improvement in resolving power of the method. A comparison of the electrophoretic pat-

terns of some of the more common hemoglobin variants using these standard techniques is shown in Figure 19.9.

Clinical Correlation

The use of isoelectric focusing (Zeineh et al., 1975; Monte et al., 1976) on horizontal polyacrylamide gels separates proteins according to differences in their isoelectric points. The resolution obtained by this technique is superior to other types of electrophoresis, and the introduction of polyacrylamide gel as a stabilizing medium has allowed the staining and densitometric scanning of the separated proteins in approximately 3 hours. This method can be applied to the characteristics and mapping of abnormal hemoglobins but, because of the time taken to complete the separation and the relative unavailability of commercial systems, it is not recommended for routine use.

Tests for Immune Disorders

Direct Antiglobulin Test

Principle

Red cells onto the surface of which either immunoglobulin or complement has been absorbed can be agglutinated by the addition of a suitable antiglobulin reagent. This combines with the antibodies bound to the surface of adjacent cells, forming a molecular bridge and producing visible agglutination.

Reagents and Equipment

1. Antiglobulin serum (broad-spectrum): This antisera should contain antibodies to both IgG and C3d complement component. If further characterization is required for positive tests, monospecific antisera to either IgG or C3d should be used.
2. Centrifuge (Serofuge).
3. Tubes: 10 × 75 mm.
4. Normal saline.
5. Anti-D.
6. Water bath, 37°C.
7. Pasteur pipettes.

Specimen

The specimen used is EDTA-anticoagulated blood. Control specimens of both positive-coated and negative-coated cells should be tested simultaneously.

Method

1. The test cells are washed four times with copious volumes of saline to remove any traces of unbound serum proteins attached to the red-cell membrane. A final 2–5% saline cell suspension is made in fresh normal saline.
2. One volume of broad-spectrum antiglobulin serum is added to one volume of the washed red-cell suspension, is mixed by tapping the tube, and is centrifuged at 3,500 rpm for 10–15 seconds.
3. To dislodge the cell button, the technologist should gently rotate the tube between the palms of both hands. The tube must not be shaken vigorously, as this may result in false-negative test results because of the disruption of weak agglutinates. The cells are observed for macroscopic agglutination; if negative, the cell suspension is checked by viewing under a low-power lens.
4. To all negative test samples, one volume of 2–5% IgG-coated red cells is added. This either can be obtained commercially under a variety of trade names or can be prepared as outlined in the following section on controls.

Results

Agglutination of the test cells in the presence of adequate controls indicates that the *cells* are coated with an antibody. If the cells are negative, the addition of the IgG-coated cells (step 4) will result in agglutination.

Controls

Both IgG and C3d control specimens should be run in parallel with the test.

Immunoglobin G. Anti-D is suitably diluted to give a 1+ reaction with heterozygote D–positive cells (e.g., CDe/cde). Equal volumes of the diluted anti-D are added to a 2–5% saline suspension of the cells, and the mixture is incubated at 37°C for 30–60 minutes. The coated cells then are tested as described in steps 1–4 in the preceding section on method. If correctly prepared, a 1+ reaction should be obtained. Negative controls for the test can be made by using the same cells without the addition of the anti-D.

C3d. In vitro preparation of C3d-coated cells can be accomplished as follows:

1. Reagent A: Sucrose, 23.1 g, along with 0.173 g sodium dihydrogen phosphate (monohydrate) and

0.395 g disodium EDTA, is dissolved in distilled water, and this mixture is diluted to 250 ml.

2. Reagent B: Sucrose, 23.1 g, disodium hydrogen phosphate, 0.178 g, and disodium EDTA, 0.395 g, are dissolved in distilled water and diluted to 250 ml. The pH of reagent A is adjusted to 5.1 by the addition of approximately 6.5 ml reagent B.

3. The pH-adjusted reagent is chilled by refrigerating for 1–2 hours, and 1 ml acid citrate dextrose whole blood is added to 19 ml cooled reagent.

4. Immediately, 0.1 ml magnesium chloride is added (81.0 g/liter). The mixture is stirred mechanically for 1 hour, keeping the reagent chilled. The cells are washed four times with chilled normal saline in a refrigerated centrifuge. The resulting cells should be coated with C3d.

Sources of Error

False-negative test results usually are caused by incorrect technique. The principal cause of false-negative findings is the inadequate washing of the cells to remove serum protein. If some unbound protein remains in the cell suspension when the antiglobulin sera is added, neutralization of the sera occurs, resulting in a negative test result. In addition, delays in testing the patient's cells could result in antibody dissociation from the cell membrane, producing false test results.

Clinical Correlation

A positive direct antiglobulin test result is caused by coating of the red-cell membrane by antibodies. Such coating can be incited by one or more of the following situations:

Autoantibodies against red-cell antigens can form, resulting in IgG or complement sensitization.

Immune complexes can form as a result of the presence of an antidrug complex (page 99).

Antibodies against drugs can attach to the red-cell membrane. A common example of this type of mechanism is that resulting from penicillin antibodies (page 99).

A nonspecific uptake of protein attached to a modified red-cell membrane can occur, such as is seen in individuals treated with cephalothin sodium.

Antibodies can result from incompatible transfusions and from hemolytic disease of the newborn.

Polyagglutination from bacterial contamination of reagents or patient's cells can occur; the outcome is exposure of T antigens to anti-T antigens.

Complement components can attach to the cells in a wide variety of disorders not associated with a hemolytic process (Freedman, 1979).

Indirect Antiglobulin Test

Principle

This modification of the direct antiglobulin test detects the presence of antibodies in the serum of sensitized individuals. Serum under investigation is added to appropriate cells and is incubated at 37°C to allow the cells to become coated with the antibody. After this sensitization has occurred, the coated cells are washed as in the direct test, and antiglobulin serum is added. The difference between this test and the direct antiglobulin test is that in the direct antiglobulin test, the *cells* are tested for in vivo antibody coating, whereas in the indirect test, the patient's *serum* is tested for the presence of the antibody.

Reagents and Equipment

1. Two pools of commercially obtained red cells are chosen so that all clinically important red-cell antigens are included.
2. The remainder of the reagents used are as described under Reagents and Equipment in the preceding section on the direct test.

Specimen

Serum is the specimen used.

Method

1. One volume of test serum is placed in each of two tubes, and an equal volume of each of the two bottles of pooled group O cells is added to the respective tubes.

2. The tubes are shaken lightly to mix their contents and are incubated at 37°C for 15 minutes to 1 hour (depending on the manufacturer's procedure).

3. Positive and negative control specimens are set up in parallel with the test sample. The positive control is composed of a dilution of 1:256 "slide test" anti-D in saline, and the negative control is saline.

4. The tubes are removed from the water bath and centrifuged at 3,500 rpm for 10–15 seconds. The cell button is resuspended gently, as described for the direct antiglobulin test, and macroscopic agglutination is sought.

5. If no agglutinates are seen, the cells are washed in copious volumes of saline three to four times to remove any unbound protein, and they are resuspended in the residual saline left after the last washing.

6. One volume of broad-spectrum antiglobulin serum is added to each tube and is mixed and centrifuged at 3,500 rpm for 10–15 seconds. The cell buttons are resuspended as previously described, and one looks for agglutination both macroscopically and by use of a low-power lens.

7. One volume of a coated control cell, either commercially obtained or made as shown on page 334, is added to each negative-cell tube.

8. The mixture is centrifuged at 3,500 rpm for 10–15 seconds, the cell button is resuspended, and agglutination is sought in the same way. The negative control sample will now show agglutination if the cells were washed adequately.

Results

A positive test result denotes the presence of a serum antibody. For the test to be acceptable, the positive and negative control tubes run concurrently have to produce acceptable results, and the coated cells added to the negative control tubes have to produce agglutination after centrifugation. Failure to show agglutination invalidates the test. Such failure is due to neutralization or contamination of the antiglobulin reagent.

Sources of Error

It is essential that the cells be washed completely with large volumes of saline for both the direct and indirect tests. Additionally, the cell buttons should be resuspended and mixed well between the additions of saline, and the residual saline should be completely decanted after centrifugation. Failure to

wash cells adequately in this test results in false-negative reactions due to neutralization of antiglobulin serum with contaminated proteins.

A positive result on the indirect antiglobulin test is nonspecific and does not serve to type or identify the antibody. Further identification can be made using a panel of genotyped red cells, but this is not a routine practice in the hematology laboratory and should be referred to an immunohematology laboratory that has experience in such identification.

EDTA Two-Stage Antiglobulin Test

Principle

EDTA is added to stored serum, which consists of chelated calcium ions necessary for the binding of the C1q-C1r-C1s complex to form bound C1. Using this chelated serum, antigen-antibody complexes are formed, but C1 is unable to attach to the antibody-combining site and is removed with the antibody by washing. Fresh compatible serum is added as a source of complement, enabling the antibody complex to bind (Polly and Mollison, 1961).

Reagents and Equipment

1. EDTA reagent: Dipotassium EDTA, 4 g, and 0.3 g sodium hydroxide are dissolved in 100 ml distilled water. The final pH of the reagent should approximate 7.0–7.4.
2. Fresh ABO-compatible normal serum (i.e., same ABO group as the patient).
3. Normal saline.
4. Pooled indicator cells as in the indirect antiglobulin test (page 335).
5. Centrifuge (Serofuge).
6. Pipettes: 1 ml, graduated; Pasteur.
7. Tubes: 10 × 75 mm.

Specimen

The specimen consists of clotted whole blood, which provides serum and free red cells.

Method

1. EDTA reagent (0.1 ml) is added to 1 ml test

serum and is allowed to stand at room temperature for 10 minutes.

2. The indicator cells are washed in saline, as described for the direct and indirect antiglobulin tests (see page 336), and four volumes of the EDTA-serum mixture (step 1) are added to one volume of dry packed cells and are mixed and incubated for 1 hour at 37°C.

3. The cells are washed in copious volumes of saline, three to four times, ensuring that the cells are resuspended completely between centrifugation. The saline is drained entirely from the cell button after the last washing, and two volumes of fresh ABO-compatible normal serum are added as a source of complement.

4. The solution is mixed and incubated at 37°C for 15 minutes and is washed three to four times as described in step 3.

5. The residual saline from the last washing is drained, and two volumes of antiglobulin serum are added to the cell button. This is mixed well and centrifuged at 3,500 rpm for 10–15 seconds.

6. The cell button is dislodged gently, as described on page 336, and is examined for the presence of agglutination in the standard way.

7. Control tubes should be set up as in the indirect antiglobulin test, including the addition of a coated cell to all negative control tests (see page 336).

Results

A positive test result denotes the presence of a serum antibody.

Clinical Correlation

This test is useful in screening sera that have been stored for a considerable time and that may have become anticomplementary. The two-stage test has proved to be very satisfactory in the detection of some antibodies, particularly those in the Lewis system, but its degree of sensitivity depends on the equilibrium constant of the particular antibody.

Elution of Antibodies, Heat Method

Principle

Antibodies are removed from the coated red-cell surface by heating (Landsteiner et al., 1925).

Reagents and Equipment

1. Normal saline.
2. Bovine albumin 6%.
3. Water bath, 56°C.
4. Centrifuge (Serofuge).
5. Tubes: 10×75 mm.
6. Pasteur pipettes.

Specimen

Clotted whole blood is used.

Method

1. Free cells are removed from the clotted test specimen and are washed five times in copious volumes of room-temperature saline.

2. An equal volume of 6% bovine albumin is added to the final washed cell button so as to make a 50% cell suspension, and the mixture is incubated at 56°C for 30 minutes. It is important to agitate the cell suspension at least every 5 minutes during the incubation.

3. The solution is centrifuged in warm buckets at 3,500 rpm for 15–30 seconds. The supernatant is removed and is tested by standard techniques for the presence of antibodies.

Elution of Antibodies, Freeze Method

Principle

Antibodies are removed from coated cells by hemolyzing the cells using a freeze-thaw procedure (Weiner, 1957).

Reagents and Equipment

1. Normal saline.
2. Ethyl alcohol 50%, chilled in freezer.
3. Water bath, 37°C.
4. Centrifuge (Serofuge).
5. Freezer: –20°C.
6. Pasteur pipettes.

Specimen

The specimen used is clotted whole blood.

Method

1. Free cells obtained from the clot are washed as in the preceding (heat) method and then are hemolyzed by alternately freezing and thawing (placing in a freezer and immersing in a 37°C water bath).

2. Ten volumes of prechilled 50% ethyl alcohol are added to one volume of the hemolyzed test cells. The solution is mixed and allowed to remain in the freezer at –20°C for 2 hours.

3. It is centrifuged at 3,500 rpm for 2–3 minutes, and the supernatant is removed. The sediment is broken up and washed in an excess of distilled water. An equal volume of saline is added to the sediment, and this is incubated in a 37°C water bath for 30 minutes.

4. It is centrifuged, the supernatant is removed, and standard tests for the presence of antibodies are performed.

Elution of Antibodies, Ether Method

Principle

Antibodies are removed from coated cells after hemolyzing the cells by the addition of ether (Rubin, 1963).

Reagents and Equipment

1. Normal saline.
2. Diethyl ether.
3. Centrifuge (Serofuge).
4. Tubes: 10×75 mm.
5. Pasteur pipettes.

Specimen

Clotted whole blood is used.

Method

1. Free cells obtained from the clot are washed as previously described (see page 337) and are made up to a 50% suspension with saline. An equal volume of ether is added to the mixture; the contents are mixed by inversion and centrifuged at 3,500 rpm for 5–10 minutes.

2. The two top layers of the supernatant are discarded, and the hemoglobin-stained bottom layer is kept to test for antibodies by standard techniques.

Qualitative Donath-Landsteiner Test

Principle

The Donath-Landsteiner hemolysin found in PCH differs from normal cold antibodies in that it is more hemolytic toward normal cells and is biphasic in its mode of action. At low temperatures, it binds affected red cells and causes hemolysis in the presence of complement when warmed to 37°C.

Reagents and Equipment

1. Refrigerator.
2. Tubes: 10×75 mm.
3. Water bath, 37°C.

Specimen

Whole blood that is not anticoagulated is used.

Method

1. Three tubes are prewarmed to 37°C, and approximately 1 ml unclotted whole blood is added directly from the syringe into each tube.

2. One tube is left undisturbed at 37°C, allowed to clot, and incubated for 1 hour.

3. The second tube is allowed to clot in the refrigerator and is left for 1 hour.

4. The third tube is allowed to clot in the refrigerator, is left for 30 minutes, and then is transferred to the 37°C water bath for 1 hour.

5. At the end of the incubation phases, all tubes are inspected for hemolysis.

Results

Hemolysis in the third tube (clotted at 4°C and warmed to 37°C), without hemolysis in the other two tubes, indicates the presence of a Donath-Landsteiner antibody. Hemolysis in either of the first two tubes indicates a hemolysin acting either in the warm or in the cold tubes.

Clinical Correlation

The presence of the Donath-Landsteiner hemolysin was first associated with syphilis but now usually is found in the presence of viral disorders or other conditions related to lymphoproliferation. The antibody is an IgG immunoglobulin that acts as an autoantibody, fixing to red cells in the presence of complement at 4–20°C. When the red-cell temperature returns to 37°C, hemolysis takes place. The antibody usually has anti-P specificity (Worlledge and Rousso, 1965).

Detection of Warm Hemolysins

Principle

Test serum is titrated in fresh ABO-compatible normal serum to provide a source of complement. The dilutions are incubated at 37°C with group O cells and are read macroscopically for the presence of hemolysis.

Reagents and Equipment

1. Normal saline.
2. Fresh ABO-compatible normal serum, free of hemolysis.
3. Pooled group O cells, commercially obtained.
4. Water bath, 37°C.
5. Tubes: 10 × 75 mm.
6. Pipettes: 1 ml, graduated; Pasteur.

Specimen

The specimen is clotted whole blood, free of hemolysis, collected in a warm syringe.

Method

1. Doubling dilutions of test serum in fresh normal serum are made, and an equal volume of a 2–5% suspension of pooled group O cells is added to each dilution.
2. The dilutions are incubated at 37°C for 1–2 hours and are inspected macroscopically for hemolysis.

Results

The highest dilution that produces hemolysis is recorded as the titer. Normal serum will not exhibit any hemolysis in any tube.

Detection of Cold Hemolysins

Principle

Test serum is titrated in fresh acidified ABO-compatible normal serum to enhance cold hemolysin activity in the presence of complement.

Reagents and Equipment

1. Hydrochloric acid, 0.1 N.
2. Other reagents and equipment as listed for the detection of warm hemolysins (see preceding section).

Specimen

Clotted whole blood, free of hemolysis, collected and stored cold.

Method

1. One volume of 0.1-N hydrochloric acid is added to nine volumes of normal serum. Doubling dilutions of test serum in fresh acidified normal serum are made, and an equal volume of 2–5% suspension of pooled group O cells is added to each dilution.

2. The dilutions are incubated at 4°C for 2 hours and are inspected macroscopically for hemolysis.

Results

The highest dilution that produces hemolysis is recorded as the titer. Normal serum may show some hemolysis at a titer of up to 1:2.

Detection of Cold Agglutinins

Principle

Group O cells are incubated at 4°C with doubling dilutions of the patient's serum.

Reagents and Equipment

1. Normal saline.
2. Group O red cells, either commercially obtained or freshly prepared. The cells are washed three times in normal saline and are resuspended to 2–5% in saline.
3. Tubes: 10 × 75 mm.
4. Pipettes: 1 ml, graduated.
5. Refrigerator.

Specimen

Five milliliters of blood are collected in a warm syringe or vacuum tube and are allowed to clot at 37°C. The serum is separated and refrigerated at 4°C until the test is performed. The blood must not be allowed to clot at room temperature.

Method

1. Doubling dilutions of test serum are made in saline, and an equal volume of a 2–5% suspension of group O cells is added to each dilution.
2. The dilutions are incubated at 4°C for at least 2 hours but preferably overnight.
3. Each tube is examined macroscopically for the presence of agglutination.

Reference Range

The reference range is less than 1:32.

Clinical Correlation

Increased titers of cold agglutinins can be found in Raynaud's syndrome, pleuropneumonia-like organism, PNH, trypanosomiasis, syphilitic or hypertrophic cirrhosis, hemolytic anemias, Hodgkin's disease, lymphomas, and febrile tuberculosis.

Detection of Antibodies to Penicillin and Cephalosporins

Principle

Drug-coated normal cells are prepared and exposed to the test serum (Spath et al., 1971; Garratty, 1972).

Reagents and Equipment

1. Barbital buffer, 0.1 M (pH 9.6): Sodium barbital, 20.6 g, is dissolved in 1 liter of distilled water. One and one-half milliliters of 0.1-N hydrochloric acid are added to 98.5 ml of the 0.1-M buffer. The pH is checked and adjusted accordingly.
2. Group O cells, freshly obtained.
3. K-benzylpenicillin G.
4. Cephalothin sodium.
5. Normal saline.
6. Water bath, 37°C.
7. Centrifuge (Serofuge).
8. Tubes: 10 × 75 mm.
9. Pipettes: 1 ml, graduated.

Specimen

The specimen is clotted whole blood.

Method

1. Penicillin-coated cells are prepared by adding 1 ml fresh, packed, washed red cells to 1×10^6 units (approximately 600 mg) of K-benzylpenicillin G dissolved in 15 ml of the 0.1-M barbital buffer.
2. This preparation is incubated at room temperature for 1 hour, being gently mixed throughout the incubation. The cells are washed three times in copious volumes of saline. Once prepared, the coated cells are stable for 1 week when refrigerated if stored in standard acid-citrate-dextrose or citrate-phosphate-dextrose-1 anticoagulant.
3. Cephalothin sodium–coated cells are prepared by adding 1 ml fresh, packed, washed red cells to 400 mg cephalothin sodium dissolved in 10 ml of the 0.1-M barbital buffer.
4. The mixture is incubated at 37°C for 2 hours with gentle mixing, and the cells then are washed as previously described.
5. An eluate is prepared from the patient's cells by one of the standard procedures (page 337), and the eluate and test serum are tested against treated and coated cells.
6. Serial dilutions of the test serum from 1:1 to 1:64 are set up.
7. One volume of a 2% saline suspension of drug-treated cells is incubated with two volumes of the eluate. This is performed for each serum dilution and is repeated using uncoated cells.

8. This mixture is incubated at room temperature for 15 minutes and centrifuged at 3,500 rpm for 30 seconds, and an aliquot from each tube is examined microscopically for agglutination.

9. The cells are resuspended and reincubated at 37°C for 30–60 minutes and are centrifuged and examined microscopically again for agglutination, as in step 8.

10. All cell suspensions are washed three to four times in copious volumes of saline, and one drop of broad-spectrum antiglobulin serum is added to each tube. The mixture is centrifuged at 3,500 rpm for 10–15 seconds and is examined for agglutination macroscopically and under a low-power lens.

Results

IgM penicillin antibodies will agglutinate saline-suspended penicillin-treated cells but will not agglutinate uncoated cells. IgG penicillin antibodies will react similarly when the test is converted to the antiglobulin phase.

Cephalothin sodium–treated cells can absorb proteins nonspecifically, causing all normal serum to produce a positive indirect antiglobulin test if incubated with the drug for extended periods of time. The reaction does not occur when the normal protein is diluted to a ratio of more than 1:20. The eluate does not cause such problems because of the low amount of protein present.

Chapter 20

Tests Useful in the Evaluation of Blood Coagulation

General Equipment

The equipment necessary to carry out blood coagulation tests is simple and limited in scope. The basic apparatus is a thermostatically controlled, well-insulated water bath and adequate timing devices. Stopwatches that operate by foot pedals are a useful adjunct, freeing the technologist's hands for manual pipetting. Many automated apparatuses are available commercially and can be divided into two principal groups: those that detect a fibrin strand photo-optically and those that mechanically sense fibrin formation. This equipment is discussed in more detail on page 447.

Glassware

All glassware used for blood coagulation tests must be either scrupulously clean or new. If glassware is reused, it should be washed with hot soapy water, followed by thorough rinsing in tap water and then in distilled water. If the tubes still are not clean enough, they should be immersed in chromic acid cleaning solution and left overnight. Pipettes that have been used with diatomaceous earth reagents should first be washed in hot tap water and then immersed in the acid cleaning solution.

After acid soaking, all glassware should be rinsed either by hand or in a pipette washer with large volumes of tap water and then rinsed at least five times in distilled water. The pH of the final distilled-water rinse should be tested; it should approximate 6.8–7.0. Glassware can be dried in a warm oven at approximately 50°C.

A chromic acid cleaning solution can be made by dissolving 10 g potassium dichromate in 2 ml concentrated sulfuric acid and slowly adding this to 75 ml distilled water.

Blood Coagulation Procedures

Blood Collection

Routine screening tests, including the one-stage prothrombin time (PT) and the partial thromboplastin time (PTT), do not require a special collection technique. If possible, however, the specimen for coagulation workups must be free of tissue juice contamination. In addition, the blood should not be hemolyzed from the actual venipuncture, from delivering the sample forcibly through the syringe needle, or from prolonged exposure to extreme temperatures.

Samples that are clotted, collected in the wrong tube, or filled to less than 90% of the expected capacity of the collection tube are unsuitable for testing. Specimens that are lipemic or have very high bilirubin levels may also interfere with the endpoint determinations in semiautomated or automated methods that use spectrophotometrically determined end points. Blood should be placed in melting ice immediately after its collection and transported as quickly as possible to the laboratory. Centrifugation of the uncapped specimen at 3,000 rpm for 10 minutes in a refrigerated centrifuge is recommended. After spinning, the plasma should be separated from the red cells and buffy coat using a plastic pipette. It should then be transferred to a clean tube and stored at 1–8°C or in melting ice. After the plasma has been separated, it is necessary to cap the tubes tightly to prevent loss of carbon dioxide from the sample, as such loss results in an increased pH level. If testing has not been carried out within 4 hours, the plasma should be frozen at –20°C or colder (National Committee for Clinical Laboratory Standards, 1986).

The two-syringe procedure is recommended when carrying out critical tests and workups, but it can be avoided for routine work. Siliconized syringes are best and should be prepared according to the manufacturer's instructions. In the absence of this information, glassware can be prepared as follows:

First, chemically clean glassware should be immersed in the silicon solution. The technologist should take care not to breathe the vapors. This procedure is best carried out under an exhaust hood. The silicon solution must not be allowed to contact skin, as it can initiate a contact dermatitis. For maximum protection, rubber gloves should be worn. After 2–3 minutes, the glassware is removed, air-dried, and immersed quickly in acetone to dissolve the silicon solvent. It is rinsed well in distilled water and allowed to dry in an incubator or oven at 37°C.

Method

1. A clean venipuncture is made with an untreated glass syringe and needle.
2. The first few milliliters of blood are withdrawn, and the tourniquet is released. The patient is instructed to open his or her hand, and the syringe is disconnected from the needle hub. This blood is discarded.
3. A clean, 20-ml, sterile siliconized syringe is attached quickly to the needle, and the patient is instructed to clench his or her fist, helping to build up pressure in the vein.
4. The syringe plunger is slowly withdrawn until 20 ml blood has been taken. Four and one-half milliliters of the blood are placed in either 0.5 ml 3.2% sodium citrate or in 0.5 ml citric acid–sodium citrate buffer (page 254). Ten milliliters of the blood are placed in a clean, graduated centrifuge tube. Another 6.7 ml of the blood is

placed in dipotassium ethylenediaminetetraacetic acid (EDTA) anticoagulant.

Storage

Blood for PTTs and for specific coagulation factor assays, with the exception of factor VII, should be centrifuged in a refrigerated apparatus and stored at 4°C or frozen if testing is not carried out within 24 hours. In the event that a factor VII assay is required, the plasma is best left at room temperature, as factor VII becomes activated when exposed to glass in the cold. However, the in vitro cold-promoting activation of factor VII and the shortening of the PT can be partially inhibited by the use of siliconized borosilicate glass collection tubes (BD no. 6418, available from Becton-Dickinson, Rutherford, NJ; Palmer and Gralnick, 1985).

Citrated blood for PT tests should not be separated from the red cells until just before use. The citrated whole blood is adequate for testing if left at room temperature or if maintained at 4°C if the stopper of the tube is not removed until just before the test is carried out. Blood that remains stoppered and is stored at room temperature is stable for PT tests for up to 24 hours (Koepke et al., 1975; Miale and Kent, 1979; Simmons, 1980). If unstoppered, the carbon dioxide loss changes the plasma pH and adversely affects factor V stability, causing false increases in the clotting time of the test. If the stopper is removed and the tests cannot be completed within 2–4 hours, aliquots of plasma are best stored frozen in plastic tubes at less than –20°C. Table 20.1 illustrates the storage time of plasma when used for coagulation tests if the stopper is removed from the anticoagulated blood.

Variables in Blood Coagulation Testing

Because blood coagulation is essentially an enzymatic process, the environmental pH of the reagents is of prime importance. All coagulation tests should be carried out at a pH range of 7.0–7.5 and at 37 ± 0.5°C.

Deionized water is best used for the reconstitution of reagents, as the diluent should be free of heavy trace metals that interfere with many tests, causing false prolongations of fibrin formation. Potassium or sodium oxalate is not recommended as the anticoagulant for PTs, because it does not

Table 20.1. Maximum Storage Time for the Common Coagulation Tests

Test	Never Unstoppered (hrs)	Unstoppered or Stopper Removed and Recapped (hrs)
Prothrombin time	12[a]	2
Partial thromboplastin time	?[b]	2

[a]This time can be lengthened if a thromboplastin reagent is used that contains excess factor V. Specimens stored for up to 48 hours can then be tested.
[b]The maximum storage time is unclear but, if the test is to be carried out longer than 4 hours after venipuncture, the specimen should be centrifuged and the plasma frozen as soon as possible.
Source: Data taken from A Simmons, M Paulo. Prothrombin time stability and precision. Lab Med Internat 10:22, 1993.

Table 20.2. Recommended Maximum Differences Between Results of Clotting Tests

Test Time (secs)	Maximum Acceptable Differences Between Duplicates (secs)
0–20	1–2
21–60	2–6
61–100	6–10
>100	10–20

results should be used for calculation purposes. To obtain valid averages, duplicate times should not differ by more than 10%. The standardization of duplicate test results shown in Table 20.2 is suggested. However, if the laboratory can demonstrate excellent precision over the expected range of test results, testing can proceed without duplication.

Coagulation Screening Tests

Activated Coagulation Time

Principle

The whole-blood clotting time is the sum of the activation of all the coagulation factors necessary to promote a fibrin clot. The activated modification adds a standard contact activation surface in the form of diatomaceous earth, which accelerates the first step in the cascade pathway. A trauma-free venipuncture is carried out, and the time interval between phlebotomy and blood coagulation is recorded (Hattersley, 1966).

Reagents and Equipment

1. Stopwatch.
2. Gray stoppered Vacutainer tubes (BD no. 3206) containing diatomaceous earth.
3. Water bath or heating block, 37°C.
4. Plastic syringe.

Method

preserve factor V, thereby causing falsely elevated results. Other significant errors can be caused by the inadequate collection of sufficient blood (short draw) or by traumatic venipuncture, which produces excesses of tissue juice.

A standard vacuum tube (Vacutainer, available from Becton-Dickinson) that will draw exactly 4.5 ml blood and contains 0.5 ml sodium citrate can be used. This will ensure the correct 9:1 blood-anticoagulant ratio. If this ratio is not maintained in a patient with a normal hematocrit value, the proportion of plasma to citrate will affect the test result adversely. The most commonly seen physiologic alterations that produce erroneous coagulation test results include polycythemia due either to stress or to a myeloproliferative cause or poor phlebotomy in which the tourniquet is left on the patient's arm for an excessive time. The blood obtained from all venipunctures on such individuals should be collected in special tubes containing proportionately less anticoagulant, thereby avoiding overcitration and excessive dilution of the plasma by the anticoagulant. In general, when the hematocrit exceeds 55%, the test specimen should be redrawn.

Most tests used in measuring hemostasis result in the formation of in vitro fibrin clots. Tests should be carried out in duplicate, and the average of the

1. The Vacutainer tube is prewarmed to 37°C, and the venipuncture is performed. The first 1–2 ml blood collected is discarded, and then 2 ml whole blood is added to a second Vacutainer tube.

2. The stopwatch is started when blood first enters the tube, and the specimen is incubated immediately at 37°C.

3. The tube is tilted after 60 seconds' incubation and thereafter at 5- to 10-second intervals so that the blood spreads along its length.

4. The time that it takes for a clot to form is recorded.

Reference Range

The reference range is 70–100 seconds.

Clinical Correlation

The activated coagulation time is a nonspecific test for any of the plasma parameters involved in fibrin formation. By using an activating agent, the test is shortened and made more sensitive to factor deficiencies than those obtained with the standard whole-blood test. The test is useful in monitoring heparin therapy (Hattersley, 1976) as well as in following the degree of hypocoagulation of patients undergoing open heart surgery (Bull et al., 1975).

Whole-Blood Coagulation Time

Principle

The principle underlying the whole-blood coagulation time test is the same as that for the activated coagulation time, except that an activating agent that accelerates the contact stage is not used. Rather, activation is achieved by exposure of the blood to a standard clean glass tube (Lee and White, 1913).

Reagents and Equipment

1. Tubes: 8-mm diameter.
2. Water bath or heating block, 37°C.
3. Plastic syringe.
4. Stopwatch.

Method

1. Five milliliters of blood are collected by a clean trauma-free venipuncture, and the first 1 ml is discarded.

2. Approximately 1 ml blood is transferred to each of three tubes, and these are incubated at 37°C. The stopwatch is begun.

3. One tube is tilted at 30-second intervals through an angle of 90 degrees until the blood has coagulated. The other two undisturbed tubes are checked to verify the results. If the blood in the other two tubes has not clotted, one tube is tilted in the same way as in step 2, and the process is repeated with the third tube if necessary.

4. The clotting times of all three tubes are averaged.

Reference Range

The reference range is 6–10 minutes.

Sources of Error

The stopwatch is started when blood first enters the tubes, *not* when it is seen in the plastic syringe. If a glass syringe is used, the time should be taken from the moment the blood becomes glass-activated. This method can be modified by the use of siliconized tubes, prepared as described on page 344. The use of such tubes slows down the contact activation and allows the test to be more sensitive to depressions of coagulation factors. However, this modification has generally been replaced by the activated test described previously.

When carrying out either of the two coagulation time procedures just described, care should be taken to always tilt the tubes in the same direction and through the same angle. The standard Lee-White method is sensitive to severe bleeding disorders only when the levels of specific coagulation factors fall to 1–2% of normal. Thus, a hemophiliac would require 98% depletion of factor VIII to produce an abnormal test result.

Prothrombin Time

Principle

The plasma coagulation time is measured in the presence of excess tissue thromboplastin and calcium. The PT test detects deficiencies in the intrinsic pathway as well as in the common pathway of blood coagulation (Quick, 1935).

Reagents and Equipment

1. Commercially obtained thromboplastin-calcium reagent.
2. Water bath, 37°C.
3. Pipettes: 5 ml, graduated; 0.1-ml and 0.2-ml micropipettes.
4. Stopwatch.
5. Tubes: 12 × 75 mm.
6. Commercially controlled trilevel plasma controls: normal, borderline, and abnormal ranges.
7. Deionized water.

Specimen

Exactly 4.5 ml blood is added to 0.5 ml 0.11-M sodium citrate. It is mixed well and centrifuged at 1,000*g* for 10–15 minutes. The plasma is removed and tested as soon as possible. If testing cannot be completed within 2 hours, the stopper should not be removed from the tube, which should be maintained at room temperature.

Method

1. The thromboplastin-calcium reagent is lyophilized with deionized water by following the manufacturer's recommendations. It is swirled briefly and allowed to stand 15 minutes at room temperature to obtain a solution.

2. The control plasma is reconstituted in a similar way and is allowed to go into solution.

3. The thromboplastin-calcium reagent and the control plasmas are prewarmed, and 0.2 ml of the reagent is pipetted into a series of warmed tubes.

4. One-tenth milliliter of one control plasma is added to the reagent, and the stopwatch is started immediately. The time required for fibrin formation is noted. The procedure is repeated in duplicate for each control and test plasma. Each of the duplicates is averaged, and the control times are compared with a previously established range derived from a statistically large number of control results. If the controls are acceptable, the test time in seconds is reported.

Reference Range

The reference range is 10–13 seconds.

Sources of Error

As this test depends on the exact ratio of blood to anticoagulant, tests that have less than 3.5–4.0 ml blood added to the 0.5 ml sodium citrate cannot be satisfactorily tested because, when small volumes of blood are drawn, the ratio of sodium citrate to plasma is excessive, resulting in both an overdilution of the coagulation factors and excessive citration. If small volumes of blood are taken, this overcitration is not compensated for by the addition of the test calcium. Similarly, in patients who are polycythemic or who have hematocrit values in excess of 55%, falsely abnormal results will be produced. In such individuals, special citrated tubes that contain less anticoagulant should be prepared.

Other in vitro factors that affect the test result involve the partial inhibition of cold-promoting activation when blood is collected in siliconized borosilicate glass tubes. Such activation is almost totally inhibited in normal blood samples and is reduced by approximately 50% in patients receiving oral anticoagulant therapy (Palmer and Gralnick, 1985). The test plasma should be tested as soon as possible after collection (within 2 hours). If this is impossible, the citrated whole blood should remain capped and be kept cool at 4°C until tested. If specimens are to be transported over long distances or if extreme time delays are encountered, the plasma should be removed within 2 hours of collection and immediately frozen.

If blood is taken into buffered citric acid–sodium citrate anticoagulant, the test can be run up to 12 hours, even if left unstoppered at room temperature (Simmons et al., 1993).

Clinical Correlation

The PT is carried out principally to monitor oral anticoagulant therapy. Although various methods have been suggested for report formats, it is common practice to report the normal control time and the test time in seconds. Anticoagulation therapy is considered adequate when the patient's PT exceeds the control by a factor of 1.5–2.0 (Wessler, 1984). It has been recommended that to standardize PT reports internationally, manufacturers of thromboplastin should indicate the relationship of each batch of their material to the World Health Organization (WHO) International Reference Preparation by a number that describes the comparative slope

(Loeliger, 1985). This is referred to by WHO as the *international sensitivity index* (ISI). The recommendation also suggests that the manufacturer provide a table or graph detailing the relationship between the conventional terms of expression of results and the international normalized ratio (INR), which is derived from the following equation:

$$INR = R^c$$

where R is the ratio of the patient's time in seconds over the mean normal time and c is the comparative slope of the thromboplastin used (Loeliger, 1985). Reports using dilution curves and percentage activity are not recommended.

If PT tests are carried out as part of a general hemostatic workup, the reference range of the procedure should be reported with the test result. The PT may be prolonged in patients with liver disease, disseminated intravascular coagulation (DIC), or a deficiency of extrinsic pathway coagulation factors (factors V, VII, and X; prothrombin; and fibrinogen), as well as in those being treated with oral anticoagulants. Like many coagulation tests, the procedure may be modified by the use of automated or semiautomated equipment (discussed on page 447). The PT test has historically been set up in duplicate to minimize test error. However, single determinations using automated equipment have proved such duplicate testing unnecessary (Morris et al., 1987).

Activated Partial Thromboplastin Time

Principle

The activated PTT is a screening test for deficiencies and inhibitors of all the coagulation factors (except factors VII and XIII) and for both qualitative and quantitative platelet abnormalities (Rodman et al., 1958). The test uses brain lipids to replace platelet phospholipids and added calcium, which, together with citrated test plasma, provide the necessary components to produce a fibrin clot. The contact stage in the intrinsic pathway is activated and standardized by a variety of materials, principally diatomaceous earths such as kaolin or celite, but surface activators such as crushed glass or chemicals such as ellagic acid can also be used.

Reagents and Equipment

1. Activated partial thromboplastin, commercially obtained.
2. Calcium chloride, 0.025 M: The anhydrous salt, 2.77 g, is dissolved in 100 ml deionized water.
3. Water bath, 37°C.
4. Stopwatch.
5. Tubes: 12 × 75 mm.
6. Pipettes: 5 ml, graduated; 0.1-ml micropipettes.
7. Controls, commercially obtained and consisting of a two-level lyophilized plasma.

Specimen

The specimen used is citrated blood. Exactly 4.5 ml blood is added to 0.5 ml sodium citrate (0.11 M), and the anticoagulated blood is centrifuged at 2,000 rpm for 15 minutes. Precautions in the drawing and handling of the specimen are detailed in the section on the PT test (page 347).

Method

1. The controls and partial thromboplastin reagent are reconstituted according to the manufacturer's instructions and are allowed to reach 37°C. Calcium chloride is also prewarmed.
2. One-tenth milliliter of partial thromboplastin reagent is pipetted into a tube, and 0.1 ml of control is added. The mixture is allowed to incubate for 3 minutes at 37°C.
3. One-tenth milliliter of calcium chloride (0.025 M) is added to the mixture, and the timer is started immediately. The tube is agitated gently, and the specimen is observed for final gel formation. The stopwatch is *not* stopped at the point of *partial* fibrin formation.
4. The procedure is repeated in duplicate for each control and test plasma specimen.
5. Each of the paired results is averaged, and the control times are compared with a previously established range derived from a statistically large number of control results. If the controls are acceptable, the test times are reported in seconds.

Reference Range

The reference range depends principally on the nature of the activator and the manufacturer of the reagent. Whenever possible, it should be determined by each laboratory. However, times of 25–35 seconds are often found in ellagic acid activation products, and 30- to 45-second times are found for many of the diatomaceous earth–activated products.

Sources of Error

A two-level control system should be run with the test. These controls should be tested at the start and end of the test run. For batches of 20 tests or more, additional controls should be run in the middle of the batch.

Whenever possible, test plasma specimen should be run within 2 hours of collection. If this is impossible, the plasma should be separated and kept frozen until tested.

Errors can be produced by a variety of technical problems, including poor venipuncture technique, an inadequate volume of blood being diluted with the standard sodium citrate volume, dirty glassware, incorrect pipetting, and failure to prewarm all reagents. All tests and controls should be run in duplicate and the paired results averaged. If the difference between paired samples exceeds 3%, a third test should be carried out and the outlier discarded. Between-run precision goals of 4% have been recommended for fresh plasma, and between-day goals of 5% have been recommended for lyophilized normal and abnormal controls (Koepke, 1986).

An abnormally long test may be due to a deficiency of one or more coagulation factors involved in the intrinsic and common pathways of blood coagulation. Among these are factors V, VII, IX, X, XI, and XII; prothrombin; and fibrinogen. The test is sensitive to decreases of factor levels to less than 25–30% of normal but will usually be normal if the factor levels are greater than this. Fibrinogen deficiencies will be detected only if the level is less than 100 mg/dl. The type of activation of the test is the principal variable in test sensitivity. Micronized silica and ellagic acid reagent systems are similar in sensitivity to factor VIII, factor IX, and factor XII deficiencies, whereas micronized kaolin reagent is significantly less sensitive to these deficiencies. Factor XI deficiency is detected equally well with all these reagents. Both the micronized silica and the ellagic acid reagents are insensitive to all but severe deficiencies in prekallikrein, but the kaolin reagent does not detect this deficiency at all. All reagents appear insensitive to all but severe deficiencies in high-molecular-weight kininogen (Turi and Peerschke, 1986).

Inhibitors such as heparin, or circulating anticoagulants against either individual factors or factor complexes also will result in prolonged PTTs. If an abnormally elevated test result is detected in the absence of a reasonable explanation for such a result, the test sample should be redrawn and the test repeated to rule out technical errors arising from traumatic venipuncture or a very high hematocrit value. In cases in which the hematocrit value is greater than 55%, the citrate concentration or volume should be adjusted so that the correct proportions of anticoagulant to plasma are maintained. Tests should not be carried out on blood samples containing less than 3.5–4.0 ml when the standard 0.5-ml citrate volume is used.

The test can be carried out using automated or semiautomated equipment, using either a photooptical or mechanical method for sensing fibrin clot formation.

Reptilase Test

Principle

Reptilase is a thrombinlike enzyme isolated from the venom of *Bothrops atrox* that is capable of clotting fibrinogen. The fibrin monomers formed by thrombin polymerize side to side, whereas the monomers formed by reptilase are capable of polymerizing end to end only. Thrombin inhibitors such as heparin, heparinoids, and hirudin do not inhibit the activity of this enzyme, and the reptilase is unabsorbed by fibrin. The enzyme does not activate plasminogen and is uninhibited by antifibrinolytics such as ε-aminocaproic acid. Inhibition of reptilase can be accomplished by specific antibodies contained in anti-*Bothrops* serum (Blomback et al., 1957).

Reagents and Equipment

1. Reptilase (Abbott, North Chicago, IL): Deionized water, 1 ml, is added to a vial of the enzyme, and the mixture is swirled and left to dissolve at room temperature. This reagent is stable for 4 weeks when reconstituted and stored at 4°C.
2. Stopwatch.
3. Water bath, 37°C.
4. Pipettes: 1 ml, graduated; 0.1-ml micropipettes.
5. Tubes: 12 × 75 mm.

Specimen

As in the PT and activated PTT tests, the test specimen is citrated blood. A normal control plasma specimen should also be obtained.

Method

1. All reagents and plasma specimens are prewarmed to 37°C for 5 minutes.
2. One-tenth milliliter of reptilase is added to 0.3 ml citrated plasma, and the timer is started immediately. The tube is agitated gently, and the technologist observes for the presence of a fibrin clot.
3. The test is repeated using normal citrated control plasma.

Reference Range

The reference range is 18–22 seconds.

Clinical Correlation

An increase of more than 25 seconds in the reptilase time is an indication of a dysfibrinogenemia, hypofibrinogenemia, or afibrinogenemia. Unlike the inhibition of thrombin-formed fibrin monomers by fibrin split products, the polymerization of monomers obtained by reptilase is influenced only slightly by fibrinogen or by the split products or is not influenced by them at all. The test is used principally for testing heparinized individuals, in lieu of the thrombin time.

Russell's Viper Venom Test (Stypven Time)

Principle

Russell's viper venom directly activates factor X, bypassing factor XII. The test is sensitive to deficiencies of factors V and X, prothrombin, and fibrinogen, but shows normal results in factor VII deficiency (Prentice and Ratnoff, 1969).

Reagents and Equipment

1. Russell's viper venom (Sigma Chemical Co., St. Louis, MO): The venom is reconstituted as directed in the manufacturer's package insert.

2. Thromboplastin (Difco, Detroit, MI) or Platelin (General Diagnostics, Morris Plains, NJ).
3. Calcium chloride, 0.025 M: Anhydrous calcium chloride, 2.77 g, is dissolved in 1 liter distilled water.
4. Stopwatch.
5. Water bath, 37°C.
6. Pipettes: 1 ml, graduated; 0.1-ml micropipettes.
7. Tubes: 12×75 mm.

Specimen

The specimen used is citrated plasma, as in the PT and activated PTT tests. A normal control plasma specimen should also be obtained.

Method

1. All reagents are prewarmed to 37°C for 5 minutes, and 0.1-ml volumes of venom, plasma, and calcium chloride are added together, and the timer is started. The clotting time of the mixture is recorded.
2. The PT of the test plasma specimen is determined as described on page 346.

Reference Range

The reference range is 11–15 seconds.

Sources of Error

A normal control should be run with the test, and an acceptable range should be established, as discussed in the section on testing the activated PTT.

Clinical Correlation

If the PT and the Russell's viper venom (Stypven) time are both abnormal, a deficiency of factor X, factor V, prothrombin, or fibrinogen is possible. However, if the test is normal with an abnormal PT, a factor VII deficiency or the presence of factor X_{FRIULI} is indicated (Girolami, 1971).

Thrombin Time

Principle

The time required for a standard thrombin solution to clot test plasma is proportional to the conversion

Table 20.3. Comparison Between the Reptilase and the Thrombin Time Test

Thrombin Time	Reptilase Test	Cause
Elevated	Elevated	Decrease in or lack of fibrinogen, antithrombin III, or fibrin split products
Elevated	Extremely elevated	Dysfibrinogenemia
Elevated	Normal	Heparin or antithrombins

rate of fibrinogen to fibrin. Besides being sensitive to fibrinogen levels, the thrombin time is affected by the presence of antithrombin III, heparin, and fibrin split products.

Reagents and Equipment

1. Thrombin (Parke Davis, Detroit, MI): 1,000 U/ml are used. Thrombin is reconstituted by adding 1 ml normal saline to the vial.
2. Stopwatch.
3. Water bath, 37°C.
4. Pipettes: 1 ml, graduated; 0.1-ml micropipettes.
5. Tubes: 12 × 75 mm.

Specimen

Citrated plasma is used, as previously described in the section on the PT test (page 347).

Method

1. All reagents and plasma specimens are pre-warmed to 37°C.
2. One-tenth milliliter of thrombin is added to 1 ml normal plasma. The stopwatch is started immediately, and the time it takes for a fibrin clot to form is recorded.
3. The procedure is repeated with a dilution of thrombin in normal saline so that the normal plasma produces a clot in 20–22 seconds. This diluted reagent is stable for 15–20 minutes at room temperature.
4. The procedure is repeated using the test plasma as well as an equal dilution of test and normal plasma.

Interpretation

Prolonged thrombin times using only test plasma may indicate hypofibrinogenemia, dysfibrinogenemia, or the presence of fibrin split products. Ele-vated test times using equal volumes of test and normal plasma probably indicate the presence of fibrin split products or, rarely, a dysfibrinogenemia. If the results of both the test plasma and the test-normal mixture are abnormal, the presence of heparin should be ruled out.

Further interpretations of the thrombin time and reptilase tests are shown in Table 20.3. Table 20.4 illustrates the ability of various screening tests to detect procoagulant deficiencies.

Standard Factor Assay

Fibrinogen

Principle

The enzyme thrombin converts the soluble plasma protein, fibrinogen, into its insoluble polymer, fibrin. At high thrombin concentrations of approximately 100 National Institutes of Health (NIH) units/ml and low fibrinogen levels of 5–80 mg/dl, the reaction rate is determined by the fibrinogen concentration. The thrombin clotting time produces a linear relationship to fibrinogen levels when plotted on double log graph paper.

Reagents and Equipment

1. Veronal buffer (Owren's), pH 7.35: Sodium barbital, 5.9 g, and 7.1 g sodium chloride are dissolved in 2.5 ml 0.1-N hydrochloric acid and 785 ml distilled water. This reagent is stable indefinitely at 4°C.
2. Thrombin: 100 NIH units/ml.
3. Fibrinogen calibration reference: This is a lyophilized, stable, normal citrated plasma that has been assayed by macro-Kjeldahl. Note that all these reagents (items 1–3) can be obtained commercially (as Data Fi) from Dade Corporation, Division of American Hospital Supply, Miami, FL.

Table 20.4. Ability of Screening Tests to Detect Procoagulant Abnormalities

Deficiency	Prothrombin Time	Activated Partial Thromboplastin	Thrombin Time
Fibrinogen	+	+	+
Prothrombin	+	+	−
Factor V	+	+	−
Factor VII	+	−	−
Factor VIII	−	+	−
Factor IX	−	+	−
Factor X	+	+	−
Factor XI	−	+	−
Factor XII	−	+	−
Factor XIII	−	−	−
Prekallikrein	−	+	−

Table 20.5. Fibrinogen Calibrate Dilutions

	Tube 1	Tube 2	Tube 3
Veronal buffer (ml)	1.6	0.8	2.8
Fibrinogen calibrate (ml)	0.4	0.4 from tube 1	0.4 from tube 2
Final dilution	1:5	1:15	1:40

4. Water bath, 37°C.
5. Stopwatch.
6. Pipettes: 1 ml, graduated; 0.1-ml micropipettes.
7. Tubes: 13 × 100 mm.

Specimen

The test specimen is sodium citrated whole blood. Four and one-half milliliters of whole blood are collected in 0.5 ml 3.8% sodium citrate. The specimen is centrifuged at 3,000 rpm for 5 minutes as soon as possible, and the plasma is removed. The specimen is stable for 72 hours when stored at 4°C. Controls composed of either fresh normal citrated plasma or commercially obtained plasma are run simultaneously with the test.

Method

1. Three tubes are set up as shown in Table 20.5. The contents of tube no. 1 are mixed, 0.4 ml is transferred to tube no. 2, and 0.4 ml is transferred to tube no. 3.
2. Duplicate determinations are run on the cali-

brated tubes using the following procedure: Each dilution is incubated at 37°C for 2 minutes. One-tenth milliliter of thrombin is added forcibly to each tube, and the stopwatch is started. By use of a hooked nickel-chromium wire, the first sign of clotting is determined. At a 1:40 dilution, only a small fibrin thread is formed but, at a 1:5 dilution, a solid clot will form after a very brief time.
3. The average of the three sets of duplicate times is plotted against the fibrinogen concentration, as illustrated in Figure 20.1. The three points are connected. The calibration curve may be extended beyond the 1:5 point to a maximum fibrinogen concentration of 800 mg/dl and beyond the 1:40 point to a concentration of 50 mg/dl. Figure 20.1 shows the fibrinogen standard curve.
4. The test plasma and control specimens are diluted 1:10 by adding 0.1 ml plasma to 0.9 ml buffer.
5. The average duplicate thrombin clotting times on these samples are determined by the method described in step 2.
6. The clotting time obtained on the 1:10 plasma is read from the calibration curve.

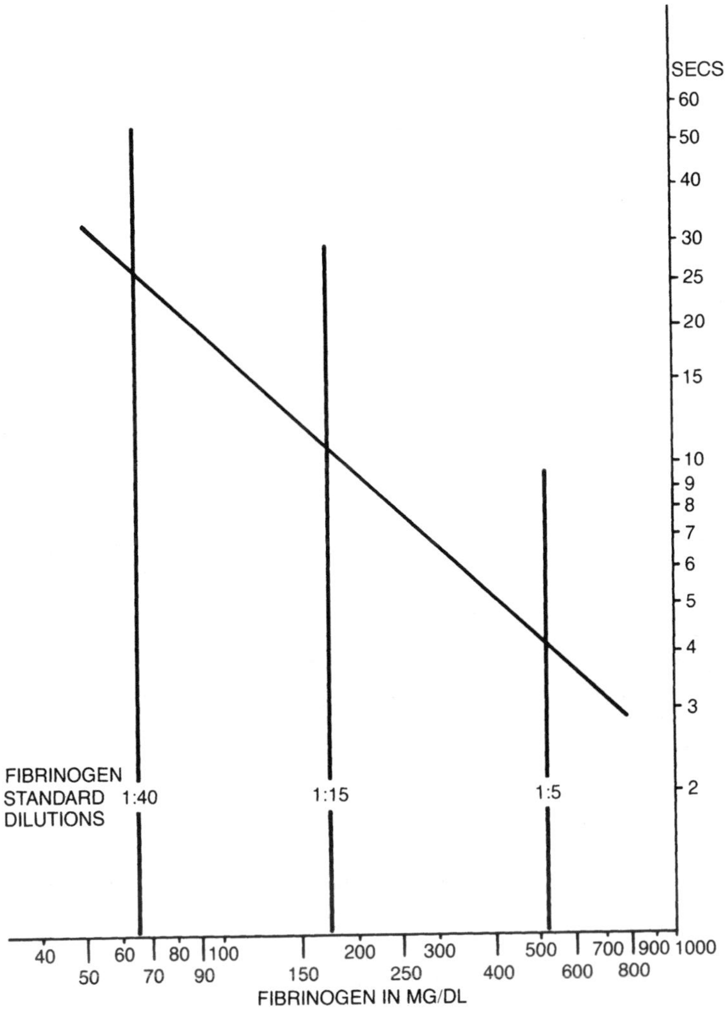

Figure 20.1. A typical fibrinogen standard curve.

Reference Range

The reference range is 200–400 mg/dl.

Sources of Error

Controls covering the expected test ranges should be run, and a statistically acceptable range for each material should be established. If a fibrinogen value greater than 800 mg/dl is present, the test plasma should be diluted 1:20 with buffer, and the result should be calculated by multiplying by two the value obtained from the calibration curve. Similarly, low fibrinogen values of less than 50 mg/dl should be repeated using a 1:5 dilution, and the result should be divided by two. This procedure can be adapted to most automated and semiautomated equipment. The procedure is not affected by usual heparin levels found in patients undergoing anticoagulation therapy or by the presence of antithrombin, owing to the great excess of thrombin used in the procedure.

Clinical Correlation

Hypofibrinogenemia can result from a wide range of acquired clinical conditions, including DIC and liver disease, or it can be an inherited disorder. Increases in fibrinogen are found in acute infections, hepatitis, nephrosis, burns, myeloma, collagen diseases, and various malignancies.

Table 20.6. Standard Dilutions Used for Coagulation Factor Assays

Tube No.	Buffer (ml)	Normal Plasma 100% (ml)	Transfer (ml)	Final Dilution	Concentration of Factors (%)
1	1.8	0.2	1.0	1:10	100
2	1.0	—	1.0	1:20	50
3	1.0	—	1.0	1:40	25
4	1.0	—	1.0	1:80	12.5
5	1.0	—	1.0	1:160	6.25
6	1.0	—	1.0*	1:320	3.12

*Discard 1.0 ml from tube no. 6.

Factor Assays Based on the Prothrombin Time

Factors V, VII, and X, and Prothrombin Assays

Principle

A PT test is carried out on the test plasma, and the degree of correction obtained when the test plasma is mixed with a factor-deficient plasma substrate is determined. This correction is compared with the correction obtained when normal plasma is substituted for the deficient plasma.

Reagents and Equipment

1. Thromboplastin or thromboplastin-calcium reagent, obtained commercially.
2. Calcium chloride, 0.025 M (if the thromboplastin-free reagent is used): Anhydrous calcium chloride, 2.77 g, is dissolved in 1 liter distilled water.
3. Normal pooled plasma or commercially obtained pooled plasma.
4. Factor-deficient substrate plasma (George King Biomedical, Overland Park, KS).
5. Veronal buffer (Owren's), pH 7.35 (see page 351).
6. Water bath, 37°C.
7. Stopwatch.
8. Pipettes: 1 ml and 5 ml, graduated; 0.1-ml and 0.2-ml micropipettes.
9. Tubes: 12 × 75 mm.
10. Log-log graph paper (two-cycle).

Specimen

As in the PT and activated PTT tests, citrated blood is used.

Method

1. Serial dilutions of either commercially obtained normal plasma or a pool of no less than five normal plasma specimens are prepared. Dilutions ranging from 1:10 to 1:100 are made using veronal buffer, as shown in Table 20.6.
2. The deficient substrates are reconstituted according to the package instructions.
3. One-tenth milliliter of the substrate is added to 0.1 ml of a 1:10 buffer dilution of the standard plasma.
4. The solution is mixed and incubated at 37°C for 2–5 minutes. Two-tenths milliliter of prewarmed thromboplastin-calcium reagent or 0.1 ml thromboplastin and 0.1 ml 0.025-M calcium chloride are added.
5. The stopwatch is started, and the clotting time is recorded.
6. Steps 3–5 are repeated for each dilution of standard plasma. The clotting times are determined in duplicate, and the individual averages of these times are plotted on log-log graph paper, with the dilutions plotted on the abscissa and the time in seconds on the ordinate. The resulting graph should be a straight line.
7. The test plasma is diluted 1:10 and 1:20 with buffer, and steps 3–5 are repeated, test plasma being substituted for standard plasma for each dilution.
8. The percentage factor deficiency is read from the graph as the point at which the 1:10 dilution of test plasma intercepts the normal (100%) curve. The result obtained with the 1:20 dilution is obtained in a similar manner, and this percentage is multiplied by two to produce the undiluted result. The percentage activity derived from each dilution should not differ by more than 10% from the actual result.

Reference Range

The reference range is 50–150%.

Sources of Error

All clotting times should be determined in duplicate. Once made up, dilutions of buffered plasma should be tested within 30 minutes, and a new standard curve should be made with each batch of assays.

Clinical Correlation

This basic assay can be used for all factors (except fibrinogen) involved in the PT test. The difference in each individual assay is only the nature of the deficient substrate, all other reagents being constant.

For example, if a factor V assay is desired, a factor V–deficient substrate would be used in step 3. Likewise, a factor X–deficient substrate would be substituted if a factor X assay were desired.

Prothrombin Assay, Two-Stage Method

Principle

Brain thromboplastin is added to citrated plasma, and the mixture is recalcified (Biggs and Douglas, 1953). Thrombin generation is assayed by adding subsamples of the mixture to a standard fibrinogen solution. The fibrinogen clotting times are converted to thrombin units, which are graphed against the subsampling times. A normal plasma specimen is assayed and compared.

Reagents and Equipment

1. Thromboplastin (Difco), 1:5 dilution in normal saline.
2. Calcium chloride, 0.025 M: Anhydrous calcium chloride, 2.77 g, is dissolved in 1 liter distilled water.
3. Fibrinogen (General Diagnostics), 300 mg/dl.
4. Thrombin (Parke Davis), 10 NIH units/ml: Normal saline, 10 ml, is added to a 1,000–NIH units/ml vial of thrombin. It is allowed to dissolve, and 1 ml of the dilution is added to 9 ml saline.
5. Water bath, 37°C.

6. Stopwatches.
7. Tubes: 10×75 mm.
8. Pipettes: 1 ml, graduated; 0.1-ml micropipettes.

Specimen

The specimen used is citrated whole blood. Anticoagulated blood is centrifuged at 3,000 rpm for 10 minutes, and the plasma is removed and stored at 4°C until assayed. A normal control plasma specimen is obtained and treated as the test plasma.

Method

1. Four-tenths milliliter of fibrinogen is added to each of 10 tubes at 37°C.
2. In a separate tube, 0.4 ml fresh normal citrated plasma is added to 0.4 ml diluted thromboplastin, and 0.4 ml 0.025-M calcium chloride then is added to this mixture. A stopwatch is begun on the addition of the last reagent, and the clotting time of the mixture is recorded.
3. The formed clot is removed with an applicator stick as quickly as possible and at 1-minute intervals. One-tenth milliliter of the thrombin-generating mixture in step 2 is removed and added to one of the fibrinogen tubes prepared in step 1.
4. A second stopwatch is started when the generating mixture is added, and the time it takes for a clot to form is recorded.
5. The process is repeated for all 10 fibrinogen tubes.
6. The entire process is repeated using test plasma in place of the normal plasma.

Standard Thrombin-Fibrinogen Curve

1. Dilutions as shown in Table 20.7 are set up.
2. One-tenth milliliter of each of the eight dilutions is drawn into a series of new tubes, and 0.4 ml fibrinogen is added to each turn. The fibrinogen clotting times of each tube are recorded.
3. The reciprocal of these times is plotted against the thrombin units using linear graph paper (Figure 20.2).

Calculation

The thrombin units of both the normal and the test plasma, obtained from the thrombin-fibrinogen

Table 20.7. Standard Thrombin-Fibrinogen Dilutions

Tube No.	Thrombin Solution, 10 U/ml (ml)	Normal Saline	Thrombin Units
1	1.0	—	10
2	0.8	0.2	8
3	0.5	0.5	5
4	0.4	0.6	4
5	0.3	0.7	3
6	0.2	0.8	2
7	0.1	0.9	1
8	0.05	0.95	0.5

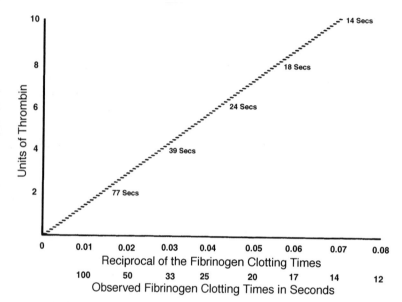

Figure 20.2. Thrombin-fibrinogen calibration curve.

curve, are plotted against the subsampling time (Figure 20.3). Then the two graphs are compared by measuring the areas under the curves, and the percentage of prothrombin is calculated by the following formula:

$$\frac{\text{Area under curve of test plasma}}{\text{Area under curve of normal plasma}} \times 100$$

$$= \% \text{ Prothrombin}$$

Reference Range

The reference range is 60–150%.

Clinical Correlation

The assay of prothrombin is of value only when investigating neonatal bleeding or the extremely rare congenital prothrombin deficiency. Most clinical situations involving a reduction in prothrombin also parallel decreases in other liver-produced coagulation factors or in vitamin K–related factors. Consequently, the utility of a prothrombin assay is strictly limited.

Newer techniques for assaying prothrombin are based on the rate of production of thrombin, which releases *p*-nitroaniline (*p*NA) from a chromogenic substrate. The *p*NA formation is spectrophotometri-

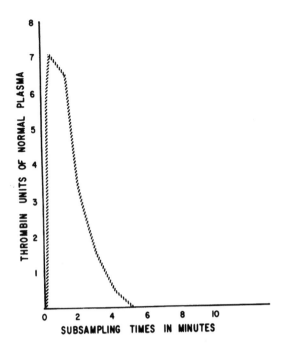

Figure 20.3. Thrombin units of normal plasma plotted against subsampling times.

cally measured at 405 nm and is proportional to the amount of prothrombin present, as there is complete prothrombin-thrombin conversion (Triplett and Harms, 1981).

Factor Assays Based on the Partial Thromboplastin Time

Factors VIII, IX, and XII Assays

Principle

A PTT is carried out on the test plasma, and the degree of correction obtained when the test plasma is mixed with a severely factor-deficient plasma substrate is determined. This correction is compared with the correction obtained when normal plasma is substituted for the deficient plasma.

Reagents and Equipment

1. Activated partial thromboplastin reagent, as described on page 348.

2. Buffered sodium citrate–citric acid anticoagulant (see page 254).
3. Factor VIII– or factor IX–deficient substrate plasma: Citrated blood is obtained from a severely deficient individual or purchased commercially (George King Biomedical).
4. Calcium chloride, 0.025 M (as described on page 348).
5. Veronal buffer, pH 7.35: Sodium diethyl barbiturate, 5.878 g, and 7.335 g sodium chloride are dissolved in 215 ml 0.1-N hydrochloric acid, and the volume is diluted to 1 liter with distilled water.
6. Water bath, 37°C.
7. Two stopwatches.
8. Tubes: 12 × 75 mm.
9. Pipettes: 0.1-ml and 0.2-ml micropipettes.
10. Two-cycle semilog graph paper.

Specimen

Citrated blood is used, as in the PT and activated PTT tests. A normal control specimen is obtained and treated in the same way.

Method

1. The activated PTT reagent and the factor-deficient substrate plasma are reconstituted. These are kept refrigerated until ready to use.
2. The calcium chloride is prewarmed.
3. Four tubes are set up as shown in Table 20.8. All tubes are kept at 4°C until ready for use.
4. The following are placed in another 37°C tube: 0.1-ml volumes of well-mixed partial thromboplastin reagent, factor-deficient plasma, and diluted control plasma from tube no. 1. The stopwatch is started immediately when the diluted control is added.
5. After exactly 3 minutes, 0.1 ml 0.25-M calcium chloride is added to the mixture, and the second stopwatch is started.
6. The contents of the tube are mixed quickly and are left at 37°C for exactly 30 seconds.
7. The tube is removed from the water bath and is tilted gently at a rate of approximately once per second. The tube is observed for gel formation. The stopwatch must not be stopped at the point of partial coalescence.
8. Steps 4–7 are repeated using the dilutions in tube nos. 2–4.

Table 20.8. Plasma Dilutions for the Partial Thromboplastin Time Assays of Factors VIII and IX

Tube No.	Veronal Buffer (ml)	Normal Plasma (ml)	Dilution	Plasma Concentration (%)
1	0.4	0.1	1:5	100
2	0.9	0.1	1:10	50
3	1.9	0.1	1:20	25
4	3.9	0.1	1:40	12.5

Table 20.9. Examples of the Calculation of Factor Assays Using the Partial Thromboplastin Time

Plasma Concentration (%)	Clotting Time (secs) Normal Plasma	Test Plasma	Equivalent Control Plasma Concentration (%)	Multiplication of Control Plasma by the Dilution Factor	Factor Activity of the Test Plasma
20	58	75	6	6×5	30
10	68	85	3	3×10	30
5	77	95	1.5	1.5×20	30
2.5	87	104	1	1×40	40

Note: Average factor assay = 32%.

9. Steps 3–7 are repeated using the patient's plasma in place of the normal plasma.

Calculation

Table 20.9 gives examples of the calculation of factor assays using the PTT.

1. The clotting time of each dilution is plotted against the plasma concentration on semilog graph paper (Figure 20.4).

2. By interpolation, the concentrations of normal control plasma that will produce the same clotting time as 20%, 10%, 5%, and 2.5% test plasma are determined.

3. The resulting control plasma concentrations are multiplied by the equivalent test plasma dilutions (i.e., 2.5% concentration × 40 = 100%, 5% concentration × 20 = 100%, and so on).

4. The four assays are averaged to give the final test result.

Reference Range

Factors VIII, IX, and XI	50–150%
Factor XII	30–200%
Mild factor VIII deficiency	5–25%
Moderately severe factor VIII deficiency	1–5%
Severe factor VIII deficiency	<1%
Von Willebrand's syndrome	1–50%

Sources of Error

All the clotting times in the assay should be determined in duplicate and the results averaged. When carrying out the test, it is essential to keep the diluted plasmas at 4°C or on crushed ice, and the test plasma should be stored frozen if there is a delay in testing.

If factor XI or factor XII assays are set up, it is essential that the test plasma not come into contact with any glass surface until step 4 of the method is reached. In addition, factor XI assays should be set up using fresh test samples only, as freezing may increase factor XI activity during storage.

There is considerable variation in the precision and sensitivity of the test depending on whether factor IX or other factor assays are involved. This is due to the type of activated PTT reagent used (Brandt et al., 1990). Two reagents (Ortho Thrombosil, available from Ortho Diagnostics Inc, Raritan, NJ; and Actin Fs, available from Baxter Healthcare Corp., McGaw Park, IL) appear more sensitive than other reagents. Increased responsiveness of a reagent in a one-stage factor VIII assay has been associated with improved precision

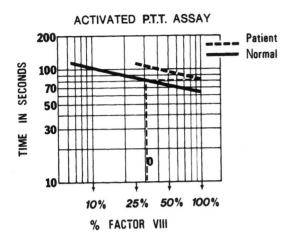

ACTIVATED P.T.T. ASSAY

Figure 20.4. The calculation of factor VIII using the PTT test.

(Brandt et al., 1988). A new assay has been described for the determination of factor XII using a chromogenic substrate and a selective inhibitor of plasma, kallikrein (Stürzebecher et al., 1989).

Factor VIII$_{VWF}$ Assay (Ristocetin Cofactor Assay)

Principle

Factor VIII ristocetin cofactor activity is the functional part of the factor VIII molecule required for platelet agglutination in the presence of the antibiotic ristocetin. Levels of this plasma factor are determined by the ability of platelet-poor plasma to cause agglutination of formalin-fixed platelets on the addition of ristocetin.

Reagents and Equipment

1. Phosphate-buffered saline (PBS), pH 7.2: Monobasic sodium phosphate, 13.8 g, is dissolved in 100 ml distilled water (1.0 M). Dibasic sodium phosphate, 3.404 g, is dissolved in 100 ml distilled water (0.5 M). For use, 13.2 ml of the 1-M monobasic sodium phosphate is added to 53.6 ml of the 0.5-M dibasic sodium phosphate. Sodium chloride, 34 g, is dissolved in the double phosphate solution with 2 liters distilled water and then diluted to 4 liters.
2. Ristocetin (Sigma Chemical Co.): Ristocetin, 0.018 g, is dissolved in 1 ml PBS. Dry ristocetin

is stored in the dark at room temperature. The made-up reagent is stored frozen at –20°C.
3. Bovine serum albumin (BSA): BSA, 0.1 g, is dissolved in 2.5 ml PBS.
4. Normal saline.
5. Formaldehyde, 2%, in PBS: Formalin, 2 ml, is added to 98 ml PBS.
6. Water bath, 37°C.
7. Formaldehyde-fixed platelets: A unit of newly expired platelet concentrate is obtained from the blood bank and is warmed to 37°C for 1 hour. The platelet concentrate is divided and placed into large plastic screw-cap tubes. It then is diluted with an equal volume of 2% formaldehyde and is mixed by gentle inversion and refrigerated at 4°C for 18–24 hours.

The mixture is centrifuged at 500 rpm for 10–15 minutes to separate possible red-cell contamination, and the platelet-rich supernatant is transferred into plastic centrifuge tubes and centrifuged at 3,000 rpm for 20–30 minutes in a refrigerated centrifuge at 4°C. The supernatant is discarded.

The platelets are resuspended gently in approximately 50 volumes of normal saline and centrifuged at 3,000 rpm for 10–15 minutes at 4°C. The saline washing is repeated two more times. The platelets are resuspended in PBS so that the concentration is approximately 500×10^9/liter.

8. Platelet aggregometer.
9. Plastic screw-cap tubes: 40-ml size.
10. Refrigerated centrifuge.
11. Two-cycle log-log graph paper.

Specimen

The test specimen is sodium citrated whole blood, which is centrifuged at 3,000 rpm for 10 minutes. The platelet-poor plasma is removed, with care taken not to remove the buffy coat.

A standard reference pool of plasma is prepared by the same method. The pool should consist of plasma obtained from 10 normal men and 10 normal women. The women should not be pregnant, and they should not be taking oral contraceptives.

Method

1. The standard normal pool plasma is diluted 1:2–1:16 in doubling dilutions with the BSA. The

undiluted plasma is considered to contain 100% factor VIII_{VWF}.

2. The test plasma is diluted 1:2 and 1:4 with BSA.

3. Five-tenths milliliter of the fixed platelet suspension and 0.1 ml plasma are added to the aggregometer cuvette and are placed in the aggregometer with a stir bar.

4. A blank is prepared by diluting four volumes of fixed platelet suspension with three volumes of BSA.

5. The aggregometer baseline is adjusted to 0%, and 0.05 ml ristocetin is added. If necessary, the aggregometer is readjusted to zero after maximum minus deflection has occurred.

6. The percentage of change in optical density is recorded, and a reference curve is prepared on arithmetic graph paper using the standard reference plasma pool dilutions.

7. One-tenth milliliter of undiluted patient plasma or plasma dilution is added. The value is read from the reference curve.

Calculation

The lag time for the addition of ristocetin is determined in minutes to the point at which agglutination is first detected. On two-cycle log-log graph paper, the percentage of activity is plotted on the abscissa and the lag time is plotted on the ordinate for each of the standard dilutions. The percentage of activity of the patient is determined by locating the point at which the patient's lag time intersects the standard curve.

Reference Range

The reference range is 50–130%.

Sources of Error

When 1:2 dilutions of plasma are used, a small amount of aggregation may occur before the addition of the ristocetin. Ristocetin should not be added to the mixture until the optical density remains constant. If a large amount of spontaneous platelet aggregation occurs, a new batch of platelets should be prepared and the old batch discarded.

Factor VIII–Related Antigen (Immunoelectrophoresis)

Principle

Factor VIII antigen is electrophoresed on agarose gel plates containing factor VIII antisera. At the junction of the antigen and the antibody, a precipitate peak is formed that is directly proportional to the level of the antigen (Laurell, 1966; Sibley, 1977).

Reagents and Equipment

1. Electrophoresis chamber and power supply.
2. Agar template.
3. Telfa (absorbent) strips (wicks).
4. Microdispenser.
5. Agarose 1% (A380, available from Fisher Scientific Co., Fairlawn, NJ).
6. Factor VIII antiserum (Behring Diagnostics, American Hoechst Corp., Somerville, NJ).
7. Buffer, TRIS(hydroxyethyl) aminomethane (TRIS)-barbital, pH 8.8, ionic strength 0.028: High-resolution buffer (Gelman Sciences Inc, Ann Arbor, MI), 17 g, is dissolved in distilled water and is diluted to 2 liters. The pH is adjusted if required. The diluted buffer is stored at 4°C.
8. Decolorizing solution: Concentrated acetic acid, 200 ml, is added to 1 liter absolute methyl alcohol and 1 liter deionized water.
9. Coomassie brilliant blue stain: 0.25 g stain (R250) is dissolved in decolorizing solution and is diluted to 1 liter. It is stored at room temperature.
10. Glass slides, 8.1 × 10 mm, Kodak, prepared as follows: The slide is precoated by quickly flooding it with hot 0.1% agarose solution. All excess agarose is drained from the slide, and the slide is cooled and stored at 4°C. Agarose (9.15 g) is added to 15 ml TRIS-barbital buffer in an Erlenmeyer flask. The agarose is dissolved by placing it in a boiling water bath for 5–10 minutes or until the solution is clear. The flask is swirled occasionally during heating. The agarose is placed in a 50°C water bath and allowed to reach that temperature. Factor VIII antiserum (0.08 ml) is added to the agarose solution, and the flask is swirled to mix. Each Kodak slide requires 15 ml agarose.

The precoated slide is warmed on a tepid hot plate, and 15 ml of the agarose antisera is applied to the slide, using a prewarmed 25-ml graduated pipette. The slide must be placed on a level surface before the addition of the agarose. It is allowed to cool for 10–15 minutes and is placed on a moistened filter paper enclosed in an airtight plastic bag. This is stored at 4°C overnight. The plates should be used within 3 days.

Three-millimeter holes are punched in the gel just before use, using the agarose template. The agarose is removed carefully by suction or a Pasteur pipette.

11. Water bath, 50°C.
12. Erlenmeyer flask: 50 ml.
13. Pipettes: 10 ml and 25 ml, graduated.
14. Refrigerated centrifuge.
15. Filter paper: Whatman no. 1.
16. Normal plasma: either a pool of five fresh normal citrated plasma specimens or commercially obtained lyophilized normal plasma.
17. Log-log graph paper.

Specimen

Citrated blood is the specimen used. By a two-syringe technique, nine volumes of blood are added to one volume of 3.2% sodium citrate in a plastic tube. The tube is covered with parafilm (plastic sheeting) and is inverted several times to mix. Then it is centrifuged at 4°C at 2,000 rpm for 20–30 minutes. The plasma is removed and is stored frozen in a plastic tube until the technologist is ready to conduct the test.

Method

1. The lyophilized normal plasma is reconstituted, or the fresh normal plasma specimens are pooled, and the dilutions shown in Table 20.10 are set up.
2. The test plasma is thawed rapidly and diluted 1:2 and 1:4 with buffer.
3. The microdispenser is used to apply 5-µl volumes of the diluted reference plasma specimens and test plasma specimens to each well. The pipette is washed out several times between each application to avoid sample contamination. All applications to the wells should be made within a 5-minute period to minimize radial diffusion.

Table 20.10. Dilutions Used in the Quantitation of Factor VIII–Related Antigen

	Tube No.			
	1	**2**	**3**	**4**
Buffer (ml)	—	0.5	0.75	0.9
Normal plasma (ml)	1.0	0.5	0.25	0.1
Reference %	100	50	25	10

4. The Telfa wicks are presoaked in buffer and placed on the cathode and anode sides of each gel. Each wick should be flat against the agarose, with the other end remaining in the buffer.
5. The slide is placed in the electrophoresis chamber with the wells situated on the cathode side of the apparatus.
6. Each side of the chamber is filled with TRIS-barbital buffer, the chamber is covered, and electrophoresis is performed for 24 hours at 8 mA per plate. The electrophoresis chamber should be set up in a cold room, or it can be placed in a refrigerator with the electrical leads being passed through the rubber gasket of the door to the power supply.
7. The power supply is turned off, and the plates are removed and soaked in deionized water overnight to remove any excess protein buildup.
8. The agarose slide is placed on a filter paper and is covered immediately with 5–10 additional filter papers. A glass side is placed on top of the filter paper, and a weight is added. This is left for 15–20 minutes to remove excess water from the plate. The filter paper is removed, and the slide is dried in a mildly warm oven or with a hair dryer.
9. The slide is placed in a jar of Coomassie blue stain for 10 minutes and then is decolorized until the background is clear, using as many different changes of decolorizing solution as needed.

Calculation

The peak heights are measured in millimeters from the top point of the application well. The reference peak heights are plotted against the relative factor VIII–related antigen concentration. A "best-fit" line is constructed, which should be linear between the extreme dilutions. The factor VIII–related antigen concentration is read, using the two test dilutions from the graph. The results are averaged.

Reference Range

The reference range is 70–150%. The factor VIII–related antigen is normal or increased in hemophiliacs and factor VIII carrier states, but it is decreased or lacking in von Willebrand's syndrome.

Prekallikrein Detection (Screening)

Principle

The activated PTT is corrected when prekallikrein deficiency plasma is incubated for a prolonged time using a diatomaceous earth activator (Hattersley and Hayse, 1976).

Reagents and Equipment

The reagents and equipment used for prekallikrein detection are those used for the activated PTT test (page 348).

Method

An activated PTT test is carried out as described on page 348. The test is then repeated and modified by lengthening the incubation time of the plasma and reagent from 3 to 10 minutes.

Interpretation

Correction of the test result to normal after the lengthened incubation is suggestive of prekallikrein (Fletcher factor) deficiency.

Sources of Error

The activator used in the partial thromboplastin reagent should be one of the diatomaceous earths. Ellagic acid activation should not be used. Alternatives to this screening test rely on mixing studies using prekallikrein-deficient substrate plasma specimens in the same way as described for other factor assays. Additionally, prekallikrein can be assayed using chromogenic substrates. The synthetic chromogenic substrate S-2302 is a chain of amino acids

that mimic the terminal portion of bradykinin, kallidin, and methionine-lysine-bradykinin, which are released by kallikrein from high-molecular-weight kininogen.

Kallikrein, formed by activation of prekallikrein with kaolin, releases the chromogen pNA, which can be measured spectrophotometrically (Egberg and Bergstrom, 1976).

Factor XIII Detection (Screening)

Principle

Normal plasma clots are insoluble in 5-M urea, whereas clots formed when factor XIII is lacking are soluble (Duckert, 1971).

Reagents and Equipment

1. Urea, 5 M: Urea, 30 g, is dissolved in 100 ml distilled water.
2. Calcium chloride, 0.025 M (as described on page 348).
3. Tubes: 12 × 75 mm.
4. Pipettes: 1 ml and 10 ml, graduated.
5. Water bath, 37°C.

Specimen

Citrated normal and test plasma constitute the specimens.

Method

1. Five-tenths milliliter each of normal and test plasma is pipetted into separate tubes.
2. Five-tenths milliliter of normal plasma is added to 9.5 ml test plasma, and a 0.5-ml volume is removed to a third tube.
3. Five-tenths milliliter of 0.025-M calcium chloride is added to each of the three tubes. These are mixed and placed in a 37°C water bath for 30 minutes.
4. Five-milliliter volumes of 5-M urea are added to each of the three tubes. The formed clots are removed from the tubes set up in step 3 and are transferred to the 5-M urea tubes. These tubes are allowed to stand at room temperature, and the clots are observed.

Results

When factor XIII is lacking, the clot will dissolve within 2–3 hours, whereas the normal clot and that obtained from the normal plasma and test plasma mixture will remain intact for at least 24 hours. Dissolution of the normal plasma–test plasma clot is suggestive of fibrinolytic activity.

Sources of Error

Factor XIII deficiency is a rare disorder. The factor is present normally in physiologic excess. As little as 1% of factor XIII is sufficient to render a clot insoluble in 5-M urea.

Physiologic Inhibitors

Circulating Anticoagulant Screening Test (Using Recalcification Time)

Principle

When platelet-rich plasma containing a circulating anticoagulant is added to normal blood, the recalcification time of the normal blood is prolonged in proportion to the strength of the anticoagulant.

Reagents and Equipment

1. Calcium chloride, 0.025 M (as described on page 348).
2. Water bath, 37°C.
3. Stopwatch.
4. Tubes: 8 × 75 mm.
5. Pipettes: 1 ml, graduated.

Specimen

Citrated test and normal blood specimens are obtained. The blood is centrifuged at 500–1,000 rpm for 2–5 minutes.

Method

1. Five tubes are set up in a 37°C water bath, as shown in Table 20.11, with care taken to use plastic or siliconized pipettes when handling the platelet-rich plasma specimens.

Table 20.11. Plasma Dilutions for Measuring Circulating Anticoagulants by Recalcification Times

Tube No.	Test Plasma (ml)	Normal Plasma (ml)
1	1.0	—
2	0.9	0.1
3	0.5	0.5
4	0.01	0.9
5	—	1.0

2. One milliliter of 0.025-M calcium chloride is added to tube no. 1, and the time to clot formation is recorded. The procedure is repeated with the remaining tubes.

Interpretation

In the presence of a circulating anticoagulant, the recalcification times of tube nos. 1–4 will be prolonged in proportion to the titer of the anticoagulant. The recalcification time of tube no. 5 will be normal.

Circulating Anticoagulant Screening Test (Using the Prothrombin or Activated Partial Thromboplastin Time)

Principle

The presence of a circulating anticoagulant against one of the factors involved in either the intrinsic or the extrinsic coagulation pathway will prolong the standard test time and also will prolong the test time when normal plasma is used. If the abnormality is due to a specific factor deficiency, the addition of the normal plasma will produce a corrected time.

Reagents and Equipment

1. Reagents and equipment as listed for the PT and the activated PTT tests (see pages 347 and 348).
2. Veronal buffer, pH 7.35: Sodium diethyl barbiturate, 5.875 g, and 7.335 g sodium chloride are dissolved in 600 ml deionized water, and 215 ml 0.1-N hydrochloric acid is added to the mixture. The mixture is adjusted to pH 7.35 and is diluted to 1 liter with deionized water.
3. Pipettes: 0.5-ml and 0.1-ml micropipettes.

Table 20.12. Plasma Dilutions for the Detection of Circulating Anticoagulants Using the Prothrombin or the Partial Thromboplastin Time Tests

Plasma	Tube No.						
	1	2	3	4	5	6	7
Normal (ml)	—	0.05	0.1	0.25	0.4	0.45	0.5
Test (ml)	0.5	0.45	0.4	0.25	0.1	0.05	—

Specimen

As for the PT test, exactly 4.5 ml blood is added to 0.5 ml 0.11-M sodium citrate. It is mixed well and is centrifuged at 1,000g for 10–15 minutes. The plasma is removed and tested as soon as possible. If testing cannot be completed within 2 hours, the stopper should not be removed from the tube, which should be maintained at room temperature.

Method

The test system used depends on the one that showed the abnormality. That is, if the original PT was abnormal, a series of PTs are carried out in step 2 that follows. Similarly, if the activated PTT was abnormal, PTTs are used in step 2.

1. Dilutions of test plasma in normal plasma are set up as shown in Table 20.12. These are kept on melting ice or are refrigerated until tested.
2. Either the PT or the activated PTT test is carried out (depending on the abnormality), and the tests are repeated after the plasma dilutions are incubated for 1 hour at 37°C.

Interpretation

The presence of an inhibitor is suggested when tube no. 4 does not correct the test to normal. This is substantiated by the finding that tube no. 6 has a significantly prolonged test time; that is, 10% of the test plasma increases the normal plasma test. If the test results appear diagnostic of an inhibitor, the test need not be repeated after incubation, but such repeat testing should be done routinely if the initial dilutions appear unhelpful.

Factor VIII Inhibitor

Principle

Inhibitors to factor VIII are assayed by mixing test plasma with a standard amount of factor VIII that is present in normal pooled plasma (Kasper, 1975). After incubation, the residual factor VIII level is measured and compared to a control. The degree of inhibition is expressed in Bethesda units, one unit being the amount of inhibitor that will inactivate 50% of the factor VIII activity present.

Reagents and Equipment

1. Veronal buffer, pH 7.35: For preparation, see page 351.
2. Activated partial thromboplastin reagent.
3. Calcium chloride, 0.025 M (as described on page 348).
4. Factor VIII–deficient plasma (as described on page 357).
5. Water bath, 37°C.
6. Stopwatch.
7. Tubes: 12 × 75 mm.
8. Two-cycle semilog graph paper.

Specimen

The test specimen is citrated blood, as described on page 347. Pooled fresh normal plasma specimens should be obtained. Lyophilized commercial plasma should not be used.

Method

1. The test plasma is diluted 1:2 and 1:4 in veronal buffer, and the tubes shown in Table 20.13 are set up.

Table 20.13. Dilutions Used to Detect Factor VIII Inhibitor

Reagent	Tube No.			
	1	2	3	4
Normal control plasma (ml)	0.2	0.2	0.2	0.2
Buffer (ml)	0.2	—	—	—
Test plasma (ml)	—	0.2	—	—
Diluted test plasma, 1:2 (ml)	—	—	0.2	—
Diluted test plasma, 1:4 (ml)	—	—	—	0.2

2. The tubes are mixed and stoppered. They are incubated at 37°C for 2 hours, and factor VIII assays are carried out on each mixture (page 357).

Calculation

The factor VIII levels are determined, and then the residual factor VIII activity (RFA) is found by using the factor VIII level of the control (tube no. 1) and the test plasma dilution that possesses a residual factor VIII level greater than 25%.

$$RFA = \frac{\text{Factor VIII level of the test}}{\text{Factor VIII level of the control}} \times 100$$
$$= \text{Thrombin inhibited (\%)}$$

This RFA then is converted to Bethesda units according to Table 20.14.

The factor VIII inhibitor in Bethesda units is calculated from the following formula:

Dilution of the test plasma used × Bethesda units (Table 20.14) = Factor VIII inhibitor (in Bethesda units/ml plasma)

Interpretation

The lack of an inhibitor produces RFA of 100%, whereas the effect of an inhibitor to factor VIII proportionally depresses the assay.

Sources of Error

If the RFA is less than 25% with the 1:4 test dilution, the test is repeated using greater dilutions until the RFA is greater than 25%. This method is used principally to compare factor VIII inhibitors found in classic hemophilia, but it may not be sufficiently sensitive to detect weak antibodies. If weak inhibitors are suspected, the test can be made more sensitive by prolonging the incubation period for 4–6 hours at 4°C.

Examples of the calculations are as follows:

Factor VIII level of control (100%)—
tube no. 1 = 70%

Factor VIII level of equal volumes of test and control—tube no. 3 = 30%

$$\text{RFA of tube no. } 3 = \frac{30}{70} \times 100 = 43\%$$

Table 20.14 shows that 43% RFA corresponds to a factor of 1.20, so the plasma dilution (1:1) times the factor is equal to the factor VIII inhibitor in Bethesda units—that is:

$$1:1 \times 1.2 = 1.2 \text{ Bethesda units}$$

Lupus Anticoagulant

Principle

Test plasma is incubated with varying dilutions of thromboplastin-calcium, and the PTs of the dilutions are determined. The lupus anticoagulant inhibits the tissue thromboplastin and consequently prolongs the PT (Margolius et al., 1961; Schleider, 1976).

Reagents and Equipment

1. Reagents and equipment as in the PT test (page 347), except that pure brain thromboplastin is reconstituted according to the manufacturer's directions (Difco).

Table 20.14. Bethesda Unit Conversion Chart for Factor VIII

Residual Factor VIII (%)	Factor	Residual Factor (%)	Factor
97	0.05	48	1.05
93	0.10	46	1.10
90	0.15	45	1.15
87	0.20	43	1.20
84	0.25	42	1.25
81	0.30	41	1.30
78	0.35	40	1.35
75	0.40	38	1.40
73	0.45	37	1.45
70	0.50	35	1.50
68	0.55	34	1.55
66	0.60	33	1.60
64	0.65	32	1.65
61	0.70	30	1.70
59	0.75	29	1.75
57	0.80	28	1.80
53	0.90	27	1.85
51	0.95	26	1.90
50	1.00	25	2.00

Table 20.15. Thromboplastin Dilutions for the Detection of Lupus Anticoagulants

Tube No.	Saline (ml)	Thromboplastin (ml)	Final Dilution
1	—	0.5	1:1
2	0.4	0.1	1:5
3	0.9	0.1	1:10
4	9.9	0.1	1:100
5	49.9	0.1	1:500
6	99.9	0.1	1:1,000

2. Calcium chloride, 0.025 M (as described on page 348).

3. Normal saline.

4. Pipettes: 10 ml, graduated; 0.1-ml micropipettes.

5. Volumetric flasks: 10 ml, 50 ml, and 100 ml.

Specimen

Citrated test and normal control plasma specimens are used (see page 347).

Method

1. The tissue thromboplastin is diluted with normal saline as in Table 20.15.

2. One-tenth milliliter of each thromboplastin dilution is added to prewarmed tubes, and the PTs of both the test and the control plasma are determined using these different thromboplastin dilutions.

Results

If an anticoagulant is present against the tissue thromboplastin (human brain) used in the test, it will produce increasing PTs as the thromboplastin becomes more diluted. Table 20.16 shows typical results found in patients with a lupus anticoagulant. The results are expressed as a ratio of test to control. Ratios of 1:1 or less are considered normal, 1:1–1:3

Table 20.16. Typical Results in the Detection of Tissue Thromboplastin Anticoagulants

Thromboplastin dilution	—	1:5	1:10	1:100	1:500	1:1,000
Prothrombin time (secs), positive result	13	25	40	65	90	150
Prothrombin time (secs), normal result	12	16	25	35	55	70

Table 20.17. Dilutions of Pooled Normal Plasma for Functional Assay to Detect Antithrombin III

	Tube No.			
Reagent	1	2	3	4
Buffered saline (ml)	2.0	1.9	1.7	1.5
Pooled normal plasma (ml)	—	0.1	0.3	0.5
Final dilution (%)	—	25	75	125

are considered borderline, and greater than 1:3 is considered abnormal.

Antithrombin III (Functional Assay)

Principle

Thrombin is neutralized by antithrombin that is present in defibrinated plasma. The neutralized plasma is then clotted with fibrinogen. A linear relationship exists between the log of the clotting time and the thrombin left after neutralization (Frigola, 1977).

Reagents and Equipment

1. Thrombin (Fibrindex, available from Ortho Pharmaceutical Co., Raritan, NJ): The thrombin is reconstituted by adding 1 ml normal saline to produce a concentration of 50 U/ml. Before testing, the stock thrombin is diluted to 4 U/ml by diluting to 12.5 ml with normal saline.
2. Fibrinogen (General Diagnostics).
3. Buffered normal saline, pH 7.4: TRIS base, 24.3 g, is dissolved in 250 ml distilled water. 42 ml of 0.1-N hydrochloric acid are added to the solution, and the volume is made up to approximately 950 ml with distilled water. The pH is adjusted to 7.4, and the mixture is diluted to 1 liter. Sodium chloride, 2.2 g, is added to the TRIS buffer, and the solution is mixed by agitation.
4. Water bath, 37°C and 56°C.
5. Stopwatch.
6. Tubes: plastic, 12 × 75 mm.
7. Pipettes: 1 ml, 2 ml, and 5 ml, graduated.
8. Normal citrated plasma: A pool made from the plasma of 15–20 normal donors is made by centrifuging each sample at 3,000 rpm for 15 minutes to obtain platelet-poor plasma. Separation should take place within 30 minutes of collection. The platelet-poor plasma is removed and stored in a plastic tube at 4°C.
9. Semilog graph paper.

Specimen

The specimen is citrated test plasma. Platelet-poor plasma is made as described in step 8.

Method

1. Dilutions of the pooled normal plasma are made as shown in Table 20.17.
2. Four-tenths milliliter of the normal plasma in tube no. 1 is added to another tube and is incubated at 37°C for 5 minutes.
3. Two-tenths milliliter of fibrinogen is added to a separate tube and is incubated at 37°C for 5 minutes.
4. One-tenth milliliter of the working thrombin reagent (4 U/ml) is added to the plasma tube (step 2) and is mixed gently and incubated at 37°C.
5. After *exactly 3 minutes*, 0.1 ml of this mixture is removed and delivered to the fibrinogen tube (step 3). The clotting time of the mixture is recorded.

Table 20.18. Expected Results with Duplicate Testing in the Functional Assay of Antithrombin III

Clotting Time (secs)	Agreement ± (secs)
7–12	1
13–25	2
26–44	3
>45	4

6. Steps 2–5 are repeated for all the plasma dilutions shown in Table 20.17. All clotting tests are carried out in duplicate. Agreement should be as shown in Table 20.18.

7. If the duplicate clotting times are not acceptable, the dilutions are retested and a third value is obtained. The two closest results are averaged, and the times are plotted against the dilutions on semi-log graph paper. This is the normal curve.

8. One milliliter of test plasma is incubated in a plastic tube at 56°C for *exactly 5 minutes.*

9. The tube is transferred immediately to an ice bath or freezer for 5 minutes.

10. It is centrifuged at 3,000 rpm for 15 minutes. The supernatant defibrinated plasma is removed to another tube.

11. Steps 2–5 are repeated using the defibrinated test plasma in place of the normal diluted plasma specimens. All tests are carried out in duplicate, and the results are averaged.

Calculation

The antithrombin III activity is determined from the normal graph.

Reference Range

The reference range is 81–120%.

Sources of Error

The use of plastic tubes and the accurate timing of all incubation periods in the procedure are essential for valid rest results. Antithrombin III neutralizes thrombin activity by the formation of a 1:1 stoichiometric complex through an interaction between arginine on the antithrombin molecule and serine on the thrombin molecule.

Besides the functional assay described previously, three other techniques can be used to measure quantitatively the presence of the antithrombin III anticoagulant: (1) radial immunodiffusion, (2) rocket electrophoresis, and (3) chromogenic or fluorogenic substrates. Of these methods, the chromogenic assays are more precise, but there may be moderate differences between reference ranges, depending on the methodology used.

Clinical Correlation

Normal levels of antithrombin III vary with age and gender. A moderate decrease in antithrombin III occurs in middle age, especially in men, whereas, in women of childbearing age, the concentration is lower than that seen in men of comparable age. Reductions in antithrombin III levels are seen in liver disease, in intravascular coagulation, and in women taking oral contraceptives.

Fluorogenic Assay of Antithrombin III

Principle

The fluorogenic assay of antithrombin III uses the synthetic substrate D-phenylalanine-proline-arginine-5-amidosiophalic acid dimethyl ester, which releases the fluorescent molecule 5-aminoisophthalic acid dimethyl ester (AIE) after thrombin interaction (Mitchell, 1978). This is measured fluorometrically, and the antithrombin III activity is determined indirectly by the incubation of thrombin with test plasma and heparin. These reactions are as follows:

Antithrombin III + thrombin →
antithrombin III–heparin complex →
(antithrombin III–heparin complex–thrombin)
+ residual thrombin

Residual thrombin + Phe-Pro-Arg-AIE →
Phe-Pro-Arg + AIE (fluorescent)

Reagents and Equipment

1. Fluorometer (Protopath, available from Dade).
2. Stopwatch.
3. Water bath, 37°C.
4. Ice bath.

5. Vortex mixer.
6. Tubes: plastic, 12 × 75 mm.
7. Pipettes: 1 ml and 2 ml, graduated; 0.2-ml, 0.1-ml, and 0.05-ml micropipettes, plunger type with plastic tips.
8. Antithrombin III substrate assay reagents (Dade):
   a. Heparin: 1 USP units/ml heparin, buffered. It must be stored at 4°C. It must not be used if cloudy.
   b. Thrombin: purified human buffered thrombin stored at 4°C. It should be reconstituted with 1 ml deionized water. The solution is stoppered and swirled gently until dissolved. The final reagent contains 1 NIH unit thrombin per milliliter. The reagent should be kept 4°C or on ice when in use. It is stable at 4°C for 72 hours. Glass pipettes should be avoided when measuring this reagent.
   c. Thrombin substrate: a lyophilized buffered preparation of 0.3 μmol of D-phenylalanine-proline-arginine-AIE in disposable cuvettes identified by the presence of a green dot. The substrate is packaged in a foil pouch and, once opened, must be used within 7 days when stored at 4°C. The substrate is reconstituted with 2 ml deionized water and contains a concentration of 0.15 μmol/ml. This reagent is stable for 4 hours at room temperature or for 8 hours at 4°C and should be protected from direct light.
9. Control (Prototrol, available from Dade).
10. Citrated pooled normal plasma: 5–10 normal citrated blood specimens obtained as described in the section on specimens. These are centrifuged, and the plasma specimens are pooled. They are stored frozen in plastic tubes.

Specimen

Nine volumes of blood are collected using a plastic syringe, and they are anticoagulated with one volume of 3.8% sodium citrate. The blood is centrifuged at 2,000 rpm for 15–20 minutes. The plasma is removed and stored frozen in plastic tubes until used. The specimen is stable for 30 days if kept frozen at −20°C.

Method

1. The fluorometer is allowed to warm up for 45 minutes. All tubes are prewarmed to 37°C.

2. One thrombin substrate cuvette is reconstituted for each blank, pooled normal plasma, Prototrol control, and test sample. The cuvettes are warmed to 37°C for 10 minutes, care being taken not to place them in the light path until the test mixture is added.

3. Two milliliters of heparin reagent and 5-ml volumes of pooled normal plasma, test plasma, and Prototrol are dispensed into three tubes, respectively. They are mixed by vortexing. These dilutions are stable for 6 hours at room temperature.

4. The fluorometer function is checked according to the manufacturer's instructions.

5. The antithrombin III reagent blank is prepared by adding 0.2 ml heparin reagent to 0.1 ml thrombin in a prewarmed tube. The stopwatch is started and, after *exactly 60 seconds,* the contents of the prewarmed cuvette are poured into the tube. The reaction mixture is immediately poured back into the cuvette, and the tube is discarded.

6. The cuvette is placed in the fluorometer. The compartment cover is closed, and the value obtained on the digital display once it has stopped flashing is recorded. It should read 95–105. The calibrator control is adjusted if the reading is outside this range.

7. Two-tenths milliliter of the dilutions made in step 3 are transferred to a prewarmed tube and are placed at 37°C for 1–2 minutes; 0.1 ml thrombin reagent is added. The stopwatch is started and, after *exactly 60 seconds,* the reaction mixture is poured back into the cuvette. The tube is discarded.

8. The cuvette is placed in the fluorometer. The sample compartment cover is closed, and digital readout values are recorded when the lag phase is completed.

Calculation

The inhibitor activity of each plasma sample is calculated from the following equation:

$$\frac{\text{Reagent blank value} - \text{test value}}{\text{Reagent blank value}} \times 100$$

$$= \text{Thrombin inhibited (\%)}$$

When the reagent blank is 100, the percentage thrombin inhibited is 100 minus the test value.

The inhibitor activity for each test is expressed as a percentage of normal activity, using the pooled normal plasma as a standard.

$$\frac{\%\ \text{Thrombin inhibited for test}}{\substack{\%\ \text{Thrombin inhibited} \\ \text{for pooled normal plasma}}} \times 100$$

$$= \text{Inhibitor activity (\%)}$$

Reference Range

The reference range is 85–115%.

Clinical Correlation

Antithrombin III determinations have been shown to be a useful aid in the diagnosis of numerous thrombohemorrhagic diseases, including hereditary antithrombin III deficiency, DIC, deep vein thrombosis, and pulmonary emboli (Bick et al., 1985). However, the choice of assay method has a direct relationship to the utility of the test, as poor correlations have been reported between the DuPont aca method and the Dade Protopath and other techniques (Bick et al., 1985), with spuriously high values being noted with the DuPont aca method.

Heparin Assay

Principle

The amount of protamine required to neutralize heparin in a test plasma is titrated using a system based on the thrombin time.

Reagents and Equipment

1. Veronal buffer, pH 7.35: Sodium diethyl barbiturate, 5.878 g, and 7.335 g sodium chloride are dissolved in 215 ml 0.1-N hydrochloric acid and are diluted to 1 liter with distilled water.
2. Thrombin reagent (Parke Davis): A 1,000-U/ml vial of thrombin is diluted with buffer until it produces a clotting time greater than 20 seconds with normal citrated plasma.
3. Protamine sulfate: 10 mg/ml.

4. Stopwatch.
5. Water bath, 37°C.
6. Tubes: 10×75 mm.
7. Pipettes: 1 ml and 5 ml, graduated; 0.1-ml micropipettes.

Specimen

Citrated blood is centrifuged at 2,000 rpm for 5 minutes. The test plasma is removed and stored at room temperature. A normal control plasma specimen is treated as the test plasma specimen.

Method

1. The stock protamine sulfate is diluted as shown in Table 20.19.
2. One-tenth milliliter of citrated plasma is pipetted into each of the five tubes, and 0.1 ml the protamine sulfate dilution (step 1) is added to each.
3. One-tenth milliliter of thrombin is added to tube no. 1, and the stopwatch is started. The time of clot formation is recorded. The procedure is repeated for the other protamine sulfate dilution.

Interpretation

The lowest concentration of protamine that completely corrects the thrombin time is the point at which the heparin has been completely neutralized by the protamine. Eighty-five units of heparin are neutralized by 1 mg protamine sulfate.

Tests Useful in the Investigation of Disseminated Intravascular Coagulopathy

Fibrinogen–Fibrin Degradation Products Staphylococcal Clumping Test

Principle

Suspensions of certain staphylococci will clump in the presence of fibrinogen, some fibrinogen degradation products, some fibrin breakdown products, and insoluble fibrin monomers or polymer complexes (Leavelle et al., 1971). To detect these breakdown products, blood is collected in the presence of excess thrombin to ensure complete conversion of fibrinogen to fibrin and its subsequent

Table 20.19. Dilutions of Stock Protamine Sulfate Reagent

Tube No.	Protamine Sulfate (ml)	Buffer (ml)	Final Concentration of Protamine Sulfate (µg/ml)	Equivalence to Heparin Units
1	1.0 stock	99.0	100	8.5
2	0.5 from the total of tube no. 1	4.5	10	0.85
3	2.0 from the total of tube no. 2	2.0	5	0.42
4	2.0 from the total of tube no. 3	2.0	2.5	0.21
5	2.0 from the total of tube no. 4	2.0	1.25	0.10

removal in the clot. Additionally, ε-aminocaproic acid (EACA) is added to inhibit conversion of plasminogen to plasmin. When excess preformed plasmin is expected, such as in patients undergoing streptokinase therapy, trypsin inhibitor is added in place of the EACA. Blood is incubated at 37°C to allow complete coagulation, clot retraction, and inactivation of excess thrombin. After centrifugation, the serum is separated and diluted in a buffered saline reagent and is mixed with the staphylococcal cell suspension.

An estimate of the degradation products present can be obtained by comparing the amount of cell clumping produced by the test serum with the clumping produced by known levels of fibrinogen.

Reagents and Equipment

1. Glass plate: 20×20 cm, marked off in approximately 2-cm squares.
2. Microdiluters: 0.5 ml.
3. Calibrated pipette droppers: 0.05 ml.
4. Water bath, 37°C.
5. Buffered saline, 0.05 M (pH 7.3): The base is made by dissolving 0.680 g imidazole (0.2-M) in distilled water and diluting to 50 ml. The buffer is made by adding 2.5 volumes of base to 2.86 volumes of 0.1-N hydrochloric acid and 5.64 volumes of distilled water to produce a concentration of 0.05 M. The pH is adjusted to 7.3. To each 100 ml buffer, 0.585 g sodium chloride is added. The working reagent is made by adding one volume of the buffer to two volumes of normal saline.
6. Phosphate-citrate-albumin buffer: Anhydrous disodium hydrogen phosphate, 3.2 g, along with 7.2 g anhydrous potassium dihydrogen phosphate, 14.7 g trisodium citrate, 4.0 g bovine albumin, and 10 ml 0.1% sodium azide, is dissolved in ap-

proximately 800 ml warm distilled water and diluted to 1 liter.

7. Soybean trypsin inhibitor 1% (Sigma): It should be stored at –20°C.
8. Thrombin: 1,000 U/ml (Parke Davis).
9. Lyophilized preparations of *Staphylococcus aureus* (Newman D_2C strain, available from Sigma): stored at –20°C. The *S. aureus* preparation is removed from the freezer 30 minutes before its use, and 1 ml distilled water is added 1 minute before use.
10. Fibrinogen, working standards: The fibrinogen level of normal plasma is determined, and the material is diluted with phosphate-citrate-albumin buffer to produce a final concentration of 10 µg/ml. This stock standard is divided into 2.5-ml volumes and is stored frozen at –20°C. The working standard is made up by thawing one of the frozen vials of stock and diluting it as shown in Table 20.20.

Specimen

Two milliliters of freshly drawn whole blood are withdrawn from the syringe and dispensed into a tube containing 1 mg soybean trypsin inhibitor. The blood is mixed and immediately transferred to a tube containing 100 units of thrombin. It is incubated at 37°C for 1–2 hours, the clotted blood is centrifuged at 2,000 rpm for 10 minutes, and the serum is removed for testing.

Method

1. A series of serum dilutions is made as shown in Table 20.21.
2. Five-tenths milliliter of each of the seven serum dilutions and 0.05 ml each of the fibrinogen dilutions are pipetted onto the glass tile, each kept

Table 20.20. Preparation of Working Fibrinogen Standards

Tube No.	Stock Standard (ml)	Phosphate-Citrate-Albumin Buffer (ml)	Final Concentration (µg/ml)
1	0.6	—	10.0
2	0.6	0.2	7.5
3	0.6	0.4	6.0
4	0.6	0.6	5.0
5	0.6	2.4	2.5
6	0.3	2.7	1.7
7	0.5 from tube no. 6	0.5	0.5
8	0.5 from tube no. 7	0.5	2.5

Table 20.21. Preparation of Test Serum in the Detection of Fibrin Degradation Products

Tube No.	Serum (ml)	Imidazole Buffered Saline (ml)	Dilution
1	0.1	0.1	1:2
2	0.1 from the total of tube no. 1	0.1	1:4
3	0.1 from the total of tube no. 2	0.1	1:8
4	0.1 from the total of tube no. 3	0.1	1:16
5	0.1 from the total of tube no. 4	0.1	1:32
6	0.1 from the total of tube no. 5	0.1	1:64
7	0.1 from the total of tube no. 6	0.1	1:128

separate from the other. With each set of sera and controls, a blank consisting of 0.05 ml imidazole-buffered saline is included.

3. Five-tenths milliliter of a freshly prepared, well-mixed staphylococcal suspension is added to each dilution and to the blank.

4. Each suspension is spread over a 2-cm area with a clean applicator stick, and the tile is rocked gently over a black nonreflective background lit indirectly from below.

5. The tile is observed for cell clumping. The blank should appear as a fairly uniform suspension. The end point is the highest dilution of each serum that shows clumping of cells.

6. The fibrinogen control that most closely matches the clumping intensity of the end point of the serum is determined.

7. The fibrinogen equivalents of the serum are obtained by multiplying the reciprocal of the dilutions of the serum end point by the micrograms of fibrinogen in the closest matching control. For example, if the serum end point occurs in the 1:64 dilution and the matching control contains 0.2 µg fibrinogen per milliliter, the micrograms of fibrinogen equivalent in the serum are $64 \times 0.2 =$ 12.8 µg/ml.

Reference Range

The reference range is less than 0.4 µg fibrinogen "equivalents" per milliliter. Results between 5 and 7 µg are considered borderline, and those that exceed 8 µg are elevated. The results are interpreted as fibrinogen equivalents per milliliter because, although the test measures fibrin–fibrinogen degradation products remaining after fibrinogen removal, the data are based on activities equivalent to known amounts of fibrinogen.

Lupus Anticoagulant by Activated Partial Thromboplastin Time Screen and Hexagonal-Phase Phospholipid Neutralization Test

Principle

Lupus anticoagulants are antibodies that inhibit one or more of the in vitro phospholipid-dependent tests of blood coagulation (activated PTT, diluted Russell's viper venom test, etc.). The antibodies specifically recognize as an antigenic epitope a hexagonal-phase phospholipid configuration. This test procedure (Staclot) is based on the principle that when lupus anticoagulant plasma is incubated with hexagonal phase phosopholipid (II), binding takes place that inhibits the antibody from interfering with the second step of the performance of an activated PTT test. Before addition of the activated PTT reagent, a normal plasma is added to the test system to correct for the variable of factor deficiency. Adding normal plasma also dilutes out a heparin- or specific factor-inhibiting effect. The activated PTT reagent is diluted to increase the test sensitivity to the lupus anticoagulant.

Reagents and Equipment

1. PTT-LA lupus anticoagulant-sensitive APTT reagent (Diagnostica Stago, catalog no. 00599): The reagent contains cephalin and a particulate activator, silica, in a buffered glycine media. This reagent is provided freeze-dried. The vial of PTT-LA is reconstituted with 2 ml ultrafiltered deionized water and is swirled gently to obtain a homogeneous suspension. The reagent in intact vials is stable until the expiratory date when stored at 2–8°C. Once reconstituted, it remains stable for 1 day at 20°C or for 5 days at 2–8°C. The reconstituted reagent must not be frozen.
2. Calcium chloride, 0.25 M.
3. Reference emulsion (IL, catalog no. 9756904).
4. Staclot-LA Kit (Diagnostica Stago, catalog no. 00599):
   a. Reagent 1: buffer. The reagent is ready for use. Once opened, it is stable for 8 hours at 20°C and for 1 day at 2–8°C.
   b. Reagent 2: freeze-dried hexagonal-phase phosphatidylethanolamine. Each vial should be reconstituted with 0.25 ml distilled water and then swirled gently until completely dissolved. The reconstituted material is allowed to stand at room temperature for 15 minutes before use. Once reconstituted, it remains stable for 8 hours at 20°C and for 1 day at 2–8°C.
   c. Reagent 3: freeze-dried normal human plasma. Each vial should be reconstituted with 0.5 ml distilled water and swirled gently. The reconstituted material is allowed to stand at room temperature for 15 minutes before use.

Once reconstituted, the plasma remains stable for 8 hours at –20°C. It must not be frozen.
   d. Reagent 4: freeze-dried PTT-LA reagent consisting of cephalin, silica activator, and a heparin inhibitor. Each vial should be reconstituted with 1 ml reagent 5 and swirled gently. The reconstituted material is allowed to stand at room temperature for 15 minutes before use. Once reconstituted, the reagent remains stable for 8 hours at 20°C and for 1 day at 2–8°C.
   e. Reagent 5: solvent for the reconstitution of reagent 4. The reagent is ready for use.
5. Ultrafiltered deionized water (Fisher, catalog no. W2-20).
6. ACL 300/3000 coagulation system.
7. ACL rotors (IL, catalog no. 6800), and thermal printer paper (catalog no. 8007504).
8. Stir bars (IL catalog no. 9746206).
9. Stago ST4 coagulation system.
10. ST4 cuvette strips (Diagnostica Stago, catalog no. 6432), ST4 thermal paper (Diagnostica Stago, catalog no. 6649), ST4 magnetic stir bars (Diagnostica Stago, catalog no. 6405), ST4 ball dispenser (Diagnostica Stago, catalog no. 6548).
11. Sample cups (IL, catalog no. 6593010).
12. Class A volumetric pipettes: 1 ml and 8 ml.
13. Disposable Beral pipettes.
14. Eppendorf Combitips, 1.25-ml (catalog no. 22261100).
15. Water bath, 37°C.
16. Stopwatch.
17. Normal plasma controls.
18. Plunger-type multipipette.

Specimen

Nine volumes of whole blood are collected into one volume of 3.8% sodium citrate. This is centrifuged immediately at 3,500 rpm for 15 minutes. The plasma is removed, and a 1-ml aliquot of plasma is placed into each of two plastic tubes and immediately frozen. If the hematocrit exceeds 55%, the following formula is used to correct for the relative lack of plasma:

$$X = (100 - \text{hematocrit}) \div (595 - \text{hematocrit})$$

where X is the volume of anticoagulant needed to prepare 1 unit volume of anticoagulated blood.

The plasma may be stored for 4 hours at 2–8°C. The plasma should be frozen at –70°C if longer storage is required. Specimens are unacceptable if they are hemolyzed, icteric, or lipemic.

Method

1. Patient specimen and controls are thawed.
2. An activated PTT test is performed on the patient specimen and controls.
3. A Staclot LA test is carried out on all patient samples with an abnormal activated PTT test.
4. A vial of 0.025-M calcium chloride is placed in the storage well of the ST4 instrument without the magnetic stirrer.
5. The 1.25-ml Combitip is fitted to the multipipette, and the volume selection dial is adjusted to position 2 to allow for a 50-μl delivery.
6. The Combitip is filled with prewarmed calcium chloride (37°C) and is inserted into the ST4 storage well.
7. A four-cuvette strip is placed in incubation column 1. A ball is dispensed to each cuvette, and the cuvettes remain in position for at least 3 minutes to reach 37°C.
8. Into each of the four cuvettes, 25 μl of the control plasma is pipetted.
9. Into cuvettes 1 and 3, 25 μl of reagent 1 (buffer) is pipetted.
10. Into cuvettes 2 and 4, 25 μl of reagent 2 (phosphatidylethanolamine) is pipetted.
11. Into all four cuvettes, 25 μl of reagent 3 (normal plasma) is pipetted.
12. Timer key 1 is depressed while 50 μl of reagent 4 (PTT-LA) is pipetted into cuvette 1 and, in 5-second intervals, into each of cuvettes 2, 3, and 4.
13. When timer key 1 reaches the 290-second mark, the ST4 will begin to beep. At this point, the cuvette strip should be transferred into the test column. The multipipette is primed once into the calcium chloride vial, and the *PIP* key is pressed to activate the ball movement in the cuvettes.
14. Calcium chloride, 50 μl, is pipetted in 5-second intervals into all four cuvettes exactly on the 300-second mark on timer 1. The ST4 will print out the clotting times of all cuvettes.
15. All steps in the method are repeated using the patient's specimen.

Calculations

Subtract the clotting time of cuvette 2 from that of cuvette 1 and that of cuvette 4 from cuvette 3.

Interpretation

If the net clotting time is 8 seconds, the test is negative. Net clotting times in excess of 8 seconds are interpreted as positive results. If the clotting time of cuvette 2 is longer than that of cuvette 1, the test result is considered negative.

Sources of Error

The presence of coagulation factor antibodies does not produce a correction in the clotting time with the Staclot LA test. Plasma containing heparin levels in excess of 1 IU/ml may interfere with the procedure.

Lipemic specimens should be ultracentrifuged and retested. The centrifugal step in the procedure is critical, as the specimen must be platelet-free. The most common cause of an unexplained prolonged activated PTT is heparin contamination: Therefore, all patients should be free of heparin.

Clinical Correlation

Lupus anticoagulants are usually IgG, IgM, IgA, or combinations of the immunoglobulins that interfere with in vitro phospholipid-dependent coagulation tests (PT, activated PTT, Russell's venom viper test, etc.). The antibodies are nonspecific in their action against coagulation factors but appear to react against anionic phospholipids. The lupus anticoagulant can be found in infections, autoimmune disorders, and malignancies, and after ingestion of some medications. The anticoagulant can be associated with arterial and venous thrombosis, recurrent abortions, thrombocytopenia, and cutaneous manifestations such as cutaneous necrosis.

Functional Protein S Assay

Principle

The cofactor activity of protein S enhances the anticoagulant action of activated protein C. This is reflected in the lengthening of the clotting time of a system enriched with factor Va, the physiologic substrate for activated protein C.

Reagents and Equipment

1. Staclot Protein S kit (Diagnostica Stago, catalog no. 00476).

2. Protein S–deficient plasma, lyophilized: Each vial is reconstituted with 1 ml ultrafiltered deionized water and is allowed to stand at room temperature for 1 hour. This must be mixed before use. Once reconstituted, the plasma is stable for 4 hours at room temperature and at 2–8°C. It must not be frozen.

3. Human activated protein C, freeze-dried: Each vial is reconstituted as in step 2.

4. Bovine factor Va, freeze-dried: reconstituted as in step 2.

5. Calcium chloride, 0.025 M (Diagnostica Stago, catalog no. 00363).

6. Owren-Koller buffer (Diagnostica Stago, catalog nos. 00358, 00364).

7. Ultrafiltered deionized water (Fisher, catalog no. W2-20).

8. ST4 coagulation system.

9. ST4 cuvette strip (Diagnostica Stago, catalog no. 6432).

10. ST4 thermal paper (Diagnostica Stago, catalog no. 6649).

11. ST4 magnetic stir bar (Diagnostica Stago, catalog no. 405).

12. ST4 ball dispensers (Diagnostica Stago, catalog no. 6548).

13. Eppendorf Combitips, 1.25-ml (Diagnostica Stago, catalog no. 22261100).

14. Adjustable mechanical pipet, 100–1,000 µl.

15. Water bath, 37°C.

16. Timer.

17. Plastic tubes: 12 × 75 mm.

18. Normal and abnormal control plasma (George King, catalog no. 0040-0).

Specimen

Whole blood, 4.5 ml, is collected into 0.5 ml 3.8% sodium citrate and centrifuged immediately at 3,500 rpm for 15 minutes. The plasma is removed, and 1-ml aliquots are placed into each of two plastic tubes and are immediately frozen. The plasma is stable at 2–8°C for 4 hours.

Method

1. All controls and patient plasmas are diluted 1:10 with Owren-Koller buffer before testing (0.1 ml plasma to 0.9 ml buffer).

2. A 1.25-ml Combitip is fitted onto the ST4 multipette, and the volume selection dial is set to position 2 for 50-ml delivery. The Combitip is filled with prewarmed calcium chloride and is placed in the storage position of the ST4.

3. From the main menu of the ST4, 1 is selected for test mode, and confirmation is effected by pressing ENT. Then 7 is pressed for inhibitors, 2 is pressed to select protein S, and ENT is pressed to allow confirmation.

4. The patient identification number is entered.

5. A 4-mm cuvette strip is placed in incubation column 1. A ball is added to each cuvette, and these are incubated at 37°C for 3 minutes.

6. Normal control specimen, 50 µl, is pipetted into cuvettes 1 and 2. Abnormal control specimen, 50 ml, is pipetted into cuvettes 3 and 4.

7. Protein-deficient plasma, 50 µl, is pipetted into all four cuvettes.

8. Activated protein C reagent, 50 µl, is pipetted into all four cuvettes.

9. Factor Va reagent, 50 µl, is pipetted into cuvette 1, and incubation timer 1 is begun immediately. A 5-second interval is allowed, and then factor Va reagent is pipetted into cuvette 2. This is repeated at 5-second intervals so that reagent is placed into the remaining cuvettes.

10. The cuvette strip is transferred to the test column when the incubation timer beeps at the 110-second mark. The multipipette is primed once into the calcium chloride vial. The PIP key is pressed to activate the ball movement in the cuvette.

11. Calcium chloride is pipetted into cuvette 1 at exactly the 120-second mark and into the remaining cuvettes at 5-second intervals.

12. The ST4 will print out the duplicate clotting times of the controls and test plasmas when all four cuvettes have clotted, together with the mean protein S activity of each sample.

Reference Range

The reference range is 65–140%.

Sources of Error

Heparin does not affect the results when present at a concentration of less than 1 IU/ml of plasma. Higher levels, however, may lead to an overestimation of the protein S level. Factor VIII does not interfere with the assay if the level is less than 250% of normal.

Clinical Correlation

In an inflammatory syndrome, the in vivo increase of C4b-BP leads to an increase of bound protein S and to a concomitant decrease of free and functional protein S levels. Decreased levels of protein S may be seen in hepatic disease, in individuals on oral anticoagulants, in patients on L-asparaginase, and in the newborn. In congenital deficiency, the total protein S concentration may vary, the diagnosis being established only by parallel determinations of protein S activity and free protein S antigen.

Protein S is a vitamin K–dependent protein that is essential for the expression of the anticoagulant activity of activated protein C. It is found in the plasma, platelets, and endothelial cells, but lacks the amino acid structure needed to form an active enzyme. It is found in two forms: 40% is free and serves as a cofactor for activated protein C, and 60% is complexed to C4b-BP and is functionally inactive.

Protein S Antigen Assay

Principle

A plastic support coated with specific rabbit antiprotein S antibody is allowed to come into contact with plasma containing the protein S to be measured. The protein S contained in the plasma binds to the plastic support by one antigenic determinant. Rabbit anti–protein S antibody coupled with peroxidase then is added, and this binds to the free remaining antigenic sites of protein S, forming a sandwich. The bound enzyme peroxidase is detected by its activity in a predetermined time on the substrate orthophenylenediamine (OPD) in the presence of hydrogen peroxide.

Reagents and Equipment

1. Protein S reagent kit (Diagnostica Stago, catalog no. 00572).
2. Precoated plate: One plate of 96 microwells precoated with specific rabbit anti–protein S F(ab')$_2$ fragments, stabilized and sealed in an aluminum pouch. The 96 wells can be divided into six strips of 16 wells.
3. Anti–protein S peroxidase conjugate: Specific rabbit anti–protein S antibody coupled with peroxidase. Each vial of anti–protein C peroxide conjugate is reconstituted with 8 ml dilution buffer. Reconstitution is performed just before use. The reconstituted material is stable for 24 hours at 2–8°C.
4. OPD substrate: 8 mg OPD, 2 ml hydrochloric acid per vial, lyophilized with buffer. The OPD substrate is prepared just before use. For two strips, two tablets of OPD are added to 8 ml ultrafiltered deionized water. Immediately after the tablets have completely dissolved, 120 μl 3% hydrogen peroxide is added. This OPD reagent is stable for 1 hour at room temperature. (The OPD must be handled with care, and contact with skin and metal surfaces must be avoided.)
5. Polyethylene glycol (PEG) 25%.
6. Dilution buffer: Tenfold concentration of phosphate buffer with bovine albumin and Tween-20. A 1:10 dilution of buffer in distilled water is prepared. The diluted buffer is stable for 15 days at 2–8°C.
7. Washing solution: Twentyfold concentration of phosphate, sodium chloride, and Tween-20. A 1:20 dilution of washing solution in distilled water is prepared. The dilution is stable for 15 days at 2–8°C.
8. Sulfuric acid, 3 M, or 1-N hydrochloric acid.
9. Hydrogen peroxide 3%: Must be pure and inhibitor-free.
10. Multichannel pipettes adjustable to deliver 50 μl and 200 μl.
11. Adjustable pipettes: 10–100 μl and 100–1,000 μl.
12. Pipette tips.
13. Washing equipment for microwell plates.
14. Plate reader set at 490 or 492 nm.
15. Ultrafiltered deionized water (Fisher, catalog no. W2-20).
16. Plastic tubes: 75 × 12 mm.
17. Disposable glass tubes: 16 × 75 mm.
18. Parafilm.
19. Reference plasma (George King, catalog no. 00807).
20. Normal and abnormal control plasma (George King, catalog nos. 0025-0 and 0040-1).

Specimen

Whole blood, 4.5 ml, is added to 0.5 ml 3.8% sodium citrate and centrifuged immediately at 3,500 rpm for 15 minutes. The plasma is removed, and 1-ml aliquots are placed into two plastic tubes and frozen immediately. If the hematocrit exceeds 55%, the ratio of anticoagulant to plasma is adjusted by the following formula:

$$X = (100 - \text{hematocrit}) \div (595 - \text{hematocrit})$$

where X is the volume of anticoagulant needed to prepare the unit volume of blood. The plasma may be stored for up to 4 hours at 2–8°C. Plasma can be stored in excess of 4 hours at –70°C.

Method

1. The free protein S is first extracted from the calibrator, controls, and test plasma by treatment with PEG. Calibrator, controls, and test plasma, 300 μl each, are placed in centrifuge tubes and warmed for 5 minutes at 37°C.

2. PEG, 50 μl, is added, and the tubes are capped, vortexed, and incubated for 30 minutes in an ice bath. The tubes are centrifuged for 10 minutes at 3,000 rpm. The supernatant, which contains only free protein S, is collected.

3. A 1:100 dilution of the free protein S (FPS) calibrator is prepared with the dilute buffer (50 μl FPS and 4.95 ml dilute buffer). This is the stock solution for the FPS, which, by definition, is the 100% calibrator.

4. Four tubes are labeled as follows for the remaining FPS calibrator curves, and then the tubes are vortexed:

Calibrator tubes (% FPS):	50	25	10	5
Diluted protein S calibrator (ml):	0.5	0.25	0.1	0.05
Diluted buffer (ml):	0.5	0.75	0.9	0.95

5. The controls and test plasmas are prepared by making a 1:200 dilution in diluted buffer (20 μl of test specimen into 3.98 ml buffer).

6. A 1:100 dilution of the protein S calibrator is prepared in dilute buffer (50 μl total protein S in 4.95 ml dilute buffer). This is the stock solution for

total protein S (TPS), which, by definition, is the 100% calibrator.

7. Four tubes are labeled as follows for the remaining TPS calibrator curve, and then the tubes are vortexed:

Calibrator tubes (% FPS):	50	25	10	5
Diluted protein S calibrator (ml):	0.5	0.25	0.1	0.05
Diluted buffer (ml):	0.5	0.75	0.9	0.95

8. The controls and test plasmas are prepared by making a 1:200 dilution in buffer (20 μl of the controls and test plasmas to 3.95 ml diluted buffer).

9. Calibrator, controls, and test specimens (200 μl each) are pipetted into separate wells, and a grid is labeled for identification.

10. The plate is covered with parafilm and incubated in the dark at room temperature for 1 hour.

11. Each well is washed five times with 300 μl buffer. The plate is then tapped dry on a paper towel.

12. The conjugate is reconstituted with 24 ml dilution buffer 10 minutes before the first incubation is over.

13. The second antibody to the protein S–peroxidase conjugate (200 μl) is pipetted to each well.

14. The plate is covered with parafilm and incubated for 1 hour at room temperature.

15. The plate is washed as in step 12 and tapped dry.

16. Six OPD tablets are reconstituted with 24 ml ultrafiltered deionized water, and 120 μl 3% hydrogen peroxide is added.

17. The OPD–hydrogen peroxide solution (200 μl) is pipetted into each well, beginning with column 1, and the timer is started, allowing 10-second intervals between each column.

18. After 5 minutes, 100 μl 1-N hydrochloric acid is pipetted into each well, beginning with column 1 and allowing 10 seconds between each column.

19. The plate should be rotated five to six times and left for 10 minutes at room temperature.

20. The optical density is measured at 491 or 492 nm.

Calculation

The optical density readings of each duplicate set are averaged and, on log-log graph paper, the average optical density values of the protein S calibrator (total

Table 20.22. Classes of Protein S Deficiency

Classification	Functional Clotting	Free Protein S Antigen	Total Protein S Antigen	C4b-BP
Congenital				
Type I	D	D	D	—
Type II	D	N	N	—
Type III	D	D	N	N
Acquired	D	D	N	I

D = decreased; N = normal; I = increased.

or free) are plotted on the y-axis, and the corresponding protein S levels (%) are plotted on the x-axis. Point-to-point curves also are plotted, one for the TPS and one for the FPS (using the respective calibrators). The optical density value for the control is interpolated on the TPS calibrator curve, and its value is determined. The optical density value of the test sample is interpolated on the corresponding TPS and FPS calibrator curves to determine their respective levels.

Reference Ranges

The reference range for total proteing is over 79%. The reference range for free proteins is over 78%.

Sources of Error

Anti-rabbit antibodies, if present, can produce a false-positive reaction. The 2-hour incubation time at room temperature allows immunologic equilibrium to be reached. This time may be shortened to 1 hour without modifying the procedure or altering the results. However, a too-low optical density at 492 nm may be compensated for by lengthening the color development time.

Clinical Correlation

Protein S is synthesized in the liver as an inactive precursor. The active form is obtained after carboxylation of glutamic residues by a vitamin K–dependent carboxylase and contains 10 carboxyglutamic residues, allowing the molecule to fix calcium. Protein S functions as an anticoagulant, as it acts as the cofactor of activated protein C. In the presence of calcium, the protein C–protein S greatly potentiates protein C anticoagulant function by increasing protein C affinity of phospholipid membranes. Protein S can be modified by

thrombin, but it then loses its anticoagulant function as a cofactor for activated protein C. In the latter state, it can displace protein S–activated protein C complexes from the phospholipid surface.

Three classes of congenital and one class of acquired protein S deficiency exist (Table 20.22).

Functional Protein C Assay

Principle

Protein C is activated in vitro by Protac (Curtis Matheson Corp., Houston, TX), which is extracted from the venom of *Agkistrodon contortix*. The anticoagulant effect is measured by the activated PTT test. The Proclot test used is a functional assay based on the prolongation of the activated PTT test.

Reagents and Equipment

1. Proclot test kit (Curtis Matheson Instrumentation Laboratory [CMS-IL], Lexington, MA, catalog no. 84683-10):
   a. Protein C activator: Each vial is reconstituted with 1.5 ml ultrafiltered deionized water. All reagents must be kept at room temperature for 30 minutes. The vials are inverted and mixed before use. This reagent is stable for 36 hours if kept at 2–8°C and for 7 days at –20°C.
   b. Protein C–deficient plasma: Each vial contains 1.0 ml freeze-dried human plasma artificially depleted of protein C by immunoabsorption. Each vial is reconstituted with 1 ml ultrafiltered deionized water and kept closed. Dissolution is effected by gentle rotation, avoiding the formation of foam. The reconstituted plasma is kept for 30 minutes

at room temperature before use. This reagent is stable for 4 hours at room temperature and for 7 days at –20°C.

c. Working diluent: IL-test Proclot diluent, 6.5 ml, is added to 1.5 ml protein C activator (Protac). This reagent is stable for 8 hours at 2–8°C. The Proclot diluent contains 100 ppm of mercuric ion, derived from thimerosal.

2. IL-test activated PTT reagent (CMS-IL, catalog no. 200060): an extract of rabbit brain phospholipids in a buffered silica solution. The reagent is supplied ready for use. Open vials are stable for 30 days when stored at 2–8°C. The reagent must not be frozen.

3. IL calcium chloride, 0.025 M (CMS-IL, catalog no. 200060).

4. Reference emulsion (CMS-IL, catalog no. 97569-04).

5. Ultrafiltered deionized water (Fisher, catalog no. W2-20).

6. Adjustable mechanical pipet: 100–1,000 μl

7. ACL 300/3,000 coagulation system.

8. ACL rotors (CMS-IL, catalog no. 68000).

9. Water bath, 37°C.

10. Cooling block.

11. Timer.

12. Plastic tubes: 12 × 75 mm.

13. Sample analyzer cups: 0.5 ml (CMS catalog no. 339788).

14. Vortex.

15. ACL macro reagent reservoirs with stir bars.

16. Calibration plasma (CMS-IL, catalog no. 200000).

17. Normal and abnormal control plasma (CMS-IL, catalog no. 20020; George King, catalog no. 0040-0).

Specimen

Whole blood, 4.5 ml, is added to 0.5 ml 3.8% sodium citrate. This is centrifuged immediately at 3,500 rpm for 15 minutes. The plasma is removed, and 1-ml aliquots are placed into plastic tubes and frozen immediately. If the hematocrit is greater than 55%, the following formula is used to calculate the anticoagulant volume:

$$X = (100 - \text{hematocrit}) \div (595 - \text{hematocrit})$$

where X is the volume of anticoagulant required.

The test plasma can be stored for 4 hours at 2–4°C. It should be stored at –70°C if kept more than 4 hours.

Method

1. The ACL is placed in the ready mode and the cursor moved to select *special test. Enter* is pressed.

2. The cursor is moved to *Proclot*, and *enter* is pressed.

3. The instructions displayed on the screen are followed.

4. Patient, control plasmas, and calibrator plasma, and the protein C–deficient plasma are diluted 1:10 with working diluent before use. Fifty microliters of the sample are diluted with 450 μl of working diluent in a 12 × 75–mm plastic tube and vortexed. The diluted sample should be stored at 2–8°C and used within 30 minutes.

5. Diluted sample aliquots are dispensed into the micro cups.

6. The diluted controls are placed in positions 1 and 2 on the ACL sample tray.

7. The diluted patient samples are placed in positions 3–14 on the sample tray.

8. The calibration plasma is placed in the *pool* position on the tray.

9. The protein C–deficient plasma is placed in the *DIL* position on the tray.

10. The undiluted protein C–deficient plasma is placed in position 18 as plasma substrate for protein C analysis.

11. The cephalin reagent is placed in macro reagent reservoir 2 with the stir bar, and the calcium chloride reagent is placed in macro reagent reservoir 3.

12. The instructions displayed on the ACL screen are followed.

Reference Range

The reference range is 74–151%.

Sources of Error

Lipemic samples may interfere with the reading of the clotting times and should be cleared before testing. The method is sensitive to heparin dosages in excess of 1 U/ml. The Proclot assay results may be affected by the presence of lupus anticoagulants and by patient samples having factor VIII concentrations in excess of 250%.

Clinical Correlation

Protein C is a vitamin K–dependent plasma protein present in the plasma as a proenzyme. Thrombin activates the proenzyme by cleaving the amino terminal dodecapeptide bound to the thrombomodulin on the vascular endothelial membrane surface. The activated protein C inhibits thrombin formation by inactivating surface-bound factors Va and VIIIa through proteolytic cleavages. Systematic defects that occur typically become manifest in young adults. Homozygous deficiencies are usually associated with a fulminant neonatal thrombotic disorder, often leading to death within a few days after birth. Heterozygotes are at increased risk for developing warfarin-induced skin necrosis due to the short half-life of the protein.

Protein C Antigen Assay

Principle

A plastic microwell coated with specific rabbit anti–protein C antibody is allowed to come into contact with test plasma. The protein C in the plasma binds to the plastic by one of its antigenic determinants. Rabbit anti–protein C antibody coupled with peroxidase is added and binds to the free remaining antigenic determinants of protein C, forming a sandwich. The bound enzyme is then detected by its activity in a predetermined time on the substrate OPD in the presence of hydrogen peroxide. The color change produced is proportional to the protein C concentration.

Reagents and Equipment

1. Protein C reagent kit (Diagnostica Stago, catalog no. 00571).
2. Precoated plates: Two plates of 96 microwells precoated with specific rabbit anti–protein C F(ab')$_2$ fragments, hermetically sealed in aluminum pouches. Each 96-well plate can be divided into six strips of 16 wells (two rows of eight).
3. Anti–protein C peroxidase conjugate: Two vials each containing (20 ml after reconstitution) specific rabbit anti–protein C antibody

coupled with peroxidase, lyophilized with stabilizers.
4. OPD substrate: Two vials, each containing 8 mg OPD, lyophilized with buffer.
5. Dilution buffer: Two vials each containing 20 ml of tenfold concentration of phosphate buffer with bovine albumin, sodium chloride, and Tween-20.
6. Washing solution: Two vials each containing 50 ml of twentyfold concentration of phosphate, sodium chloride, and Tween-20.
7. 3-M sulfuric acid or 1-N HCL.
8. Hydrogen peroxide, 30% or 3%: Must be pure and inhibitor-free.
9. Adjustable pipettes: 50 µl, 100 µl, 200 µl, and 300 µl, graduated; and 10–100 µl and 100–1,000 µl.
10. Yellow and blue pipette tips.
11. Washing equipment for microwell plates or strips.
12. Plate reader set at 490 or 492 nm.
13. Ultrafiltered deionized water (Fisher Scientific Co., catalog no. W2-20).
14. Disposable polyprolylene tubes: 17 × 10.
15. Parafilm.

Reagent Preparation. The Asserachrom Protein C kit (Diagnostica Stago, catalog no. 00571) is stable until the expiration date indicated on the box label, when stored at 2–8°C.

1. Precoated plates: Carefully cut open one end of an aluminum pouch. Pull out the plastic plate. Break off as many 16-well strips as needed. Replace unused strips back in the aluminum pouch, including the desiccant bag. Seal the aluminum pouch carefully with clear adhesive tape. The unused strips thus resealed may be stored for up to 15 days at 2–8°C, when protected from moisture.

2. Dilution buffer: Prepare a 1:10 dilution by transferring the contents of each vial (20 ml) into a 200-ml graduated flask, and then add distilled water to the 200-ml mark on the flask. The diluted buffer is stable for 15 days at 2–8°C.

3. Washing solution: Prepare a 1:20 dilution by transferring the contents of each vial (50 ml) into a 1-liter graduated flask, and then add distilled water to the 1-liter mark on the flask. The diluted washing solution is stable for 15 days at 2–8°C.

4. Antibody-enzyme conjugate: Reconstitute each vial of anti–protein C peroxidase conjugate with 21 ml dilution buffer. Reconstitute just before use.

The reconstituted reagent is stable for 24 hours at 2–8°C. If fractional use of a vial is anticipated, reconstitute each vial with 2 ml distilled water, and split the resulting solution into aliquots of convenient size for storage at –30°C or lower for a period not exceeding 1 month. When needed, each aliquot is thawed and a 1:10 dilution is prepared with dilution buffer. For example, to each thawed aliquot of 500 µl add 4,500 µl dilution buffer to make a 1:10 dilution.

5. OPD substrate: Just before use, prepare the OPD substrate. For two strips, add two tablets of OPD to 8 ml ultrafiltered deionized water. Immediately after the tablets have completely dissolved, add 120 µl 3% hydrogen peroxide. The OPD solution thus obtained is stable for 1 hour at room temperature.

The OPD tablets must be handled with great care. The technologist should wear gloves to avoid contact with skin, keep the OPD tablets in their packaging and dissolve them just before use to minimize spontaneous hydrolysis, and avoid all contacts with metallic surfaces as well as with oxidizing agents.

Calibration

The protein C calibrator (Diagnostica Stago, catalog no. 00807) is a freeze-dried, citrated human plasma intended for the calibration of protein C assays, with both immunologic and functional methods. Reconstitute each vial with exactly 0.5 ml ultrafiltered deionized water. Swirl gently until completely dissolved. Allow the reconstituted material to stand at room temperature (18–25°C) for 10 minutes before use.

The starting dilution contains the highest calibrator level, which corresponds to the value stated in the Assay Value insert. This starting dilution is used to prepare other lower calibrators. Dilutions of 5%, 10%, 25%, 50%, and 100% are used to plot a point-to-point curve for the protein C.

Quality Control

1. Cryo√ Check Normal Plasma (Precision Biologicals, Dartmouth, NS, Canada, catalog no. CCN-10) is used to monitor normal levels of immunologic and functional methods. Unopened vials should be stored at –70°C. To prepare for use, thaw in 37°C water bath for 4 minutes. Mix gently to facilitate thawing. The mixture should be used within 8 hours and will remain stable for up to 8 hours if capped and stored at 4°C when not in use.

2. Cryo√ Check Ref. Abnormal 1 (Precision Biologicals, catalog no. ARP1) is used to monitor low levels of immunologic and functional methods. Unopened vials should be stored at –70°C. To prepare for use, thaw in 37°C water bath for 4 minutes. Mix gently to facilitate thawing. The mixture should be used within 2 hours and will remain stable for up to 8 hours if capped and stored at 4°C when not in use.

3. Cryo√ Check normal and abnormal controls are assayed on each plate strip in duplicate and alternating.

Specimen

The specimen requirements and stability are similar to those in the protein S antigenic assay.

Method

1. The calibrator and the controls are reconstituted, and the test plasma is thawed at 37°C.

2. A 1:100 dilution of the test plasma is made using 30 µl of sample and 2.45 ml dilution buffer.

3. A 1:50 dilution of the calibrator is prepared (100 µl of the sample and 4.9 ml dilution buffer) to be used as the 100% calibrator.

4. Six tubes for the calibration curve are labeled as follows:

Calibration tube (%):	100	50	25	10	5	0
Protein C calibrator (ml):	1.0	0.5	0.25	0.1	0.05	0
Diluted buffer (ml):	0	0.5	0.75	0.9	0.95	1.0

The 1:50 dilution is used as the 100% calibrator for protein C.

5. Calibrators, controls, and test sample, 200 µl each, are pipetted into the respective wells, and these are labeled on a grid.

6. The plate is covered with parafilm and is incubated in the dark at room temperature for 1 hour.

7. Each well then is washed five times with 300 µl of buffer, and the plate is tapped to dry it.

8. The conjugate is reconstituted with 23 ml diluted buffer for 10 minutes before the first hour ends.

9. The second antibody of the protein C–peroxidase conjugate (200 µl) is pipetted to each well.

10. The plate is covered with parafilm and allowed to incubate at room temperature for 1 hour.

11. The plate is washed as in step 7 and tapped to dry after the last wash.

12. The OPD vial is reconstituted with 24 ml distilled water, and 120 μl 3% hydrogen peroxide is added.

13. At 10-second intervals, 200 μl OPD–hydrogen peroxide is pipetted into each well, starting with column 1.

14. One hundred microliters of 1-N hydrochloric acid are pipetted into each well at exactly 3 minutes after the introduction of the OPD–hydrogen peroxide reagent, beginning at column 1 and pipetting at 10-second intervals.

15. The plate is rotated five times on the bench and is left for 10 minutes at room temperature.

16. The optical density is measured at 490 or 492 nm.

Calculation

The optical density of each value of duplicates is averaged and, on log-log graph paper, the average optical density values of the protein C calibrator are plotted on the y-axis, whereas the corresponding values of the protein C levels (%) are plotted on the x-axis. A point-to-point curve is plotted for protein C (using the calibrator) of the test sample. The optical density value for the control is interpolated on the protein C calibrator curve, and it is ascertained that the observed value is within the acceptable limits provided with the controls. The optical density values of the test plasma are interpolated on the calibration curve to determine the results.

Reference Range

The reference range exceeds 70%.

Sources of Error

Traces of impurity in the deionized water or distilled water used will affect the results. The incubation time of 2 hours at room temperature allows the immunologic equilibrium to be reached. This time may be shortened to 1 hour if desired. A too-low optical density obtained at 492 nm may be compensated for by lengthening the color development time. It is, however, essential that this time duration be identical for all the assay points. The color change remains stable for at least 2 hours at room temperature if protected from light.

Clinical Correlation

Anti-rabbit antibodies, if present, have been reported to produce a false-positive result. In such cases, it is recommended that the test plasma first be incubated with normal rabbit serum to eliminate the interference.

Protein C levels are reduced in the newborn to approximately 35% of normal adult levels. This is the range seen in adults associated with thrombotic episodes and in inherited deficiencies. In type II protein C deficiency, the antigen level may be normal, but the functional activity is decreased. Before the diagnosis of congenital protein C deficiency, the acquired deficiency due to liver disease, coumarin therapy, DIC, renal disease, and pregnancy should be ruled out.

Venous Occlusion Test

Principle

Localized venous occlusion of an arm for a standardized time is used as a stimulus for the release of tissue-type plasminogen activator (t-PA) from the vessel wall. Pre- and postocclusion lysis times, using the euglobulin lysis time, are measured. In normal subjects, fibrinolysis is greatly enhanced by occlusion.

Reagents and Equipment

The reagents and equipment used are the same as those for the euglobulin lysis time test (see page 385).

Specimen

The specimen is sodium citrate–anticoagulated blood.

Method

1. Sodium citrated blood is obtained from the arm to be tested and is stored in an ice bath.

2. The blood pressure cuff is inflated at a point midway between the systolic and the diastolic pressure and left for 10 minutes.

3. A citrated blood sample is withdrawn from below the blood pressure cuff and placed on ice.

4. The euglobulin lysis time is measured on both specimens.

Interpretation

The postocclusion lysis time should be shorter than the preocclusion time by at least 30 minutes.

Clinical Considerations

The test is uncomfortable, and some patients may not be able to tolerate the total 10 minutes that the blood pressure cuff is on the arm. Failure to enhance lysis is seen in some cases of recurrent venous thrombosis, in obese individuals, and in postsurgical trauma or severe illness. It may also be due to the failure to release the activator because insufficient pressure was applied or the occlusion time was too short. Normal subjects vary in the degree of response. In good responders, the concentration of t-PA is increased by 300–400%, whereas poor responders may show only a slight increase of fibrinolysis even with longer occlusion times.

Thrombo-Wellcotest

Principle

A suspension of latex particles in buffer is sensitized with specific antibodies to purified fibrinogen degradation products. The sensitivity of the reagent is adjusted so that in the presence of fibrinogen concentrations of 2 µg/ml or greater, the latex particles clump together, creating macroscopic agglutination. By testing two unknown samples at different dilutions, the approximate concentration of fibrin degradation products can be determined. The agglutination pattern can be seen most clearly when the slide is viewed against a distinct dark background, with bright, diffused daylight as illumination.

Reagents and Equipment

1. Thrombo-Wellcotest kit (Burroughs-Wellcome Co., Research Triangle Park, NC).
2. Water bath, 37°C.
3. Pipettes: 1 ml, graduated.

Specimen

Two milliliters of blood are added to the blue-topped tube provided, which contains thrombin and soybean inhibitor. It is mixed well by inverting the tube, and the blood is allowed to clot and retract at 37°C for 30 minutes. The clotted sample is centrifuged, and the serum removed.

Method

1. Test serum dilutions (1:5 and 1:20) in glycine buffer are prepared.
2. One drop of each serum dilution is transferred to the test slide provided in the kit.
3. The latex suspension is mixed by vigorous shaking of the tube. One drop of the latex is added to each serum dilution on the slide.
4. Each of the serum-latex mixtures is stirred in turn, by use of a disposable mixing rod, spreading each pool of liquid to fill its respective circle.
5. The slide is rocked gently for a maximum of 2 minutes and is observed for agglutination.

Results

If there is no agglutination in the 1:5 serum dilution, there is less than 10 µg/ml fibrin degradation products. If agglutination is present at the 1:5 dilution but lacking in the 1:20 serum dilution, the level of fibrin degradation products is between 10 and 14 µg/ml. If both dilutions show agglutination, there is in excess of 40 µg/ml fibrin degradation products present.

Controls

Both the positive and negative controls provided with the kit should be tested simultaneously with the unknown blood specimens.

Reference Range

The reference range is 0–10 µ/ml fibrin degradation products.

Sources of Error

If blood is collected from patients undergoing heparin therapy, the thrombin of the sample collection tube may be inhibited to such an extent that the blood will fail to clot. In such cases, the whole blood should be treated with reptilase (Abbott Scientific, North Chicago, IL), a thrombinlike enzyme that will clot fibrinogen in the presence of heparin and other antithrombins. The content of one bottle of reptilase is reconstituted in 1 ml distilled water. One-tenth milliliter of this solution is sufficient to clot 1 ml heparinized blood at 37°C.

Additional thrombin may be required to ensure complete clotting in the blood of patients undergoing heparin or streptokinase therapy. Although heparin does not interfere with the clumping reaction, increased levels of heparin may inhibit coagulation, producing falsely elevated results caused by the presence of unconverted fibrinogen. When possible, blood should be collected before the initiation of heparin or streptokinase therapy.

Clinical Correlation

Serum fibrin degradation products are increased in primary and secondary fibrinolytic states. Primary states may arise from increased levels of circulating plasminogen, which produces plasmin, with resulting lysis of fibrinogen. Secondary fibrinolytic states are characterized by DIC and fibrinolysis. Increases in fibrin degradation products are found also in cirrhosis and following cesarean section, preeclamptic toxemia, abruptio placentae, and uterine death. Moderate to marked increases often are present in postoperative pulmonary embolism and venous thrombosis. Peripheral vascular occlusions treated with streptokinase also show marked serum fibrin degradation product elevations.

Ethanol Gel Solubility Test

Principle

The addition of ethanol to the soluble fibrin present in the plasma of individuals with intravascular coagulation causes a gel to form (Breen and Tullis, 1968).

Reagents and Equipment

1. Ethyl alcohol 50%.
2. Pipettes: 1 ml and 5 ml, graduated.

Specimen

The specimen is platelet-poor plasma. A plastic syringe is used to anticoagulate 4.5 ml blood with 0.5 ml 3.2% sodium citrate. The blood is centrifuged at 2,500 rpm for 15 minutes. Normal blood is treated in the same way as the control.

Method

1. Ethanol 50% (0.15 ml) is added to 0.5 ml of platelet-poor test plasma and to 0.5 ml of the normal control plasma.
2. The tubes are inverted to mix and are observed at 5-minute intervals at room temperature.

Results

Visible gel formation is seen within 5 minutes if the plasma contains fibrin degradation products. The presence of a granular precipitate is read as a negative test result.

Reference Range

No precipitation or a granular precipitate is seen in normal individuals.

Sources of Error

Ethanol in a final concentration of 10–15% causes soluble fibrin to gel promptly at room temperature. The reaction is independent of the fibrinogen level, and unaltered by the presence of fibrinolytic activity, heparin, or red-cell contamination. Gel formation after the first 5 minutes should be tested by adding one drop of 0.1-N sodium hydroxide and gently shaking the tube. Nonspecific precipitates will return promptly to solution, whereas the fibrin gel will remain. False-positive results on ethanol gel testing may be found in idiopathic thrombocytopenic purpura, bleeding gastrointestinal lesions, menstruation, and postoperative states.

Protamine Sulfate Test (Paracoagulation Test)

Principle

When added to citrated plasma, protamine sulfate causes polymerization of fibrin monomer complexes and visible fibrin formation (Kidder et al., 1972).

Reagents and Equipment

1. Protamine sulfate 1% (wt/vol) (Eli Lilly Co., Indianapolis, IN).
2. Water bath, 37°C.
3. Pipettes: 1 ml, graduated.

Specimen

The specimen is citrated platelet-poor plasma, as was described for the ethanol gel solubility test (page 384).

Method

1. One milliliter of plasma is prewarmed to 37°C for 3–5 minutes, and 0.1 ml protamine sulfate is added. The tube is agitated gently to mix the contents.

2. It is incubated at 37°C for 15 minutes and observed for the presence of a precipitate by gentle tilting of the tube back and forth against a concave mirror in a strong light.

Reference Range

No precipitation is seen in normal individuals.

Sources of Error

Blood samples obtained from indwelling catheters may produce a positive test result because of the clotting of blood at the catheter tip. Likewise, false-positive reactions will also be found if the plasma is not prewarmed to 37°C before the addition of protamine, as fibrinogen may be precipitated. If plasmin is present in the plasma, one or two drops of EACA (Amicar, available from Lederle Laboratories, Pearl River, NY) should be added before testing to neutralize the fibrinolysin.

Clinical Correlation

The presence of a fibrin web or strands, or an easily visible precipitate, is a positive indication of the presence of fibrin monomers. The test can be used as a rapid method for detecting fibrin monomers re-sulting from acute DIC. An isolated occurrence of a positive protamine sulfate test result, without significant abnormalities of other coagulation parameters (PT, activated PTT, fibrinogen, platelets), should not be misinterpreted as DIC. Conversely, a negative test result does not eliminate the diagnosis of DIC, because fibrin monomers are not necessarily present at each stage of the process.

The test can be modified so that fibrin monomers or fibrin degradation products, or both, can be quantitated (Niewiarowski and Gurewich, 1971). Such modifications involve serially diluting patients' plasma in saline and adding protamine sulfate to each dilution.

Tests of the Fibrinolytic System

Euglobulin Lysis Time

Principle

The euglobulin fraction of plasma contains plasminogen, plasminogen activators, and fibrinogen. Normally occurring inhibitors of the plasminogen-plasmin conversion reaction are not present in this fraction. The test is a measurement of fibrinolytic activity.

Reagents and Equipment

1. Borate solution 0.1%, pH 9.0: Sodium chloride, 9 g, and 1 g sodium borate are dissolved in distilled water and diluted to 1 liter.
2. Calcium chloride, 0.025 M (as described on page 348).
3. Acetic acid 1%.
4. Pipettes: 1 ml and 10 ml, graduated; 0.1-ml micropipettes.
5. Water bath, 37°C.
6. Stopwatch.
7. Tubes: 13 × 75 mm.

Specimen

Citrated blood, centrifuged at 2,000 rpm for 10 minutes, is the test specimen. The plasma is removed and stored at 4°C (for no longer than 30 minutes) until tested. A normal blood specimen should be obtained and treated in the same way as the test specimen.

Table 20.23. Dilutions Used for Measuring Circulating Anticoagulants by the Whole Blood Coagulation Time

Tube No.	Patient's Whole Blood (ml)	Normal Whole Blood (ml)
1	1.0	—
2	0.9	0.1
3	0.5	0.5
4	0.1	0.9
5	—	1.0

Note: The patient's and normal whole blood samples should be ABO-compatible.

Method

1. Five-tenths milliliter of plasma is diluted to 9 ml with distilled water, and 0.1 ml of 1% acetic acid is added.

2. The solution is placed at 4°C for 30 minutes to allow the euglobulin fraction to precipitate out of solution. The euglobulin is separated by centrifuging at 3,000 rpm for 5–10 minutes. The supernatant is decanted, and the tube is drained by inverting onto filter paper.

3. Five-tenths milliliter of 0.1% borate is added to the precipitate, placed in a 37°C water bath, and stirred gently with a glass rod for 5–10 minutes.

4. Five-tenths milliliter of 0.025-M calcium chloride is added, and the stopwatch is started when a fibrin clot forms.

5. The clot is inspected at hourly intervals for signs of lysis.

Reference Range

Normal clots require more than 2 hours for complete lysis.

Sources of Error

The lysis time is the time at which the clot is no longer visible and only shreds of fibrin remain. Pathologic fibrinolysis can produce lysis times as short as 5–10 minutes. The test is considered a qualitative measure of plasminogen activator and plasmin.

If the sample is not drained and the interior of the tube is wiped clean, antiplasmins drain back into the sediment, producing prolongation of the lysis time. The test can be moderately shortened by leaving the tourniquet on the patient's arm for a pro-longed period, by rubbing the vein vigorously, or by pumping the fist excessively. These activities apparently release plasminogen activator from the endothelial cells. Euglobulin lysis can also be prolonged by the presence of platelets, which contain antiplasmins and antiplasminogen activators.

Whole-Blood Clot Lysis

Principle

If blood containing a circulating anticoagulant is mixed with a normal specimen, the whole-blood coagulation time of the normal specimen is prolonged in proportion to the strength of the anticoagulant.

Reagents and Equipment

1. Siliconized syringes.
2. Unsiliconized tubes: 8 × 75 mm.
3. Water bath, 37°C.
4. Stopwatch.
5. Pipettes: 1 ml, graduated.
6. Anti-A and anti-B typing sera.

Specimen

Patient's blood and normal ABO blood group–compatible whole blood.

Method

1. Five milliliters of normal whole blood are obtained using a siliconized syringe, and the volumes shown in Table 20.23 are dispensed quickly into five unsiliconized tubes placed in a 37°C water bath.

2. Five milliliters of patient's blood are obtained, and the stopwatch is begun as soon as blood appears in the syringe. The blood is dispensed rapidly into the normal blood as shown in Table 20.23.

3. The blood is mixed by tapping the tube and is incubated at 37°C. The coagulation time of each tube is measured by the method described on page 346.

Results

In the presence of a circulating anticoagulant, which commonly is plasmin, a prolongation of the coagulation times is seen in tubes 1–4.

Clinical Correlation

The test measures the total activity of plasminogen activator, inhibitors, plasminogen, plasmin, and fibrinogen.

Plasminogen Assay

Principle

Plasma is acidified to destroy inhibitors of fibrinolysis. Streptokinase is added to convert plasminogen to plasmin. Caesin is used as a substrate for plasmin activity, and the tyrosine liberated is estimated with standard Folin-Ciocalteu reagent (Alkjaersig et al., 1959).

Reagents and Equipment

1. Streptokinase, 100,000 U/vial (Lederle Laboratories): The contents of the vial are dissolved in 10 ml normal saline to produce a solution of 10,000 U/ml. It is diluted 1:5 with saline just before use so as to make a 2,000-U/ml working solution. Unused solutions are discarded.

2. PBS, 0.15 M (pH 7.4): Sodium dihydrogen phosphate dihydrate, 23.4 g, is dissolved in distilled water and diluted to 1 liter, and 21.3 g anhydrous disodium hydrogen phosphate is dissolved in distilled water and diluted to 1 liter. Eighteen milliliters of sodium dihydrogen phosphate solution are added to 82 ml of the disodium hydrogen phosphate and diluted to 200 ml with normal saline.

3. Caesin: 15 g suspended in 175 ml PBS. This is placed in a boiling water bath for 15 minutes, and the pH is adjusted to 7.4 with 0.1-N sodium hydroxide. It is then diluted to 250 ml with the buffered saline. The solution is stored at –20°C in 20-ml aliquots.

4. Folin-Ciocalteu reagent (phosphotungstomolybdic acid complex) diluted 1:3 with distilled water before use. The concentrate is stored at 4°C.

5. Tyrosine standard, stock solution: Tyrosine, 0.036 g, is dissolved in 900 ml 0.1-N hydrochloric acid and is diluted with isopropanol to 1 liter.

6. Hydrochloric acid, 0.167 N: Hydrochloric acid, 1 N, is diluted 1:6 with distilled water.

7. Sodium hydroxide, 0.167 N and 0.5 N: Sodium hydroxide, 1 N, is diluted 1:6 with distilled water to make the 0.167-N solution and is diluted 1:2 to make the 0.5-N solution.

8. Trichloroacetic acid, 5% and 10% solutions.

9. Water bath, 37°C.

10. Stopwatch.

11. Spectrophotometer.

12. Pipettes: 1 ml, graduated.

13. Tubes: 13 × 100 mm.

Specimen

Citrated whole blood is centrifuged at 2,000 rpm for 15–20 minutes to produce platelet-poor plasma.

Method

1. Five-tenths milliliter of platelet-poor plasma is added to 0.5 ml 0.167-N hydrochloric acid. This mixture is allowed to stand at room temperature for 15 minutes.

2. Five-tenths milliliter of 0.167-N sodium hydroxide, 0.1 ml 0.15-M PBS, 0.5 ml streptokinase, and 2.0 ml caesin are added to the tube. The contents are mixed and incubated at 37°C. The stopwatch is started on the addition of the last reagent.

3. After *exactly 2 minutes*, 1 ml of the incubation mixture is pipetted to a second tube containing 1 ml 10% trichloroacetic acid. This is mixed well. It constitutes the blank tube.

4. After 1 hour, 1 ml of the incubation mixture is moved to a second tube containing 1 ml 10% trichloroacetic acid. This is centrifuged at 2,000

Table 20.24. Standard Tyrosine Dilutions for Plasminogen Assays

Tube No.	Tyrosine Stock (ml)	Distilled Water (ml)	Equivalent Plasminogen (U/ml)
1	0.5	—	4
2	0.375	0.125	3
3	0.25	0.25	2
4	0.125	0.375	1
5	—	0.5	0

rpm for 5 minutes, and 0.5 ml of the supernatant is transferred to a clean tube.

5. A series of five standards is set up as shown in Table 20.24. To each tube, 2.7 ml 0.5-N sodium hydroxide, 0.75 ml 5% trichloroacetic acid, and 0.75 ml diluted Folin-Ciocalteu reagent are added. The solution is maintained at room temperature for 30 minutes.

6. Two and one-half milliliters of 0.5-N sodium hydroxide, 0.75 ml 5% trichloroacetic acid, and 0.75 ml diluted Folin-Ciocalteu reagents are added, and the solution is allowed to stand at room temperature for 30 minutes to allow the color to develop.

7. The standard tyrosine dilutions and test color are read spectrophotometrically at 650 nm, using the blank prepared in step 4.

8. The arbitrary plasminogen values assigned to the tyrosine dilutions are shown in Table 20.24. They are graphically plotted against the optical densities obtained, and the test readings are converted to plasminogen units from the graph.

Reference Range

The reference range is 1.5–4.0 U/ml plasma.

Fluorogenic Assay of Plasminogen

Principle

This method uses the synthetic substrate D-valine-leucine-lysine-5-amidoisophthalic acid dimethyl ester (Val-Leu-Lys-ATE), which possesses a high specificity for the enzyme plasmin. Inactive plasminogen is activated to plasmin by the action of streptokinase, which cleaves the fluorescent molecule AIE from the substrate. This is fluorometrically measured and compared with assayed reference materials (Triplett, 1979).

The reactions that take place are as follows:

$$\text{Plasminogen} \xrightarrow{\text{streptokinase}}$$
$$\text{(Streptokinase - plasminogen)}$$

$$\text{Val - Leu - Lys - AIE} \longrightarrow$$
$$\text{Val - Leu - Lys - AIE (fluorescent)}$$

Reagents and Equipment

1. Fluorometer (Protopath, available from Dade).
2. Water bath, 37°C.
3. Tubes: plastic, 12 × 75 mm.
4. Vortex.
5. Pipettes: 1 ml and 5 ml, graduated; micropipettes or pipetting devices capable of measuring 0.2 ml, 0.1 ml, and 0.01 ml.
6. Plasminogen substrate kit (Dade):
   a. Plasminogen reagent: reconstituted with 0.2 ml distilled water and swirled until dissolved. It is stored at 4°C and is stable for 24 hours.
   b. Streptokinase reagent, lyophilized: stored at 4°C. The reagent is reconstituted by adding 5 ml distilled water, which produces a concentration of 2,000 U/ml. It is stored at 4°C for no more than 8 hours or is stored frozen. It is stable at −20°C for 2 weeks. This reagent may be frozen and thawed twice for use as a reference material. It is discarded after the second thawing.
   c. Plasminogen substrate: a lyophilized preparation of Val-Leu-Lys-AIE in a disposable cuvette, identified by the presence of a blue dot. The substrate is packaged in a foil pouch and, once opened, must be used within 7 days when stored at 4°C. The substrate is reconstituted with 1 ml distilled water and contains a

concentration of 0.8 mol/ml. This reagent is stable for 4 hours at room temperature or for 8 hours at 4°C, and it should be protected from direct light.

7. Control (Prototrol, available from Dade).

Specimen

Nine volumes of blood are collected using a plastic syringe and are anticoagulated with one volume of 3.8% sodium citrate. The blood is centrifuged at 2,000 rpm for 15–20 minutes, and the plasma is removed and stored frozen in plastic tubes until used. The specimen is stable for 30 days if kept frozen at –20°C.

Method

1. The fluorometer is allowed to warm up for 45 minutes. All tubes are prewarmed to 37°C.

2. One vial each of plasminogen reference, streptokinase reagent, and control are reconstituted.

3. Streptokinase reagent aliquots of 0.5 ml are dispensed into three tubes and 10 μl plasminogen reference, control, and test plasma are added to each tube, respectively.

4. The specimen is vortexed and incubated at 37°C for 10 minutes to activate plasminogen to plasmin. After incubation, the specimen must be used within 4 hours if tubes are kept at room temperature or within 8 hours if stored at 4°C.

5. A plasminogen substrate cuvette is reconstituted with 1 ml distilled water and is warmed to 37°C for 10 minutes, with care taken not to place it in the light path until the test mixture is added.

6. The fluorometer function is checked according to the manufacturer's instructions.

7. One-tenth milliliter of plasminogen reference activation mixture (step 2) is added to the prewarmed plasminogen substrate (step 5). The cuvette is placed in the fluorometer. The compartment cover is closed, and the value obtained from the digital display, once it has stopped flashing, is recorded. The rate displayed should be numerically equivalent to the plasminogen reference assay multiplied by a factor of 10. If the display does not read ×10 ± 2, the test should be repeated and the fluorometer adjusted.

8. One-tenth milliliter of the control activation mixture is added to the plasminogen substrate. The cuvette is placed in the sample well, the compartment cover is closed, and the value obtained from the digital display, once it has stopped flashing, is recorded. The fluorometer is calibrated properly if the value displayed when the lag phase is completed is within the assay range for the control.

9. One-tenth milliliter of the patient's sample activation mixture is added to the plasminogen substrate, and it is mixed by repeated rinsing of the pipette tip. The cuvette is placed in the sample well, the cover is closed, and the digital readout is recorded as described.

Calculation

Display reading × 10 = Plasminogen (U/ml).

Reference Range

The reference range is 2.4–3.8 U/ml.

Clinical Considerations

Reductions in plasminogen levels occur during thrombolytic therapy, in systemic fibrinolysis, and in DIC. Low values are found also in infants younger than 6 months.

Plasminogen can also be assayed using a synthetic chromogenic substrate, with a principle similar to the fluorometric procedure described previously.

Platelet Function Tests

Bleeding Time (Simplate Method)

Principle

A long standardized incision is made on the forearm, and the blood is removed carefully by filter paper, with care taken not to touch the skin. The duration of bleeding is recorded as the bleeding time (Mielke et al., 1969).

Reagents and Equipment

1. Simplate (General Diagnostics).
2. Sphygmomanometer.
3. Filter paper: Whatman no. 1.
4. Stopwatch.

Method

1. An area of the forearm distal to the antecubital veins and without any obvious surface vessels or scars is cleansed with alcohol and allowed to dry.

2. The sphygmomanometer cuff is placed around the arm above the elbow and inflated to a pressure of 40 mm.

3. The Simplate is placed on the clean forearm surface, and an incision 5 mm long and 1 mm deep is made by depressing the trigger. Pressure is not applied to the device.

4. The stopwatch is started immediately after the incisions are made.

5. The blood resulting from the incision is removed with filter paper, with care taken to avoid touching the wound edges or skin. The blood is blotted away every 30 seconds until it no longer stains the paper.

6. This time interval is recorded as the bleeding time.

Reference Range

Adults:	2.5–6.5 minutes
Children:	2.5–8.5 minutes

Sources of Error

Good peripheral circulation is essential if satisfactory results are to be obtained. Chilling may impair the circulation and should be avoided by allowing the patient's skin temperature to equilibrate with the ambient temperature. This may be hastened by immersing the cold limb in warm water or wrapping it in a warm towel. Many drugs interfere with the bleeding time (the most common being aspirin or aspirin-containing drugs) by impeding platelet release mechanisms.

Several methods exist for determining the bleeding time, but all suffer from a lack of standardization and, consequently, produce results that are imprecise and subject to differences in clinical interpretation. The Duke procedure, which uses capillary puncture of the ear lobe or finger, is the most inaccurate and imprecise, as it is virtually impossible to standardize adequately the depth or size of the cut. In addition, vascularity of the ear and finger varies greatly among individuals, and this affects the accuracy of the results. A better technique, although even less precise than the Duke procedure, is the Ivy method, which standardizes the blood flow and pressure by the use of a constant pressure cuff. The Ivy technique, like other methods, depends a great deal on the surface area of the incision rather than on its depth and, for this reason, the Simplate method produces a more standardized cut and, therefore, a more standardized result.

A modification of the bleeding time, the secondary bleeding time (Borchgrevink and Waaler, 1958), has been used to test the intrinsic coagulation pathway function. The method uses a standardized Ivy test, after which bleeding from the wound is started by removing the partially healed tissue and recording the bleeding time. This secondary bleeding time is believed to be sensitive to intrinsic coagulation pathway defects such as classic hemophilia (Smith et al., 1984). The procedure is not used widely as a screening test.

The bleeding time reference range should be established in the laboratory by testing a statistically large enough group of normal specimens. The test is affected by the environmental temperature as well as by a variety of other factors. The skin should be warm and dry, with a free flow of blood from the wound. Hematologically, the bleeding time is affected by quantitative reductions (less than 30×10^9/liter) and qualitative disorders of platelets.

Clinical Considerations

The clinical utility of the bleeding time is well established. It is the only test that evaluates the in vivo response to injury—that is, the sequence of events leading to the formation of the primary hemostatic plug. Primary hemostasis requires functional and numerically adequate platelets, plasma proteins, and adequate numbers of red cells, substrate collagen, and vascular response. Patients with a positive clinical history of bleeding or extensive bruising should be evaluated with a bleeding time. The most common causes of abnormal bleeding are quantitative or qualitative abnormalities of platelets, including von Willebrand's syndrome. Uremic patients, those undergoing plastic surgery and preoperative major surgery, and patients with a history of antiplatelet medication (e.g., aspirin) use should also be evaluated.

Aspirin Tolerance Test

Principle

The ingestion of aspirin has been found to prolong the bleeding time by impeding platelet release mechanisms (Quick, 1966; see page 173).

Reagents and Equipment

1. Simplate (General Diagnostics).
2. Sphygmomanometer.
3. Filter paper: Whatman no. 1.
4. Stopwatch.

Method

The bleeding time is determined both before and 2 hours after three aspirin tablets (approximately 970 mg) are taken.

Reference Range

Before aspirin ingestion: 2.0–6.5 minutes
After aspirin ingestion: 5–10 minutes

Clinical Correlation

The test result is abnormal in individuals with functional platelet release defects or abnormal capillary morphologic features. Ingestion of standard doses of aspirin often produces bleeding times in excess of twice the upper limit of normal in such situations. Patients with mild disorders, including mild von Willebrand's syndrome, may have normal bleeding times before taking aspirin but prolonged times after ingestion.

Tourniquet Test

Principle

A sphygmomanometer is placed around the arm at a pressure exactly between the systolic and diastolic blood pressures. At such a level, the blood is pumped to the arm and hand but is not allowed to return easily to the vascular tree. The net result is that the capillaries are subjected to an increased internal pressure.

Reagents and Equipment

1. Sphygmomanometer.
2. Timer.
3. Stethoscope.

Method

1. A sphygmomanometer cuff is placed around the arm above the elbow and is inflated to a point midway between the systolic and diastolic pressures. It is left at this pressure for 5 minutes.

2. The cuff is removed, and the patient is instructed to lift the arm to shoulder height. The area immediately below the antecubital fossa is tapped gently with the hand and examined for the presence of multiple petechiae. Occasionally, petechiae are also present on the dorsal surface of the hand.

Reference Range

The reference range is fewer than 10 petechiae in a circle 6 cm in diameter.

Sources of Error

Capillary resistance is subject to physiologic diurnal variations, which tend to be lower in the afternoon and evening, apparently as the result of the diurnal rhythm of adrenocortical activity. Capillary resistance may also fluctuate from day to day and show seasonal variations, with a tendency to decrease in the late winter and early spring. Other factors influencing the result include the effect of physical and emotional stress related to vasopressin and histamine release and to the level of corticosteroid production.

Clinical Correlation

The tourniquet test has limited diagnostic value. On occasion, it may be helpful in detecting von Willebrand's syndrome, but it produces inconsistent results in thrombocytopenia. The test result is usually positive in nonthrombocytopenic or anaphylactoid purpura.

Clot Retraction (Quantitative Method)

Principle

Blood is allowed to clot in a clean tube and is then left for 1 hour at 37°C to allow retraction to take place. The clot is removed, and the free cells and serum are measured and expressed as a percentage of the total blood volume.

Reagents and Equipment

1. Graduated centrifuge tube.
2. Applicator stick.
3. Water bath, 37°C.
4. Centrifuge, microhematocrit.
5. Microhematocrit tubes.

Specimen

Whole blood and EDTA-anticoagulated blood are the specimens.

Method

1. Ten milliliters of whole blood are removed directly from the syringe and placed into a clean, graduated centrifuge tube. An applicator stick is placed in the blood before it clots.
2. The blood is allowed to clot and is incubated at 37°C for exactly 1 hour after clot formation.
3. The clot is withdrawn by gentle removal of the applicator stick. The free cells and serum are drained from the clot.
4. The characteristics of the clot are noted and recorded as either complete or poor clot retraction and as firm or friable.
5. The volume of the free cells and serum produced are measured, and the hematocrit value of the patient is determined by the method described on page 256 using the EDTA-anticoagulated blood sample.

Calculation

$$\frac{\text{Volume of serum expressed from clot} \times 100}{(100 - \text{hematocrit } \%)}$$

$$= \text{Clot retraction } (\%)$$

For example, if the hematocrit is 46% and 4 ml serum is expressed from 10 ml blood, and if the retraction were 100% complete, 5.4 ml serum should have been expressed (i.e., 10 – 4.6 ml). However, because 4 ml serum was obtained, the serum represents 74% retraction—that is,

$$\frac{4.0}{5.4} \times 100 = 74\% \text{ Clot retraction}$$

Reference Range

The reference range is 58–97%.

Sources of Error

Clot retraction depends on the presence of intact platelets and small quantities of divalent cations. Retraction is often poor in thrombocytopenia, particularly when the platelet count is less than 20.0×10^9/liter (Didisheim, 1967).

Using this quantitative procedure, the red-cell mass and degree of anemia are compensated for by expressing the result as a correlation of the hematocrit. Consequently, anemia and polycythemia do not influence the test result. Qualitative clot retraction methods, in which whole blood is allowed to remain at room temperature overnight, are not recommended because of their extreme subjectivity and lack of adequate control.

Platelet Factor 3 Availability Test

Principle

During coagulation, platelets release a phospholipid that possesses a partial thromboplastin function in vitro. The activity of the phospholipids released is compared directly with that of normal platelets using a modification of the PTT (Hardisty and Ingram, 1965).

Reagents and Equipment

1. Kaolin 0.5%: Kaolin, 1 g, is suspended in 200 ml PBS (page 371), pH 7.2. This is stored at room temperature.
2. Calcium chloride, 0.025 M.

Table 20.25. Kaolin-Activated Platelet Factor 3 Availability Test

	Tube No.			
Reagent	1	2	3	4
Platelet-rich plasma, control (ml)	0.1	0.1	—	—
Platelet-rich plasma, test (ml)	—	—	0.1	0.1
Platelet-poor plasma, control (ml)	0.1	—	0.1	—
Platelet-poor plasma, test (ml)	—	0.1	—	0.1
0.5% Kaolin (ml)	0.1	0.1	0.1	0.1

3. Stopwatch.
4. Water bath, 37°C.
5. Pipettes: 0.1 ml and Pasteur pipettes.
6. Log-log graph paper.

Specimen

Both platelet-rich and platelet-poor plasma are used. *Platelet-rich plasma from normal, control, and patient's specimens* consists of 9 volumes whole blood collected in a siliconized syringe and added to 1 volume 3.8% sodium citrate. The solution is centrifuged at 1,500 rpm for 3 minutes, and the plasma is transferred into a tube using a Pasteur pipette. All glassware used should be siliconized, or the pipettes and tubes should be plastic. The platelet-rich plasma is allowed to stand at room temperature. *It must not be refrigerated.* The control platelet-rich plasma specimen should be made by pooling 5–10 normal specimens using the same technique as is described for the patient's specimen.

Platelet-poor plasma from normal, control, and patient specimens consists of 9 volumes whole blood that are collected and added to 1 volume 3.8% sodium citrate. Siliconized or plastic pipettes and tubes are *not* required. The blood is centrifuged at 3,000 rpm for 30 minutes, and the plasma is removed and stored at 4°C for up to 4 hours.

Method

1. The reagents are set up in four tubes as shown in Table 20.25.
2. All tubes are incubated at 37°C for 15–20 minutes. The contents of the tubes are mixed, and

0.1 ml 0.025-M calcium chloride is added to each tube. The clotting times are recorded.

Interpretation

The clotting times of tube nos. 3 and 4 will be within 2–5 seconds if their platelet factor 3 availability is normal. The test can be quantitated by the following modification:

1. Doubling dilutions of normal platelet-rich plasma are made in platelet-poor plasma from the same normal subject, and kaolin clotting times are carried out on these dilutions as described previously.
2. The clotting time of each dilution is plotted on a linear scale against the platelet count (calculated from that of the undiluted platelet-rich plasma), on a log scale, as shown in Figure 20.5.
3. By interpolation on this curve, the normal platelet count can be found, which gives the same kaolin clotting time as the mixture of equal parts of test platelet-rich and normal platelet-poor plasma. The test platelet factor 3 availability index then is calculated from the following:

$$\frac{\text{Platelet count of normal platelet-rich}}{\text{plasma giving same time}} \times 100$$

For example, if the clotting time of the test mixture is 50 seconds, the platelet count of the test mixture is 250×10^9/liter, and the platelet count of normal platelet-rich plasma that gives the same clotting time (from the standard curve) is 13×10^9/liter:

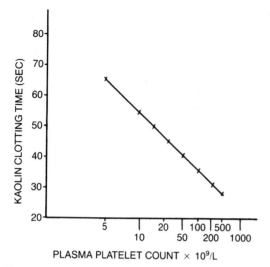

Figure 20.5. The relationship between the platelet count and the kaolin clotting time of platelet-rich plasma.

$$\frac{13}{200} \times 100 = 5.2\% \text{ Platelet factor 3 availability}$$

Reference Range

The reference range is greater than 25%.

Sources of Error

The test cannot be used to quantitate platelet factor 3 if a plasma coagulation factor defect is present, but a qualitative assessment of the clotting times of tube nos. 2 and 3 will allow for a subjective result. The test is difficult to standardize. Care should be taken in preparing the platelet-rich plasma specimens and in the use of siliconized or clean plastic hardware. As kaolin is a dense diatomaceous earth, all mixtures containing kaolin should be mixed immediately before any reagents are added to ensure that the particles are in suspension.

Platelet Aggregation

Principle

Platelet-rich plasma is interposed between a light source and a light detector, which is attached to a chart recorder that plots the transmission of light through the cuvette as a function of time. Initially, the platelets absorb and reflect light so that less light passes through the cuvette and is collected by the photomultiplier tube than would pass through a cuvette of platelet-poor plasma. If the platelets are stimulated to aggregate, the number of particles will decrease because of the aggregation, but their size will increase, thereby allowing more light to be transmitted. Maximum light transmission occurs in platelet-free plasma. The aggregometer is adjusted so that the platelet-rich plasma produces little light transmission and platelet-poor plasma gives 90–100% light transmission. The test uses various agents to stimulate platelet aggregation, and the curves obtained are compared with similar tracings from abnormal patients (Figure 20.6).

Reagents and Equipment

1. Platelet aggregometer (Payton Associates, Buffalo, NY) fitted with a Bausch & Lomb VOM5 Recorder: Other commercial aggregometers are available and can be used.
2. Disposable cuvettes (0.5-ml) with siliconized stirring bars.
3. Centrifuge.
4. Ice bath.
5. Centrifuge tubes: 10 ml, siliconized.
6. Pipettes, siliconized: 1 ml and 10 ml, graduated; 0.1-ml and Pasteur pipettes.
7. Syringes: either plastic or siliconized with 20-gauge needles.
8. Parafilm.
9. Stopwatch.
10. Preparation of siliconized apparatus: All glassware is siliconized using the technique described on page 344. Siliconization of the stirring bars should be carried out using a similar method *except* that the bars are *not rinsed* in distilled water but are dried either in a hot-air oven or at 37°C.
11. Tyrode's buffer, pH 7.35:
    a. Stock solution 1: 160 g sodium chloride, 4 g potassium chloride, 20 g sodium bicarbonate, and 1 g sodium dihydrogen phosphate dissolved in distilled water and diluted to 1 liter. The pH is adjusted to 7.35 with 0.1-N hydrochloric acid.
    b. Stock solution 2: 20.33 g of the 0.1-M magnesium chloride salt dissolved in distilled

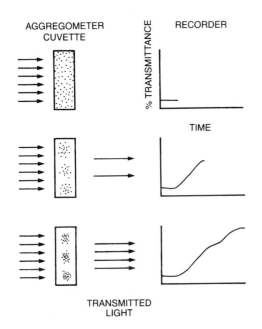

AGGREGOMETER
CUVETTE

% TRANSMITTANCE

RECORDER

TIME

TRANSMITTED
LIGHT

Figure 20.6. The principle of platelet aggregometry. (Modified from BS Coller. Platelet Aggregation by ADP Collagen and Ristocetin. A Critical Review of Methodology and Analysis. In D Seligson, RM Schmidt [eds], CRC Handbook Series in Clinical Laboratory Science: Section 1. Hematology. Vol. 1. Boca Raton, FL: CRC Press, 1979. P 381.)

water and diluted to 1 liter. This reagent is stable for 2–3 months when stored at 4°C.

c. Stock solution 3: 21.99 g of the 0.1-M calcium chloride salt dissolved in distilled water and diluted to 1 liter.

12. Tyrode's albumin: 50 ml stock buffer solution 1, 10 ml stock buffer 2, and 20 ml stock buffer 3 added together with 3.5 g bovine albumin fraction V (Pentex) and 1 g dextrose. The mixture is adjusted to pH 7.35 and diluted to 1 liter with distilled water. This reagent should be made up daily.

13. Acid-citrate-dextrose: 0.8 g anhydrous citric acid, 2.2 g anhydrous sodium citrate, and 2.45 g dextrose in 100 ml distilled water.

14. Adenosine diphosphate (ADP) stock (Dade): 0.1 g ADP dissolved in 10 ml distilled water. The resulting dilutions are divided into 0.2-ml volumes, are sealed with parafilm, and are stored immediately at –20°C. ADP stock is stable for 2–3 months if kept frozen.

15. Owren's buffer, pH 7.35: 11.75 g sodium diethyl barbital and 14.67 g sodium chloride dissolved in 430 ml 0.1-N hydrochloric acid. The mixture is diluted to 2 liters with distilled water.

16. ADP working solution: 0.01 ml stock ADP added to 10 ml Owren's buffer to produce a 1.0-µg/ml concentration of ADP. One milliliter of the 1.0-µg/ml solution is added to 1 ml Owren's buffer to produce a 0.3-µg/ml concentration of ADP. Six-tenths milliliter of the 1.0-µg/ml solution is added to 1.4 ml Owren's buffer to produce a 0.5-µg/ml concentration of ADP. Two-tenths milliliter of the 1.0-µg/ml solution is added to 1.8 ml Owren's buffer to produce a 0.1-µg/ml concentration of ADP.

17. Epinephrine chloride, stock solution, 1 mg/ml (Parke Davis): 0.1 ml diluted with 1.9 ml Owren's buffer. Stock solution is stored in the dark at 4°C. Working solution is made just before use.

18. Collagen reagent (available as cluster platelet aggregation reagents from Dade): Alternatively, collagen may be made by adding 9.4 g bovine collagen (Sigma) to 2 ml saline. It is vortexed for 5 minutes and centrifuged at 2,000 rpm for 5 minutes, and then 0.05 ml of the supernatant is added to 0.5 ml normal plasma.

19. Thrombin (Parke Davis), 1,000 U/ml: reconstituted by adding 1 ml normal saline to the vial. Additional dilutions are made with Tyrode's buffer to produce final concentrations as shown in Table 20.26.

Specimen

The collection of the specimen should be carried out using siliconized or plastic syringes. Six volumes of blood are anticoagulated with one volume of acid-citrate-dextrose, and this is centrifuged in a Sorvall RC2-B centrifuge (DuPont Medical Products, Wilmington, DE) using an HB-4 head at 750 rpm for 10 minutes. Alternatively, other centrifuges can be used at 150–160g for 10 minutes.

The platelet-rich plasma is separated into siliconized or plastic centrifuge tubes, and the total volume is recorded. Platelet counts are carried out using a standard technique. The platelet-rich plasma is recentrifuged at 5,000 rpm for 6 minutes (4,080 × g) and the plasma is removed. The platelet volume

Table 20.26. Dilutions of Stock Thrombin

Reagents	Tube No.							
	1	2	3	4	5	6	7	8
Thrombin, 1,000 U/ml	0.1	—	—	—	—	—	—	—
Tyrode's buffer (ml)	9.9	9.9	2.5	2.5	1.2	1.0	1.0	0.6
Transfer from previous tube (ml)	—	0.1 from tube no. 1	2.5 from tube no. 2	2.5 from tube no. 3	0.8 from tube no. 4	1.0 from tube no. 5	1.0 from tube no. 6	0.4 from tube no. 7
Final thrombin concentration (U/ml)	100	10	5	2.5	1.0	0.5	0.25	0.1

is recorded. The platelets are suspended in Tyrode's albumin so that the count approximates 250×10^9/liter.

Method

1. The aggregometer is allowed to warm up to 37°C for 15 minutes.
2. The apparatus is set as follows: stir bar speed, 900 rpm; range, 3; level, 0.2; output and zero, 0.
3. The recorder is set as follows: full-scale values, 0.01 volts; power, measure.
4. The pen is placed at *1* on the chart paper using the zero set control. The power set is adjusted to the standby setting.
5. Platelet-rich plasma, platelet-poor plasma, and ADP working solutions are prepared, and suspensions of collagen are diluted. All reagents are kept on ice.
6. The aggregometer is calibrated with both platelet-rich and platelet-poor plasma. Siliconized pipettes are used to transfer 0.9-ml volumes of platelet-rich plasma and platelet-poor plasma to each of two cuvettes, respectively. One stir bar is added to each cuvette.
7. The platelet-poor plasma is placed in the cuvette holder, and the aggregometer switch is turned to *measure*. The pen is set at *9* on the recorder using the aggregometer output control.
8. The recorder control is turned to *standby*, and platelet-poor plasma is removed from the apparatus and replaced with platelet-rich plasma.

9. The recorder is turned to *measure*. Using the zero control, the pen is set to *1* on the chart-paper scale.
10. The recorder control is returned to the standby setting, and step 7 is repeated, adjusting the pen to *9* if necessary.
11. Nine-tenths milliliter of platelet-rich plasma is pipetted into a cuvette, the stir bar is added, and the cuvette is placed in the holder. The recorder switch is set to *measure*. The aggregometer zero control is used to adjust the pen to *1* on the chart-paper scale.
12. The recorder switch is set to *record* to obtain a stable baseline tracing for at least 1 minute.
13. One-tenth milliliter of the collagen reagent is added to the platelet-rich plasma in the cuvette, with care taken not to let any air bubbles form in the plasma.
14. The recorder is allowed to run long enough for the reaction to reach the maximum level. A characteristic curve is obtained, with the pen returning to the baseline as the platelets disintegrate.
15. Steps 13 and 14 are repeated using the ADP and thrombin dilutions.

Interpretation

The interpretation of platelet aggregation tests is subjective and does not always produce clear-cut results. The laboratory should always determine the response to a standardized normal pool of platelets before evaluating patient status. This pool should be

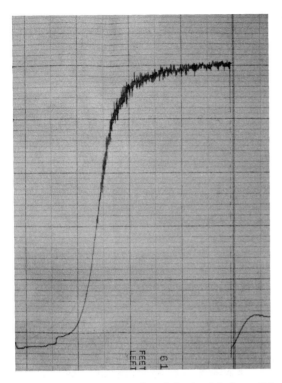

Figure 20.7. Platelet aggregation of platelet-rich plasma following the addition of collagen.

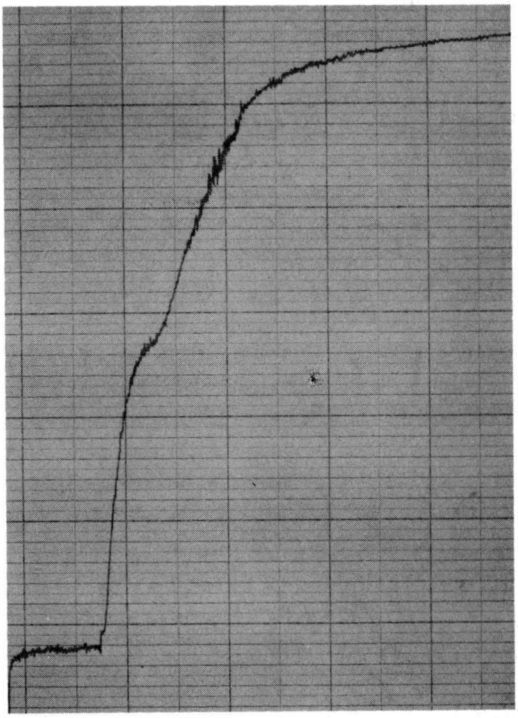

Figure 20.8. Platelet aggregation of platelet-rich plasma following the addition of 1:500 adenosine diphosphate.

selected from a group of individuals of widely varying ages and of both genders who are known not to be taking any medications.

Two waves of platelet aggregation usually are seen with ADP, epinephrine, and ristocetin. Collagen has only a secondary wave after a delay of approximately 1 minute (Figure 20.7).

The correct concentration of additives causing aggregation varies among individuals. Most normal platelets aggregate at a strength of 1.03 μM ADP (Figure 20.8), 2.5 μM epinephrine, 0.25 mg/ml collagen, and 1.2 mg/ml ristocetin. Aspirin removes the second phase of platelet aggregation by ADP and epinephrine and partially inhibits it by collagen. Because of this, aspirin should be avoided for 7–10 days before testing.

Ristocetin aggregation testing is discussed on page 359. Platelets from individuals with von Willebrand's syndrome are usually not aggregated by ristocetin in concentrations of 1.2 mg/ml or less. Platelets from patients with factor VIII deficiency demonstrate a normal response.

Acquired abnormalities of platelet aggregation are due to ingestion of many drugs; the more common among these are aspirin, phenylbutazone, indomethacin, sulfinpyrazone, chlorpromazine, antihistamines, antidepressants, cough remedies, and dipyridamole. Table 20.27 lists the inherited disorders of platelet function that relate to platelet aggregometry and bleeding time (Dreykin, 1974).

Discussion

Alternate principles have been used for measuring platelet aggregation. A sensitive measurement of the early stages of aggregation may be achieved by using continuous-flow particle counters, the degree of aggregation being inversely proportional to the number of single platelets remaining in the assay system (Gear, 1981). The use of optical fluctuations to study microaggregate formations in platelet suspensions has been described (Gabbosov et al., 1989). This method is based on the analysis of light transmission fluctuations produced by the changes in the number of platelets in the optical channel. The relative dispersion of these fluctuations is used as a parameter to estimate the degree of platelet aggregation and to

Table 20.27. Inherited Disorders of Platelet Function

Disorder	Frequency	Bleeding Time	Platelet Aggregation	
			ADP, Collagen, Epinephrine	Ristocetin
von Willebrand's syndrome	Common	N/I	N	A/P
Glanzmann's thrombasthenia	Rare	I	A	N
Bernard-Soulier disease	Rare	I	N	A
Storage pool syndrome	Rare	I	Primary wave only	N
Mild platelet disorders (abnormal release reaction)	Common	N/I	Primary wave only	N

ADP = adenosine diphosphate; N/I = normal to increased; I = increased; N = normal; A/P = absent or poor; A = absent.

analyze the aggregation kinetics. This method allows the detection of microaggregates and aggregation induced by very low concentrations of ADP in platelet-rich citrated plasma. Platelet function screening in whole blood, using an impedance lumi-aggregometer, is another alternative (Chronolog Corporation, Haverton, PA). The method uses 5 ml whole blood and does not require any centrifugation. Aggregometry by this method allows the test to be carried out up to 3 hours after phlebotomy (Sweeney et al., 1989a).

Several factors influence the final result, including pH, temperature, and the type of anticoagulant used. The control of pH is critical for accurate results. Platelet aggregation is maximal at pH 8.0 but is lacking if the pH is outside the range of 6.4–10.0 (Han and Ardlie, 1974). Increases in pH to greater than 7.7–8.0 inhibit the release reaction caused by epinephrine and ADP. If the pH level is greater than this, ADP aggregation is altered because of a reduction in available calcium ions, as citrate has an increased affinity to calcium at increasing pH levels. The principal cause of pH change is the rate of diffusion of carbon dioxide out of the plasma. The rate is influenced by the volume of platelet-rich plasma, the surface area of the air-liquid interface, mixing of the sample, and capping of the container (Coller et al., 1976). Other factors that affect the pH change are the concentration and acid-base properties of the aggregating agent, the proportion of platelet-rich plasma to the agent, and the concentration of buffer used.

Platelet aggregation is also influenced by environmental temperatures. Platelets stored at room temperature are more sensitive to various aggregating agents, particularly ADP, and should be warmed to 37°C on testing, as the release reaction is reduced at less than 33°C (Zucker, 1970). Consequently, the second phase of aggregation induced by ADP or epinephrine will not take place at temperatures of less than 30°C. Furthermore, platelet aggregation gradually decreases on storage, particularly at 37°C. Aggregation is slower at room temperature than at 37°C and shows less disaggregation. At 4°C, aggregation does not occur; the platelets lose their disc shape and form irregular spheres without visible microtubules (White and Krivit, 1967).

Platelet aggregation is influenced, too, by the ABO blood group of the patient. Factor VIII:C, von Willebrand's factor, and ristocetin cofactor levels are reduced in group O individuals. The aggregation response to collagen and ADP and the release of adenosine triphosphate are unaffected, but the response to ristocetin is better in group O than in group A individuals (Sweeney et al., 1989b).

The effect of anticoagulants on platelet aggregation is also critical. Increased concentrations of sodium citrate chelate large quantities of calcium ions, leaving an insufficient quantity to allow platelet aggregation to occur. Smaller increases in the citrate concentration inhibit aggregation, particularly affecting the epinephrine-induced reaction and only mildly affecting collagen aggregating properties. High citrate concentrations also affect the primary and secondary waves of ADP aggregation, the secondary wave being more susceptible (Ts'ao et al., 1976). Blood drawn into heparin often contains platelet aggregates, producing poor platelet yields (Zucker, 1975). In addition, heparin enhances primary aggregation by inducing the release reaction, probably because ionized calcium is available. Heparin may also inhibit ristocetin-induced aggregation (Percelen and Inceman, 1975). EDTA is unsuitable for platelet aggregation studies because of its strong chelating action. EDTA-anticoagulated platelet-rich plasma aggregates only with ristocetin and does not produce aggregation with other agents unless additional exogenous calcium ions supplement the reaction.

It has been recommended that, for efficient test use, platelet aggregation studies be reserved for those patients for whom a negative evaluation of von Willebrand's syndrome has been obtained, a repeated abnormal bleeding time is found, or uremia or drug ingestion has not been ruled out (Remaley et al., 1989).

Platelet Adhesion

Principle

A standard incision is made as for the bleeding time, and the platelet count obtained from the skin incision and that obtained from the venipuncture are compared (Borchgrevink, 1960).

Reagents and Equipment

1. Simplate apparatus, as described in the section on bleeding time (page 389).
2. Standard venipuncture equipment.

Method

1. Using the Simplate apparatus, a standard cut is made on the forearm below the elbow. The flow of blood must not be disturbed but must be allowed to accumulate until the drop is sufficiently large to fill the micropipette (Unopette). This usually takes 1 minute.
2. The blood is blotted away, with care taken not to touch the skin. The collection is repeated at 1-minute intervals until bleeding has ceased.
3. A manual platelet count is carried out on each of the dilutions, as described on page 280, and the results are averaged.
4. The platelet count is determined from a venous EDTA-anticoagulated blood sample drawn from the patient's other arm.

Calculation

$$\frac{\left(\text{Venous platelet count} - \text{Average capillary platelet count}\right)}{\text{Venous platelet count}}$$
$$\times 100 = \text{Platelet adhesiveness} (\%)$$

Reference Range

The reference range is 24–58%.

Sources of Error

Platelet adhesion methods reproduce poorly and have two disadvantages that cause the principal errors. First, they depend on differences between the results of two counts, a technique that, if done manually, is subject to a wide coefficient of variation. Second, it is assumed that the loss of platelets as a result of their passage over a foreign surface has been due to adhesion to that surface, whereas in fact the surface may have stimulated platelet disintegration without adhesion.

Several alternative procedures have been described for measuring platelet adhesion, but all appear to lack standardization. Techniques have been tried using a Harvard pump that passes blood over a column of fine beads, but the procedure is difficult to carry out because of the unavailability of the beads. The procedure calculates the standard platelet count from a venous specimen and then subjects the blood to a standard glass bead surface in a plastic column. The platelet count then is determined, and the platelet adhesion is expressed as a percentage of the native blood.

Detection of Platelet Antibodies by the Antiglobulin Consumption Test

Principle

The antiglobulin consumption test is designed to demonstrate antibodies adsorbed onto platelet surfaces by exposing antiglobulin serum to the coated platelet and then testing the anti-globulin serum for a reduction in titer (Dausset et al., 1961).

Table 20.28. Platelet Antibody Procedure

Reagent	Tube No.			
	1	2	3	4
Test platelet button (ml)	0.02	0.02	—	—
Normal platelet button (ml)	—	—	0.02	0.02
Test serum (ml)	0.02	—	0.02	—
Normal serum (ml)	—	0.02	—	0.02
Antiglobulin serum (ml)	0.15	0.15	0.15	0.15

Reagents and Equipment

1. Glassware: All glassware used in the test must either be siliconized or plastic. Siliconization should be carried out as described on page 344.
2. Water bath, 37°
3. Refrigerated centrifuge.
4. Tubes: 10 × 75 mm.
5. Pipettes: Micropipette or pipetting device capable of measuring 0.15 ml; Pasteur pipettes.
6. Platelet suspension: normal and test platelets, anticoagulant (dipotassium EDTA, 2%, in normal saline). Nine volumes of blood are obtained by a nontraumatic venipuncture carried out by siliconized or plastic syringe and are added to one volume of EDTA-saline anticoagulant. The blood is centrifuged at 1,000 rpm for 10 minutes at 10°C to obtain platelet-rich plasma. The platelet-rich plasma is removed with a siliconized pipette and is transferred to a second tube. The blood is recentrifuged at 3,000 rpm for 15–20 minutes to obtain a platelet button. The platelets are washed three to four times in the EDTA-saline solution, and the button is resuspended in one drop of the anticoagulant. Aliquots of 0.02 ml are transferred to each of two tubes.
7. Anti-D serum.
8. Coated red cells: one volume of a 50% suspension of washed, group O, Rhesus-positive cells suspended in nine volumes of high-protein anti-D serum that has been previously diluted 1:16 with saline. This suspension is incubated at 37°C for 1 hour.
9. Antihuman globulin serum (broad-spectrum), diluted 1:128 with normal saline.

Specimen

Test and control serum is obtained from blood that has been allowed to clot at 37°C. After centrifugation, 1 volume of 2% EDTA-saline anticoagulant is added to 9 volumes of serum. The specimen is stored frozen at −20°C until used.

Method

1. Four tubes are set up as shown in Table 20.28. To each tube, 0.15 ml antiglobulin serum is added. The contents of the tubes are mixed and incubated at 37°C for 15 minutes.
2. All tubes are centrifuged at 1,000 rpm for 5 minutes to obtain the "consumed" serum.
3. The antiglobulin sera obtained from step 2 are titrated in saline dilutions to 1:1,024. One volume of coated red cells is added to each tube, and the mixture is allowed to stand for 10–15 minutes at room temperature.
4. The highest dilution of the antiglobulin serum that shows a positive reaction with these cells is recorded.
5. The titration is repeated for all four tubes.

Results

The test result is considered positive if there is a three-tube or greater reduction in titer between the serum absorbed with test platelets (tube nos. 1 and 2) and the serum absorbed with normal platelets.

Clinical Correlation

The antiglobulin consumption test result is positive in 50–60% of individuals with idiopathic thrombocytopenic purpura. The procedure is difficult to carry out, and care should be taken in the preparation of the siliconized glassware and in following the method precisely.

Platelet antibodies can be found in individuals receiving large numbers of platelet transfusions, particularly those with leukemia and other neoplastic conditions. Patients whose platelet responses do not appear adequate following transfusion likely develop antibodies and consequently become refractive to therapy.

Detection of Platelet Antibodies Using a Rosette Technique: Direct Method

Principle

Platelets are fixed with paraformaldehyde and are introduced to rabbit antihuman IgG heavy-chain-specific antibody–coated polyacrylamide beads. The beads are observed microscopically for platelet rosetting (Salmassi et al., 1980).

Reagents and Equipment

1. Acid-citrate-dextrose anticoagulant: 22.0 g trisodium citrate, 8.0 g citric acid, and 24.5 g dextrose dissolved in distilled water and diluted to 1 liter.
2. Bovine albumin 30% containing 0.005% Evans blue (BSA).
3. Buffer: 0.35 g potassium dihydrogen phosphate, 0.576 g disodium hydrogen phosphate, 6.97 g sodium chloride, 2 g dextrose, 0.08 g adenosine, 0.1 g sodium hydroxide, 0.12 g α-tocopherol acetate (vitamin E acetate), and 5 ml dimethyl sulfoxide dissolved in 1 liter of distilled water.
4. Paraformaldehyde 2%, in buffer.
5. Refrigerated centrifuge.
6. Pipettes: micropipettes and Pasteur, all siliconized.
7. Tubes: 10×75 mm, siliconized.
8. Rabbit antihuman IgG heavy-chain-specific antibody–coated polyacrylamide beads (Immunobeads, available from Bio-Rad Labs, Richmond, CA).
9. Slides and coverslips.
10. Toluidine blue 0.03%, in buffer.
11. Water bath, 37°C.

Specimen

To obtain the platelets for testing, the following procedure is undertaken:

1. Blood is collected in acid-citrate-dextrose anticoagulant in a ratio of 1 volume of acid-citrate-dextrose to 6.7 volumes of blood. It is centrifuged at $200g$ for 15 minutes at 25°C. Then the platelet-rich plasma is removed with a siliconized pipette and layered over the BSA reagent in a ratio of 1 volume BSA to 6 volumes platelet-rich plasma.
2. The mixture is centrifuged at $900g$ for 15 minutes at 37°C, and the platelet zone is transferred into an equal volume of buffer. It is allowed to stand at room temperature for 5 minutes, and then an equal volume of buffer is added. This is allowed to stand at 37°C for 10 minutes.
3. The platelet suspension is mixed with 0.5 volume of 2% paraformaldehyde. It is allowed to stand at room temperature for 10 minutes. Another 0.5 volume of 2% paraformaldehyde is added to make a final concentration of 1%.
4. The platelet suspension is again layered onto 0.2 ml 30% bovine albumin and is centrifuged at $900g$ for 5 minutes.
5. Steps 2 and 3 are repeated, and the final concentration of the suspension is adjusted to 2×10^9/ml with buffer.

Method (Direct Platelet Antibody)

1. One-tenth-milliliter volumes of platelet test suspension, prepared as previously described, and antibody-coated beads at a concentration of 10–20 $\times 10^9$/liter are combined and are allowed to stand at room temperature for 15 minutes.
2. The mixture is centrifuged at $200g$ for 2 minutes and is resuspended gently by turning the tubes slowly while tilting them.
3. A drop of the mixture is placed on a slide, and one drop of 0.03% toluidine blue is added. The coverslip is placed, and the specimen is examined microscopically.

Results and Interpretation

A positive rosette sign is recognized by the presence of the Immunobeads surrounded by four or more platelets. The number of rosettes is expressed as a percentage of 200 Immunobeads.

Reference Range

The reference range is 2.5–5.0%. A result in the range of 5.0–10% is inconclusive.

Indirect Procedure for Platelet Antibody Detection

Specimen

The specimen is test serum, inactivated at 56°C for 30 minutes. Serum is frozen at –70°C overnight, is thawed, and is centrifuged at 900*g* for 30 minutes at 25°C. Platelets are prepared as they are in the direct method (see preceding section).

Method

1. Equal volumes of test serum and normal fixed platelets are mixed and incubated at 37°C for 30 minutes.
2. The platelet suspension is washed three times using buffered albumin at 900*g* for 10 minutes and is resuspended to make the final concentration approximately 2×10^8/ml.
3. One-tenth-milliliter volumes of platelet suspension and Immunobeads are added. The mixture is centrifuged at 200*g* for 2 minutes and is examined and interpreted as in the direct method.

Results, Interpretation, and Reference Range

The results, their interpretation, and the reference range all are similar to those in the direct method (refer to preceding section).

Clinical Correlation

This test is sensitive to the presence of both platelet-bound and free serum platelet antibodies. It is particularly useful in detecting antibodies in individuals with idiopathic thrombocytopenic purpura. The direct test shows rosetting of between 34 and 68%, and the indirect test shows rosetting of between 29 and 43%, when platelet antibodies are present. Of the original series tested, all individuals with idiopathic thrombocytopenic purpura demonstrated positive test results. In contrast, 71% of individuals with systemic lupus erythematosus showed positive results.

The procedure is sensitive to platelet antibodies but depends on several varying technical factors. First, increasing the Immunobead concentration in the presence of a constant number of sensitized platelets results in a yield of fewer rosettes. However, extremely low concentrations of Immunobeads compared with a constant number of platelets makes it impossible to distinguish true positive results from spontaneous rosette formation. Prolonged storage of fixed platelets also introduces a gradual diminishing of sensitivity. Storage of fixed platelets should not exceed 3 days at either room temperature or 4°C.

A quantitative enzyme-linked immunosorbent assay procedure for the measurement of in vivo bound platelet-associated IgG using intact patient platelets has been described (Lynch et al., 1985). The assay requires quantitation and standardization of the number of platelets bound to microtiter plate wells and an absorbance curve using quantitated IgG standards. Platelet-bound IgG is measured using an F(ab')$_2$ peroxidase-labeled antihuman IgG and O-phenylenediamine dihydrochloride as the substrate. This procedure appears sensitive and specific for the detection of platelet-bound IgG.

Radioactive antiglobulin tests have also been used to detect platelet antibodies. The procedure involves anti-IgG and anti-C3 antisera and appears to be valuable in the diagnosis of immune and nonimmune thrombocytopenia (Freedman et al., 1985).

The most recent methodology and the most sensitive procedure is to use fluorescent markers with flow cytometry. The principle is to label platelet concentrates with immunofluorescent dyes and to detect and quantitate those platelets that fluoresce by classic flow-cytometric methods. Both platelet-bound antibodies (analogous to a direct red-cell antiglobulin test) and free platelet antibodies in the serum (analogous to the indirect antiglobulin test) can be detected in this way.

Chapter 21

Staining Procedures

Red Cells and Hematoparasites

Siderocytes: Prussian Blue Reaction

Principle

Siderocytes are red cells containing nonhemoglobin iron granules that give a positive Prussian blue reaction when exposed to a potassium ferrocyanide–hydrochloric acid mixture (Mills and Lucia, 1949).

Reagents and Equipment

1. Absolute methyl alcohol.
2. Potassium ferrocyanide, 2% aqueous.
3. Hydrochloric acid 1% (by volume).
4. Eosin, 0.1% aqueous.
5. Water bath, 37°C.
6. Coplin jar.

Specimen

Air-dried peripheral blood or bone marrow smears are used.

Method

1. The smears are fixed in methyl alcohol for 15 minutes at room temperature and allowed to air-dry.
2. Equal volumes of 2% potassium ferrocyanide and 1% hydrochloric acid are mixed in a Coplin jar, and the smears are stained at 37°C for 10 minutes.
3. The slides are washed in running tap water and counterstained for 5–10 seconds in 0.1% aqueous eosin. They are rinsed in tap water and are allowed to air-dry.
4. The smears are examined with an oil-immersion objective.

Reference Range

The reference range is 0.4–0.6%.

Clinical Correlation

Siderocytes are found in moderate numbers in normal blood and the bone marrow but are characteristically increased in hemolytic anemias and infections and following splenectomy. When siderocytes are present in nucleated red cells, the term *sideroblast* is used. Common levels of peripheral blood siderocytosis are as follows: in infections, 6–10%; in severe burns, 3–10%; in pernicious anemia, 8–14%; in lead poisoning, 10–30%.

Staining of Malarial Parasites: Field's Stain for Thick Smears

Principle

The blood smears are unfixed. Aqueous stains are used to stain the malarial parasites and hemolyze the red cells (Markell and Voge, 1981).

Reagents and Equipment

1. Coplin jars.
2. Staining rack.
3. Phosphate buffer: Solution A consists of 1.3 g methylene blue, 0.5 g Azure I, 1.3 g anhydrous

disodium hydrogen phosphate, and 6.25 g anhydrous potassium dihydrogen phosphate dissolved in distilled water and diluted to 500 ml.

Solution B consists of 1.3 g eosin, 5 g anhydrous disodium hydrogen phosphate, and 6.25 g anhydrous potassium dihydrogen phosphate dissolved in distilled water and diluted to 500 ml.

The salts are dissolved first in the water, and the stains are then added. The Azure I in solution A is ground in a mortar before being added to the phosphate buffer. Once the stains are dissolved in the buffer, the solutions are allowed to stand at room temperature for 24 hours and are filtered. If a scum forms or the dye precipitates, the solution is refiltered. The staining solutions can be used for 3–4 weeks if stored at 4°C, but they should be renewed if the eosin in solution B becomes greenish.

Specimen

Thick, unfixed blood smears are used. Three drops of blood, each approximately the size used to make a thin smear, are placed close together near one end of a slide. With one corner of another absolutely clean slide, the blood is stirred over an area 2 cm in diameter. Stirring is continued for at least 30 seconds, and the smear is allowed to air-dry. Heat is not used.

Method

1. The slide is dipped in solution A for 1 second and is rinsed by immersion in a Coplin jar of tap water for 2–3 seconds until the stain ceases to flow from the smear.
2. The slide is dipped in solution B for 1 second and rinsed as in item 1.
3. The preparation is allowed to air-dry at room temperature.

Staining of Malarial Parasites for Thin Smears

Principle

The principle underlying staining of malarial parasites for thin smears is the same as that for differential leukocyte counts (see page 270).

Reagents and Equipment

1. Coplin jars.
2. Wright's stain (as described on page 271).
3. Phosphate buffer, pH 6.8.

Specimen

The specimen is thin blood smears.

Method

1. The smear is fixed by immersion in undiluted Wright's stain for 1 minute and then transferred to a jar containing an equal volume of stain and buffered water, pH 6.8 (see page 271), for 5–15 minutes. The length of staining should be determined by trial and error.
2. The stain is rinsed from the slide with buffer, and the smear is allowed to air-dry at room temperature.

Microfilarial Concentration and Stain

Principle

The method of microfilarial concentration and stain hemolyzes the red cells and concentrates leukocytes and microfilariae.

Reagents and Equipment

1. Centrifuge.
2. Tubes.
3. Formalin 2%.
4. Slides.
5. Wright's stain.
6. Pasteur pipettes.

Specimen

One milliliter of whole blood is delivered directly into a tube containing 10 ml 2% aqueous formalin, and the solution is mixed.

Method

1. The diluted specimen is centrifuged at 1,500 rpm for 1 minute.

2. The supernatant is decanted, and the sediment is spread out to approximately the thickness of normal blood smears. It is allowed to air-dry.

3. The specimen is stained by the routine procedure described on page 271.

Leishmania Staining Procedure

Principle

This technique uses a buffy-coat preparation obtained from blood that has been anticoagulated with ethylenediaminetetraacetic acid (EDTA).

Reagents and Equipment

1. Wintrobe tube.
2. Centrifuge.
3. Pasteur pipettes.
4. Slides.

Specimen

1. A Wintrobe tube is filled and centrifuged at 3,000 rpm for 30 minutes.
2. The buffy coat is removed with a Pasteur pipette, and smears are made by the standard technique.
3. The preparation is allowed to air-dry and is stained as for a peripheral blood smear.

Method

The method is the same as that used for Wright's stain (page 271).

Clinical Correlation

The *Leishmania* staining method is useful for the detection of *L. donovani* if present in the circulation, and it also will detect *Histoplasma capsulatum*, a fungus that is morphologically similar to *Leishmania*.

Trypanosome Staining Procedure

Principle

The parasites are concentrated by differential centrifugation and stained using a standard procedure.

Reagents and Equipment

1. Sodium citrate, 6% aqueous.
2. Centrifuge.
3. Standard staining reagents, as described on page 271.
4. Pasteur pipettes.
5. Tubes: 13×100 mm.

Specimen

Nine milliliters of blood are delivered directly into 1 ml 6% sodium citrate.

Method

1. The specimen first is centrifuged at 1,000 rpm for 10 minutes.
2. The supernatant is removed with a Pasteur pipette, delivered into another tube, and recentrifuged at 1,500 rpm for 10 minutes.
3. The supernatant is removed again, transferred to a clean tube, and recentrifuged at 2,500 rpm for 10 minutes.
4. The sediment is transferred to a slide, a smear is prepared, and this is stained using Wright's stain.

White Cells

Peroxidase Stain

Principle

Peroxidase present in the granules of myeloid and monocytic cells acts on hydrogen peroxide, liberating oxygen. This then reacts with a benzidine substitute, 3-amino-9-ethylcarbazole (Sigma Chemical Co., St. Louis, MO), to produce a red-brown precipitate at the site of peroxidase production (Graham et al., 1965).

Reagents and Equipment

1. Formalin acetone fixative (pH 6.6–6.8): Disodium hydrogen phosphate, 0.2 g, and 1.0 g potassium dihydrogen phosphate are dissolved in 300 ml distilled water. The solution is then added to 450 ml acetone and 250 ml formalin. The fixative is stored at 4°C.

2. Acetic acid, 0.02 M: Glacial acetic acid, 1.16 ml, is diluted to 1 liter with distilled water.
3. Sodium acetate, 0.02 M: Sodium acetate, 2.72 g, is diluted to 1 liter with distilled water.
4. Acetate buffer, 0.02 M (pH 5.0–5.2): Acetic acid, 0.02 M (176 ml), is added to 800 ml 0.02-M sodium acetate. This is stored at 4°C.
5. Hydrogen peroxide, 0.3%: Hydrogen peroxide 30% (0.1 ml) is diluted to 10 ml with distilled water. It should be prepared just before use.
6. Stain (pH 5.5): 3-Amino-9-ethylcarbazole, 0.01 g, is dissolved in 6.0 ml dimethyl sulfoxide and 50 ml acetate buffer (0.02 M); 0.4 ml 0.3% hydrogen peroxide then is added to the reagent. The stain is filtered before use.
7. Mayer's hematoxylin: Sodium iodate (0.5 g), hematoxylin (5.0 g), and aluminum ammonium sulfate (50 g) are dissolved in 700 ml distilled water and 20 ml acetic acid. Three hundred milliliters of glycerol are added to the solution. The reagent is stable for 3 months when stored at room temperature.
8. Glycerol gelatin: Gelatin, 20 g, is dissolved in 105 ml warm distilled water, and 125 ml glycerol is added to the mixture. The preparation is stored in a jar at 4°C. Before use, a portion of the jelly is removed and heated until liquefied.
9. Coplin jars.

Specimen

The specimen consists of fresh thin blood or bone marrow smears.

Method

1. The smears are fixed in buffered formalin-acetone for 15 seconds at room temperature and then are washed gently under running tap water.
2. The smears are immersed in a Coplin jar filled with filtered stain for 2 minutes at room temperature.
3. The smears then are washed gently under running water and counterstained for 8 minutes with Mayer's hematoxylin.
4. Excess stain is removed by rinsing under tap water. Smears are air-dried and mounted with glycerol jelly.
5. The smears are examined under a high-power oil-immersion lens.

Results

Peroxidase activity is indicated by the presence of red-brown deposits in the cytoplasm of all mature granulocytes except basophils. Monocytes and less mature granulocytes show decreasing peroxidase activity.

Clinical Correlation

Peroxidase staining for white cells uses a modification of older techniques that use the carcinogen benzidine, which is unavailable for routine use. The cytochemical demonstration of peroxidase depends on the use of an oxidizable substrate possessing brightly colored oxidation products. Besides the use of 3-amino-9-ethylcarbazole, 2,6-dichlorophenol-indophenol has been used, which produces a deep purple end color (Jacoby, 1963), and *p*-phenylenediamine and catechol have been used, which produce a brown-black reaction (Hanker et al., 1977).

Lipid Stain, Sudan Black B

Principle

The inert diazo dye Sudan black B stains a variety of lipids, including neutral fats, phospholipids, and sterols. To a lesser extent, it also stains some non-lipid cellular components. It appears to stain both azurophilic and specific granules in neutrophils, in contrast to peroxidase, which is found only in azurophilic granules. Early myeloid cells, such as myeloblasts and early promyelocytes, react with the stain (Sheehan and Storey, 1947).

Reagents and Equipment

1. Buffer diluent: Crystalline phenol, 16 g, is dissolved in 30 ml absolute ethyl alcohol and is added to 100 ml distilled water in which 0.3 g hydrated disodium hydrogen phosphate has been dissolved.
2. Sudan black B stock reagent: 0.3 g Sudan black B is dissolved in 100 ml absolute ethyl alcohol. It is shaken frequently for 1–2 days and is filtered.
3. Sudan black B working reagent: 40 ml of the buffer are added to 60 ml of the stock solution, and this reagent is filtered.
4. Wright's stain and buffer (see page 271).

5. Formalin 40%.
6. Ethyl alcohol 70%.
7. Coplin jars.

Specimen

The specimen used is air-dried blood or bone marrow smears.

Method

1. The smears are fixed by allowing them to be exposed to formalin vapor for 10–15 minutes.
2. The smears are washed in tap water for 10 minutes and stained by immersion for 1 hour in a Coplin jar filled with Sudan black B working solution.
3. They then are washed in 70% ethyl alcohol for 3 minutes to differentiate the stain and are rinsed in running tap water for 2 minutes.
4. The smears are counterstained with Wright's stain (as described on page 271) and examined microscopically under a high-power oil-immersion lens.

Results

Granulocytes show increasing distribution of lipids as they mature. Eosinophils at all stages of maturation exhibit a strong reaction at the periphery of the specific granules, which retain an unstained central core. Basophils demonstrate a variable reaction, whereas lymphocytes are usually nonsudanophilic. Monocytes and megakaryocytes show scattered lipid deposits, and red cells also normally stain negatively. In general, granules that are peroxidase-positive are also sudanophilic.

Sources of Error

Because lipids are more stable than peroxidases, the smears used for Sudan black B lipid staining need not be fresh to obtain a satisfactory reaction.

Clinical Correlation

In most cases of acute myeloid leukemia, nearly all the myeloid cells, except for blast forms, are sudanophilic. Auer bodies stain intensely. Typically,

leukemic granulocytic cells contain coarse granules, frequently in the Golgi zone of the cell. In acute monocytic leukemia, 5% of the nucleated cells contain discrete scattered granules resembling those seen in normal monocytes. In acute lymphocytic leukemia, the nucleated cells do not stain. Sudan black B is most useful in distinguishing granulocytic leukemias (acute myeloid) from nongranulocytic forms.

Nitroblue-Tetrazolium Test

Principle

Nitroblue-tetrazolium (NBT) is a colorless dye that is reduced to blue-black formazan deposits in the cytoplasm of actively phagocytizing neutrophils. A small percentage of neutrophils from normal individuals will reduce the dye but, in systemic bacterial infections and in some fungal and parasitic disorders, this dye reduction is quantitatively increased (Okamura et al., 1974).

Reagents and Equipment

1. Phosphate buffer, 0.067 M (pH 7.2): Anhydrous potassium dihydrogen phosphate, 9.08 g, is dissolved in 1 liter of distilled water, 9.47 g anhydrous disodium hydrogen phosphate is dissolved in 1 liter of distilled water, and 28 ml of the potassium phosphate solution is added to 72 ml of the sodium phosphate reagent.
2. NBT 0.1%, in normal saline: The dye is light-sensitive and should be stored in the dark. It is stable for 2–3 months and should be filtered before use.
3. Working glucose buffer: Glucose, 0.2 g, is dissolved in 100 ml of the phosphate buffer containing 0.6 g sodium chloride. This solution is filtered before use.
4. Water bath, 37°C.
5. Sterile tubes: plastic.
6. Microhematocrit centrifuge.
7. Capillary tubes: plain and sealer (see page 256).
8. Romanowsky stains and buffers (see page 271).

Specimen

Fresh heparinized blood is the specimen.

Method

1. Equal volumes of freshly filtered NBT dye and glucose-saline-buffer reagent are mixed in a disposable sterile plastic tube.

2. Two volumes of a freshly drawn heparinized blood sample are added and mixed gently with the reagent.

3. The preparation is incubated at 37°C for 15 minutes, with gentle shaking every 5 minutes.

4. The blood-dye mixture is introduced into a hematocrit capillary tube and centrifuged for 5 minutes to obtain a buffy coat.

5. The capillary tube is broken at the plasma-cell interface, and blood smears are made with the buffy coat.

6. The preparation is stained using a routine Romanowsky procedure.

7. The preparation is examined under a high-power oil-immersion lens for the presence of black deposits within the neutrophils. One hundred neutrophils are counted, and the percentage of positive neutrophils is calculated.

Reference Range

The reference range is 2–22%.

Clinical Correlation

The principal advantage of this modified procedure over the original method (Park et al., 1968) is that neutrophil morphologic characteristics are better preserved, which leads to higher NBT counts and reference ranges because of the presence of fewer smudged cells.

The reduction of NBT by neutrophils is a reflection of the activity of a cyanide-insensitive cytoplasmic pyridine nucleotide oxidase (Baehner and Nathan, 1967). This enzyme is related to the increased oxygen consumption, increased pentose shunt activity, and increased hydrogen peroxide formation associated with phagocytosis, degranulation, and intracellular destruction of bacteria.

The test is used often as a screening procedure for chronic granulomatous disease (CGD). If large numbers of formazon deposits are present in neutrophils, CGD is ruled out. If no deposits are found, confirmation by stimulation tests with endotoxins, latex particles, or bacterial filtrates should be done before an absolute diagnosis is made (Baehner and Nathan, 1968).

False-negative NBT test results are seen in the presence of bacterial infections in patients with congenital and acquired agammaglobulinemia, sickle cell disease, and kwashiorkor (Park, 1971; Seeler et al., 1972; Shousha and Kamel, 1972). False-positive reactions are seen in parasitic and fungal infections, particularly when caused by *Candida albicans* in individuals on birth control medication, in normal neonates, and in lymphoma (Park et al., 1968; Humbert et al., 1970; Matula and Paterson, 1971; Ng et al., 1972; Silverman and Reed, 1973).

Glycogen Periodic Acid–Schiff Reaction

Principle

Periodic acid specifically oxidizes glycols and related compounds, including glycogen, to produce aldehydes. These then react with the Schiff reagent (leukobasic fuchsin) to release fuchsin, which stains the cellular components pinkish red (McManus, 1946).

Reagents and Equipment

1. Formalin-alcohol fixative: Neutral formalin, 10 ml, is added to 90 ml 95% ethyl alcohol. It is stored in a stoppered bottle at 4°C.

2. Periodic acid 0.5%: Periodic acid, 0.5 g, is dissolved in 100 ml distilled water. The reagent is stable indefinitely if stored in a dark bottle at 4°C.

3. Schiff reagent: Distilled water, 200 ml, is brought to a boil. The mixture is removed from the heat, and 1 g basic fuchsin is added very slowly. When the dye has dissolved, it is allowed to cool and then filtered. Two grams of sodium metabisulfite and 10.1 ml 1-N hydrochloric acid are added. The mixture is allowed to stand for 24 hours at room temperature, and then 1 g activated charcoal is added. The reagent is shaken for 1 minute and filtered through a Whatman no. 1 filter paper. The solution should be colorless. It is stored at 4°C. The reagent is stable until it becomes a light pink. Schiff reagent is available commercially from Sigma Chemical Co.

Table 21.1. Scoring Procedure in the Periodic Acid–Schiff Staining Method

Score	Visual Interpretation
0	No staining
1+	Faint, diffuse staining tinge or fine granular staining, or both
2+	Moderately coarse granular staining
3+	Coarse granular staining
4+	One or more staining blocks present

4. Sodium metabisulfite 0.6%: Sodium metabisulfite, 0.6 g, is dissolved in 95 liters of distilled water and diluted to 100 ml with 1-N hydrochloric acid. It is prepared fresh just before use.
5. Mayer's hematoxylin: Hematoxylin, 1 g, is added to 500 ml distilled water. It is heated to boiling, and an additional 500 ml distilled water, 0.2 g sodium iodate, and 50 g aluminum potassium sulfate are added. This is shaken well, filtered, and stored at room temperature in a brown bottle.
6. Coplin jar.

Specimen

The specimen used is air-dried blood or bone marrow smears.

Method

1. The smears are fixed in formalin-alcohol for 15 minutes.
2. They are rinsed in distilled water and are transferred to a Coplin jar containing Schiff's reagent for 15 minutes. Then the smears are washed briefly in distilled water.
3. The preparation is immersed in two successive 5-minute baths of 0.6% sodium metabisulfite solution. The smears are rinsed with water and allowed to stand in distilled water for 10 minutes.
4. They are counterstained with Mayer's hematoxylin for 15 minutes.
5. The smears are rinsed five times in distilled water and allowed to stand in the final water. They are then rinsed for 5 minutes.
6. The smears are air-dried and examined under the high-power oil-immersion lens.
7. One hundred neutrophils are examined and quantitatively scored using the procedure shown in Table 21.1.

Results

A magenta staining reaction indicates the presence of glycogen.

Quality Control

Two normal slides are used as controls for the test. After fixing, one smear is covered in centrifuged human saliva for 1 hour, and both smears are carried through the staining procedure, as outlined previously. The untreated smear should show glycogen deposits, and the smear treated with saliva should be negative for glycogen.

Interpretation

Table 21.1 shows the scoring procedure in the periodic acid–Schiff (PAS) staining method. The normal reference range for the quantitative interpretation of the stain should be obtained by each laboratory.

Clinical Correlation

Typical PAS reactions in normal cells are shown in Table 21.2. Myeloblasts do not usually stain but may occasionally be seen with diffuse cytoplasmic staining. Commencing at the promyelocyte stage of maturation, the granulocytic cells gradually take on an increased positive reaction, eventually reaching the intense magenta reaction found in the mature neutrophil. Monocytes do not stain intensely, although they may contain fine or coarse PAS-positive granules. Occasional lymphocytes may show a few small positive granules. Eosinophil-specific granules stain negatively, whereas basophilic granules stain positively. Megakaryocytes and platelets are strongly positive. Normal red-cell precursors do not stain.

Table 21.2. Periodic Acid–Schiff Staining Reactions of Normal Cells

Cell	Reaction
Myeloblast	Negative
Promyelocyte	Usually negative
Myelocyte	Negative or weakly positive
Neutrophil	Positive
Monocyte	Negative or weakly positive
Lymphocyte	Usually negative
Megakaryocyte	Positive
Platelet	Positive
Nucleated red cell	Negative

In disease states, the PAS reaction is frequently positive and can be used to differentiate some hematologic neoplasms. Acute lymphocytic leukemia demonstrates variable PAS reactions. In some cases, there is a positive reaction, the cells showing fine-to-coarse granulation. Glycogen blocks are occasionally seen in some cells.

Acute myeloid leukemias show quantitative differences. The M1 forms show diffuse staining in almost all cells, and the few neutrophils present may show coarse uneven staining patterns. Lymphocytes in the peripheral blood show high scores in most cases, if there are sufficient cells to score. The M4 and M5 variants of acute myeloid leukemia demonstrate diffuse staining in some cells and granular positivity in others. Peripheral blood lymphocytes show high scores in approximately 66% of all cases. Type M6 acute myeloid leukemia (*erythroleukemia*) is characterized by the presence of a wide range of positive reactions in the immature erythroid cells, which range from a diffuse pink-red reaction to the presence of large blocks of PAS material. This finding, however, is nonspecific for type M6 leukemia, as PAS-positive red-cell precursors can also be found in iron-deficiency anemia, thalassemia, and severe acquired hemolytic anemias.

In chronic myeloid leukemia in blastic crisis, variable numbers of blast cells show reactions ranging from diffuse staining to the presence of coarse granules and large blocks of PAS-positive material. Chronic lymphocytic leukemias usually are marked by high scores that may revert to normal if the patient's disease remits or may increase if disease relapse occurs.

Leukocyte Alkaline Phosphatase

Principle

The leukocyte alkaline phosphatase reaction depends on the hydrolysis of α-naphthol phosphate by alkaline phosphatase, which liberates free naphthol. This, in turn, unites with a diazotized amine to form an insoluble color precipitate proportionate to the concentration of the enzyme present in the granulocytic cytoplasm (Kaplow, 1955, 1963).

Reagents and Equipment

1. Fixative, 10% formalin-methanol: Formalin, 10 ml, is added to 90 ml absolute methanol. The reagent is stable for 2–4 weeks if stored at –20°C.
2. Stock buffer, 0.2 M propanediol: 2-Amino-2-methyl-1,3-propanediol (21 g) is dissolved in distilled water and is diluted to 1 liter. This is stored at 4°C.
3. Working buffer, 0.05 M propanediol (pH 9.4–9.6): 3.5 ml 2-N hydrochloric acid is added to 250 ml stock buffer and is diluted to 1 liter with distilled water. The solution, which is stored at 4°C, should be warmed to room temperature before use.
4. Fast violet B.
5. Naphthol AS-B1 phosphate-sodium salt.
6. Substrate: Naphthol AS-B1 phosphate-sodium salt, 0.05 g, and 0.04 g fast violet B are added to 60 ml of the working buffer. The mixture is shaken well to dissolve the substrate and dye, is filtered, and is used immediately. This reagent cannot be stored.
7. Mayer's hematoxylin: Prepared as in the PAS staining procedure (see page 408).
8. Coplin jars.

Specimen

The specimen use is a fresh blood smear, less than 1 hour old. Once fixed, the smear is stable if kept at 4°C for 24 hours, or it can be stored at –20°C for 3–4 weeks.

Method

1. The smears are fixed in cold (0–5°C) formalin-methanol reagent for 30 seconds and washed gently in running tap water.

Table 21.3. Scoring Criteria in the Leukocyte Alkaline Phosphatase Reaction

Cell Rating	Precipitated Azo Dye in the Cytoplasm			Cytoplasm Background
	Amount (%)	Granule Size	Stain Intensity	
0	—	—	—	Unstained
1+	20–50	Small	Faint to moderate	Unstained to pale pink
2+	40–80	Small/medium	Moderate/strong	Unstained to pale pink
3+	80–100	Medium/large	Strong	Pink
4+	100	Medium/large	Brilliant	Cytoplasm not visible

Source: Data from G Cudak. Leukocyte alkaline phosphatase stain. Lab Perspect 3:9, 1983.

2. They are allowed to air-dry and placed in freshly prepared substrate that has been brought to room temperature. The smears are left in the substrate for 15 minutes.

3. The smears are rinsed again in tap water and counterstained with filtered Mayer's hematoxylin for 6–8 minutes.

4. Once again, they are allowed to air-dry. The slide is prepared by placement of a drop of water on the smear and careful application of a coverslip. It is examined with a high-power oil-immersion lens.

5. After examination, the coverslip is removed, and the smear is air-dried.

6. One hundred consecutive neutrophils are counted, and each is rated from 0 to 4+ based on the intensity of the stain. The sum of the 100 ratings is the smear score. (A convenient method of scoring is shown in Table 21.3.)

Quality Control

Positive control smears should always be stained along with the test. The most convenient source of elevated leukocyte alkaline phosphatase slides is from women in the later stages of pregnancy. Such control smears may be prepared in batches, fixed, and stored at –70°C for up to 1 year without loss of enzyme activity. If kept at –10°C, these smears are stable for 3–4 weeks, with a loss of approximately 10% enzyme activity.

Reference Range

Adults	15–100
Newborns	150–300

Sources of Error

Care should be exercised when handling naphthol and diazonium salts, as they are potentially carcinogenic. Both skin contact and inhalation should be avoided.

The smears can be fixed by storing the fixative in the freezer in a Coplin jar and placing the smears directly in the iced reagent. The leukocyte alkaline phosphatase staining procedure should be carried out in duplicate, and at least two 100-cell counts should be made. Eosinophils, basophils, monocytes, and lymphocytes should not be included in the count. Blood smears are best made directly from a capillary puncture or from blood left in the venipuncture needle. EDTA-coated blood should not be used, as it has an inhibitory effect on the reaction and will produce a falsely low result.

Clinical Correlation

Elevated leukocyte alkaline phosphatase activity is found in infections, in nonleukemic myeloproliferative disorders such as polycythemia vera, and in pregnancy, Hodgkin's disease, cirrhosis, aplastic anemia, and Down's syndrome. Low scores are often found in chronic myeloid leukemia, paroxysmal nocturnal hemoglobinuria, and infectious mononucleosis. Normal values are present in chronic lymphocytic leukemia, lymphosarcoma, multiple myeloma, and secondary polycythemia. The low activity of leukocyte alkaline phosphatase in myeloid leukemia is believed to be due to cytoplasmic immaturity (Pedersen and Hayhoe, 1971; Bondue et al., 1980).

Leukocyte Acid Phosphatase with Tartrate Resistance

Principle

Under normal conditions, acid phosphatase is present in granulocytes, lymphocytes, and platelets. The cellular enzyme hydrolyzes a substrate, naphthol AS-B1 phosphoric acid, releasing naphthol, which couples with "hexazotized" pararosaniline, producing a colored precipitate within the cytoplasm. In the presence of L(+) tartaric acid, the acid phosphatase isoenzymes are inhibited in all cells, with the exception of those found in leukemic reticuloendotheliosis, or hairy-cell leukemia (Katayama and Yang, 1977).

Reagents and Equipment

1. Fixative, buffered formalin-acetone (pH 6.6–6.8): Disodium hydrogen phosphate, 0.2 g, and 1.0 g anhydrous potassium dihydrogen phosphate are dissolved in 300 ml distilled water. 450 ml and 250 ml formalin are added to the buffer. The solution is stored at 4°C.
2. Sodium nitrite, 4% aqueous.
3. Pararosaniline reagent: Pararosaniline, 1.0 g, is dissolved in 20 ml distilled water and 5 ml concentrated hydrochloric acid. The reagent is mixed well to ensure that the dye is in solution, and it is then stored in the dark at room temperature.
4. Acetic acid, 1 N: Glacial acetic acid, 6 ml, is diluted with distilled water to 1 liter.
5. Acetate buffer, 0.1 M (pH 5.0): Sodium acetate, 4.797 g, is added to 14.75 ml 1-N acetic acid and is diluted with distilled water to 1 liter.
6. Solution A: Immediately before use, 2.4-ml volumes of 4% sodium nitrite and pararosaniline reagent are mixed.
7. Solution B: Naphthol AS-B1 phosphoric acid, 0.04 g, is dissolved in 4 ml 1 N, N-dimethylformamide and 71.2 ml 0.1-N acetate buffer. The reagent is mixed just before it is used.
8. Incubation reagent 1: The entire volume of solution B is added to solution A and mixed well. A 40-ml aliquot is removed, and the pH of the mixture is adjusted to 5.1 with saturated sodium hydroxide. It is filtered directly into a Coplin jar and used immediately.
9. Incubation reagent 2: L(+) tartaric acid, 0.3 g, is dissolved in the 40-ml aliquot of incubation mixture no. 1 and is adjusted to pH 5.1 with saturated sodium hydroxide. This is then filtered directly into a Coplin jar and used immediately.
10. Methyl green 1%: 1 g of the dye is dissolved in 100 ml of 0.1-N acetate buffer. The mixture is adjusted to pH 4.2–4.5 with either 1-N sodium hydroxide or 1-N hydrochloric acid.
11. Polyvinylpyrrolidone (PVP) mounting media: PVP, 8 g, is dissolved in 10 ml distilled water over a 12- to 16-hour period.
12. Incubator.
13. Coplin jar.

Specimen

The specimen of choice is fresh air-dried peripheral blood or bone marrow smears.

Method

1. Two smears are fixed by immersion in the buffered formalin-acetone reagent at 4°C for 30 seconds. They are rinsed in distilled water.
2. One of the smears is incubated in incubation reagent 1 for 1 hour at 37°C. It is washed in a stream of distilled water.
3. The second smear is incubated in incubation reagent 2 for 1 hour at 37°C. It is washed in a stream of distilled water.
4. Both smears are counterstained with 1% methyl green for 2 minutes and rinsed quickly under running tap water.
5. They are allowed to air-dry and are mounted and coverslipped in PVP medium. The smears are examined microscopically using a high-power oil-immersion lens.

Results

Acid phosphatase is identified by a red cytoplasmic reaction.

Interpretation

All nucleated cells and platelets will show the presence of acid phosphatase in the smear incubated in incubation reagent 1 and either will be devoid of any enzyme activity or will show a marked reduction after treatment in incubation reagent 2. Hairy cells will show marked acid phosphatase reaction after treatment with either of the incubation reagents.

Clinical Correlation

The most common use of the tartrate-resistant acid phosphatase stain is in identifying hairy cells formed in leukemic reticuloendotheliosis. However, tartrate-resistant acid phosphatase can also be found in other conditions, including variant lymphocytes from infectious mononucleosis and other lympho-proliferative disorders. The presence of tartrate-resistant acid phosphatase does not appear to be specific for T- and B-cell lines of malignant lymphocytes, as it has been described in cells with either type of cell marker (Utsinger et al., 1977). The enzyme has also been found in the blast cells of children with acute lymphocytic leukemia (Loffler et al., 1977; Morse et al., 1980). Its presence seems most useful in differentiating lymphocytic malignancies from monocytic and histiocytic disorders.

Seven different tissue and phosphatase isoenzymes have been reported (Katayama et al., 1972). Isoenzyme 0 is found only in macrophage storage cells in Gaucher's disease; isoenzymes 1, 2, and 4 predominate in neutrophils; isoenzymes 1 and 4 are found in monocytes; isoenzyme 3 is present in lymphocytes and platelets; and isoenzyme 3b is found in primitive blast cells. All these isoenzymes are inhibited by tartrate. Isoenzyme 5 is tartrate-resistant and is the fraction present in hairy cells and in the blast cells of children with acute lymphocytic leukemia.

Leukocyte Esterases: Naphthol AS-D Chloroacetate Esterase (Specific Esterase)

Principle

Naphthol AS-D chloroacetate esterase, a leukocyte esterase, hydrolyzes a synthetic substrate that liberates naphthol, which, in turn, couples with a diazonium salt to produce a blue precipitate at or near the site of enzyme activity (Yam et al., 1971).

Reagents and Equipment

1. Fixative: 10 ml of 40% formalin are added to 90 ml absolute methyl alcohol.

2. Michaelis buffer (pH 7.4):
   a. Stock solution A: Anhydrous sodium acetate, 11.7 g, and 29.42 g sodium diethyl-barbiturate are dissolved in 1 liter of distilled water.
   b. Stock solution B: Concentrated hydrochloric acid, 8.4 ml, is diluted to 1 liter with distilled water.
   c. Working solution: 10-ml volumes of stock solution A and stock solution B are diluted with 26 ml fresh distilled water.
3. Naphthol AS-D chloroacetate reagent: 0.02 g of the reagent is dissolved in 1.6 ml acetone.
4. Incubation mixture: The following are added, in order: 20 ml distilled water, 20 ml working buffer, 1 ml propylene glycol and naphthol AS-D chloroacetate reagent, and 0.04 g fast blue RR (Sigma Chemicals). These are mixed well to dissolve the dye and are filtered through Whatman no. 1 filter paper.
5. Harris hematoxylin.
6. Coplin jar.

Specimen

Specimens are fresh blood or bone marrow smears, which should be air-dried for at least 30 minutes before staining. The smears may be stored unfixed at room temperature for up to 2 weeks without appreciable loss of enzymatic activity.

Method

1. The smears are fixed by placement in the formalin-alcohol for 30 seconds at 4°C. They are rinsed in tap water for 5–10 seconds.

2. The smears are placed in the incubation mixture for 10 minutes and washed gently in running water for 30 seconds.

3. They are counterstained in Harris hematoxylin for 10 minutes and rinsed in water for 1 minute and allowed to air-dry.

4. The smears are examined under the high-power oil-immersion lens.

Interpretation

The esterase is demonstrated by a blue hue in the specific and nonspecific granules of the cell.

Clinical Correlation

Cells belonging to the myeloid series usually show strong reactions for chloroacetate esterase. Promyelocytes and myeloblasts are also frequently positive. Monocytes and basophils show only minimal activity, and eosinophils, lymphocytes, plasma cells, megakaryocytes, and nucleated red cells are uniformly negative.

Chloroacetate esterase is very weak in myeloblasts found in acute leukemia. This is in contrast to the activity found in normal myeloblasts. Auer bodies, if present, are strongly positive, and the nucleated red cells seen in erythroleukemia may exhibit weak reactions. Leukemic lymphocytes and lymphoblasts are negative for this specific esterase. The reactions of chloroacetate esterase parallel those seen of Sudan black B and peroxidase, both in normal granulocytes and in the acute leukemias. These staining reactions are more sensitive than chloroacetate esterase in granulocytic cells, but the specific esterase is more consistently negative in monocytic cells (Flandrin and Daniel, 1973).

α-Naphthol Acetate Esterase (Nonspecific Esterase)

Principle

The α-naphthol acetate esterase technique is similar to the naphthol AS-D chloroacetate esterase method, except that the reaction is carried out with and without an inhibitory reagent, sodium fluoride (Yam et al., 1971).

Reagents and Equipment

1. Fixative: 40% formalin.
2. Phosphate buffer, 0.1 M (pH 6.1): Disodium hydrogen phosphate, 14.2 g, is dissolved in 1 liter of distilled water, and 13.6 g potassium dihydrogen phosphate is dissolved in 1 liter of distilled water. For use, 60 ml of the disodium phosphate is added to 40 ml of the potassium phosphate.
3. Naphthol AS-D acetate reagent: Naphthol AS-D acetate, 0.016 g, is dissolved in 3 ml acetone, and 2 ml propylene glycol is added. This is mixed by inversion.
4. Fast blue RR.
5. Sodium fluoride.

6. Incubation mixture: Fast blue RR, 0.2 g, is added to 5 ml naphthol AS-D acetate reagent and 100 ml phosphate buffer. It is mixed well with a magnetic stirrer for 3–4 minutes to ensure complete dissolution of the dye. 50 ml of this reagent are filtered directly into a Coplin jar, using Whatman no. 1 filter paper. This is the *plain incubation reagent*.

Sodium fluoride, 0.075 g, is dissolved in the remaining incubation mixture from step 6, and is filtered into a second Coplin jar, as described previously. This is the *sodium fluoride incubation reagent*.

Specimen

Fresh blood or bone marrow smears should be air-dried for at least 30 minutes before being stained. The preparations may be stored unfixed at room temperature for up to 2 weeks without appreciable loss of enzymatic activity.

Method

1. Two smears are fixed in formalin vapor for 10 minutes and then are washed gently under running tap water for 10–15 seconds. They are allowed to air-dry.
2. One smear is placed in the plain incubation reagent, and the second slide is placed in the sodium fluoride incubation reagent.
3. Both slides are incubated for 70 minutes at room temperature.
4. The slides are removed and washed under a gentle stream of tap water and are counterstained with Harris hematoxylin for 10 minutes.
5. They are rinsed as described previously and are air-dried.
6. The smears are examined under the high-power oil-immersion lens.

Interpretation

The esterase is demonstrated by the presence of blue granules.

Clinical Correlation

α-Naphthol acetate esterase is strongest in monocytes, megakaryocytes, and platelets, but it can also be weakly demonstrated in plasma cells, basophils, lymphocytes, and granulocytes. Increased activity may also be seen in nucleated red cells in erythroleukemia, in normal and leukemic promyelocytes, and in hairy cells. Nonspecific esterase activity in monocytes, megakaryocytes, platelets, plasma cells, and macrophages is inhibited by sodium fluoride, but that in lymphocytes and granulocytes is unaffected.

α-Naphthol Butyrate Esterase

Principle

The principle underlying the α-naphthol butyrate esterase technique is similar to that described for the α-naphthol acetate esterase procedure (see page 414).

Reagents and Equipment

1. Fixative: 40% formalin.
2. Phosphate buffer, 0.067 M (pH 6.4): 27 ml 0.067-M disodium hydrogen phosphate is added to 73 ml 0.067-M potassium dihydrogen phosphate as described on page 272.
3. Hexazotized pararosaniline, freshly prepared: Pararosaniline hydrochloride, 1 g, is dissolved in 20 ml distilled water and 5 ml concentrated hydrochloric acid. It is warmed gently to dissolve the dye. It is then cooled and filtered and stored at room temperature. Equal volumes of the pararosaniline solution are mixed with 4% sodium nitrite immediately before use. The sodium nitrite should be prepared fresh for optimal results, but it can be up to 7 days old if stored at 4°C.
4. α-Naphthol butyrate: α-Naphthol butyrate, 0.05 g, is dissolved in 2.5 ml ethylene glycol monomethyl ether.
5. Incubation reagent: The hexazotized pararosaniline–sodium nitrite reagent, 0.25 ml, is added to 47.5 ml buffer and 2.5 ml α-naphthol butyrate. It is mixed well and filtered before use.
6. Harris hematoxylin.
7. Ammonium hydroxide 10%.
8. Coplin jars.

Specimen

Fresh blood or bone marrow smears should be air-dried for at least 30 minutes before being stained.

Smears may be stored unfixed at room temperature for up to 2 weeks without appreciable loss of enzymatic activity.

Method

1. Smears are fixed in formalin vapor for 10 minutes and then are washed gently under running tap water for 10–15 seconds. They are allowed to air-dry.
2. The smears are immersed in the incubation reagent for 45 minutes at room temperature.
3. They then are washed under a gentle stream of tap water and are counterstained with Harris hematoxylin for 10 minutes.
4. They are rinsed in running tap water and then in diluted ammonium hydroxide until the color of the smear changes from red to blue.

Interpretation

The esterase is demonstrated by the presence of an orange or orange-brown cytoplasm.

Clinical Correlation

This esterase is strongly reactive in monocytes and macrophages. Although it is less sensitive than α-naphthol acetate esterase, it has the advantage of being more specific in its reactions with most hematopoietic cells. Table 21.4 illustrates some of the cytochemical esterase reactions found in normal and abnormal cells.

DNA: Feulgen's Reaction

Principle

Feulgen's reaction is based on the capacity of fuchsin–sulfurous acid to develop a red color with the aldehyde group produced by acid hydrolysis of DNA.

Reagents and Equipment

1. Feulgen's stain: Basic fuchsin, 1 g, is dissolved in 200 ml boiling distilled water. It is cooled to room temperature and filtered. 20 ml 1-N hydrochloric acid and 1 g anhydrous sodium bisul-

Table 21.4. Cytochemical Reactions of the Esterases

Cell/Disorder	Naphthol AS-D Chloroacetate (Specific Esterase)	α-Naphthol Acetate (Nonspecific Esterase Without Inhibition)	α-Naphthol Acetate with Sodium Fluoride Inhibition (Nonspecific Esterase with Inhibition)	α-Naphthol Butyrate (Nonspecific Esterase)
Myeloblast	–	–	–	1+
Promyelocyte	4+	1+/–	1+/–	–
Neutrophil	3+	1+	3+	–
Eosinophil	–	1+	1+	1+
Basophil	1+	1+	1+	–
Monocyte	1+	3+	–/1+	3+
Lymphocyte	–	–	–	–
Plasma cell	–	1+	–	2+
Acute myeloid leukemia				
M1	2+	–	–	–
M2	2+	–	–	–
M3	2+	1+	1+	–
M4	1+	1+/2+	1+/2+	1+/2+
M5	1+/2+	1+/3+	–	3+
M6	2+	3+	3+	2+
Acute lymphocytic leukemia				
L1	–	2+	–	–
L2	–	2+	–	–
L3	–	–	–	–

– = negative; 1+ = weakly positive; 2+ = positive; 3+ = strongly positive; 4+ = intensely strongly positive.

fite are added. The mixture is allowed to react for 24 hours. It is stored in the dark.

2. Formalin-methanol fixative : Glacial acetic acid, 5 ml, is added to 10 ml 40% formalin and 85 ml methanol.
3. Hydrochloric acid, 1 N.
4. Wright's stain and buffers (see page 271).
5. Water bath, 37°C.
6. Coplin jars.

Specimen

The specimen used is blood or bone marrow smears. Once fixed, the preparation is stable indefinitely.

Method

1. Smears are fixed in formalin-methanol for 10 minutes and rinsed under running tap water.
2. They are hydrolyzed in 1-N hydrochloric acid at 37°C for 1 hour, after which they are rinsed well in tap water for 2–3 minutes.
3. The smears are immersed in Feulgen's stain for 30 minutes, rinsed in running tap water, and counterstained in Wright's stain (see page 271).

Interpretation

Leukocytes and nucleated red cells stain in proportion to the amount of DNA present in the nucleus. The cytoplasm and mature red cells do not stain. The nuclei of mature cells stain pale pink, and the nucleoli can be differentiated as unstained areas in the nucleus.

Clinical Correlation

The stain distinguishes between mature and immature cells in that it is helpful in separating nucleoli.

RNA: Unna-Pappenheim Reaction

Principle

The Unna-Pappenheim stain is a combination of pyronin and methyl green. The pyronin stains the

RNA cell components, whereas the methyl green stains the chromatin (Dimmock, 1977).

Reagents and Equipment

1. Stain: Pyronin, 0.3 g, and 0.7 g methyl green are dissolved in 20 ml glycerol and 2.5 ml absolute ethanol. The stain is diluted to 100 ml with 0.5% aqueous phenol. For optimal results, the stain should be ground with the glycerol and alcohol before the addition of the phenol. The resulting reagent is boiled for 2 minutes and is filtered through Whatman no. 1 filter paper.
2. Fixative: Glacial acetic acid, 10 ml, is added to 30 ml chloroform and 60 ml ethanol.
3. Coplin jars.

Specimen

Blood or bone marrow air-dried smears constitute the specimens.

Method

1. Smears are fixed for 5 minutes, rinsed in tap water, and allowed to air-dry.
2. The smears are immersed in the staining solution for 45 seconds and rinsed briefly in water. Once again, they are allowed to air-dry.

Interpretation

In general, pyroninophilia parallels the cytoplasmic basophilia of routine stains. Immature cell cytoplasm stains bright red, with decreasing intensity as the cell matures. Plasma cells are intensely pyroninophilic, reflecting the high RNA content associated with immunoglobulin synthesis. Likewise, variant lymphocytes found in infectious mononucleosis are strongly pyroninophilic.

Terminal Deoxynucleotidyl Transferase (TdT)

Principle

TdT is a DNA polymerase present in lymphocytes. Rabbit antibody to TdT is incubated with cold methyl alcohol. Fixed calf cells and fluorescein isothiocyanate conjugate–labeled goat antirabbit antibody is then incubated with these cells. If TdT is present, the nuclei of positive cells fluoresce (Coleman and Hutton, 1981).

Reagents and Equipment

1. Antiserum: (Kit no. 9311s.b., available from Bethesda Research Laboratories, Rockville, MD).
2. Phosphate buffer (pH 7.4): Sodium dihydrogen phosphate, monohydride (0.4 g), disodium hydrogen phosphate (1.6 g), and sodium chloride (8.0 g) are diluted in distilled water to 1 liter.
3. Mounting media, buffered: Glycerol, 90.0 ml, and 0.05-M Trizma, 9.0–10.0 ml, are combined.
4. Controls
   a. Blood smears are made from known acute lymphocytic leukemia patients who test positively for TdT.
   b. The smears are air-dried and wrapped in plastic and then stored at –70°C. Before they are used, the smears must be thawed with the plastic cover in place.
   c. The positive control smear is treated exactly as are the test smears.
5. Absolute methanol.
6. Petri dishes.
7. Fluorescent microscope, with a barrier filter.

Specimen

Nonheparinized blood smears or bone marrow aspirate may be used. All slides should be stored at 4°C in the dark and should be stained within 2 days of preparation.

Method

1. An area of nucleated cells on the slide is circled with a diamond marker.
2. The slide is fixed in methanol at 4°C for 30 minutes.
3. The slide is rinsed well with phosphate-buffered saline to remove all the fixative, but it is not allowed to dry.
4. The slide is hydrated in phosphate-buffered saline for 5 minutes at room temperature.
5. The sample on the slide is wiped off, with care taken to leave the cells within the diamond etching.
6. Ten microliters of rabbit anti–calf TdT are added to the cells, and these are incubated for 30

minutes at room temperature in a humid chamber (under a moist Petri dish). Once again, the cells are not allowed to dry.

7. To remove excess antibody, the slide is washed with three changes of phosphate-buffered saline for 15 minutes. All the excess buffer is then wiped from around the cells, with care taken not to let the specimen dry.

8. Fifteen microliters of secondary antibody (goat anti–rabbit IgG) are added to the cells, and these are incubated for 30 minutes at room temperature in a humid chamber as previously.

9. Step 7 is repeated.

10. The specimen is mounted with buffered glycerol mounting media and is covered with a coverslip.

11. The nuclei are examined for fluorescence at 495-nm excitation with a barrier filter. The intensity of the fluorescence, on a scale of 0–4+, and the percentage of positive cells seen are recorded. The preparation can be stored in the dark at 4°C for 2–3 days.

Interpretation

Most patients with T- and null-cell acute lymphocytic leukemia and lymphoma show TdT activity. In addition, patients with pre-B-cell acute lymphocytic leukemia, 50% of patients with acute undifferentiated leukemia, and 30% of patients with chronic myeloid leukemia in blastic crisis have TdT activity. Approximately 5% of patients with acute myeloid leukemia also demonstrate TdT activity.

Chapter 22

Miscellaneous Tests

Bone Marrow Biopsy

Bone marrow biopsy is an integral part of hematologic investigation and testing. Besides identification of the cellularity of the specimen and the makeup of the cellular components, the architecture, cytochemistry, and chromosomal culture of the specimen can be determined.

Samples of bone marrow can be obtained by three main methods: (1) an open surgical biopsy or open trephine, (2) percutaneous trephine using a Jamshidi or comparable needle, and (3) aspiration using a special needle and syringe. Most specimens are obtained by needle aspiration, using a needle similar in style to the University of Illinois sternal needle. Because the collection of the bone marrow specimens is carried out entirely by physicians, the clinical details are not included in this text, but it should be emphasized that only approximately 0.25–0.50 ml should be aspirated to avoid hemodiluting the specimen and complicating the bone marrow differential cell count if undertaken. Various sites may be used for aspiration. In adults, both the iliac crest and the sternum at the second intercostal space are commonly used. Other satisfactory sites include the posterosuperior iliac spine and the spinous process of the rib in adults and the head of the tibia in infants.

Preparation of Bone Marrow Smears

The preparation of satisfactory smears requires speed and good technique. Two principal approaches

to smear preparation can be used, the method of choice depending on the personal preference of the hematologist reading the slide.

The first procedure, the *coverslip method*, uses a macroscopic marrow particle placed between two coverslips, to which gentle pressure is applied so that the marrow is squashed. The coverslips are then pulled apart so that bone marrow is smeared on both of them. To facilitate the placing or identification of such particles, the contents of the syringe can be expelled into a watch glass and the particles removed by pipette. Forceps can also be used if the particles are sufficiently large. The placement of an anticoagulant in the watch glass may help in allowing sufficient time to carry out this procedure: Both heparin and ethylenediaminetetraacetic acid (EDTA) have been used with some success. However, all available anticoagulants introduce some artifactual change in cell morphologic features and, if possible, should be avoided.

The second procedure, the *slide method*, is more commonly used, despite the fact that, in general, it produces inferior preparations when compared with the coverslip crush procedure. This is because coverslips are intrinsically more difficult to stain, store, and handle than are regular microscope slides. The procedure is similar to that used in the coverslip method. The first of two possible techniques is identical to the coverslip crush method except that two slides are used instead of the coverslip. The second technique is to expel bone marrow spicules from the syringe onto the slides and prepare them in the same way as a conventional peripheral blood smear. The key to this technique is to use only the smallest amount of material on each slide and to make many smears as rapidly as possible.

In assessing the macroscopic adequacy of the bone marrow tap and smear preparation, two principal criteria are used: the presence of fat spaces seen when the preparation is held up to the light and the presence of bone marrow fragments at or near the tail of the smear. If, on inspection of the smear, these criteria appear to be lacking, the remainder of the marrow can be pipetted from the watch glass, if anticoagulated, and concentrated by centrifugation in Wintrobe tubes.

Preparation of Bone Marrow Sections and Special Handling Techniques

The histologic characteristics of bone marrow fragments provide a clearer impression of the cellularity and architecture of the specimen, although they do not afford as detailed a picture of the individual cell morphologic features and infrastructure as does the conventional smear preparation. The fragments can be expelled onto a siliconized or anticoagulated watch glass, and marrow spicules can be pipetted up and fixed in a formalin-alcohol solution or mercury-based fixative. Histologic processing then is carried out as detailed on page 421.

Bone marrow can also be processed for electron microscopy studies by immediate fixation in 4% glutaraldehyde in phosphate buffer (pH 7.4) for 1 hour in the cold and treatment with 1% osmium tetroxide for an additional hour before dehydration and embedding. Similarly, aspirated bone marrow can be cultured for cytogenic studies by immediate placement in a tissue culture nutrient straight from the syringe. Marrow obtained from autopsy specimens requires different handling because of the rapid postmortem autolysis of the specimen. The most effective procedure is to express the marrow into 5% bovine albumin and to centrifuge the specimen gently. The cells are resuspended in approximately an equal volume of the albumin, and smears are prepared by one of the previously described techniques (Berenbaum, 1956).

Examination of Bone Marrow Specimens

Absolute nucleated cell counts from aspirates or buffy-coat preparations are of little value because of the differences in cellularity among the various sites that may be aspirated. Additionally, the collection technique greatly influences the apparent cellularity, as hemodiluted specimens may falsely appear hypocellular, and the examination of one cellular spicule may give the impression of hypercellularity.

Routine staining of both smear preparations and sections commonly involves a standard Romanowsky dye such as a Wright's or Giemsa stain. The number of megakaryocytes should be estimated by low-power scanning of the smear at the tail and at the periphery of the preparation and by complete review of the section. At this time, the low-power scan should also detect the presence of any tumor cell clusters or granulomas. More intense scanning with a higher-power lens should be carried out to estimate the presence and approximate numbers of cells undergoing mitosis.

Morphologic examination of the bone marrow smear preparation can be undertaken in two ways. The first is by subjective overview, the cellularity, numbers of mitotic figures, and distribution and morphologic features of all leukocytes, erythroid cells, and megakaryocytic elements being taken into account. The second approach is to carry out a differential count of all formed elements. Useful interpretive data are obtained if at least 500–1,000 cells are counted under an oil-immersion lens. Care must be taken to avoid areas in which ruptured cells predominate because of the trauma of the smear preparation.

The wide ranges found in normal values reflect the difficulty in obtaining accurate morphologic identification, differences in cellularity of tissue samples, and the statistical considerations of counting too few cells. Table 22.1 shows the reference range for differential bone marrow counts from smears of adult patients.

Besides Romanowsky staining, iron and glycogen stains should be carried out routinely. A sufficient number of smears should be left fixed and available for other special stains, such as peroxidase and both specific and nonspecific esterases. The hematologist conducting the routine examination should have full knowledge of the patient's hematologic history, which includes a laboratory evaluation of the complete blood cell count and reticulocyte count as well as pertinent iron and ferritin data, if necessary.

Table 22.1. Reference Ranges for Adult Differential Bone Marrow Counts

Cells	Range ± 2 SD (%)
Undifferentiated blasts	0.1–1.0
Myeloblasts	0.1–3.5
Promyelocytes	0.5–5.0
Neutrophilic myelocytes	5.0–20.0
Eosinophilic myelocytes	0.1–3.0
Basophilic myelocytes	0–0.5
Metamyelocytes	10.0–30.0
Neutrophils	7.0–25.0
Eosinophils	0.2–3.0
Basophils	0–0.5
Lymphocytes	5.0–20.0*
Monocytes	0–2.0
Megakaryocytes	0.1–0.5
Plasma cells	0.1–3.5
Rubriblasts	0.5–5.0
Prorubricytes	2.0–5.0
Rubricytes	2.0–20.0
Metarubricytes	2.0–10.0
Myeloid-to-erythroid ratio	2.5–5.0:1

*Lymphocytes present mainly as a result of peripheral blood contamination.

Histologic Processing and Staining of Bone Marrow Smears and Sections

Principle

The bone marrow is fixed and decalcified. The mercury deposits from the fixative are removed with iodine, which, in turn, is removed with sodium thiosulfate. The tissue is then overstained with heated Wright's stain diluted in an acidic buffer and is differentiated and dehydrated.

Reagents and Equipment

1. Zenker's fluid: Mercuric chloride, 5 g, and 2.5 g potassium dichromate are dissolved in distilled water and are diluted to 100 ml. 5 ml of glacial acetic acid are added immediately before use.
2. Formic acid.
3. Sodium sulfate, 5% aqueous.
4. Lugol's iodine: Iodine crystals, 1 g, and 2 g potassium iodide are dissolved in distilled water and are diluted to 100 ml.
5. Sodium thiosulfate, 5% aqueous.
6. Wright's stain (see page 271).
7. Methanol.
8. Phosphate buffer, pH 5.2 (see page 272).
9. Coplin jars.
10. Xylene substitute.

Specimen

The specimen is bone marrow biopsy material obtained from an open surgical biopsy or needle biopsy or from the concentrated particles obtained from a bone marrow aspiration.

Method

1. The bone marrow fragments are fixed as soon as possible in Zenker's fluid for 24 hours.
2. They are decalcified by transferring to formic acid for 24–72 hours.
3. The formic acid is removed by placement of the specimen in 5% sodium sulfate for 1–2 hours. The specimen is washed well under running tap water and embedded in paraffin wax and sectioned.
4. The sections are soaked in a xylene substitute for 3–5 minutes to remove the wax and are washed in 95% alcohol to remove the xylene substitute.
5. They are rinsed in distilled water for 5–10 seconds, and the mercuric salts present in the fixative are removed by placing in Lugol's iodine for 5–10 minutes.
6. The iodine is removed by placing the sections in 5% sodium thiosulfate for 4–10 minutes. They are then rinsed under running tap water for 10 minutes.
7. The smears are placed in a Coplin jar filled with warmed diluted Wright's stain (1 volume of Wright's stain diluted with 2 volumes of buffer, pH 5.2). They are allowed to stain for 1–15 minutes.
8. The sections are differentiated and dehydrated by rapid rinsing in absolute methanol for 10–15 seconds. They are cleared by rinsing in a xylene substitute for 30 seconds and mounted permanently in a neutral medium.

Staining of Bone Marrow Smears

Principle

The principle underlying the staining of bone marrow smears is the same as that for peripheral blood smears (see page 270).

Reagents

1. Phosphate buffer, pH 6.4 (see page 272).
2. Methanol.
3. Others as described for peripheral blood smears (see page 271).

Specimen

Air-dried bone marrow smears that have macroscopically visible fat droplets and bone marrow fragments are used.

Method

1. The smears are fixed in absolute methyl alcohol for 5–10 minutes.
2. One volume of Wright's stain is diluted with two volumes of buffer (pH 6.4), and the smears are allowed to stain for 15–20 minutes.
3. They are differentiated by transferring to a Coplin jar of buffer for 1–2 minutes.
4. The smears are air-dried and examined microscopically.

Serum Muramidase (Lysozyme) Assay

Principle

When added to a substrate suspension of *Micrococcus lysodeikticus*, lysozyme hydrolyzes the $\beta_{1,4}$ linkages between *N*-acetylmuramic acid and 2-acetyl-amino-2-deoxy-D-glucose residues in mucopolysaccharides, causing the cloudy suspension to clear. The rate of clearing is proportional to the amount of lysozyme present (Syren and Raeste, 1971).

Reagents and Equipment

1. Lysozyme assay kit (Worthington Biochemical, Freehold, NJ). Alternatively, the substrate can be made by suspending 100 µg *M. lysodeikticus* in 1 ml 0.06-M sodium phosphate (pH 2.0) containing 0.15-M sodium chloride.
2. Standard egg-white lysozyme, 40 µg/ml, in distilled water.
3. Spectrophotometer with cuvette capable of holding a 3-ml sample.

Table 22.2. Standard Dilutions of Egg-White Lysozyme

Standard (ml)	Distilled Water (ml)	Lysozyme Concentration (µg/ml)
0.5	0.5	20
0.4	0.6	16
0.3	0.7	12
0.2	0.8	8
0.1	0.9	4
0.05	0.95	2

4. Pipettes: 1 ml and 10 ml, graduated.

Specimen

The specimen is serum of EDTA-anticoagulated plasma.

Method

1. The standard egg-white lysozyme is diluted as shown in Table 22.2. It is stable for several months if stored at 4°C.
2. Three milliliters of the bacterial substrate are pipetted into a cuvette and allowed to come to room temperature for 5 minutes.
3. Three milliliters of serum are added to the substrate, and the solution is mixed.
4. The specimen is read spectrophotometrically at 600 nm after exactly 30 seconds and again after 180 seconds, the instrument first having been blanked with distilled water.
5. The difference in the optical densities is recorded.
6. A standard curve is prepared using the dilutions shown in Table 22.2. Three milliliters of bacterial substrate are added to 0.3-ml volumes of each dilution, and the optical density is read after exactly 30 seconds and again after 180 seconds.
7. On linear graph paper, the differences in optical density for each standard are plotted against the concentration.
8. The test concentration is read from the standard graph.

Reference Range

The reference range is 5–15 µg/ml.

Clinical Correlation

Urine lysozymes can be estimated by substituting a 24-hour aliquot of urine for the serum. Urine levels of lysozyme usually are less than 2 µg/ml.

Lysozyme is a powerful bacteriolytic hydrolase associated with the lysosomes of granulocytes and monocytes. It is present in small amounts in the serum and urine of normal individuals. The enzyme is present in all stages of granulocytic maturation and in monocytes. However, it is not present in myeloblasts, mature eosinophils, and basophils. Lysozyme also is absent from lymphocytes, red cells, and platelets.

Serum and urine lysozyme levels are increased in most myeloproliferative diseases and are higher in Philadelphia chromosome–negative (Ph^1-negative) chronic myeloid leukemia than in the Ph^1-positive form. Elevated levels are found also in monocytic leukemia, polycythemia vera, acute myeloid leukemia, Hodgkin's disease, multiple myeloma, and renal disorders. The serum lysozyme assay can be used as a marker of cellular breakdown. Decreased values are found in neutropenia with bone marrow hypocellularity, but values are normal if the bone marrow is active.

Schilling Test

Principle

The Schilling test is designed to detect the malabsorption of vitamin B_{12} either in pernicious anemia or in malabsorption syndromes (Schilling, 1953).

Reagents and Equipment

1. Scintillation counter.
2. Vitamin B_{12}, 1,000 µg/ml.
3. ^{57}Co vitamin B_{12}.

Method

1. The patient is instructed to fast overnight. All urine voided in the morning is discarded.

2. The patient is instructed to drink 25 ml radioactive vitamin B_{12} in water (1.0 µg/25 ml distilled water).

3. A 1,000-mg dose of "cold" vitamin B_{12} is injected to act as the flushing or saturating agent, and all urine is collected for the next 24 hours.

4. Step 3 is repeated, and a second 24-hour urine specimen is collected.

5. A 15-ml aliquot of urine is removed from each of the two specimens, and the radioactivity of each specimen is analyzed.

6. The percentage of radioactivity absorbed is calculated from the following: The total counts per minute in each of the 24-hour urine samples are calculated by dividing the total 24-hour volumes by 15 and multiplying by the counts per minute of the 15-ml samples.

Reference Range

When a 1-µg dose of labeled vitamin B_{12} is used, normal individuals excrete 7% or more of the administered radioactive agent in the first 24 hours.

Clinical Correlation

In pernicious anemia or vitamin B_{12} deficiency associated with malabsorption, the radioactive excretion in the urine is less than 5%. The simultaneous administration of intrinsic factor causes this value to become normal in pernicious anemia, whereas it remains subnormal in malabsorption disorders. The test reflects the vitamin B_{12} status and absorption reliability, although it is time consuming and requires the complete collection and accurate measurement of each 24-hour urine output.

Plasma Cryofibrinogen

Principle

The plasma cryofibrinogen test demonstrates the presence of plasma fibrinogen, which precipitates between 0° and 4°C and is reversible on warming (Smith and Arkin, 1972).

Reagents and Equipment

1. Tubes: 12×75 mm.

2. Centrifuge.

3. Pipettes: 1 ml, graduated.

Specimen

EDTA-anticoagulated blood is the specimen used.

Method

1. The anticoagulated sample is centrifuged at 2,000 rpm for 5 minutes.

2. One milliliter of plasma is added to each of two tubes. One tube is placed at 4°C and the other is left at room temperature for 24 hours.

3. The refrigerated plasma sample is compared against the plasma left at room temperature for the presence of discrete white particles or gel formation.

4. If a gel or precipitate is present, the specimen is incubated at 37°C for 30 minutes. A true positive test result is indicated if the gel disappears.

Results

The reference outcome is negative.

Clinical Correlation

Cryofibrinogens are fibrinogen complexes that precipitate at 4°C. They are occasionally present in carcinoma, myeloma, and acute and chronic leukemia. Cryofibrinogens may be produced in part by factor XIII, which forms cross-links between fibrin and cold-insoluble globulin enzymatically. Monomers may remain in solution in an uncomplexed form.

Cryoglobulin Detection

Principle

The principle underlying cryoglobulin detection is the same as that for plasma fibrinogen detection, except that serum is used in place of plasma (Henry, 1965).

Reagents and Equipment

The reagents and equipment needed for this test are the same as those described in the section on plasma cryofibrinogen (see above).

Specimen

Clotted whole blood is centrifuged, and serum is used in place of plasma.

Method

The method for this test is the same as that for plasma cryofibrinogen detection (see above).

Results

The reference outcome is negative.

Clinical Correlation

Cryoglobulins are serum proteins that precipitate irreversibly on cooling. They occur most frequently in association with multiple myeloma or with Waldenström's macroglobulinemia, but they may also be found in rheumatoid arthritis, collagen disorders, and cirrhosis.

Cryoprecipitation depends on the formation of noncovalent bonds between gamma-globulin molecules when exposed to low temperatures. It has been suggested that this cold precipitation may result from a decreased tyrosine and an increased tryptophan content of the proteins (Middaugh, 1978). Three main types of cryoglobulins are recognized.

Type 1 is a monoclonal protein associated with myeloma, macroglobulinemia, and other lymphoproliferative diseases. The protein usually is associated with a monoclonal IgG form, but both IgA and Bence-Jones protein have been reported (Varriale, 1962; Grey and Kohler, 1973; Moroz and Rose, 1977).

Type 2 proteins are composed of mixed immunoglobulins in which the monoclonal components possess specificity for polyclonal IgG. This type of cryoglobulin has been associated with autoimmune diseases, lymphoproliferative disorders, and hepatitis (Abramsky and Slavin, 1974).

Type 3 cryoglobulins are made up of one or more classes of polyclonal immunoglobulins. In most cases, the IgM molecule has antibody activity against polyclonal IgG molecules. This type of cryoprotein is associated with a wide variety of infections and autoimmune disorders.

Sia Test

Principle

Some serum globulins, such as macroglobulins, have a lower solubility when the serum electrolyte level is reduced by water (Waldenström, 1954).

Reagents and Equipment

1. Water.
2. Pasteur pipette.

Specimen

The specimen is serum.

Method

Two drops of serum are added to a tube containing distilled water.

Results

Normally, no cloud or precipitate is seen.

Sources of Error

In the presence of macroglobulinemia, a heavy precipitate forms in the tube. The test is nonspecific for macroproteins and can produce both false-positive and false-negative results.

Determination of Serum Viscosity

Principle

Serum viscosity is the ability of serum to resist flow. The time required for serum to pass between two points on a capillary glass bulb is compared with the time required for distilled water to pass between the same two points (Wright and Jenkins, 1970).

Reagents and Equipment

1. Ostwald viscosimeter: The apparatus consists of a U-shaped capillary tube, with one arm approximately 7.5 cm long and a second arm 2.5 cm long. The end of the longer arm is funnel-shaped, allowing blood to be introduced more readily into the tube. The short arm contains a bulb with a mark *1* directly under it and a mark *2* directly above it.
2. Stopwatch.
3. Water bath, 37°C.

Specimen

Serum is the specimen used. A normal control serum also is required.

Method

1. The viscosimeter is immersed in a 37°C water bath.
2. Five milliliters of serum are introduced through the funnel opening of the capillary stem.
3. The time required for the serum to travel from mark 1 to mark 2 is recorded.
4. The viscosimeter is cleaned and dried, and steps 1 and 2 are repeated, distilled water being used in place of serum.

Results

The viscosity is expressed as a ratio of the time required for serum to flow between two points in comparison with the time it takes distilled water to travel the same distance.

Reference Range

The reference range is 1.2–1.8.

Clinical Correlation

The viscosity of serum is mainly a function of the concentration of the individual proteins present. This, in turn, is influenced by the molecular size and shape and the interaction between these proteins and the cellular elements in the blood. IgM proteins have a large molecular weight, have a structural tetragonal shape, and produce increased viscosity when present in large amounts. Thus macroglobulinemia, characterized by an increase in IgM immunoglobulins, typically produces increased serum and blood viscosity. IgA components are also commonly asso-

Table 22.3. Serum Dilutions and Reagents Used in the Presumptive Heterophil Test

Tube	Saline (ml)	Serum (ml)	2% Sheep Cells (ml)	Final Titer
1	0.8	0.2	0.2	1:7
2	0.5	0.5 from tube no. 1	0.2	1:14
3	0.5	0.5 from tube no. 2	0.2	1:28
4	0.5	0.5 from tube no. 3	0.2	1:56
5	0.5	0.5 from tube no. 4	0.2	1:112
6	0.5	0.5 from tube no. 5	0.2	1:224
7	0.5	0.5 from tube no. 6	0.2	1:448
8	0.5	0.5 from tube no. 7	0.2	1:896
9	0.5	0.5 from tube no. 8	0.2	1:1,792
10	0.5	0.5 from tube no. 9	0.2	1:3,584
11	0.5	0.5 from tube no. 10*	0.2	1:7,168
12	0.5	—	0.2	Negative control

*Discard 0.5 ml from the total volume of tube no. 11 before adding the sheep cells.

ciated with hyperviscosity because of their tendency to aggregate, forming true polymers. Other diseases associated with increased viscosity include multiple myeloma and the lymphomas.

Heterophil Antibodies: Presumptive Test

Principle

High-titered antibodies against sheep cells are often found in the sera of patients with infectious mononucleosis (Davidsohn and Nelson, 1974). Normal titers do not exceed 1:56.

Reagents and Equipment

1. Sheep cells: a 2% saline suspension between 1 and 7 days old.
2. Normal saline.
3. Tubes: 13 × 100 mm.
4. Pipettes: 1 ml, graduated.
5. Water bath, 56°C.

Specimen

Serum is the specimen used. Test serum is inactivated at 56°C for 30 minutes to destroy complement.

Method

1. Tubes are set up as shown in Table 22.3.
2. Eight-tenths milliliter of normal saline is added to the first tube, and 0.5 ml is added to the remaining tubes.
3. Two-tenths milliliter of inactivated serum is pipetted in tube no. 1. The contents are mixed, and 0.5 ml is transferred to tube no. 2. Mixing and transferring 0.5-ml aliquots to each of the next tubes is continued through tube no. 11.
4. Half-milliliter volumes are transferred from tube no. 11. Tube no. 12 is the negative control.
5. One-tenth milliliter of 2% sheep cells is added to each tube. The tubes are shaken to mix the contents and are allowed to stand at room temperature for 2 hours.
6. Each tube of sedimented cells is resuspended gently and observed macroscopically for the presence of agglutination. The highest dilution of the serum showing agglutination is recorded as the titer.

Reference Range

The reference outcome is less than 1:56.

Clinical Correlation

The presumptive test for heterophil antibodies is nonspecific in nature. An elevation of the anti–sheep cell titer is known to occur in various other disorders, including Epstein-Barr virus (EBV) infections, Burkitt's lymphoma, postimmunization reactions involving vaccines produced using horse serum, and hepatitis. A titer exceeding 1:224 indicates infectious mononucleosis, but this should be confirmed serologically by the differential test or the Monospot test

Table 22.4. Serum Dilutions and Reagents Used in the Differential Absorption Heterophil Test

Tube	Saline (ml)	Absorbed Serum (ml)	2% Sheep Cells (ml)	Final Dilution
1	—	0.25	0.1	1:7
2	0.25	0.25	0.1	1:14
3	0.25	0.25 from tube no. 2	0.1	1:28
4	0.25	0.25 from tube no. 3	0.1	1:56
5	0.25	0.25 from tube no. 4	0.1	1:112
6	0.25	0.25 from tube no. 5	0.1	1:224
7	0.25	0.25 from tube no. 6	0.1	1:448
8	0.25	0.25 from tube no. 7	0.1	1:896
9	0.25	0.25 from tube no. 8	0.1	1:1,792
10	0.25	0.25 from tube no. 9*	0.1	1:3,584
11	0.25	—	0.1	Negative control

*Discard 0.25 ml from the total volume of tube no. 10 before adding the sheep cells.
Note: This scheme should be set up in duplicate, one row of tubes for each absorbed serum tested (guinea-pig kidney and beef cells).

(Wampole Laboratories, Inc, Cranbury, NJ) and by reviewing the peripheral blood smear for the presence of variant lymphocytes.

Differential Absorption Test for Infectious Mononucleosis

Principle

The Forssman antibody present in the serum of normal individuals is absorbed completely by tissues containing Forssman antigens (Davidsohn and Nelson, 1974). Examples of such tissues are guinea-pig kidney and horse kidney. The antibody is absorbed only partially by beef cells.

The infectious mononucleosis antibody is not absorbed to the same extent by Forssman antigens but is completely absorbed by beef cells. Heterophil antibodies in high titer are present in patients with serum sickness but can be differentiated from those found in infectious mononucleosis and from the Forssman antibody by their absorption by both beef cells and Forssman antigens.

Reagents and Equipment

1. Sheep cells: A 2% saline suspension between 1 and 7 days old.
2. Guinea-pig kidney antigen (commercially available as a desiccated reagent): It is stored at 4°C.
3. Beef-cell antigen (commercially available as a desiccated reagent). It is stored at 4°C.

4. Normal saline.
5. Water bath, 56°C.
6. Tubes: 12 × 75 mm.
7. Pipettes: 1 ml, graduated.
8. Centrifuge.

Specimen

The specimen used is serum. Test serum is inactivated at 56°C for 30 minutes to destroy complement.

Method

1. Two 0.2-ml aliquots of test serum are pipetted into separate tubes. Into one tube 0.8 ml of guinea-pig kidney antigen is added, and to the second tube 0.8 ml of beef-cell antigen is added.
2. The contents of the tubes are mixed and are allowed to stand at room temperature for 3 minutes. They are centrifuged at 1,500 rpm for 3–5 minutes, after which time the supernatants are transferred to tubes labeled *absorbed guinea-pig kidney* and *absorbed beef cells*.
3. Two rows of tubes are set up as shown in Table 22.4.
4. Normal saline (0.25 ml) is added to all the tubes except the first tube in each row.
5. One-fourth milliliter of the supernatant labeled *absorbed guinea-pig kidney* is added to the first tube in one row, and 0.25 ml of the supernatant labeled *absorbed beef cells* is added to the first tube of the other row.

6. A 0.25-ml aliquot of the serum-saline dilutions from tube no. 2 is transferred to tube no. 3. Mixing and transferring 0.25-ml volumes is continued serially through tube no. 10.

7. The final 0.25-ml volume from tube no. 10 is discarded.

8. One-tenth milliliter of a 2% saline suspension of sheep cells is added to each tube. The tubes are shaken to mix and incubated at room temperature for 2 hours. The cells are resuspended after 15 minutes by gently mixing and are allowed to stand undisturbed for the remainder of the incubation period.

9. Each tube of sedimented cells is resuspended gently and observed macroscopically for the presence of agglutination. The highest dilution of absorbed serum showing agglutination is recorded as the titer.

Interpretation

The antibody in normal serum is completely absorbed by exposure to guinea-pig kidney antigen but only partially absorbed by exposure to beef-cell antigen. In serum sickness, the antibody is absorbed completely by both guinea-pig and beef-cell antigens and, in infectious mononucleosis, the antibody is removed by the beef-cell antigen and usually shows a slight reduction in titer when exposed to the guinea-pig antigen.

Clinical Correlation

Heterophil antibodies usually, but not always, are present in individuals with infectious mononucleosis. During the first 2 weeks of EBV infection, approximately 60% of patients exhibit a positive heterophil test result, with titers exceeding 1:56. By 1 month, 80–90% of the sera are positive, and this rate decreases until the test result is found to be negative by 3–6 months following exposure.

Slide Test for the Detection of Heterophil Antibodies (Monospot Test)

Principle

The Monospot test is based on the agglutination of horse cells by the heterophil antibody found in the sera of individuals with infectious mononucleosis.

Because horse red cells contain both Forssman and infectious mononucleosis antigens, a differential absorption of the patient's serum is necessary to distinguish the specific heterophil antibody. This procedure is carried out by absorbing the serum or plasma with both guinea-pig kidney and beef red-cell stroma.

Guinea-pig kidney contains only the Forssman antigen, whereas beef red cells contain the antigen associated with infectious mononucleosis. Consequently, guinea-pig kidney will absorb only heterophil antibodies of the Forssman type, whereas beef red cells will absorb only the heterophil antibody of infectious mononucleosis. Agglutination of horse red cells by patient's absorbed serum is indicative of a positive reaction.

Reagents and Equipment

1. Guinea-pig kidney suspension, 11% (reagent 1): It is stored at 4°C.
2. Beef red-cell stroma, 11% (reagent 2): It is stored at 4°C.
3. Stabilized horse red cells, 20% (reagent 3): These are stored at 4°C. Reagents 1–3 are available from Ortho Pharmaceuticals, Raritan, NJ.
4. Stopwatch.
5. Pipettes: microcapillary, 10 μl.
6. Applicator sticks.
7. Glass slides (Monospot).

Specimen

Serum or EDTA-anticoagulated plasma is tested.

Method

1. All the reagent-cell suspensions are shaken to mix.

2. The Monospot slide is placed on a flat surface under direct light, and 10 μl of horse cells is added to one corner of each of the two squares (1 and 2) on the slide.

3. One drop of guinea-pig kidney antigen (reagent 1) is placed in the center of square 2, and one drop of beef red-cell suspension (reagent 2) is placed in the center of square 1.

4. A disposable plastic pipette is used to add one drop of the test serum to the center of each square on the slide. The test serum is mixed with the guinea-pig kidney and beef cells on each square.

5. With no more than 10 stirring motions, the horse cells are blended with each mixture.

6. The stopwatch is started when the final mixing has been completed.

7. Evidence of agglutination is sought for no longer than 1 minute after the final mixing. *The slide must not be picked up or moved during the reaction period.*

Results

Stronger agglutination in square 1 (test serum, guinea-pig kidney, and horse cells) indicates a positive result. Stronger agglutination in square 2 (test serum, beef red cells, and horse cells) indicates a negative result. If there is no agglutination on either square, or if the agglutination is equally strong in both areas, the test is considered negative.

Clinical Correlation

Horse agglutinins are present in higher titer than sheep-cell agglutinins in individuals with infectious mononucleosis. This affords the test greater sensitivity than the heterophil differential absorption or presumptive methods. The Monospot test produces a 2% false-negative rate and a 6–13% false-positive rate, in contrast to a 10% false-negative rate found in the classic heterophil test. The test remains positive at a titer of 1:40 or greater for 1 year or more in approximately 75% of cases, compared with 3–6 months for the classic procedure. False-positive test results have been reported with Burkitt's lymphoma, Hodgkin's disease, lymphocytic lymphoma, viral hepatitis, pancreatic carcinoma, rubella, and rheumatoid arthritis (Sadoff and Goldsmith, 1971; Phillips, 1972; Horwitz et al., 1973).

Infectious mononucleosis can also be detected by immunofluorescent techniques. EBV infects only human lymphoid cells with B-cell characteristics (Niederman, 1968). Infection of lymphoid B cells by EBV results in the expression of four different groups of EBV-related antigens to which the infected host responds with appropriate antibodies.

In infectious mononucleosis, the antibodies to viral capsid antigen (VCA) peak about the second week of the disease and then gradually decline to lower titers, which then persist for life. These antibodies are not influenced by the age of the patient. This differs from the heterophil antibodies, which are relatively short-lived and fail to develop in approximately 10% of adults, in some children, and in most infants (Henle et al., 1974).

Antibodies to the EBV–nuclear antigen (EBV-NA) can also be used in the diagnosis of infectious mononucleosis. Although IgM and IgG antibodies to EB-VCA rise during the acute stage of the disease, the antibody to EBV-NA may not be detected for 3 weeks to 6 months after the onset of the disease (Gallo et al., 1982). EBV-NA antibodies persist for years—probably for life—after they initially are detected. The majority of sera with antibodies to EB-VCA contain antibodies to EBV-NA, except for sera from patients with IgM antibody in early infectious mononucleosis and in patients with immunologic defects (Henle et al., 1979).

A specific serologic diagnosis of a primary EBV infection can be made by demonstration of high titers of IgM and IgG antibodies to EB-VCA and absent or low antibody titer to EBV-NA. Conversely, an EB-VCA IgM-negative and an EBV-NA-positive serum reaction is interpreted as indicating infection with EBV at some undetermined previous time.

Both EB-VCA and EBV-NA can be detected by fluorescent methods—EB-VCA usually by an indirect immunofluorescence assay and EBV-NA by a more sensitive anticomplement immunofluorescence test. Both procedures are available as kits through commercial sources.

Demonstration of Lupus Erythematosus Cells Using Heparinized Blood

Principle

The patient's leukocytes and plasma, containing the lupus erythematosus (LE) factor, are incubated. A buffy coat is obtained, and the smears are stained and examined for the presence of LE cells (Zinkham and Conley, 1956).

Reagents and Equipment

1. Rotator.
2. Centrifuge.
3. Wintrobe tubes.
4. Pasteur pipettes.
5. Tubes: 10×75 mm.

Specimen

Heparinized whole blood is drawn into a Vacutainer tube (BD no. 3835) containing 60 USP units of heparin and 10 glass beads, each 3 mm in diameter.

Method

1. Approximately 10 ml blood is drawn into heparin, and the tube is tilted gently to mix.
2. The specimen is placed on a rotator for 30 minutes to allow the beads to defibrinate the sample. It is allowed to remain at room temperature for an additional 30 minutes.
3. The specimen then is centrifuged at 1,500 rpm for 5 minutes, and supernatant plasma is removed and discarded.
4. The buffy coat and some accompanying red cells are withdrawn with a Pasteur pipette, and a Wintrobe tube is filled. It is centrifuged at 2,000 rpm for 5–10 minutes.
5. An aliquot of buffy coat is removed, and thin smears are prepared and stained. They are examined for the presence of LE bodies using a high-power oil-immersion lens.

Demonstration of Lupus Erythematosus Cells Using Normal Leukocyte Suspensions

Principle

Normal leukocytes provide a source of DNA material to produce LE cells in the presence of the LE factor in the test serum.

Reagents and Equipment

1. Normal leukocyte suspension: Heparinized group O blood, 5 ml, is centrifuged at 2,000 rpm for 10 minutes. Half of the red-cell column is removed with a Pasteur pipette and discarded. The remaining cells and plasma are remixed and are allowed to settle at 37°C until 1–2 ml of the plasma can be withdrawn. The plasma, rich in leukocytes and platelets, is centrifuged and washed three times in normal saline at 500–1,000 rpm. The leukocytes are resuspended in approximately 0.5 ml saline.
2. Wintrobe tube.

3. Incubator, 37°C.
4. Centrifuge.
5. Pasteur pipettes.
6. Slides.

Specimen

Ten milliliters of blood are allowed to clot at room temperature. The blood is centrifuged, and the serum is removed and stored frozen at –20°C until tested.

Method

1. Equal volumes of test serum and normal leukocyte suspension are added together and incubated at 37°C for 3–4 hours.
2. The specimen is centrifuged at 1,000 rpm for 5 minutes, and an aliquot of the buffy coat is removed with a Pasteur pipette. Thin smears are made and are stained with Wright's stain.
3. The smears are examined for the presence of LE cells using a high-power oil-immersion lens.

Discussion

An LE cell is a neutrophil containing a basophilic opaque homogeneous mass within its cytoplasm. The nucleus usually is displaced and sometimes appears as a crescent around the ingested material, which shows no evidence of chromatin arrangement. The LE cell exhibits a positive Feulgen reaction, demonstrating its nuclear origin.

The presence of LE cells depends on three factors: (1) viable phagocytic leukocytes, (2) nuclear protein, and (3) the LE factors. The phagocytes most commonly implicated in the reaction are neutrophils, although monocytes and, rarely, eosinophils have been known to be involved. The nuclear protein source is derived from either granulocytes or lymphocytes, and the LE factor is composed of IgG antibodies to nucleoprotein. These serum antibodies combine with the cell nuclei to produce swelling and subsequent rupture of the cell membrane. If sufficient antibody is attached to the nuclei, they are phagocytosed by neutrophils to produce the typical LE cell.

These structures are frequently confused with tart cells, which can be distinguished in two principal ways. They are usually monocytes that have phagocytosed another structure, not neutrophils, and their nuclear mass is not homogeneous but is distinguished by chromatin aggregates and threads. Additionally, most LE cells approximate 15–18 μ in diameter, in contrast to tart cells, which are smaller, on average 8–10 μ in diameter.

Preparations of LE cells may include extracellular globular material, and rosettes are also occasionally seen. These comprise ingested nuclear masses that are surrounded by several phagocytic cells. Aside from being positive in 60–75% of patients with systemic lupus erythematosus (SLE), LE cells are found in response to various medications, such as hydralazine (Apresoline) and procainamide.

Not only is the test for LE cells using heparinized blood fairly insensitive in detecting SLE, it also suffers from technical vagaries and lack of standardization. Other procedures more suited to making a diagnosis of SLE are immunofluorescence and latex agglutination. However, a recommended approach in the diagnosis of SLE and related disorders is the antinuclear antibody test, for which two or three different cell substrates should be used. If the test result is positive, follow-up tests using a variety of specific antigens are recommended to characterize the antibody (Tan, 1983).

Demonstration of the Lupus Erythematosus Phenomenon Using Latex Particles

Principle

Polystyrene latex particles are coated with deoxyribonucleoprotein (DNP) extract from fetal calf thymus. Agglutination takes place in the presence of antibodies to DNP.

Reagents and Equipment

1. Latex test reagents (Fisher Scientific Co., Orangeburg, NY).
2. Stirrer.
3. Glass slide.
4. Stopwatch.

Specimen

Hemolysis-free serum is the specimen used.

Method

1. Equal volumes of test serum and latex suspension are placed on a slide, the mixture is spread evenly over the slide, and the slide is rotated for 1 minute.
2. The specimen is observed for macroscopic agglutination over a dark background in reflected light. The results are read after 1 minute.

Results

Agglutination appearing in 1 minute is considered a positive result.

Exudate and Transudate Leukocyte Cell Counts: Standard Procedure

Principle

The principle underlying exudate and transudate leukocyte cell counts is the same as that described for manual blood cell counts (see page 265).

Reagents and Equipment

1. Diluting fluid: Methyl violet, 0.2 g, is dissolved in 10 ml glacial acetic acid and diluted to 100 ml with distilled water. This fluid is filtered before use.
2. Pipettes: As described under manual cell counting (see page 265).
3. Hemocytometer: Improved Neubauer or Fuchs-Rosenthal type.

Specimen

The specimen is EDTA-anticoagulated transudate or exudate.

Method

1. The diluting fluid is pipetted to the *1* mark of the Thoma pipette, and the specimen is pipetted to the *11* mark. Alternatively, the Unopette system is used.
2. The pipette is shaken, and the first few drops of fluid are discharged.
3. The hemocytometer is set up as described on page 258, and the cells are allowed to settle for 5 minutes at room temperature.

4. All the cells seen in the entire side of the hemocytometer are counted.

Calculation

Using the *improved Neubauer* rulings, the calculation is as follows:

> The dimension of the entire ruled area is 3×3 mm = 9 mm^2.
>
> The depth of the chamber is 0.1 mm.
>
> The total volume of the diluted fluid within the ruled area then is $3 \times 3 \times 0.1$ mm = 0.9 µl.
>
> If n number of cells are counted in the total volume of 0.9 µl of dilution, the number of cells in 1 µl of dilution is n/0.9.
>
> The dilution of the specimen fluid is 1.1, so there are n/0.9 $\times$ 1.1 cells in 1 µl of undiluted sample.
>
> The number of cells counted in the entire ruled area is multiplied by 1.22 to calculate the number of cells per unit volume.

Using the *Fuchs-Rosenthal* hemocytometer, the calculation is as follows:

> The dimension of the ruled area is 4×4 mm = 16 mm^2.
>
> The depth of the chamber is 0.2 mm.
>
> The total volume of the diluted fluid within the ruled area is then $4 \times 4 \times 0.2$ mm = 3.2 µl.
>
> If n number of cells are counted in the total volume of 3.2 µl of dilution, the number of cells in 1 µl of dilution is n/3.2.
>
> The dilution of the specimen fluid is 1.1, so there are n/3.2 $\times$ 1.1 cells in 1 µl of undiluted sample.
>
> The number of cells counted in the entire ruled area is multiplied by 0.34 to calculate the number of cells per unit volume.

Exudate and Transudate Leukocyte Cell Counts in a Purulent Specimen

Principle

The principle underlying exudate and transudate leukocyte cell counts in a purulent specimen is the same as that for the standard procedure.

Reagents and Equipment

1. Diluting fluid: Acetic acid, 2% aqueous solution, or hydrochloric acid.
2. Pipettes: As described previously (see page 265).
3. Hemocytometer: Improved Neubauer type.

Specimen

EDTA-anticoagulated transudate or exudate is used.

Method

1. The specimen is diluted, by use of a manual Thoma pipette or an Unopette, to a dilution of 1:10 or 1:20, depending on the extent of the specimen cellularity.
2. Steps 2–4 are repeated as described for the standard procedure, and all the cells in the four corner squares of the improved Neubauer chamber are counted.

Calculation

> The dimension of each of the squares counted is $1 \times 1 = 1$ mm^2.
>
> The depth of the chamber is 0.1 mm.
>
> The total volume of the diluted fluid within the ruled area counted then is $1 \times 1 \times 0.1$ mm $\times 4$ = 0.4 µl.
>
> If n number of cells are counted in the total volume of 0.4 µl of dilution, the number of cells in 1 µl of dilution is n/0.4.
>
> If the dilution used is 1:20, there are n/0.4 $\times$ 20 cells in 1 µl of undiluted sample. The number of cells counted in the four corner squares is multiplied by 50 to calculate the number of cells per unit volume.
>
> If the 1:10 dilution is used, the number of cells is multiplied by a factor of 25.

Comment

For all purulent fluids, a smear should be made and stained using the same procedure as outlined for blood smears (see page 271). A differential cell count should be carried out as far as possible, separating mononuclear cells from granulocytes, and the report should reflect these data.

E Rosettes for T-Cell Evaluation

Principle

Washed lymphocytes are incubated with washed sheep red cells. The percentage and population of cells forming the rosettes is calculated.

Reagents and Equipment

1. Culture media (RPMI 1640, available from Microbiological Associates, Walkersville, MD).
2. Heat-inactivated fetal calf serum (Microbiological Associates): Thawed and divided into 1-ml aliquots and stored at –20°C.
3. Sheep red cells less than 2 weeks old (R Kent Richards, Salt Lake City, UT).
4. Trypan blue 0.2%: Trypan blue, 1.0 g, is mixed with distilled water to a solution of 500 ml.
   Sodium chloride 4.25%: 21.25 g of 4.25% sodium chloride is added to distilled water to a solution of 500 ml.
   Working solution: This is made fresh immediately before its use and is made up of 4.25% sodium chloride, 100 µl, and 0.2% trypan blue, 400 µl.

Specimen

The test specimen may be EDTA-anticoagulated blood, bone marrow, or aspirated fluids less than 48 hours old.

Method

1. Sheep red cells are washed three times with RMPI culture media.

2. Fifty microliters of the sheep red-cell pellet are added to 5 ml RMPI. The suspension is mixed and added to an equal volume of a 4,000 cell/µl lymphocyte suspension.
3. The specimen is incubated at 37°C for 15 minutes.
4. It then is centrifuged at 1,000 rpm for 10 minutes.
5. Half of the supernatant is removed and replaced with an equal volume of heat-inactivated fetal calf serum, with care taken not to disturb the cell button.
6. This is incubated for 2 hours or overnight at 4°C.
7. The cell button is resuspended with a Pasteur pipette, leaving small visible clumps of cells.
8. One hundred microliters of the cell suspension are added to 100 µl fresh trypan blue.
9. A standard wet preparation is made, and the percentage of viable cells that have three or more sheep red cells attached is recorded.
10. Two drops of the resuspended button from step 7 are removed and stained with a standard Romanowsky stain (e.g., Wright's stain).

Comment

Normal specimens should be run as a control for this method. Viable cells do not stain with trypan blue; dead cells cannot exclude the dye and, consequently, stain blue.

True rosettes are surrounded by sheep red cells that appear to be stretched. The Wright's-stained smear is useful in determining which population of cells is rosetting.

Chapter 23

Apparatus and Automation

The ever-expanding number of automated apparatus currently available make a textbook discussion of equipment immediately outdated. In the area of particle counting, the laboratory staff has the choice of many counting devices, some with automated sample trays and printout capabilities and some that are strictly manual and designed for the smaller hospital or physician's office laboratory. Some have "walk-away" capabilities, whereas others remain strictly semiautomated devices. It is impossible to present here adequate coverage of modern equipment because of the increasing number of new models and the emergence of new companies that would render this discussion immediately obsolete. However, the basic principles of automated hematologic analyzers are unchanged, and they are discussed in this chapter.

Cell Counters

Multichannel Cell Counters

Principle

The principal manufacturer of multichannel cell counters is Coulter Electronics in Hialeah, FL. Coulter manufactures a wide range of cell counters, most of which use the principle of electrical resistance. This principle relies on individual cells moving through a small, constricted electrical current path when suspended in a diluting fluid. Detection of these cells is based on the differences in electrical conductivity between the cells and the suspending fluid. In passing through the electrical current path, the individual cell changes the electrical resistance in the circuit and causes a change in the voltage. The boundary of the current path is the bore of a small, submerged orifice in the wall of an insulated vessel. Figure 23.1 illustrates this orifice in a simplified form.

A diluted suspension of blood cells is allowed to pass through the orifice. By means of a current source and a pair of relatively large area electrodes placed in isotonic fluid, an electrical current is allowed to flow through the orifice. This fluid carries the cells to be counted through the opening, and the external fluid connects the electrical current to its electrode. Typically, the orifice is 100 µ in diameter, but smaller apertures can be used if smaller particles are counted. For example, 70-µ apertures often are used to enumerate platelets. The orifice may be considered as a minute conductivity cell, with the fluid volumes at each end of the aperture serving as electrodes that make contact with the contents of the bore. Cells may be suspended in any of the commonly used diluting fluids. The diluents, being electrolytes, are good conductors, whereas the cells are very poor electrical conductors. As the suspending fluid carries a cell through the orifice, the cell displaces a volume of the relatively good electrical conducting fluid, and this slightly raises the electrical resistance of the total contents of the orifice. Time of passage through the orifice varies, depending on the orifice's length and the pressure

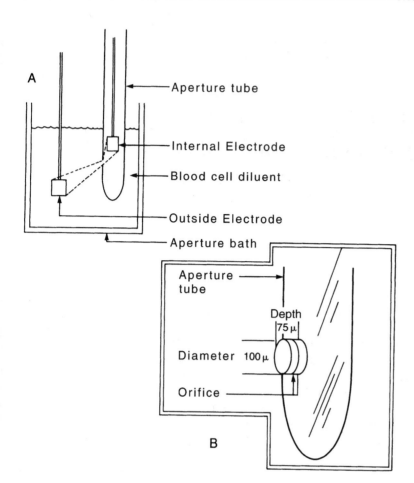

A

Aperture tube

Internal Electrode

Blood cell diluent

Outside Electrode

Aperture bath

Aperture tube

Depth
75 μ

Diameter 100 μ

Orifice

B

Figure 23.1. The principle of electronic impedance. A. The relative positions of the electrodes to the aperture tube. B. A magnified view of the orifice of the aperture tube.

differential exerted on the diluted blood. Usually, the cell is present in the orifice between 0.00002 second and 0.00001 second, and because of the brevity of this stay, very high current densities may be used without vaporizing the fluid. The slight increase in resistance during this time increases the voltage appearing across the orifice, and the voltage pulses that are produced are amplified for display on an oscilloscope screen. These readings can then be fed to a pulse-height discriminator and converted to a measurement of cell size.

Figure 23.1A shows the aperture and orifice with connecting electrodes, and Figure 23.1B shows the orifice in three dimensions. The oscilloscope, showing a variety of pulse-height displacements, is illustrated in Figure 23.2.

Irrespective of the degree of blood dilution, there are occasions when more than one cell will pass through the orifice at one time. In this event, the pulse produced will be disproportionately large and will reflect the total displacement of all the cells in the orifice at the same time. This will produce a single increased pulse display instead of a series of smaller impulses, thus causing a count loss. Such coincidental errors are corrected for all counts, either automatically in the more updated counters or manually by means of correction charts in older electrical impedance instruments.

For example, when the standard 100-μ–diameter orifice is used and there is a concentration of 50,000 cells in a 0.5-ml sample volume, the count loss and required correction is approximately 12.2%. Figure 23.3 graphically displays the percentage of coincidental correction for various cell counts using different-sized apertures.

For cell size distribution studies, the pulse-height spread seen on the oscilloscope is a guide for determining the threshold levels at which the counts

Figure 23.2. A typical oscilloscope pattern seen in electrical
impedance counters. Each pulse
height represents a red cell or
particle passing through the orifice. The height of the impulse
is proportional to the cell volume. (RBC = red blood cell;
MCV = mean cell volume.)

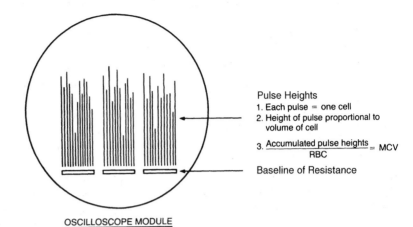

Figure 23.2. A typical oscilloscope pattern seen in electrical
impedance counters. Each pulse
height represents a red cell or
particle passing through the orifice. The height of the impulse
is proportional to the cell volume. (RBC = red blood cell;
MCV = mean cell volume.)

Pulse Heights
1. Each pulse = one cell
2. Height of pulse proportional to
   volume of cell
3. $\dfrac{\text{Accumulated pulse heights}}{\text{RBC}} = \text{MCV}$

Baseline of Resistance

OSCILLOSCOPE MODULE

Figure 23.3. Coincidence correction chart for 500-μl sampling volumes using various
aperture diameters.

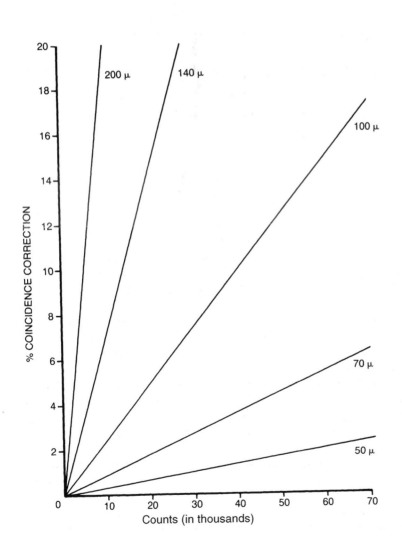

should be taken. This sizing procedure can be translated directly into cell volume measurement and, in the case of red cells, it can be used to determine the mean cell hemoglobin (MCH) and to calculate the hematocrit value. The calculated hematocrit value is defined from the following equation:

$$\text{Hematocrit} = \frac{V}{Vt} \times 100,$$

where Vt is the volume of blood and V is the volume of red cells in the blood. Because the pulse height (ei) is proportional to the volume of the blood cell,

$$ei = K \times Vi,$$

where K is a constant and Vi is the volume of one cell.

The volume V of n blood cells suspended in the volume Vt of the blood is expressed as

$$V = \sum_{i=1}^{n}; \quad V_i = \frac{1}{K} \sum_{i=1}^{n} ei.$$

By satisfying this formula for the hematocrit value,

$$\frac{V}{Vt} \times 100,$$

becomes

$$\text{Hematocrit} = \frac{1}{K \times Vt} \times \sum_{i=1}^{n} ei \times 100.$$

Examples of multichannel counters include those produced by Coulter Electronics, Sysmex (Los Alomitos, CA), Abbott Diagnostics (Abbott Park, IL), and Miles Laboratory (Technicon) (Tarrytown, NY). The various models of Coulter and Sysmex instruments are basically similar in design and in the principle of operation. They differ in the sophistication of sample handling, statistical manipulation of data, speed of analysis, and reagents used, although they all use the same electrical impedance principle. Some models allow for a display showing cell size histograms, although none of them can discriminate leukocytes from other nucleated particles in the counting procedure.

Most multichannel counters determine leukocyte and red-cell counts, hemoglobin, and mean cell volume (MCV) values. Hemoglobin is measured directly by a colorimetric cyanmethemoglobin method. From these values, MCH and mean cell hemoglobin concentration (MCHC) results are calculated mathematically and either are printed out on paper tape or cards or are fed directly into a computer terminal by way of an interface. Some of the more sophisticated instruments also routinely separate platelets by use of a histogram derived through a pulse-height analyzer.

With pulse-height analysis, leukocytes can also be displayed according to their various proportions of granulocytes, lymphocytes, and mononuclear cells. This last category includes not only monocytes but also undifferentiated immature cells, and thus this aspect of the counter may be used as a differential leukocyte screening apparatus. However, no provision is made for detecting very small numbers of immature cells, as they will automatically be included with the "mononuclear" monocyte classification (Bollinger et al., 1987).

The large multichannel instruments, such as the Coulter model, dilute the whole-blood sample automatically. A lysing agent is added to one dilution, and the hemolyzed blood is separated into two pathways: One segment is read spectrophotometrically at 540 nm to produce the hemoglobin value by a cyanmethemoglobin method, and the other segment is passed through an aperture and the particles are counted by the electrical impedance method previously discussed. The exact physical layout and schematics of the instrumentation vary from one manufacturer to another; some use more than one counting orifice and average the results, whereas others use different diluents at different points in the analysis (Figure 23.4).

The remainder of the primary dilution is then usually rediluted to remove statistically any nucleated cells. This is accomplished by greatly diluting the specimen so that the effect of leukocytes is proportionally insignificant when compared with the number of red cells present. This dilution is then passed through a similar orifice, and the voltage pulse-heights are displayed and recorded as previously explained. More advanced counters can produce red-cell distribution width (RDW) data and platelet counts, as well as differential white cell counts, by using the pulse-height analyzer. By least-

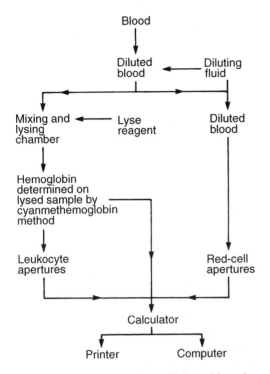

Figure 23.4. Flow diagram of a multichannel impedance counter.

squares fitting, an algorithm based on the logarithmic normal size distribution of platelets can be produced that will separate platelets from red cells and other fragmented particles and artifacts. These cell width distribution analyses can graphically produce a picture of the degree of anisocytosis and of two or more red-cell populations, if present, and, as such, are extensions of the Price-Jones plots used in the past. An example of a blood-cell histogram produced on the Coulter Counter Model S-Plus IV is shown in Figure 23.5.

Platelet counting, although precise, presents problems with accuracy unless the data are statistically and electronically manipulated. Because these multichannel cell counters count only particles, cytoplasmic fragments, microcytic red cells, and debris can masquerade as platelets if they are sufficiently small (Savage, 1982; Savage et al., 1983). The problem is resolved by a curve-fitting computed analysis that counts particles of between 2 and 20 fl. The resulting raw data are tested against a set of mathematic criteria and fitted to a logarithmic normal curve from 0 to 70 fl. By "stretching" the curve along the x-axis—that is, the cell size—

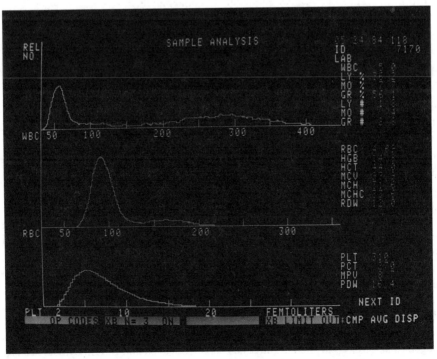

Figure 23.5. White-cell, red-cell, and platelet histograms produced by the Coulter Model S-Plus IV. (Courtesy of Coulter Electronics, Hialeah, FL.)

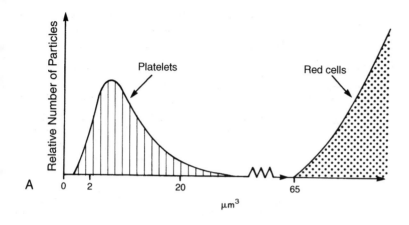

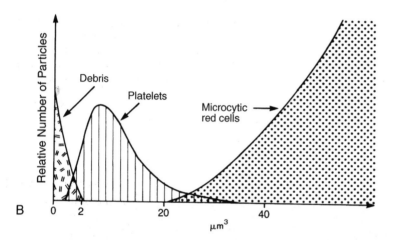

Figure 23.6. A normal (A) and abnormal (B) cell size distribution curve. A. A normal distribution graph, showing the relative platelet and red-cell positions. B. An abnormal cell distribution, showing overlaps of cell stroma and debris with platelets and large platelets with red-cell fragments and microcytes.

the platelets can be electronically separated from other smaller particles such as microcytic red cells. This is illustrated in Figure 23.6.

The same size-referenced system based on nuclear volume is used in the analysis of leukocytes, which can be grouped into three populations: lymphocytes, mononuclear cells, and granulocytes. Mononuclear cells include promyelocytes, myelocytes, and monocytes. In normal individuals, mononuclear cells represent only monocytes but, in abnormal situations, an increase in these groups could indicate cellular immaturity. Figure 23.7 illustrates the subpopulations produced by such sample histograms.

The leukocyte sizing is made possible by the use of a new reagent that gives controlled erythrolysis and stable and reproducible biphasic distributions of leukocyte volumes. Cell residues falling between

45 and 99 fl are thought to derive from lymphocytes, whereas particles larger than 99 fl are believed to be nonlymphocytic cells, including granulocytes and monocytes. Comparisons between this method of estimating differential leukocyte counts (using a computed image analyzer) and conventional manual counts generally show good correlation for lymphocytes and granulocytes, but poor correlation has been reported for mononuclear cells (Allen and Batjer, 1985; Cornbleet and Kessinger, 1985; Nelson et al., 1985; Kalish and Becker, 1986; Miers et al., 1987; Barnard et al., 1989).

Red-Cell Distribution Width

Anisocytosis and poikilocytosis are recognized as morphologic markers of anemia, but they are, by their very nature, subjective in assessment. The

Figure 23.7. Cell size distribution in the separation of leukocytes.

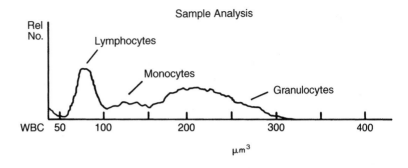

Sample Analysis

Table 23.1. Classification of Anemia Based on the Mean Cell Volume and Red-Cell Distribution Width

Mean Cell Volume	Red-Cell Distribution Width	
	Normal	**High**
Low	Heterozygous thalassemia	Iron-deficiency anemia, hemolytic anemia
Normal	Anemia of chronic disease, anemic hemoglobinopathy (heterozygous forms)	Early megaloblastic anemia, nonmixed nutritional deficiencies, hemoglobinopathies (homozygous forms)
High	Aplastic anemia, preleukemic syndrome, alcohol-induced macrocytosis	Megaloblastic anemia, autoimmune hemolytic anemia, cold agglutinins

RDW, as provided by many multichannel cell counters, provides quantitative information by counting particles in the range of 36–360 fl (Coulter, 1979), according to the following equation:

$$RDW = \frac{\left(\dfrac{\text{20th percentile}}{\text{volume}} - \dfrac{\text{80th percentile}}{\text{volume}} \right)}{\left(\dfrac{\text{20th percentile}}{\text{volume}} + \dfrac{\text{80th percentile}}{\text{volume}} \right)} \times \text{constant}$$

The classification of anemias based on both the MCV and RDW is shown in Table 23.1.

In normal and most abnormal individuals, red-cell size is distributed in an apparently gaussian manner. As long as the red-cell volume distribution histogram is unimodal, the red-cell size is described by the MCV and the coefficient of variation (RDW) of the red-cell size. In normal individuals, the RDW on the Coulter S-Plus IV ranges from 11.5 to 14.0%.

An increase in RDW is proportional to the degree of anisocytosis found in the peripheral blood smear. The quality control of red-cell size is optimal in normal individuals and can vary only in the direction of greater heterogeneity or increased RDW. As the RDW is the coefficient of variation of the red-cell size distribution, an increased value may be found with a reduced MCV. Increases are found in anemia of nutritional cause, such as iron depletion, and folate and vitamin B_{12} deficiencies, irrespective of the MCV data (England and Down, 1979). An increased RDW is an earlier sign of a nutritional anemia than is provided by the MCV. The RDW is usually normal in aplastic anemia and other hypoplastic anemias, but it is increased in proportion to the degree of anemia in hemoglobinopathies and thalassemia (Schweiger, 1981; Kaye and Alter, 1982). A particularly valuable distinction based on the RDW is that between iron deficiency and anemia of chronic disease and thalassemia. Iron-deficiency anemia characteristically produces high RDW data and a normal or low MCV; anemia of chronic disease characteristically shows a normal RDW and a normal or low MCV; and thalassemia produces a normal or slightly elevated RDW and low MCV results (Bessman and Feinstein, 1979).

The level of reticulocyte response affects the RDW, as do elevated leukocyte and platelet counts (Roberts and El Badawi, 1985).

istribution Width
ı Platelet Volume

Platelet size is distributed widely in normal individuals, with a mean value of 8.5–9.0 fl. The platelet distribution width (PDW) increases nonlinearly as the mean platelet volume (MPV) increases. PDW is increased in megaloblastic or aplastic anemia, in leukemic patients receiving chemotherapy, and in chronic myeloid leukemia (Bessman et al., 1981; Bessman, 1983a). The PDW may also be erroneously increased if fragmented red cells or leukocyte fragments broaden the cell distribution population. The causes of a true increased PDW are unclear, but they are believed to be related to megakaryocytic ploidy (Bessman, 1983b).

In immune thrombocytopenic purpura, there is both an increase in the number of circulating megathrombocytes and an elevation of the MPV. The inverse relationship of the platelet count to the MPV is preserved during recovery and relapse. Three mechanisms for thrombocytopenia have been proposed: (1) immunologic destruction (Kelton et al., 1979), (2) disseminated intravascular coagulopathy, and (3) bone marrow suppression (Cohen and Gardner, 1961). Consequently, a high MPV during sepsis-induced thrombocytopenia indicates peripheral platelet destruction with bone marrow compensation. The smaller the MPV, the greater is the bone marrow suppression. Citrated blood samples are preferred to samples anticoagulated with ethylenediaminetetraacetic acid (EDTA) for detecting an increased platelet size in idiopathic thrombocytopenic purpura (Boneu et al., 1986). When tripotassium EDTA is used as the anticoagulant, the MPV increases by approximately 10% in the first 2 hours, this increase being inversely related to the osmolarity (Thompson et al., 1985; Evans and Smith, 1986).

The MPV is normal in chronic lymphocytic leukemia, atherosclerotic heart disease, and diabetes mellitus, but it is reduced in individuals treated with cytotoxic chemotherapy for acute nonlymphocytic leukemia, in megaloblastic anemia, and in aplastic anemia. Individuals with chronic myeloid leukemia exhibit an increased MPV (Bessman et al., 1982; Table 23.2).

Platelet volume is influenced by both platelet production in the bone marrow and by platelet activation or sequestration in the circulation. In thrombocytopenic patients, it is often possible to differentiate between megakaryocytic and amegakaryocytic disease states on the basis of platelet volume analysis. In patients with thrombocytosis, a myeloproliferative disorder may be suspected if the platelet distribution width is high. However, the conditions of sample preparation and storage still give rise to considerable inaccuracy in the determination of platelet volume parameters. In vitro platelet volume is affected principally by the anticoagulant, the most pronounced effect being associated with EDTA. The platelet's swelling is likely due to chelation of membrane calcium (White, 1968). To a lesser degree, the volume increases when sodium citrate and glutaraldehyde are used. Low concentrations of glutaraldehyde, however, inhibit platelet swelling for up to 2 hours. (Wehmeier and Schneider, 1989). This suggests that there is a rapid increase in platelet volume during or immediately after venipuncture, which can be prevented if the blood is drawn promptly into a cross-linking agent.

Sources of Error

Besides the coincidence errors that occur when multiple cells simultaneously pass through the orifice, most impedance systems (particularly older models) also produce carryover errors, especially when leukopenic or anemic specimens are counted following normal or elevated cell counts. This carryover error can result in mistaken counts as high as 2–5% over the true value (Brittin and Brecher, 1971). Consequently, the laboratory staff should determine for itself at which level counts should be repeated, and this policy should be stated in the laboratory's standard operational procedure manual and should be strictly followed.

Nonetheless, with some of the newer instrumentation now available, it has been determined that carryover is negligible (Coulter S-Plus, Ortho ELT-8) and can be ignored (Drewinko et al., 1982). Hemoglobin errors can be produced by turbidity associated with leukocytosis, particularly if the count is in excess of 30×10^6/liter. The MCV and red-cell count can also be falsely elevated in such situations because of the large numbers of cells counted and the proportional increase in the average cell size. This, in turn, falsifies the hematocrit and the remaining cell indices. Precipitation of IgM plasma proteins by the quaternary ammonium salts

Table 23.2. Classification of Platelet Disorders Based on the Platelet Count and Mean Platelet Volume

Mean Platelet Volume	Platelet Count		
	Low	Normal	High
Low	Bone marrow hypoplasia due to drugs or sepsis, hypersplenism, aplastic anemia, megaloblastic anemia	Mild bone marrow depression	—
Normal	—	—	—
High	Immune platelet destruction, other platelet consumptive disorders	—	Myelofibrosis, primary thrombocytosis, post-splenectomy, chronic myeloid leukemia

contained in the lysing agents used in the Coulter Model S-Plus IV has also been reported and can result in whole-blood hemoglobin blank values as high as 7.3 g/dl (Nicholls, 1985).

Other errors found in multichannel counts relate to the osmolarity of the diluting fluid and the blood being tested. High blood glucose levels, particularly those in excess of 400 mg/dl, and hyperosmolarity due to other causes can create erroneously high MCV and hematocrit values and low MCHC results (Nevius, 1963; Beautyman and Bills, 1982; Holt et al., 1982;). This is a result of the diluent being relatively hypertonic compared to the hypotonic blood sample being tested, thus inciting the red cells osmotically to take up water and swell. Prediluting the specimen and allowing it to stand for approximately 10 minutes at room temperature before counting can eliminate this problem.

Hypertonicity can also be exaggerated by the choice of anticoagulant. Routine use of the tripotassium salts of EDTA yields lower values for the hematocrit and MCV than when the disodium salt of EDTA is used. This has been attributed to the lower pH found in the disodium EDTA–anticoagulated blood and the consequent swelling of the red cells (Sears et al., 1985).

Cold agglutinins, if present in high titer, can also cause erroneous results. They are introduced through the orifice as large red-cell masses that produce falsely elevated MCV data and reduced red-cell counts, as well as extremely high MCHC results. This problem can be eliminated or reduced, depending on the titer of the antibody. If a moderate titer exists, warming the blood to 37°C before

diluting in the counter will usually suffice but, on rare occasions when the titer is extremely high, the problem cannot be resolved merely by warming. As the prewarmed blood is introduced into the instrument, the effect of the room-temperature saline or diluent will cause spontaneous agglutination of the cells.

Erroneous leukocyte counts can be seen in these types of counting apparatus and usually occur in leukemic patients undergoing chemotherapy. In such situations, the cells often are more fragile than normal and disintegrate during their pressurized passage through the counting orifice. The count will vary, depending on the final size of the fragmented cells or particles produced. If the fragments are large enough to be counted, a false leukocytosis will result but, if the particles are small enough to be below the counting threshold, a false leukopenic count will be produced. Pseudoleukocytosis has been reported in paraproteinemia, due to IgG and IgM forms of cryoproteins, and in pseudothrombocytopenia, due to platelet satellitism (Taft, 1973; Gulliani et al., 1977).

Plasma turbidity caused by hyperlipidemia results in errors too—mainly elevated hemoglobin and the calculated MCH and MCHC results (Nosanchuk et al., 1974). The problem may be so severe that the complete blood cell count (CBC) can be carried out only manually, but it is most often corrected by determining the hemoglobin value on a prediluted specimen. If the CBC is done manually, the patient's plasma is diluted and used as a blank to "zero" the spectrophotometer. To calculate the correct volume of cyanmethemoglobin to use in such situations when 20 µl plasma is added as a blank, the following formula can be used:

$$N = \frac{5 \text{ ml}}{1 - \text{hematocrit}}$$

Alternatively, the following procedure can be carried out: Lipemic whole blood is run on the counter in the usual way, and a printout of the data is obtained. Two microhematocrit tubes are spun, the tubes are broken off at the plasma–buffy coat interface, and a 44.7-µl pipette is filled with the plasma. Dilution takes places in the normal manner, as in a capillary blood specimen, and the plasma blank is run immediately after the counter diluent. The hemoglobin is calculated from this formula:

$$Hb_c = Hb_s - \text{plasma} \ (1.00 - \text{hematocrit})$$

where Hb_c is the corrected hemoglobin, Hb_s is the original hemoglobin, *plasma* is the reading of the plasma blank, and *hematocrit* is the hematocrit expressed as a decimal.

Interinstrument bias between electrical impedance methodologies is well established, even among instruments produced by the same manufacturer. Particularly noticeable are MCV data variations, with differences of as much as 11 fl being reported between Coulter S-Plus II and Coulter S models on the same blood sample (Koepke, 1982). This is probably the result of several factors. The MCV as measured on Coulter instruments is very dependent on cell deformability as the cell passes through the aperture. How much the cell becomes deformed or remains more rigid plays an important role in the pulse generated and, therefore, in the final MCV. Small differences in the Coulter S and S-Plus results are probably caused by differences in the aperture size (100 µ for the model S compared to 50 µ for the S-Plus), the sweep flow added to the S-Plus to help produce a clean flow of particles through and away from the aperture, and the pulse editing added to the S-Plus to delete atypical pulses such as those cells that do not go through the center of the apertures.

The reasons for lower MCV data as revealed by the S-Plus II are more obscure, but two explanations exist. The MCV in the S-Plus II model is determined from the histogram generated by the computer, in contrast to the histogram for the S-Plus and

S, which is generated by analog means. In addition, the reagent system is different on the S-Plus II, causing the control cells to react differently in the modified diluent. When S-Plus and S-Plus II counters are compared using Isoton II and Isoton +, changes in MCV have been observed that are a result solely of the diluent used (Savage, 1984), and such changes are reflected in MCV reference range lower-limit shifts of 76–79 fl when Isoton III is used in place of Isoton +.

Quality Control

Impedance counters can be controlled by a variety of commercially available control materials that cover the expected range of test results. Many trilevel controls are available for all parameters of the CBC, including platelet counts but usually excluding differential leukocyte counts. These controls are usually composed of fixed human red cells and platelets fortified by fixed nucleated avian red cells to mimic leukocytes. Such materials should not be used as a primary calibrate but only as controls to ensure that test performance is adequate. Primary calibration of most electrical impedance devices can be carried out by one of two methods—either by the use of a laboratory-established calibrator and an acceptable primary technique or by the use of a primary commercial calibrate (S-Cal, available from Coulter Electronics).

Primary calibrates are made in the laboratory, and the data are assigned using reference methods. Those used are cyanmethemoglobin for hemoglobin, Coulter Model F or ZB1 for cell counts, and the microhematocrit procedure for hematocrits. At least 20 normal blood specimens are tested using these procedures. Each test should be carried out in triplicate and the results averaged. To correct for the trapped plasma present, the hematocrit values are adjusted by subtracting 3% (England et al., 1972) of the centrifuged value. For example, a spun microhematocrit of 41% (0.41) would be adjusted to 39.8% (0.410–0.012). The red-cell indices of each of the 20 specimens are calculated. Each of the specimens is analyzed in triplicate on the impedance counter, and these results are averaged. The difference between the counter to be calibrated and the reference method for each of the 20 normal blood specimens is subtracted, and those differences are averaged for each test parameter. Each value is adjusted accordingly on the instrument being calibrated. For example, if hemoglobin values averaged 7% higher on the instrument than by reference methods, a normal blood specimen run by the reference procedure would be adjusted by a factor of 0.93. If the result was 7% lower, the result would be adjusted by a factor of 1.07. Table 23.3 shows a suggested format that can be used in the primary calibration of electrical impedance instrumentation.

The calibration settings should not be changed unless a major equipment malfunction takes place. Unless this occurs, once the reference values are established, they should be rechecked at monthly intervals for verification. Machine drift throughout a specimen run is best detected using commercial controls, as previously described. Such controls should contain blood specimens that have low, normal, and high values for each test and should be run every shift. If the number of patient specimens is sufficiently large, a full set of controls should be run at least every 50–100 samples according to the individual laboratory's operational procedures.

Some particle counters are available that automatically produce statistical data based on Bull's formula of moving averages (see page 239). This is an invaluable aid in monitoring the quality control of test specimens and makes use of the fact that, for every set of 20 patient samples, the average data should remain within a 3% spread provided that there have been no obviously abnormal groups of blood specimens run, such as those from oncologic or hemodialysis patients. A change of moving averages of greater than 3% signifies a possible loss of calibration and should be immediately checked using a full set of controls. Companies that produce electrical impedance counters include Coulter Electronics, Toa Instruments, and Clay-Adams, Inc.

Laser Flow Cytometers

Flow cytometers are instruments that make simultaneous multiple measurements on single cells entrained in fluid flow. (Figure 23.8 illustrates the schematics of a flow cytometer.) Ortho Instruments (Raritan, NJ) is the principal manufacturer of laser flow-cytometric equipment. One of the major advantages of flow cytometry is that it is capable of making more than one measurement on every cell during the few milliseconds that the cell spends passing through the sensing area. The principle of the instrument is that of the optical detection of cells in a liquid suspension that scatters light at a low forward angle. The intensity of the scattered light is detected by a photodetector for the conversion to electrical impulses of height and width equivalent to the intensity of the scattered light. This, in turn, is proportional to the cell volume.

The technology involved is the hydrodynamic focusing of a narrow stream of cells through a flow channel 250 μ in diameter. Focusing is achieved by a liquid laminar sheath flow that is coaxial to the sample flow. This method isolates the cell suspension, confining particles to the central portion of a liquid jet. A helium neon laser beam is focused on this stream of cells, forming a minute cylindric sensing zone, 20 μ in diameter and 7 μ high. This zone is in the center of the sample stream and allows for an almost single-file array of cells for sensing and detection. Leukocytes are enumerated after lysis of the red cells. Discrimination between platelets and red cells depends on three cell variables: volume, refractive index, and the time the cells take to pass through the sensing zone.

Each cell generates a pulse, the height and width of which is proportional to all three discriminating parameters of that cell. A voltage value is assigned to that pulse and is compared with an integral voltage. A value greater than the integral voltage is classified as a red blood cell, and a lower value is classified as a platelet. Hemoglobin concentration is measured spectrophotometrically using the cyanmethemoglobin method. The hematocrit value is determined from the area under the curve generated by the red-cell pulses, and the MCV, MCH, and MCHC are computed internally from the measured parameters.

The errors associated with laser flow cytometers are similar to those described for the electrical resistance methods. They include patterns of spurious red-cell parameters caused by serum cold agglutinins, showing increases in MCV, and a discrepancy between the hemoglobin and the hematocrit values, producing a falsely elevated MCHC (Solanki and Blackburn, 1985). Spuriously elevated platelet counts secondary to in vivo bacteremia have also been reported (Gloster et al., 1985).

Table 23.3. Example of the Primary Calibration of Automated Equipment

	Hemoglobin			Red-Cell Count			Mean Cell Volume			White-Cell Count		
	Counter (g/dl)	Ref (g/dl)	% Difference	Counter (×10⁹/liter)	Ref (×10¹²/liter)	% Difference	Counter (fl)	Ref (fl)	% Difference	Counter (×10⁹/liter)	Ref (×10⁹/liter)	% Difference
1	14.1	14.0	+0.7	5.6	5.2	+7.7	86	88	−2.3	5.9	5.9	0
2	15.2	15.2	0	6.4	5.9	+8.5	82	86	−4.7	5.1	5.0	+2.0
3	13.6	13.5	+0.7	4.4	4.4	0	87	91	−4.6	7.8	8.4	−7.2
4	14.6	14.7	−0.7	5.4	5.3	+1.9	83	84	−1.2	8.8	9.3	−6.4
5	15.9	15.6	+1.9	4.9	4.6	+6.5	84	88	−4.6	7.7	7.3	+5.5
6	12.8	12.8	0	3.9	3.9	0	89	89	0	7.3	7.1	+2.8
7	13.9	14.0	−0.7	5.4	5.4	0	87	93	−6.5	6.5	6.8	−4.4
8	14.1	14.0	+0.7	5.3	4.9	+8.2	82	82	0	8.4	8.3	+1.2
9	18.9	18.7	+1.1	6.5	5.9	+10.2	84	85	−1.2	7.2	7.2	0
10	15.4	15.3	+0.6	5.7	5.3	+7.5	84	84	0	8.4	8.4	0
11	15.0	15.1	−0.7	4.6	4.7	+2.7	83	84	−1.2	6.8	6.9	−0.3
12	14.7	14.6	+0.7	4.8	5.1	−5.9	89	88	+1.1	7.5	7.4	+2.4
13	15.3	15.4	−0.6	5.2	5.0	+4.0	77	81	−5.0	7.1	7.0	+3.9
14	12.9	12.9	0	4.4	4.3	+2.3	84	87	−4.5	6.7	6.8	−1.5
15	13.8	14.0	−1.5	5.0	5.0	0	83	91	−8.8	8.8	9.0	−3.7
16	14.1	14.1	0	4.9	4.8	+2.1	88	93	−5.4	8.1	8.2	−1.2
17	15.0	15.1	−0.7	5.5	5.3	+3.8	89	94	−5.3	8.8	8.5	+3.5
18	15.4	15.2	+1.3	5.8	5.9	−1.7	91	90	+1.1	7.9	7.7	+2.6
19	14.8	14.7	+0.7	4.9	4.7	+1.3	83	87	−4.6	6.9	7.1	−2.8
20	16.3	16.2	+0.6	5.0	4.6	+8.7	87	88	−1.2	7.3	7.4	−1.4
Means	14.79	14.75	+0.3	5.18	5.01	+3.1	85.1	86.6	−2.9	7.45	7.48	−0.4
Action taken	None required			Adjust counter down 3.1% for red-cell counts			Adjust counter up 2.9% for mean cell volume			None required		

Ref = reference value.

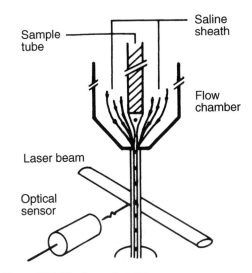

Figure 23.8. The flow cytometer.

Optical Cell Counters

The principal manufacturer of optical cell counters is Miles Company, which markets the H1, H2, and H3 counters.

Pattern Recognition Differential Leukocyte Counters

Pattern recognition differential leukocyte counters use a uniformly made and stained blood smear that is placed on a motor-driven computer-controlled microscope stage. When a stained leukocyte is viewed, the stage stops, and the optical images of the cell are recorded by a television camera and analyzed for nuclear and cytoplasmic size, density, shape, and color. These features are stored and compared with a known value for each cell class. The cell then is classified according to which class is closest to those of a standard cell. Controls consisting of coverslipped slides with known percentages of the cells of interest are run on a routine basis. The precision of the instrumental result is equated with the closeness of agreement between results of each run of these slides and the white-cell distribution previously determined by a reference method.

Some pattern recognition methods use either conventional wedge-shaped blood smears or spun smears. Red-cell and platelet morphologic features can be determined by manually viewing the smear and entering the data on a console. The procedure has precision problems similar to those associated with manual counts, as 100 or 200 cells are counted routinely, but it does provide less subjective results associated with eye counting. Automation has, however, improved the apparatus speed as later models now are available that have slide cassettes which allow the operator to walk away. These walk-away models also can detect both red-cell and platelet morphologic features.

Because conventional or spinner slides can be prepared from EDTA-anticoagulated blood, the problems of platelet satellitism seen in manual differential counting persist with these instruments. In addition, it has been reported that because of subtle changes in the properties of the stain and in instrumental factors undetected by routine quality control, pattern recognition apparatus can produce band counts on the same slides that are several multiples higher than those actually present when viewed by conventional manual techniques (Winkelman et al., 1983).

Pattern recognition counters can produce biased data, as a consequence of failure to carry quality control slides through the same procedure as the unknown specimens. Quality control slides do not necessarily present optical properties identical to those from specimens of patients that are stained and examined on each day of use. The best practical solution to this quality control problem is to prepare new control slides each day, using the same materials and staining procedures with which the unknown slides are prepared. An accurate manual differential cell count should be carried out on these controls, involving a statistically valid number of cells.

Blood Coagulation Instrumentation

Two main principles are used for the instrument detection of fibrin clots: electromechanical and optical.

Electromechanical Instrumentation

Electromechanical semiautomated coagulation instruments detect clot formation by means of an electromechanical probe. The test is performed in a plastic cup held in a thermostatically controlled block. A gun-type measuring pipette is used to introduce the unknown plasma rapidly into the reagent mixture. An electric switch activated by the pipette plunger causes a timer to start and also causes a mixing head to lower over the cup.

Two small sensing agitators mix the test solution at a regular rate until coagulation occurs. Normally, the coagulum appears quickly, causing a sudden change in the conductivity of the test solution, which, in turn, causes the timer to stop.

The problems associated with electromechanical devices principally involve routine maintenance and attention to technical detail. The probes should be wiped clean of fibrin and carefully rinsed in a saline stream between tests. Failure to do this can result in fibrin cross-contamination of subsequent specimens and, therefore, in markedly shortened test clotting times. The most commonly used electromechanical instrument is the fibrometer manufactured by Becton-Dickinson Company, Rutherford, NJ.

Optical Coagulation Instruments

Clot-detecting devices make use of changes in light transmission when fibrin is formed from fibrinogen in test plasma samples. The increase in optical density is converted to an electrical signal and compared with a reference level. If the signal exceeds the reference, a timing mechanism is stopped.

Optical systems offer some advantages to the electromechanical-based systems, as no cross-contamination is possible, and there is less chance of error because of calibration of distances between electrodes (Walenga et al., 1983). Manufacturers of optical coagulation apparatus include MLA Incorporated, Pleasantville, NY (Electra series); Organon TeKnik Corp., Morris Plains, NJ (Coag-a-mate); Ortho Diagnostics, Raritan, NJ (Koagulab); and Coulter Electronics, Hialeah, FL (ACL).

Electromagnetic Systems

Another concept in clot detection is the use of electromagnetic forces. Plasma containing a magnet is placed in a reservoir surrounded by an electromagnetic field. The reservoir continually moves but, because the plasma is a liquid, the magnet contained therein will always align itself with the poles of the electromagnetic field. However, when a clot is formed, the magnet cannot turn to align itself, and thus a change in the electromagnetic field is detected.

Kinetic Detectors

Two principal kinetic detectors are manufactured. One, manufactured by BioData Corporation (Horsham, PA) photo-optically detects the complete process of clot formation and provides information on the type of clot formed, the progress in time of clot formation, and the presence of any fibrinolysis.

Another instrument, the thromboelastograph (Vol-U-Sol Corporation, Las Vegas, NV) measures the kinetic formation of a clot in whole blood. A pin attached to a recording pen is immersed in whole blood contained in a rotating cup. The pin remains motionless in the blood until a fibrin clot is formed. The fibrin sticks to the cup and the pin, so that the two parts move as one. The pen continually records the motion or lack of motion of the pin. The thromboelastograph will monitor the time of clot formation, type of clot formed, and fibrinolysis if it occurs. Because whole blood is used, the apparatus provides a measure of the combined platelet, red-cell, whole-cell, and coagulation protein function.

Sources of Error

The principal source of error in the electromechanical apparatus has already been described and relates to the contamination of the mixing probes with traces of thrombin from previous testing. The presence of thrombin will produce accelerated coagulation times that are as short as 5 seconds in many cases. Additional errors may be introduced if the heating block is cooler than 36.5°C. Care should be taken to ensure that operating temperatures are correct by monitoring the temperature with a mercury thermometer placed in a tube of saline in one of the wells. If a plunger-type pipette gun is used to dispense reagents and plasma, great care must be exercised to ensure the pipette tips are inserted firmly in the pipette body. Also, when the plunger is depressed, care should be taken to ensure that air bubbles are not aspirated and delivered to the reaction well.

Optical coagulation instruments frequently are available as fully automated units in which patient specimens can be loaded on a refrigerated sample tray and presented sequentially for analysis. If such equipment is not used, and if large numbers of plasma specimens are to be tested, a bowl of crushed ice should be kept available so that plasma specimens waiting to be tested can be stored at 0°C to avoid coagulation factor lability. Optical instrumentation can also produce erroneous results in the presence of clots of poor quality. Such results are often found in hypofibrinogenemia. A clear-cut relationship cannot be documented between the fibrinogen level and test result, but it appears that, for some automated optical systems, fibrinogen levels of approximately 125 mg/dl are the minimum acceptable level, below which erroneous results may occur. Errors have been noted in testing specimens from hypoalbuminemic patients, who usually have elevated levels of IgM (Gutman et al., 1980).

Platelet Aggregometers

Platelet aggregation studies can be carried out using three types of instrumentation: optical aggregometers, luminescence aggregometers, and whole-blood aggregometers. The simple aggregometers measure the optical density changes in platelet-rich plasma that are proportional to the aggregation of the platelets. Many of these are single-channel aggregometers, although some have two- to four-channel simultaneous capabilities.

A modified form of the optical aggregometer is a luminescence apparatus, which measures both luminescence and aggregation simultaneously. Examples of this type of platelet aggregometer are the Lumiaggregometer (Payton Associates, Buffalo, NY) and the Chronolog Lumiaggregometer (Chronolog Corporation, Havertown, PA). Because platelet aggregation is associated with the release of adenosine diphosphate (ADP), these instruments monitor the luminescence created by the action of ADP on a luciferin-luciferase complex. This is measured in relative units. The release reaction and aggregation response are generated simultaneously.

Whole-blood aggregometers measure the charge transition on the platelet surface after an aggregating agent is added to whole blood. Because this instrument measures impedance changes, it is basically an impedometer. Little information on the clinical diagnostic efficacy of this instrument is available (Fareed et al., 1984).

Aggregometers work on a basic spectrophotometric principle. Platelet-rich plasma is obtained by centrifuging citrated whole blood at 1,500g for 3 minutes. The platelet-rich plasma is placed in a glass cuvette, and aggregating agents are added. As the platelets aggregate, more light is transmitted and is collected and measured by a photodetector, producing an aggregation tracing. Platelet aggregometry is discussed in more detail on page 394.

Glossary

Acanthocyte An erythrocyte characterized by irregularly spiculated projections that vary in length and position. This cell is associated with abetalipoproteinemia, liver disease, and postsplenectomy states.

Achlorhydria The absence of free hydrochloric acid in gastric juice.

Adenosine triphosphate A nucleotide that occurs in all cells, in which it functions as the major source of energy.

Albinism The congenital lack of normal pigment caused by a defect of melanin precursors.

Allele One of two or more alternate forms of a gene at the same site in a chromosome.

Alloantibody A term used to describe an antibody produced by one individual that reacts with antigens of another individual of the same species.

Aminopterin An antimetabolite of folic acid originally used in cancer therapy.

Anaphylaxis The manifestation of an immediate hypersensitivity reaction to a foreign antigen.

Angina pectoris A sensation of discomfort felt in the chest that typically appears on exertion. The pain is often caused by a discrepancy between oxygen demand and supply to the myocardium caused by atherosclerosis of the coronary arteries.

Anisocytosis A variation in the size of red blood cells. It is found commonly in most anemias.

Anorexia The loss of appetite.

Anuria The cessation of urine output from the kidneys.

Aplasia The failure of an organ or tissue to develop. Aplastic anemia results from the failure of the bone marrow to produce hematopoietic cells, although the granulocytic, thrombocytic, and erythrocytic elements may not always be affected equally.

Apoferritin A colorless protein found in the mucosal cells of the small intestine. Apoferritin functions by absorbing divalent iron from the gastrointestinal tract into the mucosal cells. The iron then is oxidized to the trivalent ferric form and binds with apoferritin to form ferritin.

Arachidonic acid A naturally occurring fatty acid that is a precursor of prostaglandin and is involved principally in platelet biochemistry.

Asynchronous Not occurring at the same time, as in asynchronous cell maturation, in which the cytoplasm and nuclear maturation take place independently.

Atypical lymphocyte A lymphocyte possessing abnormal morphologic features, principally in the cytoplasm, in which increased basophilia is usually present. Immaturity of the nuclear protein is sometimes also seen. Atypical lymphocytes are now more commonly termed *variant lymphocytes*.

Autosome Any non–sex-linked chromosome.

B lymphocyte A lymphocyte that is bone marrow–derived, migrating to the tissues without being influenced by the thymus. B lymphocytes play a major role in humoral immunity. When stimulated by a specific antigen, they mature into plasma cells capable of synthesizing humoral antibodies.

Basophilic stippling The presence of small basophilic granules in red cells that have been stained by a Romanowsky dye. Increased stippling is found in lead poisoning, thalassemia, and many severe anemias.

Bence-Jones protein An abnormal protein found in the urine of patients with multiple myeloma. The protein is characterized by unusual solubility properties. When heated, it precipitates at 40–60°C and then redissolves on further heating to 80–100°C. The Bence-Jones protein is a monomer or dimer of immunoglobulin light chains, having a molecular weight of 25,000 or 50,000 d.

Biliverdin The first bile pigment formed in the breakdown of heme. Biliverdin is reduced to bilirubin by the enzyme biliverdin reductase, which usually is present in such excess that biliverdin is not found in the plasma, even in severe hemolysis.

Blood island cells Clusters of primitive hematopoietic cells produced in the mesenchyme of the yolk sac.

Carcinoma A malignant neoplasm specified according to its cell of origin.

Ceruloplasmin A copper-containing glycoprotein occurring in the α_2-globulin fraction. Ceruloplasmin is the primary vehicle for copper transport in the tissues. The protein is considered an acute-phase reactant and is increased in physiologic stress, infectious disease, and pregnancy.

Codominant genes The expression of both alleles in a gene pair in the heterozygote in the absence of any influence by the other gene. For example, in individuals of blood group AB, genes that produce A and B antigens are expressed equally.

Collagen A connective tissue protein formed by fibroblasts and other mesenchymal cells.

Colony-forming unit (CFU) A hematopoietic stem cell identified by its ability to produce monoclonal colonies of cells. Included in this class are the pluripotential myeloid stem cell (CFU_S) and the precursors of neutrophils and monocytes (CFU_{NM}), eosinophils (CFU_{EOS}), erythrocytes (CFU_E), and megakaryocytes (CFU_{MEG}).

Conjugated bilirubin Water-soluble bilirubin that has been conjugated in the liver. After formation in the reticuloendothelial cells, bilirubin is transported to the liver in the form of a bilirubin-albumin complex. Here, most of it reacts with D-glucuronate to form water-soluble mono- and diglucuronides.

Deoxyuridine suppression test A test that can determine a lack of 5,10-methylene tetrahydrofolate, caused by either folate or vitamin B_{12} deficiency. Deoxyuridine normally is incorporated into DNA in place of thymidine, so inhibiting the rate of incorporation of ^{3}H-thymidine. With folate or vitamin B_{12} deficiency, the deoxyuridine uptake is inhibited and, consequently, there is less suppression of the ^{3}H-thymidine incorporation.

Diapedesis The passage of erythrocytes and leukocytes from the lumen of a blood vessel to extravascular tissue spaces, without damage to the vessel itself.

Dimorphic Occurring in two different forms.

Disseminated intravascular coagulation (DIC) A disturbance in the hemostatic balance by a procoagulant stimulus that produces the release of tissue factors into the circulation. This syndrome can also be produced by endothelial cell injury and coagulation factor activation. In DIC, platelets and coagulation factors are consumed, fibrin is deposited in small vessels, and the fibrinolytic system is activated, with the subsequent accumulation of fibrin degradation products in the plasma. These products inhibit clot formation. The syndrome is associated with severe hemorrhage resulting from the consumption of many blood coagulation factors (factor VIII, factor V, fibrinogen, platelets), and red-cell fragmentation.

Dyshematopoietic Abnormal hematopoietic activity.

Dyspnea Difficulty in breathing.

Ecchymosis A skin hemorrhage, usually greater than 3 mm in diameter.

Echinocyte A spiculated red cell possessing multiple small projections evenly distributed over the cell surface. Echinocytes occur as artifacts in the preparation of blood smears, but they are also found as true in vivo morphologic changes in patients with renal disease and in individuals on heparin therapy.

Epistaxis Nosebleed.

Erythron An inclusive term for the circulating red cells in the blood, their precursors, and the elements of the body involved in their production.

Erythropoiesis The formation and maturation of erythrocytes.

Erythropoietin A heat-stable glycoprotein produced by the action of renal erythropoietic factor from the kidneys on a liver-produced plasma substrate. The most important action of erythropoietin is to induce erythropoietin-responsive stem cells to differentiate into developing erythrocytes and thereby regulate the rate of cellular production.

Etiology The cause of a disease.

Extracellular Outside the cell. For example, extracellular hemolysis is hemolysis produced by factors external to the cell, such as antibodies.

Folic acid A water-soluble vitamin found principally in leafy green vegetables, eggs, milk, yeast, liver, whole-grain cereals, and fruits. A deficiency of folic acid results in an impairment of nucleic acid synthesis and, consequently, megaloblastic red-cell and leukocyte changes.

Gametocyte A cell that produces gamete; an oocyte or spermatocyte.

Glossitis Inflammation of the tongue.

Glycocalyx A glycoprotein that covers free cell surfaces, seen principally as the outer surface of platelets.

Glycolysis The splitting of glucose into smaller fragments with its conversion to pyruvic acid and, finally, to lactate. By this reaction, 1 mol glucose yields 2 mol lactate anaerobically, with the concomitant production of energy in the form of adenosine triphosphate.

Golgi apparatus An organelle that is found in most cells and functions in secretion and glycoprotein synthesis.

Granulomatous A tissue that is composed of granulomas, which are nodular aggregates of macrophages and lymphocytes involved in organized phagocytic and immune activities, often accompanied by fibroblasts producing collagen tissue.

Granulopoiesis The production and maturation of granulocytic cells.

Haptoglobin A plasma glycoprotein that is produced by liver cells, the principal function of which is to defend against the loss of body iron during intravascular hemolysis. Haptoglobin irreversibly binds to free hemoglobin, forming large complexes that are unable to pass through the glomerular membrane of the kidney. The complex is removed from the circulation by reticuloendothelial cells.

Heinz bodies Heinz bodies are intracellular inclusions attached to the red-cell membrane, producing increased red-cell fragility. The inclusions are 0.3–2.0 μ in diameter and consist of denatured hemoglobin. They are found in thalassemia, in enzymopathies of the hexose monophosphate shunt, following ingestion of primaquine or other drugs precipitating hemolysis, after administration of phenylhydrazine and chlorates, in some unstable hemoglobins (Köln, Zurich), and following splenectomy.

Hemarthrosis   A hemorrhage into the joint, commonly seen in congenital bleeding disorders such as hemophilia.

Hematoma   A collection of extravascular blood localized within a tissue or cavity.

Hematopoiesis   The formation and development of blood cells.

Heme   The non-protein-insoluble iron protoporphyrin constituent of hemoglobin.

Hemoglobin   The oxygen-carrying pigment of red cells. A molecule of hemoglobin contains four different polypeptide chains, each composed of multiple amino acids linked to the heme prosthetic group. The iron of the heme group is responsible for the reaction with oxygen.

Hemoglobinemia   The presence of free hemoglobin in the plasma.

Hemoglobinopathy   A disorder caused by an alteration in the normal molecular structure of hemoglobin, which results in a characteristic complex of clinical and laboratory abnormalities. Examples of hemoglobinopathies include sickle cell anemia and hemoglobin C disease.

Hemoglobinuria   The presence of free hemoglobin in the urine, often caused by intravascular hemolysis.

Hemopexin   A serum protein that possesses an affinity for free heme. It acts as a scavenger and as a transporter of heme, recycling it for hemoglobin synthesis.

Hemosiderin   Iron-containing granules composed of ferric ions that may be aggregates of ferritin. Hemosiderin is found when iron intake is greater than the amount that can be stored in the liver as ferritin. It can be demonstrated in the urine when the centrifuged deposit is stained by an iron stain such as Perls' reaction.

Hepatosplenomegaly   An enlarged liver and spleen, seen in many hematologic disorders.

Heterozygote   An individual who is heterozygous for a particular gene—that is, who possesses two different alleles of a particular gene. A heterozygote has the ability to pass either allele on to an offspring.

Homozygote   An individual who is homozygous for a particular gene—that is, who possesses two identical alleles of a particular gene. A homozygote has the ability to pass this allele on to all offspring.

Howell-Jolly bodies   Small, purple, round or oval inclusion bodies 1 μ in diameter, found in red cells and formed from nuclear fragments. Howell-Jolly bodies are seen after splenectomy, in megaloblastic anemias and, occasionally, in severe hemolytic anemia.

Humoral immunity   A component of the immune system that relates to the production and presence of antibodies and complement.

Hydrophobic   The parts of a molecule that are pushed to the interior of proteins or membranes to be away from water.

Hydrops fetalis   The accumulation of fluid within fetal tissues, as may be seen in severe hemolytic disease of the newborn and α-thalassemia disease (hemoglobin Bart's).

Hyperuricemia   An excess of uric acid in the blood.

Hypochromia   A term used to describe an abnormally low staining intensity of red cells, usually denoting a reduced mean cell hemoglobin concentration. Hypochromic red cells are often seen in iron-deficiency anemia and other severe anemias.

Hypoplastic   A term used to denote incomplete development, such as in hypoplastic bone marrow.

Idiopathic   A term used to describe a disease occurring without known cause.

Intima   A general term used to denote the innermost structure, most frequently describing blood vessels.

Intracellular   A structure situated within a cell.

Intrinsic factor   A glycoprotein secreted by the parietal cells of the gastric mucosa and necessary for the absorption of vitamin B_{12} from the gastrointestinal tract.

Jaundice   A state characterized by yellow discoloration of the skin, mucous membranes, and sclerae, caused by the accumulation of bilirubin. Jaundice is symptomatic of a variety of disorders, including liver disease, gallbladder disease, hemolytic disease, and biochemical abnormalities.

Karyorrhexis   A necrotic process in which the nucleus of a cell breaks down into fragments of variable size that are usually small and round.

Karyotypes   The character of a cell as determined by the nature of the chromosomes in the nucleus. In a nucleated organism, the chromosomes are studied most frequently when the cell is in the metaphase stage of mitosis. Each species has its own characteristic chromosome number and morphologic features. Karyotypes are the systematic display of all the chromosomes in a single somatic cell.

Lymphadenopathy   A general term used to denote any disease of the lymph nodes.

Lymphoma   A term used to describe a neoplastic disorder of the lymphoid tissue.

Lymphopoiesis   The formation and maturation of lymphoid cells.

Lyonization   The phenomenon in which X chromosomes in excess of one in a cell are inactivated. The Lyon hypothesis theorizes that only one of the two X chromosomes in females is active; the other is condensed as sex chromatin. The inactivation occurs in every cell during female embryonic development, although a portion of the short arm remains active on the inactive X chromosome.

Lysosome   A cytoplasmic organelle of a membrane-bound sac of lytic enzymes, which functions as the digestive organ of the cell.

Macrophage   A large bone marrow–produced cell derived from a circulating monocyte. Macrophages are involved in both nonspecific and specific immune responses.

Megaloblast   A large nucleated red blood cell most often associated with deficiencies of vitamin B_{12} or folic acid. Megaloblasts are characterized by asynchronous maturation of the nucleus and cytoplasm. This abnormality is seen as delayed nuclear development together with normal cytoplasmic development.

Menorrhagia   Excessive uterine bleeding.

Mesenchyme Embryonic connective tissue derived from the mesoderm that later becomes the connective tissue and vessels of the body.

Methemoglobin Hemoglobin with iron in the ferric form. This pigment is unable to transport oxygen and is valueless as a respiratory protein. In normal blood, 1% of the total circulating hemoglobin normally is converted to the ferric state each day, with a balance maintained between spontaneous methemoglobin formation and reconversion to deoxyhemoglobin by the methemoglobin reductase system.

Methemoglobinemia The presence of increased amounts of methemoglobin in the blood. This renders the hemoglobin incapable of binding oxygen at physiologic partial pressure. Methemoglobinemia often produces cyanosis.

Methotrexate A folic acid antagonist used in the treatment of neoplasms.

Micropinocytosis A process in which a cell engulfs fluids in a manner similar to that in which a phagocyte engulfs foreign material.

Mitochondria Organelles found in the cytoplasm of most cells. These structures function by producing energy derived from the high-energy phosphate bond of adenosine triphosphate by a process of oxidative phosphorylation.

Myeloma A malignant disease arising from a single clone of plasma cells, leading to the overproduction of specific immunoglobulins.

Myelophthisic anemia An anemia that arises following infiltration of the bone marrow by abnormal cells, most often caused by metastatic carcinoma or myelofibrosis. Such infiltration reduces the hematopoietic function of the bone marrow and results in the release of immature cells into the peripheral blood.

Myelopoiesis The formation and maturation of myeloid cells.

Neoplasm The formation of an abnormal mass of cells typically exhibiting uncontrolled and progressive growth.

Oliguria The finding of decreased urine output in an individual.

Opsonin A factor present in body fluids that can render microorganisms susceptible to phagocytosis. An opsonin may be an antibody capable of binding both a microorganism and a phagocyte.

Pappenheimer bodies Phagosomes formed in red cells that contain iron granules.

Parenchymal cells The cells that make up the parenchyma—that is, the functional elements of an organ as distinguished from its supporting structures.

Parietal cell A large spheroid epithelial cell that is present in the gastric mucosa and secretes hydrochloric acid.

Pathogenesis The biochemical and physiologic mechanisms by which disease progresses.

Pentose-phosphate shunt A branch of the Embden-Meyerhof pathway of carbohydrate metabolism occurring in the cytoplasm of cells.

Petechiae Small hemorrhages into the skin, usually less than 3 mm in diameter.

Pinocyte A cell that engulfs fluid by phagocytic-like action.

Pluripotential cells Hematopoietic stem cells that can give rise to all cells of the myeloid series.

Poikilocytosis The presence of abnormally shaped red cells, most often pear-shaped or tear drop–shaped. This abnormality is seen often in severe anemias, particularly in hemolytic disorders.

Polychromasia Blue gray–tinged red cells seen when the blood is stained by a Romanowsky dye. The appearance of these cells suggests early release from the bone marrow and, consequently, increased erythropoietic activity. Most polychromatic cells are reticulocytes.

Prostaglandins One of a group of fatty acids having numerous biologic functions. For example, PGH_2 is a prostaglandin that possesses vasoconstrictor properties and that also is involved in platelet aggregation.

Protozoa A phylum consisting of simple unicellular organisms made up of four subphyla, Sarcodina (amebae), Mastigophora (flagellates), Ciliophora (ciliates), and Sporozoa.

Prussian blue reaction The colored product formed in the reaction to demonstrate ferric iron.

Pyrexia Fever.

Reactive lymphocyte Synonym for atypical lymphocyte, seen frequently in infectious mononucleosis and other viral diseases.

Renal ischemia The reduction of blood supply to the kidneys.

Reticuloendothelial system Tissues having both endothelial and phagocytic properties. The system includes the spleen, liver, and phagocytes.

Rigors Chills.

Rouleaux formation An aggregate of red cells stacked like a pile of coins and seen in dysproteinemias.

Sarcoma A malignant soft-tissue tumor of mesodermal origin.

Schilling test A nuclear medicine procedure that is used to differentiate macrocytic anemias. This division includes those anemias resulting from an inability to absorb vitamin B_{12} because of a lack of intrinsic factor and those that result from malabsorption disorders, including bacterial overgrowth and fish tapeworm infestation.

Schistocytes An abnormally shaped red blood cell resulting from its entrapment in a fibrin mesh. Schistocytes can be seen in microangiopathic anemias, in disseminated intravascular coagulopathy, in uremic-hemolytic syndrome, in patients with cardiac valve or other prostheses, and in severe burns.

Schizogony The asexual life cycle of Sporozoa (e.g., *Plasmodium*).

Sequela A condition that follows or occurs as a consequence of another event.

Serine protease A proteolytic enzyme that possesses an affinity for amino acid serine.

Serotonin A vasoconstrictor found in the serum and in many tissues including platelets. Serotonin is stored in platelets and released during aggregation.

Sickle cells Red blood cells that have undergone shape deformation resulting from deoxygenation and semisolid gelation of hemoglobin. These changes are reflected in spiculated, holly-leaf, and elongated cells, which, on oxygenation, resume their normal biconcave shape.

Siderocytes Red blood cells containing nonhemoglobin iron (ferritin) either in siderosomes or within the mitochondria. Siderocytes are not visible after staining with Romanowsky dyes and can be observed only if treated first with an iron stain.

Spectrin A structural protein found at the inner surface of the erythrocyte membrane, which serves also as part of a contractile apparatus.

Spherocytosis The presence of biconvex-shaped red cells recognized by their smaller diameter and lack of central pallor. Spherocytes usually have an increased mean cell hemoglobin concentration and also exhibit increased osmotic fragility. The cells most often are seen as a result of red-cell fragmentation, in hereditary spherocytosis, and in other congenital and acquired hemolytic anemias.

Splenomegaly A condition characterized by an enlarged spleen.

Sporozoa A subphylum of protozoa characterized by a lack of organelles for locomotion in the adult stage and a complex life cycle with alternating asexual (schizogony) and sexual (sporogony) multiplication.

Sprue A disease of the small intestine characterized by impaired absorption.

Steatorrhea The excessive loss of fat by way of the feces.

Stomatocyte A cup-shaped red blood cell having a slitlike zone of central pallor. Stomatocytes are seen in hereditary spherocytosis, alcoholism, red blood cell sodium pump defects, and Rh_{null} cells. They can also be seen as artifacts resulting from drug transformation of normal red cells and following a decrease in the blood pH level.

Syncope Fainting or loss of consciousness.

T lymphocyte A lymphocyte that arises in the bone marrow, differentiates in the thymus and, finally, migrates to the lymph nodes and spleen, at which point it is available for cell-mediated immunity. T lymphocytes can be subclassified into those that enhance a B-cell response (helper T cells) and those that inhibit the response (suppressor T cells).

Tachycardia A term referring to a rapid heart rate.

Target cells Hypochromic red cells possessing an increased surface-volume ratio. Target cells commonly are found in thalassemia, iron-deficiency anemia, hemoglobin C disease, and other anemias.

Thymus A bilobed gland involved in the maturation of lymphocytes. Bone marrow–derived lymphocytes migrate to the thymus, at which point they proliferate to become T lymphocytes capable of participating in cell-mediated immune responses.

Totipotential cells Primitive cells from which all cells of the blood are formed.

Transferrin A glycoprotein that functions in the transport of iron from the intestinal tract to the sites of hemoglobin synthesis.

Trophozoites The active stage of a protozoan organism. In the malarial parasite, it is the stage of schizogony between the merozoites and the mature schizont. In the red blood cell, a trophozoite is uninucleated, ring-shaped, ameboid, and vacuolated. As it grows, its nucleus divides by mitosis and matures to become a schizont.

Uricosuria Increased levels of uric acid in the urine.

Urobilin An oxidized form of urobilinogen present in the feces and also seen occasionally in the urine.

Urobilinogen A colorless product of bilirubin formed by the action of intestinal microorganisms. Increased levels of urobilinogen occur in early hepatitis and hemolytic jaundice, and decreases are found in obstructive jaundice and liver disease.

Variant lymphocyte A preferred synonym for atypical or reactive lymphocyte.

Vitamin B_6 A group of water-soluble vitamins found in most foods, especially meats, liver, vegetables, whole-grain cereals, and egg yolks. These vitamins function as coenzymes and participate in the metabolism of amino acids.

Vitamin B_{12} A red hematopoietic vitamin found in the liver, kidneys, and heart muscle. A deficiency of this nutrient arising from the lack of intrinsic factor is termed *pernicious anemia*.

Yolk sac A sac of extraembryonic tissue that is continuous with the embryonic gastrointestinal tract. Primitive blood cells develop within its walls, giving rise to immature erythrocytes.

Appendix I
Common Hematologic Abbreviations

AChE	acetylcholinesterase	**CPD**	citrate-phosphate-dextrose
ADA	adenosine deaminase	**CSF**	cerebrospinal fluid
ADP	adenosine diphosphate	**CV**	coefficient of variation
AIHA	autoimmune hemolytic anemia		
ALA	aminolevulinic acid	**DIC**	disseminated intravascular coagulation
ALL	acute lymphocytic leukemia	**dl**	deciliter
AML	acute myeloid leukemia	**DNA**	deoxyribonucleic acid
AMML	acute myelomonocytic leukemia	**DPG**	diphosphoglycerate
AMoL	acute monocytic leukemia	**dU**	deoxyuridine
AMP	adenosine monophosphate		
ANA	antinuclear antibodies	**EACA**	ε-aminocaproic acid
APL	acute promyelocytic leukemia	**EBV**	Epstein-Barr virus
APTT	activated partial thromboplastin time	**EDTA**	ethylenediaminetetraacetic acid
AT III	antithrombin III	**EM**	electron microscope
ATP	adenosine triphosphate	**ESR**	erythrocyte sedimentation rate
BFU$_E$	burst-forming unit, erythroid	**FDP**	fibrin degradation products
		FEP	free erythrocyte protoporphyrin
C	complement	**FIGlu**	formiminoglutamide
C1, C2	complement fractions	**fl**	femtoliter
cAMP	cyclic adenosine monophosphate		
CDA	congenital dyserythropoietic anemia	**G3PD**	glucose-3-phosphate dehydrogenase
CFU	colony-forming unit	**G6PD**	glucose-6-phosphate dehydrogenase
CFU$_C$	colony-forming unit–culture	**GPI**	glucose phosphate isomerase
CFU$_E$	colony-forming unit–erythroid	**GR**	glutathione reductase
CFU$_{NM}$	colony-forming unit–neutrophil-monocyte	**GSH**	reduced glutathione
		GSSG	oxidized glutathione
CFU$_S$	colony-forming unit–spleen		
CGD	chronic granulomatous disease	**Hb**	hemoglobin
CGP	circulating granulocytic pool	**HbCO**	carboxyhemoglobin
CLL	chronic lymphocytic leukemia	**HbO$_2$**	oxyhemoglobin
CML	chronic myeloid leukemia	**HCD**	heavy-chain disease
CMV	cytomegalovirus	**Hct**	hematocrit

HD	Hodgkin's disease		**ng**	nanogram
HDN	hemolytic disease of the newborn		**NHL**	non-Hodgkin's lymphoma
HE	hereditary elliptocytosis			
HEMPAS	hereditary erythroblastic multinuclearity with positive acidified serum		**PAS**	periodic acid–Schiff
			PCH	paroxysmal cold hemoglobinuria
HK	hexokinase		**PCT**	prothrombin consumption test
HLA	human leukocyte antigen		**6PD**	6-phosphogluconate dehydrogenase
Hp	haptoglobin		**PFK**	phosphofructokinase
HPFH	hereditary persistence of fetal hemoglobin		**pg**	picogram
			PGE,	prostaglandins
			PGF,	
IF	intrinsic factor		**PGD**	
Ig	immunoglobulin			
IRSA	idiopathic refractory sideroblastic anemia		**PHA**	phytohemagglutinin
ITP	idiopathic thrombocytopenic purpura		**PK**	pyruvate kinase
IU	international unit		**PNH**	paroxysmal nocturnal hemoglobinuria
			PT	prothrombin time
LAP	leukocyte alkaline phosphatase		**PTT**	partial thromboplastin time
LDH	lactate dehydrogenase		**PV**	polycythemia vera
MAF	macrophage-activating factor		**RBC**	red blood cell (count)
MAHA	microangiopathic hemolytic anemia		**RES**	reticuloendothelial system
MCD	mean cell diameter		**Retic**	reticulocyte
MCH	mean cell hemoglobin		**RNA**	ribonucleic acid
MCHC	mean cell hemoglobin concentration			
MCV	mean cell volume		**SD**	standard deviation
mEq	milliequivalent		**SLE**	systemic lupus erythematosus
MetHb	methemoglobin		**SR**	sedimentation rate
mg	milligram			
MGP	marginal granulocytic pool		**TC I,**	transcobalamins
MIF	migration inhibitory factor		**TC II,**	
mIU	milli-international unit		**TC III**	
ml	milliliter		**TdT**	terminal deoxynucleotidyl transferase
mmol	millimole		**TF**	transfer factor
μg	microgram		**TIBC**	total iron-binding capacity
μl	microliter		**TPI**	triose phosphate isomerase
			TTP	thrombotic thrombocytopenic purpura
NAD	nicotinamide adenine dinucleotide			
NADP	nicotinamide adenine dinucleotide phosphate		**WBC**	white blood cell (count)
NBT	nitroblue-tetrazolium test		$\bar{X}$	mean

Appendix II
Reference Ranges

Antihuman Globulin Test

Direct method	Negative
Indirect method	Negative

Antithrombin III

Functional method	81–120%
Fluorogenic method	85–115%

Aspirin Tolerance Test

Before aspirin	2–6.5 mins
After aspirin	5–10 mins

Autohemolysis

Initial	0–0.94% lysis
Incubated	0.2–2.7% lysis
Incubated with 10% glucose	0–2.2% lysis
Incubated with 0.4-M ATP	0.5–2.3% lysis

Bleeding Time

Ivy method:

Adults	2–7 mins

Simplate method:

Adults	2.5–6.5 mins
Children	2.5–8.5 mins

Blood Volume

Men	52.2–83.4 ml/kg
Women	59.3–74.5 ml/kg

Bone Marrow Differential

Reticulum cells	0.1–2.0%
Hemocytoblasts	0.1–1.0%
Myeloblasts	0.1–3.5%
Promyelocytes	0.5–5.0%
Myelocytes, neutrophil	5.0–20.0%
Myelocytes, eosinophil	0.1–3.0%
Myelocytes, basophil	0–0.5%
Metamyelocyte	10.0–30.0%
Segmented, neutrophil	7.0–25.0%
Segmented, eosinophil	0.2–3.0%
Segmented, basophil	0–0.5%
Lymphocytes	5.0–20.0%
Monocytes	0–0.2%
Megakaryocytes	0.1–0.5%
Plasma cells	0.1–3.5%
Rubriblasts	0.5–5.0%
Prorubricytes	0–0.5%
Rubricytes	2.0–20.0%
Metarubricytes	2.0–10.0%
Myeloid-to-erythroid ratio	2:1–5:1

Clot Retraction

58–97%

Coagulation Time

Activated	70–100 secs
Lee/White method	6–10 mins

Cold Agglutinin
<1:32

Euglobulin Lysis Test
<2 hrs for complete lysis

Differential Leukocyte Count
Adults: Manual method

Neutrophils	50–75% (2.5–7.5 × 10⁹/liter)
Bands	2–6% (0.1–0.6 × 10⁹/liter)
Eosinophils	1–5% (0.05–0.40 × 10⁹/liter)
Basophils	0–2% (0–0.2 × 10⁹/liter)
Monocytes	2–9% (0.1–0.9 × 10⁹/liter)
Lymphocytes	20–40% (1.0–4.0 × 10⁹/liter)

Infants:

Neutrophils	21–81% (2.1–20.3 × 10⁹/liter)
Eosinophils	0–5% (0–1.3 × 10⁹/liter)
Basophils	0–1% (0–0.3 × 10⁹/liter)
Monocytes	0–6% (0–1.5 × 10⁹/liter)
Lymphocytes	8–38% (0.8–9.4 × 10⁹/liter)

Children:

Neutrophils	33–45% (1.5–6.5 × 10⁹/liter)
Eosinophils	0–5% (0–0.6 × 10⁹/liter)
Basophils	0–2% (0–0.2 × 10⁹/liter)
Monocytes	0–7% (0–0.8 × 10⁹/liter)
Lymphocytes	33–45% (1.5–6.5 × 10⁹/liter)

Adults: Cytochemical method

Neutrophils	47.6–74.6% (2.1–7.8 × 10⁹/liter)
Eosinophils	0.3–5.5% (0.04–0.39 × 10⁹/liter)
Basophils	0.1–1.5% (0.01–0.136 × 10⁹/liter)
Monocytes	1.4–11.6% (0.13–0.86 × 10⁹/liter)
Lymphocytes	15.9–38.6% (1.25–3.38 × 10⁹/liter)
Large unclassified cells	<2.5% (<0.22 × 109/liter)

Erythrocyte Sedimentation Rate
Westergren method:

Men	0–10-mm fall in 1 hour
Women	0–20-mm fall in 1 hour

Wintrobe method:

Men	0–7-mm fall in 1 hour
Women	0–15-mm fall in 1 hour

Zeta sedimentation rate:

Adults	40–51%

Micro method:

Men	0–10-mm fall in 1 hour
Women	0–20-mm fall in 1 hour

Ethanol Gel Test
Negative

Factor II
50–150%

Factor V
50–150%

Factor VII
50–150%

Factor VIII
50–150%

Factor VIII$_{RA}$
70–150%

Factor VIII$_{VW}$
50–130%

Factor IX
50–150%

Factor X
50–150%

Factor XI
50–150%

Factor XII
30–200%

Fibrin Degradation Products

Plasma	0.4 µg fibrinogen equivalents/ml
Urine	<0.25 µg/ml
Thrombo-Wellcotest	0–10 µg/ml

Fibrinogen
2.0–4.0 g/liter

Glucose-6-Phosphate Dehydrogenase
$6.5–7.9$ units $\times 10^9$ red cells

Glutathione
600–900 mg/liter red cells

Haptoglobin, Plasma
60–270 mg/dl

Hematocrit
Male adult	0.365–0.520
Female adult	0.330–0.470
Newborn	0.400–0.644
Child, 1 month old	0.256–0.427
Child, 1 year old	0.270–0.450
Child, 10 years old	0.331–0.484

Hemoglobin
Male adult	13.0–18.2 g/dl
Female adult	11.0–16.3 g/dl
Newborn	13.6–19.6 g/dl
Child, 1 month old	9.5–12.5 g/dl
Child, 1 year old	11.0–13.0 g/dl
Child, 10 years old	11.5–14.8 g/dl

Hemoglobin A
Cellulose acetate electrophoresis method	97–100%

Hemoglobin A_2
Column chromatography method	1.7–3.5%

Hemoglobin Bart's
Cord blood	0–1%

Hemoglobin F
Alkali denaturation method	0–2%

Heterophil Antibody
<1:56

Leukocyte Alkaline Phosphatase Stain
Adults	15–100
Newborn	150–300

Mean Cell Hemoglobin
27.0–35.0 pg

Mean Cell Hemoglobin Concentration
31.0–37.0 g/dl

Mean Cell Volume
75–100 fl

Methemoglobin
0–2%

Muramidase, Serum
5–15 µg/ml

Nitroblue-Tetrazolium Reduction Test
2–22%

Osmotic Fragility Test
Saline (%)	Immediate (%)	Incubated (%)
0.2	97–100	95–100
0.3	90–97	85–100
0.35	50–95	75–100
0.4	5–45	65–100
0.45	0–6	55–100
0.5	0	40–85
0.55	0	15–70
0.6	0	0–40
0.65	0	0–10
0.7	0	0–5

Partial Thromboplastin Time (Activated)
Ellagic acid activators	25–35 secs
Diatomaceous earth activators	35–45 secs

Plasma Hemoglobin
10–70 mg/liter

Plasma Volume
Men   25.2–43.2 ml/kg
Women 28.0–45.2 ml/kg

Plasminogen
Chemical method	1.5–4.0 U/ml plasma
Fluorogenic method	2.4–3.8 CTA U/ml

Platelet Adhesion Test
24–58%

Platelet Count
$150–450 \times 10^9$ /liter

Platelet Factor 3 Activity
>25%

Protamine Sulfate Test
Negative

Prothrombin Consumption Test
0–30%

Prothrombin Time
10–13 secs

Protein C
Functional	74–151%
Antigen	>70%

Protein S
Functional	65–140%
Antigen, total	>79%
Antigen, free	>78%

Pyruvate Kinase
1.2–2.2 IU/ml red cells

Red-Blood-Cell Count
Male adult	$4.20–6.10 \times 10^{12}$/liter
Female adult	$3.70–5.50 \times 10^{12}$/liter
Newborn	$4.00–5.60 \times 10^{12}$/liter
Child, 1 month old	$3.20–4.50 \times 10^{12}$/liter
Child, 1 year old	$3.60–5.20 \times 10^{12}$/liter
Child, 10 years old	$4.20–5.20 \times 10^{12}$/liter

Red-Cell Volume
Men	20.2–36.2 ml/kg
Women	19.3–31.0 ml/kg

Reptilase Test
18–22 secs

Reticulocytes
Adults	0.5–1.5% ($25–75 \times 10^9$/liter)
Infants	2.0–6.0% ($96–288 \times 10^9$/liter)

Russell's Viper Venom Test
11–15 secs

Siderocytes
0.4–0.6%

Système International D'Unités (SI Units)
See Table 1.

Thrombin Time
11–13 secs

Tourniquet Test
<10 petechiae in 6-cm diameter circle

Unstable Hemoglobin
<5% normal hemoglobin precipitated at 50°C

Viscosity, Serum
1.2–1.8 × water

White-Blood-Cell Count
Adult	$3.9–10.9 \times 10^9$/liter
Newborn	$10.0–25.0 \times 10^9$/liter
Child, 1 month old	$7.0–15.0 \times 10^9$/liter
Child, 1 year old	$6.0–15.0 \times 10^9$/liter
Child, 10 years old	$4.5–12.0 \times 10^9$/liter

Table 1. Système International D'Unités (SI Units)

Entity	Abbreviation	Recommended Units	Obsolete Units
Differential leukocyte count	—	Ratio (i.e., 0.5 = 50%) or 10^9/liter	%
Hemoglobin	Hb	g/dl	g/100 ml
Mean cell diameter	MCD	μ	—
Mean cell hemoglobin	MCH	pg	μμg
Mean cell hemoglobin concentration	MCHC	g/dl	%
Mean cell volume	MCV	fl	cuμ
Packed cell volume (hematocrit)	PCV (Hct)	Ratio (no unit needed; 1:1 implied)	%
Partial thromboplastin time	PTT	s	sec
Platelet count	—	10^9/liter	10^3/mm^3
Plasma fibrinogen	—	g/liter	mg/100 ml
Plasma hemoglobin	Plasma Hb	mg/liter	mg/100 ml
Prothrombin time	PT	s	sec
Red blood cell count	RBC	10^{12}/liter	10^6/mm^3
Reticulocyte count	—	% or 10^9/liter	mm^3
Sedimentation rate	ESR	mm/hr	—
White blood cell count	WBC	10^9/liter	10^3/mm^3

References

Abildgaard CF, Harrison J. Fletcher factor deficiency: family study and detection. Blood 43:641, 1974.

Abildgaard CF, Sidzucki Z, et al. Serial studies in the von Willebrand's disease variability versus "variants." Blood 56:712, 1980.

Abrahamson S, Miller RG, et al. The identification in adult bone marrow of pluripotential and restricted stem cells of the myeloid and lymphoid systems. J Exp Med 145:1567, 1977.

Abramsky O, Slavin S. Neurologic manifestations in patients with mixed cryoglobulinemia. Neurology 24:245, 1974.

Adams JG, Steinberg M. Alpha thalassemia. Am J Hematol 2:317, 1977.

Aledort LM. Causes of death in hemophilia. National Institutes of Health Workshop on unsolved problems in hemophilia. Bethesda, MD, March 1976.

Alkjaersig N, Fletcher AD, et al. The mechanism of clot dissolution by plasmin. J Clin Invest 38:1086, 1959.

Allen JK, Batjer JD. Evaluation of an automated method for leukocyte differential counts based on electronic volume analysis. Arch Pathol Lab Med 109:534, 1985.

Allen RH, Majerus PW. Isolation of vitamin B_{12}-binding proteins using affinity chromatography III. Purification and properties of human plasma transcobalamin II. J Biol Chem 247:7709, 1972.

Allen RR, Wadsworth LD, et al. Congenital erythroleukemia: a case report with morphological, immunophenotypic and cytogenetic findings. Am J Hematol 31:114, 1989

Amador E. Quality control by the reference sample method. Am J Clin Pathol 50:360, 1968.

Andrew M, Bhogal M, et al. Factors XI and XII and prekallikrein in sick and healthy premature infants. N Engl J Med 305:1130, 1981.

Anselstetter M, Horstmann HT, et al. Congenital dyserythropoietic anemia, types I and II: aberrant pattern of erythrocyte membrane proteins in CDAII, as revealed by two dimensional polyacrylamide gel electrophoresis. Br J Haematol 35:209, 1977.

Axline SG. Functional biochemistry of the macrophage. Semin Hematol 7:142, 1970.

Babior BM, Woodman RC. Chronic granulomatous disease. Semin Hematol 27:247, 1990.

Baehner RI, Nathan DG. Leukocyte oxidase, defective activity in chronic granulomatous disease. Science 155:835, 1967.

Baehner RI, Nathan DG. Quantitative nitroblue tetrazolium test in chronic granulomatous disease. N Engl J Med 278:971, 1968.

Baele G, DePalpe M, et al. Pseudothrombocytopenia. Acta Clin Belg 33:303, 1978.

Baglioni C. Abnormal human hemoglobins: X. A study of hemoglobin Lepore$_{BOSTON}$. Biochim Biophys Acta 97:37, 1965.

Banez E, Triplett D, et al. Laboratory monitoring of heparin therapy—the effect of different salts of heparin on the activated partial thromboplastin time. An analysis of the 1978 and 1979 CAP hematology survey. Am J Clin Pathol 74:569, 1980.

Barbui T, Finazzi G, et al. Hereditary dysfunctional protein C (protein C Bergamo) and thrombosis. Lancet 6:819, 1984.

Barnard DF, Barnard SA, et al. Detection of important abnormalities of the differential count using the Coulter STKR blood counter. J Clin Pathol 42:772, 1989

Barrett BA, Hill PI. A micromethod for the erythrocyte sedimentation rate suitable for use on venous or capillary blood. J Clin Pathol 33:1118, 1980.

Barrow EM, Graham JB. Blood coagulation factor VIII (antihemophilic factor) with comments on von Willebrand's disease and Christmas disease. Physiol Rev 54:23, 1974.

Barrow GH. Application of DNA probes to hematology: an overview with selected examples. Ann Clin Lab Sci 19:139, 1989.

Barrowcliffe TW. Studies on the binding of heparin to ATIII by crossed immunoelectrophoresis. Thromb Haemost 42:1434, 1979.

Baumgarten W, Wegner A, et al. Calla-positive acute leukemia with t(5q;14q) translocations and hypereosinophilia—a unique entity. Acta Haematol 82:85, 1989.

Beautyman W, Bills T. Osmotic error in erythrocyte volume determinations. Am J Hematol 12:383, 1982.

Beck JR, Cornwell GG. "The iron screen" modification of standard laboratory practice with data analysis. Hum Pathol 12:118, 1981.

Beck WS. Hematology (3rd ed). Cambridge, MA: MIT Press, 1982a. P 15.

Beck WS. Hematology (3rd ed). Cambridge, MA: MIT Press, 1982b.

Becker W. Determination of antisera titres using the single radial immunodiffusion method. Immunochemistry 6:539, 1969.

Beeson PB, Bass DA. The Eosinophil. In Major Problems in Internal Medicine. Vol 14. Philadelphia: Saunders, 1977.

Begtrup H, Leroy S, et al. Average of normals used as a control of accuracy, and a comparison with other controls. Scand J Clin Lab Invest 27:247, 1971.

Beller FK, Graeff H. Equipment and General Requirements of the Coagulation Laboratory. In NU Ban, FK Beller, et al. (eds), Thrombosis and Bleeding Disorders: Theory and Methods. New York: Academic, 1971.

Bennett B, Ratnoff OD. Detection of the carrier state for classic hemophilia. N Engl J Med 288:342, 1973.

Bennett B, Ratnoff OD, et al. Hageman trait (factor XII deficiency): a probable second genotype inherited as an autosomal dominant characteristic. Blood 40:412, 1972.

Bennett JM, Catovsky D, et al. Proposals for the classification of acute leukemias. Br J Haematol 33:451, 1976.

Bennett JM, Catovsky D, et al. A variant form (M3) of hypergranular promyelocytic leukemia. Br J Haematol 44:169, 1980.

Bennett JM, Catovsky D, et al. The morphological classification of acute lymphoblastic leukemia: concordance among observers and clinical correlations. Br J Haematol 47:553, 1981.

Bennett JM, Catovsky D, et al. Proposals for the classification of the myelodysplastic syndromes. Br J Haematol 51:189, 1982.

Bennett JM, Catovsky D, et al. Criteria for the diagnosis of acute leukemia of megakaryocytic lineage (M7). Ann Intern Med 103:460, 1985.

Bennett JM, Catovsky D, et al. Proposals for the classification of chronic (mature) B & T lymphoid leukemia. J Clin Pathol 42:567, 1989.

Benson PF, Chisholm JJ. A reliable qualitative urine coproporphyrin test for lead intoxication in young children. J Pediatr 56:759, 1960.

Berenbaum MC. The use of bovine albumin in the preparation of marrow and blood films. J Clin Pathol 9:381, 1956.

Berlin NJ. Diagnosis and classification of the polycythemias. Semin Hematol 12:339, 1975.

Bernard P, Dashary D, et al. Acute nonlymphocytic leukemia with marrow eosinophilia and chromosome 16 abnormality: a report of 18 cases. Leukemia 3:740, 1989.

Bertazonni U, Brusamolino E, et al. Prognostic significance of terminal transferase and adenosine deaminase in acute and chronic myeloid leukemia. Blood 60:685, 1982.

Bertina RM, Brockmans AW, et al. Protein C deficiency in a Dutch family with thrombotic disease. Thromb Haemost 48:1, 1982.

Bessman JD. Prediction of platelet production during chemotherapy for acute leukemia. Am J Hematol 13:219, 1983a.

Bessman JD. New parameters on automated hematology instruments. Lab Med 14:488, 1983b.

Bessman JD, Feinstein DI. Quantitative anisocytosis as a discriminant between iron deficiency and thalassemia minor. Blood 53:288, 1979.

Bessman JD, Williams LJ, et al. Mean platelet volume: inverse relation between platelet count and size in normal subjects and an artifact of other particles. Am J Clin Pathol 76:289, 1981.

Bessman JD, Williams LJ, et al. Platelet size in health and hematologic disease. Am J Clin Pathol 78:150, 1982.

Betke K, Marti HQ, et al. Estimation of small percentages of foetal hemoglobin. Nature 184:1877, 1959.

Beutler E. A series of new screening procedures for pyruvate kinase deficiency, glucose-6-phosphate dehydrogenase deficiency, and glutathione reductase deficiency. Blood 28:553, 1966.

Beutler E. Red cell enzyme defects as nondiseases and as diseases. Blood 54:1, 1979.

Beutler E, Duron O, et al. Improved method for the determination of blood glutathione. J Lab Clin Med 61:882, 1963.

Beutler E, Hartman G. Age-related red cell enzyme in children with transient erythroblastopenia of childhood and with hemolytic anemia. Pediatr Res 19:44, 1985.

Bick RL. Clinical relevance of antithrombin III. Semin Thromb Hemost 8:276, 1982.

Bick RL. Disseminated Intravascular Coagulation and Related Syndromes. In Disseminated Intravascular Coagulation. Boca Raton, FL: CRC Press, 1983. P 31.

Bick RL, Kovacs I, et al. A new two-stage functional assay for antithrombin III: clinical and laboratory evaluation. Thromb Res 8:745, 1976.

Bick RL, Murano G. Primary Hyperfibrino(geno)lytic Syndromes. In Basic Concepts of Hemostasis and Thrombosis. Boca Raton, FL: CRC Press, 1985. P 181.

Bick RL, Wheeler A, et al. A comparative study of the DuPont antithrombin III and fibrinogen assay systems. Am J Clin Pathol 83:541, 1985.

Bierenbaum ML, Fleischman AI, et al. Effect of cigarette smoking upon in vivo platelet function in man. Thromb Res 12:1051, 1978.

Biggs R, Douglas AS. The measurement of prothrombin in plasma. J Clin Pathol 6:15, 1953.

Biggs R, Nossel HL. Tissue extract and the contact reaction in blood coagulation. Thromb Diath Haemorrh 6:1, 1961.

Bizzaro N, Brandalise M. EDTA-dependent pseudothrombocytopenia. Am J Clin Pathol 103:103, 1995.

Bjerrum OW, Philip P, et al. Acute lymphocytic leukemia with t(4;11): a clinical subentity. Scand J Haematol 35:96, 1985

Bjornsson T, Nash PV. Variability in heparin sensitivity of APTT reagents. Am J Clin Pathol 86:199, 1986.

Block MH. Ferritin [letter to the editor]. Lab Man, 10:4, 1980.

Blomback B, Blomback M, et al. Coagulation studies on "Reptilase," an extract of the venom from *Bothrops jararaca*. Thromb Diath Haemorrh 1:1, 1957.

Bockenstedt P, Greenberg JM, et al. Structural basis of Von Willebrand factor binding to platelet glycoprotein Ib and collagen. J Clin Invest 77:743, 1986.

Boggs DR, Boggs SS. The pathogenesis of aplastic anemia. Blood 48:71, 1976.

Bollinger PB, Drewinko B, et al. The Technicon H-1: an automated hematology analyzer for today and tomorrow. Am J Clin Pathol 87:71, 1987.

Bond VP. Proliferative potentials of bone marrow and blood cells studied by in vitro uptake of H^3-thymidine. Acta Haematol 21:1, 1959.

Bondue H, Machin D, et al. The leucocyte alkaline phosphatase activity in mature neutrophils of different ages. Scand J Haematol 24:51, 1980.

Boneu B, Sie P, et al. Macrothrombocytose et purpura thrombocytopenique idiopathique effect de l'anticoagulant et de la fixation prealable sur la plaquettaire par le systeme Coulter. Nouv Rev Fr Hematol 28:15, 1986.

Boneventura J, Riggs A. Polymerization of hemoglobins of mouse and man: structural basis. Science 158:800, 1967.

Bookchin RM, Davis RP. Hemoglobin C-Harlem: a sickling variant containing amino acid substitutions in two residues of the β-polypeptide chain. Biochem Biophys Res Commun 23:122, 1968.

Borchgrevink CF. A method for measuring platelet adhesiveness in vivo. Acta Med Scand 168:157, 1960.

Borchgrevink CF, Waaler BA. The secondary bleeding time. Acta Med Scand 162:361, 1958.

Böttiger LE, Svedberg CA. Normal erythrocyte sedimentation rate and age. Br Med J 2:85, 1967.

Boyer SH, Graham JB. Linkage between the X-chromosome loci for glucose-6-phosphate dehydrogenase electrophoretic variant and hemophilia. Am J Hum Genet 17:320, 1965.

Boyer WH. CRC Handbook of Tables for Probability and Statistics. Boca Raton, FL: CRC Press, 1966.

Brandt J, Triplett D. Laboratory monitoring of heparin. Effects of reagents and instruments on the activated partial thromboplastin time. Am J Clin Pathol 76(suppl):530, 1981.

Brandt J, Triplett D. The sensitivity of different coagulation reagents to the presence of lupus anticoagulants. Arch Pathol Lab Med 111:120, 1987.

Brandt JT, Arkin CF, et al. Evaluation of APTT reagent sensitivity to Factor IX and Factor IX assay performance. Arch Pathol 114:135, 1990.

Breen FA, Tullis JL. Ethanol-gelation: a rapid screening test for intravascular coagulation. Ann Intern Med 69:1197, 1968.

Briddell RA, Brandt JE, et al. Characterization of the human burst-forming unit—megakaryocyte. Blood 74:145, 1989.

Brill AB, Tomonoga M, et al. Leukemia in man following exposure to ionizing irradiation: summary of findings in Hiroshima and Nagasaki and comparison to other human experience. Ann Intern Med 56:590, 1962.

Brinkhous KM, Roberts HR, et al. Prevalence of inhibitors in hemophilia A and B. Thromb Diath Haemorrh 51(suppl):315, 1972.

Brittin GM, Brecher GB. Instrumentation and automation in clinical hematology. Prog Hematol 7:299, 1971.

Brittin GM, Brecher GB, et al. Stability of blood in commonly used anticoagulants. Am J Clin Pathol 52:690, 1969.

Brittenham G, Lozoff B, et al. Sickle Cell Disease Among the Veddoid Groups of South India. In JI Hechter, AW Schechter, et al. (eds), Proceedings of the First National Symposium on Sickle Cell Disease (pub no. 75-723). Washington, DC: Department of Health, Education and Welfare, 1974. P 257.

Brody JI, Pickering NJ, et al. Coronary artery deposition of factor VIII–related antigen in ischemic heart disease. Am J Clin Pathol 86:269, 1986.

Brouet JC, Seligmann M. The immunological classification of acute lymphoblastic leukemia. Cancer 42(suppl): 817, 1978.

Brown GO, Herbig FK, et al. Leukopenia in negroes. N Engl J Med 275:1410, 1966.

Broxmeyer H, Van Zant G, et al. Mechanisms of leukocyte production of release: XII. A comparative assay of the leukocytosis-inducing factor (LIF) of the colony stimulating factors (CSF). Proc Soc Exp Biol Med 145:1262, 1974.

Bruckner DA, Garcia LS, et al. Babesiosis: problems in diagnosis using autoanalyzers. Am J Clin Pathol 83:520, 1985.

Brunangelo F, Schwarting R, et al. The differential diagnosis of hairy cell leukemia with a panel of monoclonal antibodies. Am J Clin Pathol 83:289, 1985.

Buchanon CR, Holtkamp GA. Prolonged bleeding time in children and young adults with hemophilia. Pediatrics 66:951, 1980.

Budzynski AZ, and Marder VJ. Degradation pathway of fibrinogen by plasmin. Thromb Haemost 38:793, 1977.

Bull BS, Brailsford JD. The zeta sedimentation rate. Blood 40:550, 1972.

Bull BS, Brecher G. An evaluation of the relative merits of the Wintrobe and Westergren sedimentation methods, including hematocrit correction. Am J Clin Pathol 62:502, 1974.

Bull BS, Elashoff RM, et al. A study of various estimators for the derivation of quality control procedures from patient erythrocytic indices. Am J Clin Pathol 61:475, 1974.

Bull BS, Hay KL. Are red blood cell indexes international? Arch Pathol Lab Med 109:604, 1985.

Bull MH, Huse WM, et al. Evaluation of tests used to monitor heparin therapy during extracorporeal circulation. Anesthesia 43:346, 1975.

Bunn F, Schechter AN. Hemoglobinopathies [educational program]. Chicago: American Society of Hematologists, 1983. P 8.

Bunn HF, Forget BG, et al. Human Hemoglobins. Philadelphia: Saunders, 1977.

Burger RK, Schneider RJ, et al. Human plasma R-type vitamin B_{12}-binding proteins: I. Isolation and characterization of transcobalamin I, transcobalamin III, and normal granulocytic vitamin B_{12}-binding protein. J Biol Chem 250:7700, 1975.

Burka ER, Weaver Z, et al. Clinical spectrum of hemolytic anemia associated with glucose-6-phosphate dehydrogenase deficiency. Ann Intern Med 64:817, 1966.

Burkart PT, Hay TCS. IgM cold-warm hemolysins in infectious mononucleosis. Transfusion 19:535, 1979.

Butterworth AE, David JR. Eosinophil function. N Engl J Med 304:154, 1981.

Caimo A, Parodi CM, et al. A new unusual translocation involving the short arms of chromosome 19 in Ph^1-positive chronic myeloid leukemia. Acta Haematol 71:124, 1984.

Calam RR, Cooper MH. Recommended "order of draw" for collecting blood specimens into additive-containing tubes. Clin Chem 28:1299, 1982.

Caramihai E, Karayalcin G, et al. Leukocyte count differences in healthy white and black children. J Pediatr 86:252, 1975.

Carrell RW, Kay R. A simple method for the detection of unstable hemoglobin. Br J Haematol 23:615, 1972.

Carstairs KC, Breckenridge A. Incidence of a positive direct Coombs' test in patients on methyldopa. Lancet 2:133, 1966.

Cassidy PG, Triplett DA, et al. Use of the agarose gel method to identify and quantitate factor VIII:C. Am J Clin Pathol 83:697, 1985.

Catovsky D. The Leukemic Cell. Edinburgh: Churchill Livingstone, 1981.

Catovsky D, O'Brien M, et al. Ultrastructural cytochemical and surface marker analysis of cells during blastic crisis of CGL. Boll 1st Sieroter Milan 57:344, 1978.

Catovsky D, Shaw MT, et al. Sideroblastic anaemia and its association with leukaemia and myelomatosis: a report of five cases. Br J Haematol 20:385, 1971.

Cembrowski GS, Westgard JO. Quality control of multichannel hematology analyzers: evaluation of Bull's algorithm. Am J Clin Pathol 83:337, 1985.

Champlin RE, Golde DW. Chronic myelogenous leukemia: recent advances. Blood 65:1039, 1985.

Chanarin I. The Megaloblastic Anemias. Philadelphia: Davis, 1969.

Chanarin I, James D. Humoral and cell-mediated intrinsic factor antibody in pernicious anemia. Lancet 1:1078, 1974.

Chandler D, Daniel SJ. Isoimmune neonatal thrombocytopenia: a case report and review. Am J Clin Pathol 83:766, 1985.

Chang JC, Van der Hoeven LH, et al. Glutathione reductase in the red blood cells. Ann Clin Lab Sci 8:23, 1978.

Chavin SI. Factor VIII: structure and function in blood clotting. Am J Hematol 16:297, 1984.

Chen KTK, Marsh H. Philadelphia chromosome–negative myelogenous leukemia with prominent eosinophilic component. Am J Clin Pathol 81:789, 1984.

Chervenick PA, LoBuglio AF. Human blood monocytes: stimulation of granulocyte and mononuclear colony formation in vitro. J Lab Clin Med 86:112, 1975.

Ching-Hai P, Behm FG, et al. Secondary acute myeloid leukemia in childhood treated for acute lymphoid leukemia. N Engl J Med 321:136, 1989.

Chisholm E. *Babesia microt* infection in man: evaluation of an indirect immunofluorescent antibody test. Am J Trop Med Hyg 27:14, 1978.

Church MK, Holgate ST. The Basophil Leucocyte: Morphological, Immunological, and Biochemical Considerations. In S Roath (ed), Topical Reviews in Haematology. Vol 1. Bristol, UK: Wright, 1980.

Cline MJ, Le Fevre G, et al. Organ interactions in the regulation of hematopoiesis. In vitro interactions of bone, thymus, and spleen with bone marrow stem cells in normal S1/S1^d and W/W^v mice. J Cell Physiol 90:105, 1977

Clouse LH, Comp PC. The regulation of hemostasis: the protein C system. N Engl J Med 314:1298, 1986.

Cohen P, Gardner FH. The thrombocytopenic effect of sustained high dosage prednisone therapy in thrombocytopenic purpura. N Engl J Med 265:611, 1961.

Cohen PR, Kurzrock R. Chronic myelogenous leukemia and Sweet syndrome. Am J Hematol 32:134, 1989.

Cohle SD, Saleem A, et al. Effects of storage of blood on stability of hematologic parameters. Am J Clin Pathol 76:67, 1981.

Coleman MS, Greenwood MF, et al. Adenosine deaminase, terminal deoxynucleotidyl transferase (TdT) and cell surface markers in childhood acute leukemia. Blood 52:1125, 1978.

Coleman MS, Hutton JJ. Terminal Transferase. In D Catovsky (ed), Methods in Haematology: 2. The Leukemic Cell. London: Churchill Livingstone, 1981. P 203.

Coller BS, Franza BR, et al. The pH dependence of quantitative ristocetin-induced platelet aggregation: theoretical and practical implications—a new device for maintenance of platelet-rich-plasma pH. Blood 47:841, 1976.

Comp PC, Esmon CT. Generation of fibrinolytic activity by infusion of activated protein C into dogs. J Clin Invest 68:1221, 1981.

Comp PC, Esmon CT. Recurrent venous thromboembolism in patients with a partial deficiency of protein S. N Engl J Med 31:1525, 1984.

Conlan M, Haire WD. Low protein S in essential thrombocytopenia. Am J Hematol 32:88, 1989.

Cook JD, Finch CA. Assessing iron states of a population. Am J Clin Nutr 32:2115, 1979.

Cornbleet J, Kessinger S. Evaluation of Coulter-S-Plus three-part differential in populations with a high prevalence of abnormalities. Am J Clin Pathol 84:620 1985.

Coulter Diagnostics. A closer look at the method. Coulter Currents 9:7, 1981.

Coulter Instruments. Coulter Counter Model S-Plus: Instruction Manual (2nd issue). Hialeah, FL: Coulter Instruments, April 1979.

Council on Food and Nutrition. Iron deficiency in the United States. JAMA 203:407, 1968.

Counts RB. Acquired Bleeding Disorders. In JE Menitove, LJ McCarthy (eds), Hemostatic Disorders and the Blood Bank. Arlington, VA: American Association of Blood Banks, 1984. P 41.

Cowan DH, Haut MJ. Platelet function in acute leukemia. J Lab Clin Med 79:893, 1972.

Cox JC, Endes-Brook J, et al. The effect of ABO blood groups on the diagnosis of von Willebrand disease. Blood 69:1691, 1987.

Criel A, Collen D, et al. A case of IgM antibodies which inhibit the contact activation of blood coagulation. Thromb Res 12:883, 1978.

Crook L, Liu PI, et al. Erythrocyte sedimentation, viscosity, and plasma proteins in disease detection. Ann Clin Lab Sci 10:368, 1980.

Crosby W. Reticulocyte counts. Arch Intern Med 141:1747, 1981.

Cruikshank JM. The effects of parity on the leucocyte count in pregnant and non-pregnant women. Br J Haematol 185:31, 1970.

Cudak G. Reticulocyte counting. Lab Perspect 1:17, 1982.

Cudak G. Leukocyte alkaline phosphatase stain. Lab Perspect 3:9, 1983.

Cullen MH, Rees GM, et al. The effect of nitrous oxide on the cell cycle in human bone marrow. Br J Haematol 42:527, 1979.

Cuttner J, Seremetis S, et al. TdT positive acute leukemia with monocytoid characteristics: clinical, cytochemical, cytogenetic, and immunologic findings. Blood 64:237, 1984.

Dacie JV (ed). Secondary or Symptomatic Haemolytic Anemias: The Haemolytic Anemias. New York: Grune & Stratton, 1967. P 908.

Dacie JV, Lewis SL. Practical Haematology (5th ed). Edinburgh: Churchill Livingstone, 1975.

da Prada A, Jakabova R, et al. Subcellular localization of the heparin neutralizing factor in blood platelets. J Physiol 257:495, 1976.

Dausset J, Colombari J, et al. Studies of leukopenias and thrombocytopenias by the direct antiglobulin test on leukocytes and/or platelets. Blood 18:672, 1961.

Davey FR, Nelson DA. Leukocyte Disorders. In JB Henry (ed), Clinical Diagnosis and Management by Laboratory Methods (17th ed). Philadelphia: Saunders, 1984. P 734.

David O, Vota MG, et al. Pyrimidine 5' nucleotidase acquired deficiency in β thalassemia: involvement of enzyme-SH groups in the inactivation process. Acta Haematol 82:69, 1989.

Davidsohn I, Nelson DA. In Clinical Diagnosis by Laboratory Methods (15th ed). Philadelphia: Saunders, 1974. P 262.

Davie EW, Fujikawa K. Basic mechanisms in blood coagulation. Annu Rev Biochem 44:799, 1975.

Davson J, Mallick NP, et al. Heterophile antibody and histiocytic medullar reticulosis. Clin Lab Haematol 3:77, 1981.

DeMarco L, Girolami A, et al. Von Willebrand factor interaction with the glycoprotein IIb/IIIa complex. J Clin Invest 77:1272, 1986.

Denburg JA, Temesuari P. Basophilic mast cell precursors in human blood. Blood 61:775, 1983.

Denson KWE, Lurie A, et al. The factor X defect: recognition of abnormal forms of factor X. Br J Haematol 18:371, 1970.

Deubelbeiss KA, Dancey JT, et al. Neutrophil kinetics in the dog. J Lab Invest 55:833, 1975.

Dexter TM, Allen TD, et al. Conditions controlling the proliferation of haematopoietic stem cells in vitro. J Cell Physiol 91:355, 1977.

Deykin D, Cochios F. Hepatic removal of activated factor X by the perfused rabbit liver. Am J Physiol 214:414, 1968.

Didisheim P. Screening tests for bleeding disorders. Am J Clin Pathol 47:622, 1967.

Didisheim P, Lewis JH. Congenital disorders of the mechanism for coagulation of blood. Pediatrics 22:478, 1958.

Di Donato C, Croci C, et al. Chronic neutrophilic leukemia: description of a new case with karyotypic abnormalities. Am J Clin Pathol 85:369, 1986.

Diess A, Kurth D. Experimental production of siderocytes. J Clin Invest 45:353, 1969.

DiGiovanni S, Valentini G, et al. Beta-2-microglobulin is a reliable tumor marker in chronic lymphocytic leukemia. Acta Haematol 87:181, 1989.

Dimmock V. Methyl-green pyronin staining of blood and bone marrow smears. Med Lab Sci 173:34, 1977.

DiScipio RG, Hermodson MA, et al. A comparison of human prothrombin, factor IX (Christmas factor), factor X (Stuart factor), and protein S. Biochemistry 16:698, 1977.

Doig R, O'Malley CJ, et al. An evaluation of 200 consecutive patients with spontaneous or recurrent thrombosis for primary hypercoagulable states. Am J Clin Pathol 102:797, 1994.

d'Onofrio G, Mango G. Non-Hereditary Myeloperoxidase Deficiency. In E Simson (ed), Hematology Beyond the Microscope. Tarrytown, PA: Technicon Instruments Corp, 1984. P 58.

Doyle CT. The effect of blood volume and choice of anticoagulant on the PCV, MCHC, and total white cell count. Ir J Med Sci 6:429, 1967.

Dozy AM, Kan YW, et al. α-Globin gene organization on blacks precludes the severe form of α-thalassemia. Nature 280:605, 1979.

Drewinko B, Bollinger P, et al. Eight-parameter automated hematology analyzers: comparison of two flow cytometric systems. Am J Clin Pathol 78:738, 1982.

Dreykin D. Emerging concepts of platelet function. N Engl J Med 290:144, 1974.

Duckert F. Assays for Fibrin Stabilizing Factor (Factor XIII). In NU Bang (ed), Thrombosis and Bleeding Disorders. New York: Academic, 1971. P 262.

Duncan SC, Winkelmann RK. Circulating Sèzary cells in hospitalized dermatology patients. Br J Dermatol 99:171, 1978.

Dunn NL, Mauer HM. Enzyme alterations in leukemic cells. Am J Hematol 13:343, 1982.

Efremov GD. Microchromatography of hemoglobin: II. A rapid microchromatographic method for the determination of hemoglobin A_2. J Lab Clin Med 83:657, 1974.

Egberg N, Bergstrom K. Determination of plasma kallikrein-like enzymes with a new synthetic chromogenic tripeptide substrate. Presented at the Second European Congress of Clinical Chemistry, Prague, October 1976.

Eisenberg S. The effect of positive pressure and position of the venous sampling site on the hematocrit and serum protein concentration. J Lab Clin Med 51:755, 1963.

Ekelund LG, Ekelund B, et al. Time course for the change in hemoglobin concentration with change in posture. Acta Med Scand 190:335, 1971.

Elion J, Wajeman H, et al. Hémoglobine J Amiens β17(A14) Lys→Asn. Coincidence d'une novelle hémoglobine abnormale sans retentissment fonctionnel et d'une polyglobulie primitive. Nouv Rev Fre Hematol 21:347, 1979.

Elking MP, Kabat HF. Drug induced modifications of laboratory test values. Am J Hosp Pharm 25:485, 1968.

Ellis RF. The distribution of active bone marrow in the adult. Phys Med Bull 5:255, 1961.

Elson EC, Ivor L, et al. Substitution of a non-hazardous chromogen for benzidine in the measurement of plasma hemoglobin. Am J Clin Pathol 69:354, 1978.

England JM, Down MC. Comparison of methods for analyzing red cell and platelet volume distribution curves. Clin Lab Haematol 1:47, 1979.

England JM, Walford DM, et al. Reassessment of the reliability of the haematocrit. Br J Haematol 23:247, 1972.

Engstrom AW. Effect of hemolysis on the one-stage prothrombin time. Am J Clin Pathol 49:742, 1968.

Esmon CT, Esmon NL. Protein C activation. Semin Thromb Hemost 10:122, 1984.

Evans AS. The spectrum of infections with EB virus: a hypothesis. Infect Dis 124:330, 1971.

Evans GO, Smith DEC. Further observations concerning MPV measurements. Am J Clin Pathol 86:126, 1986.

Exner T. Comparison of two simple tests for the lupus anticoagulant. Am J Clin Pathol 83:215, 1985.

Eyster ME, Gordon RA, et al. The bleeding time is longer than normal in hemophilia. Blood 58:719, 1981.

Fairbanks VF. Nonequivalence of automated and manual hematocrit and erythrocytic indices. Am J Clin Pathol 73:55, 1980.

Faramarz Naeim MD, Capostangno VJ, et al. Sèzary syndrome: tartrate-resistant acid phosphatase in the neoplastic cells. Am J Clin Pathol 71:528, 1979.

Fareed J, Bermes EW, et al. Automation in coagulation testing. J Clin Lab Automat 4:415, 1984.

Federal Register. No. 163, 184. Washington, DC: US Government Printing Office, 1976. P 35.

Feinstein DI. Acquired inhibitors of factor V. Thromb Haemost 39:663, 1978.

Fenton JW II. Thrombin interactions with hirudin. Semin Thromb Hemost 15:265, 1989.

Figueiredo MS, Pinto BO, et al. Dapsone-induced hemolytic anemia and agranulocytosis in a patient with normal glucose-6-phosphate dehydrogenase activity. Acta Haematol 82:144, 1989.

First International Workshop on Chromosomes in Leukemia. Chromosomes in Ph-1 positive chronic granulocytic leukemia. Br J Haematol 39:305, 1978.

First International Workshop on Chromosomes in Leukemia. Chromosomes in acute non-lymphocytic leukemia. Br J Haematol 39:311, 1981.

Flandrin G, Daniel MT. Practical Value of Cytochemical Studies for the Classification of Acute Leukemias. In G Mathè, P Pouillart, et al. (eds), Recent Results in Cancer Research: Acute Leukemia. New York: Springer, 1973. P 43.

Fleming AJ. Malaria and other parasitic diseases. Clin Haematol 10:983, 1981.

Forscher CA, Sussman II, et al. Pseudothrombocytopenia masking true thrombocytopenia. Am J Hematol 18:313, 1985.

Franklin AJ. Cytomegalovirus infections presenting as acute haemolytic anemia in an infant. Arch Dis Child 47:474, 1972.

Freedman J. False positive antiglobulin tests in healthy subjects and in hospital patients. J Clin Pathol 32:1014, 1979.

Freedman J, Cheong T, et al. Use of the indirect platelet radioactive antiglobulin test with anti-IgG and anti-C3 in immune and nonimmune thrombocytopenia. Am J Hematol 18:297, 1985.

Fried K, Kaufman S. Congenital afibrinogenemia in 10 offspring of uncle-niece marriages. Clin Genet 17:223, 1980.

Frigola A. Standardization of a simple method for the determination of antithrombin activity. J Clin Pathol 30:881, 1977.

Froom P, Margaliot S, et al. Significance of erythrocyte sedimentation rate in young adults. Am J Clin Pathol 82:198, 1984.

Fujii H, Watada M, et al. Pseudothrombocytopenia. Acta Haematol Jpn 41:523, 1978.

Fujimua Y, Tritani K, et al. Von Willebrand factor. J Biol Chem 261:381, 1986.

Fulwood R, Johnson CL, et al. Hematological and Nutritional Biochemistry Reference Data for Persons Six Months to 74 Years of Age: United States, 1976–1980. Vital and Health Statistics, series 2, no. 232, Department of Health and Human Services pub no. (PHS) 83-1682. Washington, DC: US Government Printing Office, December 1982.

Gabbasov ZA, Popov EG, et al. Platelet agglutination: the use of optical density fluctuations to study microaggregate formation in platelet suspensions. Thromb Res 54:215, 1989.

Gabig TG. Leukocyte abnormalities. Med Clin North Am 64:647, 1980.

Galen RS. Tips on technology. Meal Lab Obs 6:13, 1981.

Gallagher RE, Gallo RC, et al. Type C RNA tumor virus isolated from cultured human acute myelogenous leukemia cells. Science 187:350, 1975.

Gallo D, Walen KH, et al. Improved immunofluorescence antigens for detection of immunoglobulin M antibodies to Epstein-Barr viral capsid antigen and antibodies to Epstein-Barr virus nuclear antigen. J Clin Microbiol 15:243, 1982.

Gambino SR, Dike JJ, et al. The Westergren sedimentation rate using K_3 EDTA. Am J Clin Pathol 43:173, 1965.

Ganguly P, Sutherland SB, et al. Defective binding of thrombin to platelet in myeloid leukemia. Br J Haematol 39:599, 1978.

Garratty G. Drug-Related Problems. In RH Walker (ed), Problems Encountered in Pretransfusion Tests. Chicago: American Association of Blood Banks, 1975. P 50.

Garratty G. Immune hemolytic anemia: II. Drug-induced immune hemolytic anemia. Adv Immunohematol Spectra Biolog Oxnard 3:2, 1975b.

Gear ARL. Pre-aggregation reactions of platelets. Blood 58:477, 1981.

Geary CG, Testa NG. Pathophysiology of Marrow Hypoplasia. In C Geary (ed), Aplastic Anemia. London: Baillière Tindall, 1979. P 2.

George RP, Depratti VJ. Aplastic Anemia. In AJ Silvergleid (ed), Clinical Hematology for Blood Banks. Washington, DC: American Association of Blood Banks, 1979. P 45.

Gerrard JM, Stoddard SF, et al. Platelet storage pool deficiency and prostaglandin synthesis in chronic granulocytic leukemia. Br J Haematol 40:597, 1978.

Gerwitz AM. Human megakaryocytopoiesis. Semin Hematol 23:27, 1986.

Gerwitz AM, Hoffman R. Megakaryocytopoiesis. In DW Golde, F Takaiku (eds), Hematopoietic Stem Cells. New York: Marcel Dekker, 1984. P 81.

Gilbert HS, Ornstein L. Basophil counting with a new staining method using Alcian blue. Blood 46:279, 1975.

Girolami A. Further studies on the abnormal factor X (factor X Friuli) coagulation disorder: a report of another family. Blood 37:534, 1971.

Girolami A, Molaro G, et al. A "new" congenital haemorrhagic condition due to the presence of an abnormal factor X (factor X Friuli): study of a large kindred. Br J Haematol 19:179, 1970.

Gloster E, Strauss RA, et al. Spurious elevated platelet counts associated with bacteremia. Am J Hematol 18:329, 1985.

Goldberg A. Lead poisoning as a disorder of heme synthesis. Semin Hematol 5:424, 1968.

Golde DW, Byers LA, et al. Chronic myelogenous leukemia cell growth and maturation in liquid culture. Cancer Res 34:419, 1974.

Golde DW, Stevens RH, et al. Immunoglobulin synthesis in hairy cell leukemia. Br J Haematol 35:359, 1977.

Golomb HM, Rowley JD, et al. "Microgranular" acute promyelocytic leukemia: a distinct clinical ultrastructural and cytogenic entity. Blood 55:25, 1980.

Gombert MD, Goldstein EJC, et al. Human babesiosis: clinical and therapeutic considerations. JAMA 248:3005, 1982.

Gouldsmit R. Congenital Dyserythropoietic Anaemia, Type III. In R Gouldsmit (ed), Dyserythropoiesis. London: Academic, 1977. P 83.

Gowland E, Kay H, et al. Agglutination of platelets by a serum factor in the presence of EDTA. J Clin Pathol 22:460, 1969.

Graber SE, Krantz SB. Erythropoietin and the control of red cell production. Annu Rev Med 29:51, 1978.

Graham RC Jr, Lundholm U, et al. Cytochemical demonstration of peroxidase activity with 3-amino-9-ethylcarbazole. J Histochem Cytochem 13:150, 1965.

Gralnick HR, Coller BS. Molecular defects in hemophilia A and von Willebrand's disease. Lancet 1:837, 1976.

Gralnick HR, Galton D, et al. Classification of acute leukemia. Ann Intern Med 97:740, 1977.

Grasbeck R, Salonen E-M. Vitamin B_{12}. Prog Food Nutr Sci 2:193, 1976.

Grette K. The mechanism of thrombin catalyzed hemostatic reactions in platelet. Acta Physiol Scand Suppl 195:1, 1962.

Grey HM, Kohler PF. Cryoimmunoglobulins. Semin Hematol 10:87, 1973.

Griffin JH, Cochrane CG. Recent advances in the understanding of contact activation reactions. Semin Thromb Hemost 5:254, 1979.

Griffin JH, Evatt B, et al. Deficiency of protein C in congenital thrombotic disease. J Clin Invest 68:1370, 1981.

Griggs RC. Lead Poisoning: Hematologic Aspects. In CV Moore, EB Brown (eds), Progress in Hematology. Vol 4. New York: Grune & Stratton, 1964. P 117.

Grimaldi JC, Meeker TC. The t(5;14) chromosome translocation in a case of acute lymphocytic leukemia joins the interleukin-3 gene to the immunoglobulin heavy chain gene. Blood 73:2081, 1989.

Gulliani GL, Hyun BH, et al. Falsely elevated automated leukocyte counts on cryoglobulinemic and/or cryofibrinogenemic blood samples. Lab Med 8:14, 1977.

Gunz FW. Epidemiology and Aetiology of the Leukemias. In Leukemia: Documenta Geigy. Basel: Ciba-Geigy, 1973.

Gutcher GR, Raynor WJ, et al. An evaluation of vitamin E status in premature infants. Am J Clin Nutr 40:1078, 1984.

Gutman SI, Didisheim P, et al. Two new artifacts in automated coagulation testing. Am J Clin Pathol 73:583, 1980.

Hackett M, Hinchliffe RF, et al. Erythrocyte sedimentation rate: evaluation of a commercial capillary-ESR tube in a paediatric haematology laboratory. Med Lab Sci 40:183, 1983.

Hagler L, Pastore RA, et al. Aplastic anemia following viral hepatitis. Medicine 54:139, 1975.

Hall R, Malia RG. Medical Laboratory Haematology. London: Butterworth, 1984. P 405.

Hallberg L. Menstrual blood loss and iron deficiency. Scand J Haematol 22:17, 1979.

Halsted CH, Griggs RC, et al. The effect of alcohol on the absorption of folic acid (3H-PGA) evaluated by plasma levels and urinary excretion. J Lab Clin Med 69:116, 1967.

Ham TH, Castle WB. Studies on destruction of red blood cells. Proc Am Phil Soc 82:411, 1940.

Hamberg M. Isolation and structure of two prostaglandin endoperoxidases that cause platelet aggregation. Proc Natl Acad Sci U S A 71:345, 1974.

Hamilton LD, Gubler CJ, et al. Diurnal variation in plasma iron level of man. Proc Soc Exp Biol Med 75:65, 1950.

Han P, Ardlie NG. The influence of pH, temperature and calcium on platelet aggregation. Maintenance of environmental pH and platelet function for *in vitro* studies in plasma stored at 37°C. Br J Haematol 26:373, 1974.

Hanker JS, Yates PE, et al. A new specific sensitive and non-carcinogenic reagent for the demonstration of horseradish peroxidase. Histochem J 9:789, 1977.

Hardisty RM, Ingram GIC. Bleeding Disorders, Investigation and Management. Oxford: Blackwell, 1965. P 272.

Harlan J. Leukocyte-endothelium interaction. Blood 65:513, 1985.

Harrington DS, Weisenburger DD, et al. Epstein-Barr virus associated lymphoproliferative lesions. Clin Lab Med 8:97, 1988.

Harris ED. Case records of the Massachusetts General Hospital. N Engl J Med 301:256, 1979.

Hartmann JR, Jenkins DE, et al. Diagnostic specificity of sucrose hemolysis test for paroxysmal nocturnal hemoglobinuria. Blood 35:462, 1970.

Hathaway HS, Lubs ML, et al. Carrier detection in classical hemophilia. Pediatrics 57:251, 1976.

Hathaway WE, Belhasen LP, et al. Evidence for a new plasma thromboplastin factor. Case report, coagulation studies, and physiochemical properties. Blood 26:521, 1965.

Hattersley PG. Activated coagulation of whole blood. JAMA 196:436, 1966.

Hattersley PG. Erroneous values on the Model S Coulter due to high titer cold agglutinins. Am J Clin Pathol 55:442, 1971.

Hattersley PG. Progress report: the activated coagulation time of whole blood (ACT). Am J Clin Pathol 66:899, 1976.

Hattersley PG, Hayse D. The effect of increased contact activation time on the activated partial thromboplastin time. Am J Clin Pathol 66:479, 1976.

Hawkins RI. Smoking, platelets, and thrombosis. Nature 236:450, 1972.

Hayhoe FGJ, Quaglino D. Haematological Cytochemistry. London: Churchill Livingstone, 1980. P 131.

Hayhoe FGJ, Quaglino D, et al. The Cytology and Cytochemistry of Acute Leukemia: A Study of 140 Cases. MRC special report series, no. 304. London: Her Majesty's Stationery Office, 1964.

Hazelton JJ. Erythrocyte sedimentation rate: some observations under adverse conditions. J Med Lab Tech 25:370, 1968.

Healy GR. Babesiosis. Clin Micro News 4:33, 1982.

Healy GR, Ruebush TK. Morphology of Babesia microti in human blood smears. Am J Clin Pathol 73:107, 1980.

Heimpel H. Congenital Dyserythropoietic Anaemia, Type I. In Dyserythropoiesis. London: Academic, 1977. P 55.

Henle WG, Henle GA, et al. Epstein-Barr virus specific diagnostic tests in infectious mononucleosis. Hum Pathol 5:551, 1974.

Henle WG, Henle GA, et al. Infectious Mononucleosis and Epstein-Barr Virus Associated Malignancies. In CH Lennette, NJ Schmidt (eds), Diagnostic Procedures for Viral, Rickettsial, and Chlamydial Infections (5th ed). Washington, DC: American Public Health Association, 1979. P 441.

Henry JB. Clinical Chemistry: Principles and Techniques. New York: Hoeber, 1965. P 241.

Henry JB (ed). Clinical Diagnosis and Management by Laboratory Methods (17th ed). Philadelphia: Saunders, 1984.

Henson J, Carver J, et al. CM-cellulose microchromatography for the quantitation of hemoglobin Bart's ($\gamma4$) and its use in the detection of the α-thalassemia conditions. J Chromatogr 198:443, 1980.

Herbert V. Recommended dietary intakes (ROI) of vitamin B_{12} in humans. Am J Clin Nutr 45:671, 1987.

Herbert V, Tisman G, et al. The dU-suppression test using ^{125}I-UdR to define biochemical megaloblastosis. Br J Haematol 24:713, 1973.

Hernandez JA, Steane SM. Erythrophagocytosis by segmented neutrophils in paroxysmal cold hemoglobinuria. Am J Clin Pathol 787:82, 1984.

Hersko C, Bar-Or D, et al. Diagnosis of iron deficiency anemia in a rural population of children. Relative usefulness of serum ferritin, red cell protoporphyrin, red cell indices, and transferrin saturation determinations. Am J Clin Nutr 34:1600, 1981.

Higgy KE, Burns GF, et al. Discrimination of B, T, and null lymphocytes by esterase cytochemistry. Scand J Haematol 18:437, 1977.

Hill FGH, Enayat MS, et al. Investigation of a kindred with a new autosomal dominantly inherited variant type von Willebrand's disease (possible type IID). J Clin Pathol 38:665, 1985.

Hillman RS, Finch CA. Erythropoiesis: normal and abnormal. Semin Hematol 4:327, 1967.

Hirsh J. Basis for the therapeutic range for anticoagulant therapy. Presented at the Dade Corporation Thrombosis-Hemostasis Conference, Atlanta, GA, 1984.

Hodges RE. Hemopoietic studies in vitamin A deficiency. Am J Clin Nutr 31:876, 1978.

Hoffbrand AV. The Megaloblastic Anaemias. In A Goldberg, MC McBrain (eds), Recent Advances in Haematology. London: Churchill Livingstone, 1971a. P 40.

Hoffbrand AV. The Megaloblastic Anaemias. In A Goldberg, MC McBrain (eds), Recent Advances in Haematology. London: Churchill Livingstone, 1971b. P 45.

Hoffbrand AV, Chanarin I. Megaloblastic erythropoiesis in myelosclerosis. Q J Med 37:493, 1968.

Hoffbrand AV, Ganeshagarn K, et al. Megaloblastic anaemia: initiation of DNA synthesis in excess of DNA chain elongation as the underlying mechanism. Clin Haematol 5:727, 1976.

Hoffbrand AV, Janossy G. Enzyme and membrane markers in leukaemia: recent developments. J Clin Pathol 34:254, 1981.

Hoffbrand AV, Walters AH. Observations on the biochemical basis of megaloblastic anaemia. Br J Haematol 23(suppl):109, 1972.

Hoffman RG, Waid ME. The "average of normals" method of quality control. Am J Clin Pathol 43:134, 1965.

Holmberg L, Ljung R, et al. The effects of plasmin and protein C on factor VIIIC and VIIIC Ag. Thromb Res 31:41, 1983.

Holmberg L, Nilsson IM. Two genetic variants of von Willebrand's disease. N Engl J Med 288:595, 1973.

Holmsen H. Prostaglandin endoperoxidase-thromboxane synthesis and dense granule secretion as possible feedback loops in the propagation of platelet responses in the basic platelet reaction. Thromb Haemost 38:1030, 1977.

Holt JT, DeWandler MJ, et al. Spurious elevation of the electronically determined mean corpuscular volume and hematocrit caused by hyperglycemia. Am J Clin Pathol 77:561, 1982.

Horwitt MK. Riboflavin: Niacin. In RS Goodhart, ME Stuls (eds), Modern Medicine in Health and Disease (6th ed). Philadelphia: Lea & Febiger, 1980.

Horwitz CA, Polesky H, et al. Persistent haemagglutination for infectious mononucleosis in rheumatoid arthritis. Br Med J 1:591, 1973.

Hougie C, Twomey JJ. Haemophilia B$_m$: a new type of factor-IX deficiency. Lancet 1:698, 1967.

Hoyer LW. The factor VIII complex: structure and function. Blood 58:1, 1981.

Huang MJ, Li C-Y, et al. Acute leukemia with megakaryocytic differentiation: a study of 12 cases identified immunocytochemically. Blood 64:427, 1984.

Huang TW, Lagunoff D, et al. Nonaggregative adherence of platelets to basal lamina in vitro. Lab Invest 31:156, 1974.

Hudson P. The Activated Partial Thromboplastin Time Test. Miami: American Dade, 1983.

Hull R, Hirsch J, et al. Different intensities of oral anticoagulant therapy in the treatment of proximal vein thrombosis. N Engl J Med 27:1676, 1982.

Humbert JR, Kurtz ML, et al. Increased reduction of nitroblue tetrazolium by neutrophils of newborn infants. Pediatrics 5:125, 1970.

Hutchinson D. Platelet Function, Disorders, and Testing. In D Hutchinson, The Hemophilias. Miami: American Dade, 1983.

Hutton RA, MacNab AJ, et al. Defective platelet function associated with chronic hypoglycemia. Arch Dis Child 51:49, 1976.

Hyun BH, Ashton JK, et al. Practical Hematology. Philadelphia: Saunders, 1975.

Inle JN, Rebar L, et al. Interleukin-3. Possible roles in the regulation of lymphocyte differentiation and growth. Immunol Rev 63:5, 1982.

International Committee for Standardization in Haematology. Recommendation for measurement of erythrocyte sedimentation rate of human blood. Am J Clin Pathol 68:505, 1977.

International Committee for Standardization in Haematology. Recommendations for reference method for hemoglobinometry in human blood and specifications for international hemoglobin cyanide reference preparation. J Clin Pathol 31:139, 1978.

International Committee for Standardization in Haematology. Recommended methods for the characterization of red-cell pyruvate kinase variants. Br J Haematol 43:275, 1979.

International Committee for Standardization in Haematology. Expert panel on blood cell sizing: recommendations for reference method for determination of packed cell volume of blood. J Clin Pathol 33:1, 1980.

Inwood MI, Thompson S. Principles of Hematology. In SJ Raphael (ed), Medical Laboratory Technology (4th ed). Philadelphia: Saunders, 1983. P 670.

Isager H, Hagerup L. Relationship between cigarette smoking and high packed cell volume and hemoglobin levels. Scand J Haematol 8:241, 1971.

Issitt PD. Autoimmune hemolytic anemia. Am J Med Tech 40:479, 1974.

Issitt PD, Pavone BG. Critical re-examination of the specificity of auto-anti-Rh antibodies in patients with a positive direct antiglobulin test. Br J Haematol 38:63, 1978.

Italian Working Group. Spectrum of von Willebrand's disease: a study of 100 cases. Br J Haematol 35:101, 1977.

Jacobs HS, Jandl JH. A simple visual screening test for glucose-6-phosphate dehydrogenase deficiency employing ascorbate and cyanide. N Engl J Med 274:1162, 1966.

Jacoby F. Staining techniques. In EM Darmady, SGT Davenport (eds), Haematological Technique (3rd ed). New York: Grune & Stratton, 1963. P 127.

Jaffe EA. Endothelial cells and the biology of factor VIII. N Engl J Med 296:377, 1977.

Javid J. Hemoglobin SO Arabia disease in a black American. Am J Med Sci 265:266, 1973.

Johnson AJ, Kline DL, et al. Assay methods and standard preparations for plasmin, plasminogen, and urokinase in purified systems. Thromb Diath Haemorrh (Stuttg) 21:259, 1969.

Jones JD. Factors that affect clinical laboratory values. J Occup Med 22:316, 1980.

Jonxis JHP, Huisman THJ. A Laboratory Manual on Abnormal Hemoglobins (2nd ed). Oxford: Blackwell Scientific, 1968. P 37.

Jordan MC, Rousseau WE, et al. Spontaneous cytomegalovirus mononucleosis: clinical and laboratory observations in nine cases. Ann Intern Med 79:153, 1973.

Jordans GH. The familial occurrence of fat containing vacuoles in the leukocytes diagnosed in two brothers suffering from dystrophia musculorum progressiva. Acta Med Scand 145:419, 1953.

Josso F, Prou-Wartelle O. Interaction of tissue factor and factor VII at the earliest phase of coagulation. Thromb Diath Haemorrh Suppl 17:35, 1965.

Kalish RJ, Becker K. Evaluation of the Coulter S-Plus V three-part differential in a community hospital, including criteria for its use. Am J Clin Pathol 86:751, 1986.

Kan YW, Dozy AM, et al. Deletion of α-globulin genes in hemoglobin-H disease demonstrates multiple α-globin structural loci. Nature 255:255, 1975.

Kantarjiam HM, Kurzrock R, et al. Philadelphia chromosome–negative chronic myelogenous leukemia and chronic myelomonocytic leukemia. Hematol Oncol Clin North Am 4:389, 1990.

Kaplan SS, Penchansky L, et al. Simultaneous evaluation of terminal deoxynucleotidyl transferase and myeloperoxidase in acute leukemias using an immunocytochemical method. Am J Clin Pathol 87:732, 1987.

Kaplow LS. A histochemical procedure for localizing and evaluating leukocyte alkaline phosphatase activity in smears of blood and marrow. Blood 10:1023, 1955.

Kaplow LS. Cytochemistry of leukocyte alkaline phosphatase. Am J Clin Pathol 39:439, 1963.

Karanas A, Silver RT. Characteristics of the terminal phase of chronic granulocytic leukemia. Blood 32:445, 1968.

Kasper C. A more uniform measurement of factor VIII inhibitors. Thromb Diath Haemorrh 34:869, 1975.

Kasturi J, Basha HM, et al. Hereditary sideroblastic anemia in 4 siblings of a Libyan family—autosomal dominant. Acta Haematol (Basel) 68:321, 1982.

Katayama I, Li CY, et al. Histochemical study of acid phosphatase isoenzyme in leukemic reticuloendotheliosis. Cancer 29:157, 1972.

Katayama I, Yang JPA. Reassessment of a cytochemical test for differential diagnosis of leukemic reticuloendotheliosis. Am J Clin Pathol 68:268, 1977.

Kaufman RM, Airo R, et al. Circulating megakaryocytes and platelet release in the lung. Blood 26:760, 1965.

Kay NE, Johnson JD, et al. T-cell subpopulations in chronic lymphocytic leukemia: abnormalities in distribution and in vitro receptor maturation. Blood 54:540, 1979.

Kaye FJ, Alter BP. Red cell size distribution analysis: a new noninvasive evaluation of microcytosis. Blood 60(suppl):36a, 1982.

Kelton JG, Blanchette V, et al. Neonatal thrombocytopenia due to passive immunization. N Engl J Med 302:1401, 1979.

Koepke JA. A statistical system of quality control in hematology. Med Lab Obs 11:83, 1981.

Keshgegian AA, Mann JM, et al. Is duplicate testing for prothrombin time and activated partial thromboplastin time necessary? Arch Pathol Lab Med 110:520, 1986.

Kidder WR, Logan LJ, et al. The plasma protamine paracoagulation test. Clinical and laboratory evaluation. J Lab Clin Med 58:675, 1972.

Kilgariff M, Owen JA. An assessment of the "average of normals" quality control method. Clin Chim Acta 19:175, 1968.

Kingdon HS, Lundblad RL. Factors affecting the evolution of factor XIa during blood coagulation. J Lab Clin Med 85:826, 1975.

Kinoshita S, Harrison J, et al. A new variant of dominant type II von Willebrand's disease with aberrant multimetric patterns of factor VIII related antigen (type IID). Blood 63:1369, 1984.

Kirkwood TBL, Rizza CR, et al. Identification of sources of inter-laboratory variation in factor VIII assay. Br J Haematol 37:559, 1977.

Kisiel W, Canfield WM, et al. Anticoagulant properties of bovine plasma protein following activation by thrombin. Biochemistry 16:5824, 1977.

Kitahara M, Eyre LIJ. Familial leukocyte myeloperoxidase deficiency. Blood 57:888, 1981.

Kjeldsberg CR, Hershgold EJ. Spurious thrombocytopenia. JAMA 227:628, 1974.

Kleihauer E, Hildegard B, et al. Demonstration of fetal hemoglobin in erythrocytes of a blood smear. Klin Wochenschr 35:637, 1957.

Knight GJ, Hesse HDV, et al. Diagnosis of iron-deficiency: mean corpuscular hemoglobin (MCH) as a predictor of iron-deficiency in infants. Pediatr Res 16:168, 1982.

Koenig JM, Christensen RD. Incidence, neutrophil kinetics, and natural history of neonatal neutropenia associated with maternal hypertension. N Engl J Med 321:557, 1989.

Koepke JA. A delineation of performance criteria for the differentiation of leukocytes. Am J Clin Pathol 68:202, 1977.

Koepke JA. Tips on technology. Med Lab Obs 10:22, 1979.

Koepke JA. Why survey red cell indices. Summing Up 11(4):7, 1982.

Koepke JA. Partial thromboplastin time test—proposed performance guidelines. ICSH panel on the PTT. Thromb Haemost 55:143, 1986.

Koepke JA, Bull BS, et al. Hematology. In SL Inhorn (ed), Quality Assurance Practice for Health Laboratories. Washington, DC: American Public Health Association, 1978. P 695.

Koepke JA, Protextor TJ. Quality assurance for multichannel hematology instruments—four years' experience with patient mean erythrocyte indices. Am J Clin Pathol 75:28, 1981.

Koepke JA, Rodgers JL, et al. Pre-instrumental variables in coagulation testing. Am J Clin Pathol 64:591, 1975.

Krutihof EKO, Tran-Thang C, et al. Fibrinolysis in pregnancy: a study of plasminogen activator inhibitors. Blood 69:460, 1967.

Kubota M, Akiyama Y, et al. Acute nonlymphocytic leukemia with basophilic differentiation and t(9,11)(p22, q23) in a child. Am J Hematol 31:133, 1980.

Kubota T, Tanone K, et al. Autoantibody against platelet glycoprotein IIb/IIIa in a patient with non-Hodgkin's lymphoma. Thromb Res 53:379, 1989.

Kushner JP. Idiopathic refractory sideroblastic anemia. Medicine 50:139, 1971.

Lackner H, Javid JP. The clinical significance of the plasminogen level. Am J Clin Pathol 60:175, 1973.

La Croix KA, David GL. A review of protein C and its role in hemostasis. J Med Tech 2:95, 1985.

Lalezari P. Serologic profile in autoimmune hemolytic disease: pathophysiologic and clinical interpretations. Semin Hematol 13:291, 1976.

Lampasso JA. Changes in hematologic values induced by storage of ethylenediaminetetraacetate human blood for varying periods of time. Am J Clin Pathol 49:443, 1968.

Landsteiner K, Miller CP, et al. Serological studies on the blood of the primates: II. The blood groups in anthropoid apes. J Exp Med 42:853, 1925.

Lanham GR, Bollum FJ, et al. Detection of terminal deoxynucleotidyl transferase in acute leukemias using monoclonal antibodies directed against natured and denatured sites. Am J Clin Pathol 86:88, 1986.

Lanham GR, Melvin SL, et al. Immunoperoxidase determination of terminal deoxynucleotidyl transferase in acute leukemia using PAP and ABC methods: experience in 102 cases. Am J Clin Pathol 83:366, 1985.

Lassen M. Heat denaturation of plasminogen in the fibrin plate method. Acta Physiol Scand 27:371, 1952.

Lau P, Sererat S. Paroxysmal cold hemoglobinuria in a patient with *Klebsiella* pneumonia. Vox Sang 44:167, 1983.

Lauf PK, Joiner CH. Increased potassium transport in human Ph_{Null} red blood cells. Blood 48:457, 1976.

Laurell CB. Quantitative estimation of proteins by electrophoresis in agarose gel containing antibodies. Anal Biochem 15:45, 1966.

Lay WH, Mendes HF, et al. Binding of sheep red blood cells to a large population of human lymphocytes. Nature 230:531, 1971.

Leavelle DE, Mertens BF, et al. Staphylococcal clumping on microtiter plates: a rapid simple method for measuring fibrinogen split products. Am J Clin Pathol 75:452, 1971.

Lechnor K. Lupus Anticoagulants and Thrombosis. In M Verstraete, J Vermylen, et al. (eds), Thrombosis and Haemostasis 1987. Leuven, Belgium: International Society of Thrombosis and Haemostasis, Leuven University Press, 1987. P 525.

Lee GR. Nutritional Factors in the Production and Function of Erythrocytes. In GR Lee, TC Bithell, et al. (eds), Wintrobe's Clinical Hematology (9th ed). Philadelphia: Lea & Febiger, 1993. P 170.

Lee RI, White PD. A clinical study of the coagulation time of blood. Am J Med Sci 145:495, 1913.

Leitner A, Bidwell E, et al. An antihaemophilic globulin (factor VIII) inhibitor: purification characterization and reaction kinetics. Br J Haematol 9:245, 1963.

Leone G, Accorra F, et al. Circulating anticoagulants against factor XI and thrombocytopenia with platelet aggregation inhibition in systemic lupus erythematosus. Acta Haematol 58:240, 1977.

Lewis SM. Red cell abnormalities and haemolysis in aplastic anaemia. Br J Haematol 29:545, 1975.

Li CY. Leukemia identification by immunochemistry. Mayo Med Lab Commun 9:6, 1984.

Li CY, Lam KW, et al. Esterases in human leukocytes. J Histochem Cytochem 21:1, 1973.

Lieberman JE, Gordon-Smith EC. Red cell P5'N and glutathione in myeloproliferative and lymphoproliferative disorders. Br J Haematol 44:425, 1980.

Lie-Injo LE. Hemoglobin "Bart's" and the sickling phenomenon. Nature 191:1314, 1961.

Liepman M. The chronic leukemias. Med Clin North Am 64:705, 1980.

Liley AW. Liquor amnii analysis in management of pregnancy complicated by rhesus sensitization. Am J Obstet Gynecol 82:1359, 1963.

Lin MJ, Nagel RL, et al. Acceleration of hemoglobin C crystallization by hemoglobin S. Blood 74:1823, 1989.

Loeliger EA, International Committee for Standardization in Haematology—International Committee on Thrombosis and Haemostasis. ICSH/ICTH recommendations for reporting prothrombin time in oral anticoagulant control. Thromb Haemost 53:155, 1985.

Loeliger EA, van den Besselaar AMMP, et al. Reliability and clinical impact of the normalization of the prothrombin times in oral anticoagulant control. Thromb Haemost 53:148, 1985.

Loffler H, Graubner R, et al. Prolymphocytic Leukemia with T Cell Properties and Tartrate Resistant Acid Phosphatase. In S Thierfelder, H Rodt, et al. (eds), Immunological Diagnosis of Leukemia and Lymphomas. New York: Springer, 1977. P 177.

Lofsness KG, Kohnke ML, et al. Evaluation of automated reticulocyte counts and their reliability in the presence of Howell-Jolly bodies. Am J Clin Pathol 101:85, 1994.

Lohr GW, Waller HD. Glucose-6-Phosphate Dehydrogenase. In HU Bergmeyer (ed), Methods of Enzymatic Analysis. New York: Academic, 1963. P 11.

Loos H, Rood D, et al. Familial deficiency of glutathione reductase in human blood cells. Blood 48:53, 1976.

Loukas DF. Leukemic reticuloendotheliosis: a medical technologist's diagnosis. Am J Med Tech 42:367, 1976.

Lubbe WF, Liggins GC. Role of lupus anticoagulant and autoimmunity in recurrent pregnancy loss. Semin Reprod Endocrin 6:181, 1988.

Lugton RA. The ESR re-examined. Med Lab Sci 44:207, 1987.

Luke RG, Koepke JA, et al. The effects of immunosuppressive drugs and uremia on automated leukocyte counts. Am J Clin Pathol 56:503, 1971.

Lux SE. Spectrin-actin membrane skeleton of normal and abnormal red blood cells. Semin Hematol 16:21, 1979.

Lynch DM, Lynch JM, et al. A quantitative ELISA procedure for the measurement of membrane-bound platelet-associated IgG (PAIgG). Am J Clin Pathol 83:331, 1985.

Ma X, Beguin S, et al. Importance of factor IX dependent prothrombinase formation—the Josso pathway—in clotting plasma. Haemostasis 19:301, 1989.

MacKenzie MR, Fundenberg HH. Macroglobulinemia: an analysis of forty patients. Blood 39:874, 1972.

Mannuci PM, Vigano S. Deficiencies on protein C, an inhibitor of blood coagulation. Lancet 28:463, 1982.

Manotti C, Quintavaller R, et al. Thromboembolic manifestations and congenital factor V deficiency: a family study. Haemostasis 19:331, 1989.

Marchand A, Galen RS. The predictive value of serum haptoglobin in hemolytic anemia. JAMA 243:1909, 1980.

Marciniak E, Greenwood MF. Acquired coagulation inhibitor delaying fibrinopeptide release. Blood 53:81, 1979.

Marcus AJ. The role of lipids in platelet function with particular reference to the arachidonic acid pathway. J Lipid Res 19:793, 1978.

Marder VJ, Mannucci PM, et al. Standard nomenclature for Factor VIII and von Willebrand factor: a recommendation by the International Committee on Thrombosis and Haemostasis. Thromb Haemost 54:871, 1985.

Margolius A Jr, Jackson DP, et al. Circulating anticoagulants: a study of 40 cases and a review of the literature. Medicine 40:145, 1961.

Markell EK, Voge M. Medical Parasitology (5th ed). Philadelphia: Saunders, 1981.

Marks SM, Baltimore D, et al. Terminal transferase as a predictor of initial responsiveness to vincristine and prednisone in blastic chronic myelogenous leukemia. N Engl J Med 298:812, 1978.

Marlar RA, Endres-Brooks A, et al. Serial studies of protein C and its plasma inhibitor in patients with disseminated intravascular coagulation. Blood 66:59, 1985.

Marlar RA, Griffin JH. Alternative pathways of thromboplastin-dependent activation of human factor X in plasma. Ann N Y Acad Sci 370:325, 1981.

Massini P, Käser-Glanzmann R. Movement of calcium ions and their role in the activation of platelets. Thromb Haemost 40:212, 1978.

Mattler LE, Bang NU. Serine protease specificity for peptide chromogenic substrates. Thromb Haemost 38:776, 1977.

Matula G, Paterson PY. NBT tests in a patient on steroids. Lancet 1:803, 1971.

Mayrovitz H, Wiedeman M, et al. Factors influencing leukocyte adherence in microvessels. Thromb Haemost 38:823, 1977.

McCallum CJ, Peake JR, et al. Factor VIII levels and blood group antigens. Thromb Haemost 50:757, 1985.

McCann SR, Firth R, et al. Congenital dyserythropoietic anaemia type II (HEMPAS): a family study. J Clin Pathol 33:1197, 1980.

McClennan JE, Maddox JC. Acute megakaryocytic leukemia. Am J Clin Pathol 92:700, 1989.

McDevitt NB, McDonagh J. An acquired inhibitor to factor XIII. Arch Intern Med 130:772, 1972.

McIntosh S, O'Brien R, et al. Neonatal isoimmune purpura: response to platelet infusions. J Pediatr 82:1020, 1973.

McManus JFA. Lipid morphology of tubercle. Nature 157:722, 1946.

McPhedran P, Clyne LP, et al. Prolongation of the activated partial thromboplastin time associated with poor venipuncture technic. Am J Clin Pathol 62:16, 1974.

Meier J, Coleman MS, et al. Adenosine deaminase activity in peripheral blood cells of patients with haematological malignancies. Br J Cancer 33:312, 1976.

Mengel CE, Metz E. Anemia during acute infections: role of glucose-6-phosphate dehydrogenase deficiency in negroes. Arch Intern Med 119:287, 1967.

Mentzer WC. Hereditary stomatocytosis: membrane and metabolism studies. Blood 46:659, 1975.

Meyer D, Larrieu MJ. Factor VIII and IX variants: relationships between hemophilia B_M and hemophilia B[+]. Eur J Clin Invest 1:425, 1971.

Miale JB. Laboratory Medicine—Hematology (6th ed). St Louis: Mosby, 1982.

Miale JB, Kent JW. Standardization of the technique for the prothrombin time test. Lab Med 10:612, 1979.

Middaugh CR. Molecular basis for the temperature dependent insolubility of cryoglobulins. Immunochemistry 15:171, 1978.

Mielke CH, Kaneshiro MM, et al. The standardized normal Ivy bleeding time and its prolongation by aspirin. Blood 34:204, 1969.

Miers MK, Fogo AB, et al. Evaluation of the Coulter S-Plus IV three-part differential as a screening tool in a tertiary care hospital. Am J Clin Pathol 87:745, 1987.

Mijovic A, Rolovic Z, et al. Chronic myeloid leukemia associated with pure red cell aplasia and terminating in promyelocytic transformation. Am J Hematol 31:128, 1989.

Miller A, Green M, et al. Simple rule for calculating normal erythrocyte sedimentation rate. Br Med J 286:266, 1984.

Miller JL, Castella A. Platelet-type von Willebrand's disease: characterization of a new bleeding disorder. Blood 60:790, 1982.

Miller RM, Garbus J, et al. A modified leukocyte nitroblue tetrazolium test in acute bacterial infection. Am J Clin Pathol 66:905, 1976.

Miller RW. Deaths from childhood cancer in sibs. N Engl J Med 279:122, 1968a.

Miller RW. Relation between cancer and congenital defects: an epidemiological evaluation. J Natl Cancer Inst 40:1079, 1968b.

Mills H, Lucia SP. Familial hypochromic anemia associated with postsplenectomy erythrocyte inclusion bodies. Blood 4:891, 1949.

Milner PF. The sickling disorders. Clin Haematol 3:289, 1974.

Mitchell GA. Fluorescent substrate assay for antithrombin III. Thromb Res 12:219, 1978.

Mollison PL. Blood Transfusion in Clinical Medicine (4th ed). Oxford: Blackwell Scientific, 1967. P 89.

Mollison PL. Blood Transfusion in Clinical Medicine (7th ed). Oxford: Blackwell Scientific, 1983. P 240.

Moncrieff RE. Alloimmune neonatal thrombocytopenia. West J Med 128:52, 1978.

Monte M, Bevzard Y, et al. Mapping of several abnormal hemoglobins by horizontal polyacrylamide gel isoelectric focusing. Am J Clin Pathol 66:753, 1976.

Montgomery RR, Otsuka A. Hypoprothrombinemia: case report. Blood 51:29, 1978.

Mori PG, Pasino M, et al. Hemophilia "A" in a 46,X,i(Xq) female. Br J Haematol 43:143, 1979.

Morisaki T, Fugii H, et al. Adenosine deaminase (ADA) in leukemia: clinical value of plasma ADA activity and characterization of leukemic cell ADA. Am J Hematol 19:37, 1985.

Moroz LA, Rose B. The Cryopathies. In M Samter (ed), Immunological Diseases (2nd ed). Boston: Little, Brown, 1977. P 570.

Morris MW, Brooker DW, et al. Single versus duplicate prothrombin time assays. Lab Med 18:524, 1987.

Morrison SA, Jesty J. Tissue factor dependent activation of tritium-labelled factor IX and factor X in human plasma. Blood 63:1338, 1984.

Morse EE, Quinn J, et al. The use of leucocyte acid phosphatase in the diagnosis of malignant disease. Ann Clin Lab Sci 10:143, 1980.

Moscinski LC, So AL, et al. Myeloperoxidase-positive acute megakaryoblastic leukemia. Am J Clin Pathol 91:607, 1989.

Muntean W, Leschnick B. Factor VIII influences binding of factor IX and factor X to intact human platelets. Thromb Res 55:537, 1989.

Murphy JR. Erythrocyte metabolism. III. Relationship of energy metabolism and serum factors in the osmotic fragility following incubation. J Lab Clin Med 60:86, 1962.

Murphy S, Iland H, et al. Essential thrombocytopenia: an interim report from the Polycythemia Vera Study Group. Semin Hematol 23:177, 1986.

Murray JL, Penz-Soler R, et al. Decreased adenosine deaminase (ADA) and 5' nucleotidase (5NT) activity in peripheral blood T cells in Hodgkin's disease. Am J Hematol 21:57, 1986.

Myhre LD, Dill DB, et al. Blood volume changes during three-week residence at high altitude. Clin Chem 16:7, 1970.

Nalbandian RM, Nichols RM, et al. Dithionite tube test—a rapid inexpensive technique for the detection of hemoglobin S and non-S sickling hemoglobins. Clin Chem 17:1028, 1971.

Nathan DM, Siegel AJ, et al. Acute methemoglobinemia and hemolytic anemia with phenazopyridine. Arch Intern Med 137:1636, 1977.

National Committee for Clinical Laboratory Standards. Standardized Method for the Human Erythrocyte Sedimentation Rate (ESR) Test. Villanova, PA: National Committee for Clinical Laboratory Standards, 1978.

National Committee for Clinical Laboratory Standards. Collection, Transportation, and Preparation of Blood Specimens for Coagulation Testing and Performance of Coagulation Assays. Villanova, PA: National Committee for Clinical Laboratory Standards, 1986.

National Committee for Clinical Laboratory Standards. H 18A: Procedures for the Handling and Processing of Blood Specimens: Approved Standard. Villanova, PA: National Committee for Clinical Laboratory Standards, 1990.

National Committee for Clinical Laboratory Standards. Reticulocyte Counting by Flow Cytometry: Proposed Guidelines. Villanova, PA: National Committee for Clinical Laboratory Standards, 1993.

Needleman P. Thromboxanes: selective biosynthesis and distinct biological properties. Science 193:163, 1976.

Nelson DA, Davey FR. Erythrocytic Disorders. In JB Henry (ed), Clinical Diagnosis and Management by Laboratory Methods (17th ed). Philadelphia: Saunders, 1984. P 652.

Nelson DA, Morris MW. Basic Methodology. In JB Henry (ed), Clinical Diagnosis and Management by Laboratory Methods (17th ed). Philadelphia: Saunders, 1984. P 578.

Nelson DS. Immunobiology of the Macrophage. New York: Academic, 1976. P 84.

Nelson L, Charache S, et al. Laboratory evaluation of the Coulter[R] "three-part electronic differential." Am J Clin Pathol 83:547, 1985.

Nemerson Y. Biological control of factor VII. Thromb Haemost 35:96, 1976.

Nemerson Y, Bach R. Tissue factor revisited. Prog Hemost Thromb 6:237, 1982.

Nevius DB. Osmotic error in electronic determinations of red cell volume. Am J Clin Pathol 39:38, 1963.

Ng RP, Chan TK, et al. NBT test—false negative and false positive results. Lancet 2:1341, 1972.

Nicholls PD. Haemoglobin measurement and blood protein precipitation with automated cell counters. Med Lab Sci 42:196, 1985.

Niederman JC. Infectious mono-nucleosis: clinical manifestations in relation to EB virus antibodies. JAMA 203:205, 1968.

Nierwiarowski S, Gurewich V. Laboratory identification of intravascular coagulation: the serial protamine sulfate test for the detection of fibrin monomer and fibrin degradation products. J Lab Clin Med 77:665, 1971.

Nilsson T, Norberg B. Thrombocytopenia and pseudothrombocytopenia: a clinical and laboratory problem. Scand J Haematol 37:341, 1986.

Nishimura RN, Barranger JA. Neurologic complications of Gaucher's disease, type 3. Arch Neurol 37:92, 1980.

Nosanchuk JS, Roark MF, et al. Anemia masked by triglyceridemia. Am J Clin Pathol 62:838, 1974.

Okamura K, Kato H, et al. An improved nitroblue tetrazolium test and its correlation with toxic neutrophils. Am J Clin Pathol 62:27, 1974.

Olofsson T, Olsson I, et al. Granulopoiesis in infantile genetic agranulocytosis: in vitro cloning of marrow cells in agar culture. Scand J Haematol 16:18, 1976.

Orfanakas NG, Ostlund RE, et al. Normal blood leukocyte concentration values. Am J Clin Pathol 53:647, 1970.

Orkin SH, Old J. The molecular basis of α-thalassemia: frequent occurrence of dysfunctional loci among non-Asians with HbH disease. Cell 17:33, 1979.

Orstavik KH, Stormorken H, et al. Hemophilia B_M in a female. Thromb Res 37:561, 1985.

Oshita AK, Rothstein G, et al. cGMP stimulation of stem cell proliferation. Blood 49:585, 1977.

Østerud B, Rapaport S. Activation of factor IX by the reaction products of tissue factor and factor VII: additional pathway for initiating blood coagulation. Proc Natl Acad Sci U S A 74:5250, 1977.

O'Sullivan MB. Blood Collection. In D Seligson, RM Schmidt (eds), CRC Handbook Series in Clinical Laboratory Science: Vol 1. Hematology. Boca Raton, FL: CRC Press, 1979. P 10.

Owen CA, Bowie EJW, et al. The Diagnosis of Bleeding Disorders (2nd ed). Boston: Little, Brown, 1975. P 171.

Owen WG, Wagner RH. Antihemophilic factor: separation of an active fragment following dissociation by salts or detergents. Thromb Diath Haemorrh 27:502, 1972.

Ozsoylu S. Homozygous haemoglobin D Punjab. Acta Haematol 43:353, 1976.

Pachter MR, Johnson SA. Bleeding platelets and macroglobulinemia. Am J Clin Pathol 31:467, 1959.

Palkuti H. Laboratory monitoring of anticoagulant therapy. J Med Tech 2:81, 1985.

Palmer RN, Gralnick HR. Inhibition of the cold activation of factor VII and the prothrombin time. Am J Clin Pathol 81:618, 1984.

Palmer RN, Gralnick HR. Inhibition of cold-promoted activation of the prothrombin time: studies of new siliconized borosilicate collection tubes in normals and patients receiving warfarin. Am J Clin Pathol 83:492, 1985.

Pandolfi M, Ehinger B. Conjunctival bleeding in Osler's disease with associated platelet dysfunction. Acta Ophthalmol 56:75, 1978.

Panlilio AL, Reiss RF. Therapeutic platelet pheresis in thrombocythemia. Transfusion 19:147, 1979.

Papayannopoulou T, Stamatoyannopoulos G. Stains for Inclusion Bodies. In RM Schmidt, THJ Huisman, et al. (eds), The Detection of Hemoglobinopathies. Cleveland: CRC Press, 1974. P 32.

Park BH. The use and limitations of the nitroblue tetrazolium test as a diagnostic aid. J Pediatr 78:376, 1971.

Park BH, Fifring SM, et al. Infection and nitroblue tetrazolium reduction by neutrophils, a diagnostic aid. Lancet 11:532, 1968.

Parker C. Systemic mastocytosis. Am J Med 61:671, 1976.

Pasvol G, Weatherall DG. The red cell and the malaria parasite. Br J Haematol 46:165, 1980.

Patrick CW, Stamatoyannopoulos G, et al. Genetics: Hematology. Chicago: American Society of Clinical Pathologists, 1975.

Pearson ES, Hartley HO. Biometrika Tables for Statisticians (3rd ed). Vol 1. Cambridge, UK: Cambridge University Press, 1966.

Pearson TC, Guthrie DL. Trapped plasma in the microhematocrit. Am J Clin Pathol 78:770, 1982.

Pedersen B, Hayhoe FG. Relation between phagocytic activity and alkaline phosphatase content of neutrophils in chronic myeloid leukemia. Br J Haematol 21:257, 1971.

Peebles DA, Hochberg A, et al. Analysis of manual reticulocyte counting. Am J Clin Pathol 76:713, 1981.

Pegels JG, Brynes ECA, et al. Pseudothrombocytopenia: an immunologic study on platelet antibodies dependent on ethylene diamine tetra-acetate. Blood 59:157, 1982.

Penington DG. Formation of Platelets. In JL Gordas (ed), Platelets in Biology and Pathology. Vol 2. Amsterdam: Elsevier, 1981. P 19.

Pepper OH. Observations on vitally stainable reticulation and chromatic granules in erythrocytes preserved in vitro. Arch Intern Med 30:801, 1922.

Percelen Y, Inceman S. Heparin and ristocetin-induced platelet aggregation. Br J Haematol 4:101, 1975.

Peters SP, Lee RE, et al. Gaucher's disease: a review. Medicine (Baltimore) 56:425, 1977.

Phillips GS. False positive Monospot test results in rubella. JAMA 222:585, 1972.

Pierce LE, Rath CE. A new hemoglobin variant with sickling properties. N Engl J Med 268:862, 1963.

Piovella F, Nalli G. The ultrastructural localization of factor VIII antigen in human platelets, megakaryocytes, and endothelial cells utilizing a ferritin-labelled antibody. Br J Haematol 39:209, 1978.

Pochron SP, Mitchell GA, et al. A fluorescent substrate assay for plasminogen. Thromb Res 13:733, 1978.

Poller L. Oral Anticoagulant Therapy. In AL Bloom, DP Thomas (eds), Haemostasis and Thrombosis. Edinburgh: Churchill Livingstone, 1981. P 734.

Polly MJ, Mollison PL. Use of complement in the detection of blood group antibodies: special reference to the antiglobulin test. Transfusion 1:9, 1961.

Potolsky A, Creger A, et al. Radiation and drug therapies and leukemia. Annu Rev Med 25:75, 1982.

Prchal JF, Axelrod AA. Bone marrow responses in polycythemia vera. N Engl J Med 290:1382, 1974.

Prentice CRM. Studies on blood coagulation, fibrinolysis, and platelet function following exercise in normal and splenectomized people. Br J Haematol 23:541, 1972.

Prentice CRM, Ratnoff OD. The action of Russell's viper venom on factor V and the prothrombin-converting principle. Br J Haematol 16:29, 1969.

Pressens WT, Schur PH, et al. Lymphocyte surface immunoglobulins: distribution and frequency in lymphoproliferative diseases. N Engl J Med 288:176, 1973.

Pressley MB, Higgs MB, et al. A new genetic basis for hemoglobin H disease. N Engl J Med 303:1383, 1980.

Preud'homme JL, Gourdin MF, et al. Human lymphoid cell lines with pre-B cell characteristics. In B Serron, C Rosenfeld (eds), Inserm Symposium 8. Amsterdam: Elsevier, 1978. P 345.

Priest JB, Tjien OO, et al. Exercise-induced changes in common laboratory tests. Am J Clin Pathol 77:285, 1982.

Prieto E, Egozcue J, et al. Identification of the Philadelphia (Ph-1) chromosome. Blood 35:23, 1970.

Prindull G, Tillmann W. Fanconi's anaemia developing erythroleukemia. Scand J Haematol 23:59, 1979.

Prisco D, Paniccia R, et al. Euglobulin lysis time in fresh and stored samples. Am J Clin Pathol 102:794, 1994.

Quick AJ. The prothrombin time in hemophilia and in obstructive jaundice. J Biol Chem 109;73, 1935.

Quick AJ. Salicylates and bleeding: the aspirin tolerance test. Am J Med Sci 252:265, 1966.

Raccuglia G. Gray platelet syndrome: a variety of qualitative platelet disorders. Am J Med 51:818, 1971.

Rachmilewitz B, Rachmilewitz M. The synthesis of transcobalamin II, a vitamin B_{12} transport protein, by stimulated mouse peritoneal macrophages. Biomedicine 27:213, 1977.

Radcliffe RD, Nemerson Y. Mechanism of activation of bovine factor VII. J Biol Chem 251:4797, 1976.

Raff MC. Surface antigenic markers for distinguishing T and B lymphocytes in mice. Transplant Rev 6:52, 1971.

Rafnsson V, Bengtsson C, et al. Erythrocyte sedimentation rate in a population sample of women with special reference to its clinical and prognostic significance. Acta Med Scand 206:207, 1979.

Ralfkiaer E, Waltzin GL, et al. Phenotypic characterization of lymphocyte subsets in *Mycosis fungoides*. Am J Clin Pathol 84:610, 1985.

Ramot B. Haemoglobin O in an Arab family: sickle cell haemoglobin O trait. Br Med J 2:1262, 1960.

Rana SR, Castro OL, et al. Leukocyte counts in 7739 healthy black persons: effect of age and sex. Ann Clin Lab Sci 15:51, 1985.

Rapaport SI, Proctor RR, et al. The mode of inheritance of PTA deficiency: evidence for the existence of major PTA deficiency and minor PTA deficiency. Blood 18:149, 1961.

Rapport H. Tumors of the Hematopoietic System. Fasc 8. Washington, DC: Armed Forces Institute of Pathology, 1966.

Ratnoff OD. The Molecular Basis of Hereditary Clotting Disorders. In TH Spaet (ed), Progress in Hemostasis and Thrombosis. Vol 1. New York: Grune & Stratton, 1972. P 39.

Ratnoff OD. The Surface Mediated Initiation of Blood Coagulation and Related Phenomena. In D Ogston, B Bennett (eds), Haemostasis: Biochemistry, Physiology, and Pathology. London: Wiley, 1977. P 25.

Ratnoff OD, Jones PK. The laboratory diagnosis of the carrier state for classical hemophilia. Ann Intern Med 86:521, 1977.

Ratnoff OD, Saito H. Interactions among Hageman factor, plasma prekallikrein, high molecular weight kininogen, and plasma thromboplastin antecedent. Proc Natl Acad Sci U S A 76:958, 1979.

Ratnoff OD, Steinberg AG. Inheritance of fibrin-stabilizing factor deficiency. Lancet 1:25, 1968.

Rattazzi MC, Corash LM, et al. G6PD deficiency and chronic hemolysis: four new mutants. Relationships between clinical syndrome and enzyme kinetics. Blood 38:205, 1971.

Ray M, Noteboom G. A modification of the erythrocyte osmotic fragility test. Am J Clin Pathol 54:711, 1970.

Reisner HM, Roberts HR, et al. Immunochemical characterization of a polyclonal human antibody to factor IX. Blood 50:11, 1977.

Reiss M, Roos D. Differences in oxygen metabolism of phagocytosing monocytes and neutrophils. J Clin Invest 61:480, 1978.

Remaley AT, Kennedy JM, et al. Evaluation of the clinical utility of platelet aggregation studies. Am J Hematol 31:188, 1989.

Reno WJ, Rotman M, et al. Evaluation of the BART test (a modification of the whole blood activated recalcification time test) as a means of monitoring heparin therapy. Am J Clin Pathol 61:78, 1974.

Reynafarje C, Ramos J. The hemolytic anemia of human bartonellosis. Blood 17:562, 1961.

Rimington C. Qualitative determination of porphobilinogen and porphyrin in urine and feces. Broadsheet no. 70. London: Association of Clinical Pathologists, 1971.

Rimon A, Schiffman S, et al. Factor XI activity and factor XI antigen in homozygous and heterozygous factor XI deficiency. Blood 48:165, 1976.

Rinehart JJ, Sagone AL, et al. Effects of corticosteroid therapy on human monocyte function. N Engl J Med 292:236, 1975.

Ritzmann WE, Daniels JC. Serum Protein Abnormalities: Diagnostic and Clinical Aspects. Boston: Little, Brown, 1975. P 331.

Rizza CR, Eipe J. Exercise, factor VIII and the spleen. Br J Haematol 20:269, 1971.

Roberts GT, El Badawi SB. Red blood cell distribution width index in some hematological diseases. Am J Clin Pathol 83:222, 1985.

Roberts HR, Cederbaum AI. Molecular Variants of Factor IX. In KM Brinkhous, HC Heinker (eds), Handbook of Hemophilia. New York: American Elsevier, 1975. P 237.

Rodman NF, Barrow EM, et al. Diagnosis and control of the hemophiloid states with the partial thromboplastin test. Am J Clin Pathol 29:525, 1958.

Rogers BB, Wessels RA, et al. High-performance liquid chromatography in the diagnosis of hemoglobinopathies and thalassemias. Am J Clin Pathol 84:671, 1985.

Rogers CH. Blood sample preparation for automated differential systems. Am J Med Tech 39:435, 1973.

Rosse WF. Variation in the red cells in paroxysmal nocturnal haemoglobinuria. Br J Haematol 24:327, 1973.

Rosse WF. Paroxysmal nocturnal hemoglobinuria—present status and future prospects. West J Med 132:219, 1980.

Roth GJ, Stanford N, et al. Acetylation of prostaglandin synthetase by aspirin. Proc Natl Acad Sci U S A 72:3073, 1975.

Rothchild BM. The role of antithrombin III in clinical management of pulmonary embolization. Am J Med 74:529, 1983.

Rotoli S, Luzzatto L. Paroxysmal nocturnal hemoglobinuria. Semin Hematol 26:201, 1989.

Rowley JD. A new consistent chromosomal abnormality in chronic myelogenous leukaemia identified by quinacrine fluorescence and Giemsa staining. Nature 243:290, 1973.

Rubin H. Antibody elution from red cells. J Clin Pathol 16:70, 1963.

Ruebush TK II, Juranek DD, et al. Human babesiosis on Nantucket Island: clinical features. Ann Intern Med 86:6, 1977.

Ruggeri ZM, Nilsson IM, et al. Aberrant structure of von Willebrand factor in a new variant of von Willebrand's disease (Type IIC). J Clin Invest 70:1124, 1982.

Rümke CL. Variability of results in differential counts on blood smears. Triangle 4:156, 1960.

Saad STO, Braga GS, et al. Decreased C-peptide secretion in sickle cell anemia. Acta Haematol 82:81, 1989.

Sacker LS. Specimen Collection. In SM Lewis, JF Coter (eds), Quality Control in Haematology. London: Academic, 1975. P 211.

Sadoff L, Goldsmith O. False positive infectious mononucleosis spot test in pancreatic carcinoma. JAMA 218:1297, 1971.

Saito H, Ratnoff OD. Alterations of factor VII activity by activated Fletcher factor (a plasma kallikrein): a potential link between the intrinsic and extrinsic blood-clotting systems. J Lab Clin Med 85:405, 1975.

Sala N, Borell M, et al. Dysfunctional activated protein C (PC Cadiz) in a patient with thrombotic disease. Thromb Haemost 57:183, 1987.

Salmassi S, Mitsuo M, et al. Detection of platelet antibody using Rosette Technique with anti-IgG antibody-coated polyacrylamide gel. Vox Sang 39:264, 1980.

Salzman EW, MacIntyre DE, et al. Enhancement of platelet activity by inhibition of adenylate cyclase. Thromb Haemost 38:6, 1977.

Sarji KE, Stratton RD, et al. Nature of von Willebrand factor: a new assay and a specific inhibitor. Proc Natl Acad Sci U S A 72:2937, 1974.

Savage RA. Red cell stroma confuses laser counters. Summing Up 12:1, 1982.

Savage RA. Yet more on MCVs. Summing Up 14:9, 1984.

Savage RA, Lucas FV, et al. Spurious thrombocytosis caused by red blood cell fragmentation. Am J Clin Pathol 1:144, 1983.

Sbarra AJ, Selvaraj RJ, et al. Granulocytic, Biochemistry, and Hydrogen Peroxide Dependent Microbicidal System. In TJ Greenwalt, GA Jamieson (eds), Progress in Clinical and Biological Research: Vol 13. The Granulocyte: Function and Clinical Utilization. New York: Liss, 1977. P 29.

Schilling RF. Intrinsic factor studies in the effect of gastric juice on the urinary excretion of radioactivity after the oral administration of radioactive vitamin B_{12}. J Lab Clin Med 42:860, 1953.

Schjetlein R, Wisloff F. An evaluation of the commercial test procedure for the detection of lupus anticoagulant. Am J Clin Pathol 103:108, 1995.

Schleider MA. A clinical study of the lupus anticoagulant. Blood 48;488, 1976.

Schmelzer CH, Ebert RF, et al. Fibrinogen Baltimore IV: Congenital dysfibrinogenemia with a δ_{275} (Arg→Cys) substitution. Thromb Res 56:307, 1989.

Schmidt RM, Brosious EM. Basic Laboratory Methods of Hemoglobinopathy Detection (pub no. 77-8266). Atlanta: US Department of Health, Education and Welfare, 1976.

Schmitz H, Scherer M. IgM antibodies to Epstein-Barr virus in infectious mononucleosis. Arch Gesamte Virusforsch 37:332, 1972.

Schneider RG. Differentiation of electrophoretically binular hemoglobins as S, D, G, and P; or A_2, C, E, and O, by electrophoresis of the globin chains. Clin Chem 20:111, 1974.

Schneider RG, Hightower BJ, et al. Laboratory identification of the hemoglobinopathies. Lab Management 8:29, 1982.

Schneider RG, Janik B, et al. Proposed Guidelines for Citrate Agar Electrophoresis for Confirming Identification of Mutant Hemoglobins. Vol 1, no. 15. Villanova, PA: National Committee for Clinical Laboratory Standards, 1981.

Schneider RG, Veda S. Hemoglobin D Los Angeles in two Caucasian families: hemoglobin SD disease and hemoglobin D thalassemia. Blood 32:250, 1968.

Schorr JB, Menaché D. Clinical use of antithrombin III concentrate. Thromb News 9:7, 1983.

Schwab MLL, Lewis AE. An improved stain for Heinz bodies. Am J Clin Pathol 51:673, 1969.

Schwartz HP, Fisher M, et al. Plasma protein S deficiency in familial thrombotic disease. Blood 64:1297, 1984.

Schwartz IR. Sickling of erythrocytes with I-A electrophoretic hemoglobin pattern. Fed Proc 16:115, 1957.

Schweiger DJ. Red cell distribution width in sickle cell anemia. Am J Med Tech 47:231, 1981.

Scott BD, Esmon CT, et al. The natural anticoagulant protein S is decreased in male smokers Am Heart J 122:76, 1991.

Sears D, Charache S, et al. Electronic blood cell counters. Arch Pathol Lab Med 109:247, 1985.

Seeler RA, Metzger W, et al. *Diplococci pneumoniae* infections in children with sickle cell anemia. Am J Dis Child 213:8, 1972.

Seip M. Reticulocyte studies: the liberation of red blood corpuscles from the bone marrow into the peripheral blood and the production of erythrocytes elucidated by reticulocyte investigations. Acta Med Scand (suppl):282, 1953.

Seligsohn U, Berger A, et al. Homozygous protein C deficiency manifested by massive venous thrombosis in the newborn. N Engl J Med 310:559, 1984.

Seligsohn U, Kasper CK. Activation of human factor VII in plasma and in purified systems. J Clin Invest 64:1056, 1979.

Selwyn J, Dacie JV. Autohemolysis and other changes resulting from the incubation in vitro of red cells from patients with congenital hemolytic anemia. Blood 9:414, 1954.

Seshadri RS, Brown EJ, et al. Leukemic reticuloendotheliosis: a failure of monocyte production. N Engl J Med 295:181, 1976.

Shapiro SS. Characterization of factor VIII antibodies. Ann N Y Acad Sci 240:350, 1975.

Shapiro SS, Anderson DB. Thrombin Inhibition in Normal Plasma. In RL Lundblad, JW Fenton, et al. (eds), Chemistry and the Biology of Thrombin. Michigan: Ann Arbor Science, 1977. P 361.

Sheehan HL, Storey GW. Improved method of staining leucocyte granules with Sudan black B. J Pathol Bacteriol 59:336, 1947.

Sherman LA, Gaston LW, et al. Fibrinogen "St Louis": a new inherited fibrinogen variant coincidentally associated with hemophilia A. J Clin Invest 51:590, 1972.

Shevach E, Edelson R, et al. A human leukemia cell with both B and T cell surface receptors. Proc Natl Acad Sci U S A 71:863, 1974.

Shillitoe AJ. The common causes of lymphopenia. J Clin Pathol 3:21, 1950.

Shousha S, Kamel K. Nitroblue tetrazolium test in children with kwashiorkor with a comment on the use of latex particles in the test. J Clin Pathol 25:494, 1972.

Shreiner DR, Bell WR. Pseudothrombocytopenia: manifestations of a new type of platelet agglutinin. Blood 42:541, 1973.

Shulman IR, Branch DR, et al. Autoimmune hemolytic anemia with both cold and warm autoantibodies. JAMA 253:1746, 1985.

Sibley C. Procedures Used in the Thrombosis and Hemostasis Laboratory. In RM Schmidt (ed), Hematology Procedure Manual. Vol 3. Atlanta: US Department of Health, Education and Welfare, 1977. P 47.

Silverman EM, Reed RE. The nitroblue tetrazolium test in lymphoma. Am J Clin Pathol 60:198, 1973.

Simmons A. Technical Hematology (3rd ed). Philadelphia: Lippincott, 1980.

Simmons A. Blood storage. Am J Clin Pathol 77:116, 1982.

Simmons A, Chin T. Data base of National Health Laboratories, Inc. Plainview, NY: National Health Laboratories, 1987.

Simmons A, Paulo M. Prothrombin time stability using buffered sodium citrate. Lab Medica Int 10:6, 1993.

Simmons A, Wiseman JD, et al. The stability of hematological parameters when tested by the Coulter Model S. Presented at the International Society of Haematology Meeting, Paris. FPS 371:056, 1978.

Singer K, Chernoff AI, et al. Studies on the abnormal hemoglobins: their demonstration in sickle cell anemia and other hematologic disorders by means of alkali denaturation. Blood 6:413, 1951.

Skendzel LP, Hoffman GC. The Pelger anomaly of leucocytes: forty-one cases in seven families. Am J Clin Pathol 37:294, 1962.

Smith JR, Landow SA. Smoker's polycythemia. N Engl J Med 298:6, 1978.

Smith PS, Baglini R, et al. The prolonged bleeding time in hemophilia A: comparison of two measuring technics and clinical associations. Am J Clin Pathol 83:211, 1984.

Smith RP, Olson MV. Drug-induced methemoglobinemia. Semin Hematol 10:253, 1973.

Smith S, Arkin C. Cryofibrinogenemia. Am J Clin Pathol 58:524, 1972.

Smithies O. Zone electrophoresis in starch gels: group variations in the serum proteins of normal human adults. Biochem J 61:629, 1955.

Smyth JF, Poplack DG, et al. Correlation of adenosine deaminase activity with cell surface markers in acute lymphoblastic leukemia. J Clin Invest 62:710, 1978.

Soffer D, Yamanaka T, et al. Central nervous system involvement in adult onset Gaucher's disease. Acta Neuropathol 49:1, 1980.

Sokol RJ, Hewitt S, et al. Autoimmune haemolysis: mixed warm and cold antibody type. Acta Haematol 69:266, 1983.

Sokol RJ, Hewitt S, et al. Erythrocyte autoantibodies, autoimmune haemolysis and myelodysplastic syndromes. J Clin Pathol 42:1088, 1989.

Solani FG, Cunningham MT, et al. Plasma hemoglobin determination by recording derivative spectrophotometry. Am J Clin Pathol 85:342, 1986.

Solanki DL, Blackburn BC. Spurious red cell parameters due to serum cold agglutinins: observations on Ortho ELT-8 cell counter. Am J Clin Pathol 83:218, 1985.

Solum NO, Hagen I, et al. Platelet membrane glycoproteins and the interaction between bovine factor VIII related protein and human platelets. Thromb Haemost 38:914, 1977.

Sondergaard-Petersen H. The Di Guglielmo syndrome: a study of 17 cases: I. Clinical and hematological manifestations. Acta Med Scand 198:165, 1975.

Soslan G, Brodsky I. Hereditary sideroblastic anemia with associated platelet abnormalities. Am J Hematol 32:298, 1989.

Soulier JP, Gozin D. Assay of Fletcher factor (plasma prekallikrein) using artificial clotting reagent and a modified chromogenic assay. Thromb Haemost 42:538, 1979.

Spath P, Garratty G, et al. Studies on the immune response to penicillin and cephalothin in humans. I. Optimal conditions for titrating of hemagglutinating penicillin and cephalothin antibodies. J Immunol 107:854, 1971.

Spielman A. Human babesiosis on Nantucket Island, USA: description of the vector Ixodes (Ixodes) dammini nsp (Acarina: Ixodidae). J Med Entomol 15:218, 1979.

Spier CM, Kjeldsberg CR, et al. Chronic lymphocytic leukemia in young adults. Am J Clin Pathol 84:675, 1985.

Stass SA, Schumacher HR, et al. Terminal deoxynucleotidyl transferase immunofluorescence of bone marrow smears. Am J Clin Pathol 72:898, 1979.

Statland BE, Winkel P, et al. Evaluation of biologic sources of variation of leucocyte counts and other hematologic quantities using very precise automated analyzers. Am J Clin Pathol 69:48, 1978.

Stecher VS. Synthesis of Proteins by Mononuclear Phagocytes. In R von Furth (ed), Mononuclear Phagocytosis. Philadelphia: Davis, 1970. P 133.

Stenflo J. Structural Comparison of Normal and Dicoumarol-Induced Prothrombin. In HC Hemker, JJ Veltkamp (eds), Prothrombin and Related Coagulation Factors. London: Leiden University Press, 1975. P 12.

Stenflo J. Structure and function of protein C. Semin Thromb Hemost 10:109, 1984.

Stockbower JM. Blood Collection Problems: Factors in Specimen Collection That Contribute to Laboratory Error. In Therapeutic Drug Monitoring: Continuing Education Program. Washington: American Association of Clinical Chemistry, 1982.

Storrie B, Goldstein G, et al. Differentiation of thymocytes: evidence that induction of the surface phenotype requires transcription and translocation. J Immunol 116:1358, 1976.

Strauss HS. Acquired circulating anticoagulants in hemophilia. N Engl J Med 281:866, 1969.

Stürzebacher J, Sveridsen L, et al. A new assay for the determination of factor XII in plasma using a chromogenic substrate and a selective inhibitor of plasma kallikrein. Thromb Res 55:709, 1989.

Stutman LJ, Shinowara GY, et al. Coagulation factors in human lymph and plasma. Am J Med Sci 250:292, 1965.

Sullivan LW, Luhby AL, et al. Studies in the daily requirements for folic acid in infants and the etiology of folate deficiency in goat's milk with megaloblastic anemia. Am J Clin Nutr 18:311, 1966.

Sunderman FW. Effect of drugs upon hematological tests. Annu Clin Lab Sci 2:2, 1972.

Sweeney JD, Hoernig LA, et al. Whole blood aggregometry: influence of sample collection and delay in study performance on test results. Am J Clin Pathol 92:676, 1989.

Sweeney JD, Labuzetta JW, et al. Platelet function and ABO group. Am J Clin Pathol 91:79, 1989.

Sweet RD. An acute febrile neutrophilic dermatosis. Br J Haematol 76:349, 1964.

Syren DD, Raeste AM. Identification of blood monocytes by demonstration of lysozyme and peroxidase activity. Acta Haematol 45:29, 1971.

Szymanski IO, Araszkiewicz P, et al. Decreased amount of the Rh antigen D in hereditary spherocytosis (HS). Br J Haematol 73:537, 1989.

Taft EG. Pseudoleukocytosis due to cryoprotein crystals. Am J Clin Pathol 60:669, 1973.

Takada M. The establishment of cultured cell lines from the patients with Izumi fever and infectious mononucleosis–like disease. J Exp Med 43:209, 1973.

Takahashi H, Nagayama R, et al. Botrocetin and Polybrene-induced platelet aggregation in platelet-type von Willebrand disease. Am J Hematol 18:179, 1985.

Talstad I, Haugen HF. The relationship between the erythrocyte sedimentation rate (ESR) and plasma proteins in clinical materials and models. Scand J Clin Lab Invest 39:519, 1979.

Tamura J, Kurabayashi H, et al. Clinical features of common acute lymphoblastic leukemia antigen (CALLA) positive myeloma: report of four cases. Blut 58:229, 1989.

Tan EM. Antinuclear antibodies in diagnosis and management. Hosp Pract 18:79, 1983.

Telon MJ, Rao N. Recent advances in immunohematology: current opinion in hematology. Curr Sci 1(2):143, 1994.

Territo MC, Cline MJ. Mononuclear phagocyte proliferation, maturation, and function. Clin Haematol 4:685, 1975.

Testa JR, Golomb HM, et al. Hypergranular promyelocytic leukemia (APL): cytogenic and ultrastructure specificity. Blood 52:272, 1978.

Thangaveln M, Le Beau MM. Chromosomal abnormalities in Hodgkin's disease. Hematol Oncol Clin North Am 3:221, 1989.

Thomas WJ, Koenig HM, et al. Free erythrocyte protoporphyrin: hemoglobin ratios, serum ferritin, and transferrin saturation levels during treatment of infants with iron deficiency anemia. Blood 49:455, 1977.

Thompson CB, Diaz DD, et al. The role of anticoagulation in the measurement of platelet volume. Am J Clin Pathol 80:327, 1985.

Tichelli A, Gratwohl A, et al. Evaluation of the Sysmex R-1000. Am J Clin Pathol 93:70, 1990.

Tombridge TL. Effect of posture on hematology results. Am J Clin Pathol 49:491, 1968.

Tonks DB. A quality control program for quantitative clinical chemistry estimation. Can J Med Tech 30:38, 1968.

Tosteson DC, Shea C. Potassium and sodium of red blood cells in sickle cell anemia. J Clin Invest 31:406, 1952.

Tranzer JP, Baumgartner HR. Filling gaps in the vascular endothelium with blood platelets. Nature 216:1126, 1967.

Triplett DA. Clinical studies of the use of a fluorogenic substrate assay method for the determination of plasminogen. Thromb Haemost 42:50, 1979.

Triplett DA. Anticoagulant therapy: monitoring technique. Lab Manag 1:20, 1982.

Triplett DA, Harms CS. Procedures for the Coagulation Laboratory. Chicago: American Society of Clinical Pathologists, 1981. P 31.

Triplett DA, Harms CS, et al. The effect of heparin on the activated partial thromboplastin time. Am J Clin Pathol 70:556, 1978.

Ts'ao CH, Lo R, et al. Critical importance of citrate-blood ratio in platelet aggregation studies. Am J Clin Pathol 85:43, 1976.

Tsuda I, Tatsumi N. Reticulocytes in human preserved blood as control material for automated reticulocyte counters. Am J Clin Pathol 93:109, 1990.

Turi DC, Peerschke EI. Sensitivity of three activated partial thromboplastin time reagents to coagulation factor deficiencies. Am J Clin Pathol 85:43, 1986.

Ungar B. Antibody to gastric intrinsic factor in blood donors of hospital patients. Aust Ann Med 17:107, 1968.

Utsinger PD, Yount WJ, et al. Hairy-cell leukemia, B-lymphocyte and phagocytic properties. Blood 49:19, 1977.

Vainchenker W, Guichard J, et al. Morphological abnormalities in cultured erythroid colonies (BFU-E) from the blood of two patients with HEMPAS. Br J Haematol 42:363, 1979.

Valentine WM. The molecular lesion of hereditary spherocytosis (HS): a continuing enigma. Blood 49:241, 1977.

Valentine WM, Tanaka KR, et al. A specific glucolytic enzyme defect (pyruvate kinase) in three subjects with congenital non-spherocytic hemolytic anemia. Trans Assoc Am Physicians 74:100, 1961.

Van Biervliet JP. Glucose phosphate isomerase deficiency in a Dutch family. Acta Paediatr Scand 64:868, 1975.

Van der Merwe T, Bernstein R, et al. Acute promyelocytic transformation of chronic myeloid leukaemia with an isochromosome 17q. Br J Haematol 64:751, 1986.

Van Mourik JA, Bouma BN, et al. Factor VIII, a series of homologous oligomers and complex of two proteins. Thromb Res 4:155, 1974.

Van Royen EA, Lohmans S, et al. The inactivation and cold promoted activation of factor VII. J Lab Clin Med 152:92, 1978.

Varriale P. A urinary cryoprotein in multiple myeloma. Am J Intern Med 57:819, 1962.

Vasse M, Borg JY, et al. Protein C: roven A new hereditary protein C abnormality with low anticoagulant but normal amidolytic activities. Thromb Res 56:387, 1989.

Veehoven WA, Vander-Schans GS, et al. Pseudothrombocytopenia due to agglutinins. Am J Clin Pathol 72:1005, 1979.

Vella E, Lehmann H. Haemoglobin D Punjab (D Los Angeles). J Med Genet 11:341, 1974.

Veltkamp JJ, Meilof J, et al. Another genetic variant of haemophilia B: haemophilia B Leyden. Scand J Haematol 7:82, 1970.

Verwilghen RL. Congenital Dyserythropoietic Anaemia Type II (HEMPAS). In Congenital Disorders of Erythropoiesis (Ciba Symposium). Amsterdam: Elsevier, 1976. P 151.

Vettoro L, Zanella A, et al. A new test for the laboratory diagnosis of spherocytosis. Acta Haematol 72:258, 1984.

Vives Corron JI, Pujades MA, et al. Pyrimidine 5'–nucleotidase and several other cell enzyme activities in β-thalassemia trait. Br J Haematol 56:483, 1984.

Vupio P, Härkönen M, et al. Red cell glucose-6-phosphate dehydrogenase deficiency in Finland. Ann Clin Res 5:168, 1973.

Wajcman H, Mrad A, et al. Hemoglobin Villejuif ($β_{123}(Ch_1)Thr$ 11e): a new variant found in coincidence with polycythemia vera. Am J Hematol 32:294, 1989.

Walach B, Heddle N, et al. Transient Donath Landsteiner hemolytic anemia. Br J Haematol 48:425, 1981.

Waldenstrom J. Pathological globulins and protein synthesis. Exp Med Surg 12:187, 1954.

Walenga J, Fareed J, et al. Automated instrumentation and the laboratory diagnosis of bleeding and thrombotic disorders. Semin Thromb Hemost 9:172, 1983.

Waller HD. Glutathione Reductase Deficiency. In E Beutler (ed), Hereditary Disorders of Erythrocyte Metabolism. Vol 1. New York: Grune & Stratton, 1968. P 185.

Walls WD, Losowsky MS. Congenital deficiency of fibrin stabilizing factor. Coagulation 1:11, 1968.

Walsh PN. Oral anticoagulant therapy. Hosp Pract 1:101, 1985.

Watkins SP Jr, Shulman NR. Platelet cold agglutinins. Blood 16:153, 1970.

Watson CJ, Schwartz S. A simple test for urinary porphobilinogen. Proc Soc Exp Biol Med 47:393, 1941.

Weatherall DJ, Clegg JB. The α-chain termination mutants and their relationship to α-thalassemia. Philos Trans R Soc London (Biol) 271:411, 1975.

Wehmeier A, Schneider W. Platelet volume parameters as a diagnostic tool: the influence of anticoagulation and storage conditions on platelet impedance volume. Klin Wochenschr 67:980, 1989.

Weiner W. Eluting red-cell antibodies: a method and its application. Br J Haematol 3:276, 1957.

Weinstein IM. A correlation study of the erythrokinetics and disturbances in iron metabolism associated with the anemia of rheumatoid arthritis. Blood 14:950, 1959.

Weiss AE. The Hemophilias. Miami: American Dade, Division American Hospital Supply, 1983.

Weiss HJ. Platelet physiology and abnormalities of platelet function. N Engl J Med 293:580, 1975.

Weiss HJ, Aledort LM. The effect of salicylates on the hemostatic properties of platelets in man. J Clin Invest 47:2169, 1968.

Weiss HJ, Hawiger J, et al. Fibrinogen-independent platelet adhesion and thrombosis formation on subendothelium mediated by glycoprotein IIb/IIIa complex at high shear rate. J Clin Invest 83:288, 1989.

Weiss HJ, Sussman II. Synthesis of high-molecular-weight antihemophilic factor in von Willebrand's disease. Lancet 11:402, 1974.

Weiss HJ, Sussman II. A new von Willebrand variant (type I New York): increased ristocetin-induced platelet aggregation and plasma von Willebrand factor containing the full range of multimers. Blood 68:149, 1986.

Wermeier A, Scharf RE, et al. Bleeding and thrombosis in chronic myeloproliferative disorders: relation of platelet disorders to clinical aspects of the disease. Haemostasis 19:251, 1989.

Wessler S. A Guide to Anticoagulant Therapy (3rd ed). Dallas: American Heart Association, 1984.

Westergren A. Studies of the suspension stability of the blood in pulmonary tuberculosis. Acta Med Scand 54:247, 1920.

Westgard JO, Barry PL, et al. A multi-rule Shewhart chart for quality control in clinical chemistry. Clin Chem 27:493, 1981.

Wheby MS. Site of iron absorption in man. Scand J Haematol 7:5, 1970.

Whelton A, Donadio JV. Acute renal failure complicating rickettsial infection in glucose-6-phosphate dehydrogenase deficient individuals. Ann Intern Med 69:323, 1968.

White GC, Shoemaker CB. Factor VIII gene and hemophilia A. Blood 73:1, 1989.

White JG. Effects of ethylenediamine tetra acetic acid (EDTA) on platelet structure. Scand J Haematol 5:241, 1968.

White JG. Scanning electron microscopy of erythrocyte deformation: the influence of a common ionophore A 2387. Semin Hematol 13:121, 1976.

White JG, Krivit W. An ultrastructural basis of the shape changes induced in platelets by chilling. Blood 30:625, 1967.

Whittaker DL, Copeland DL, et al. Linkage of color blindness to hemophilias A and B. Am J Hum Genet 14:149, 1962.

Wiggins RC, Bounds W, et al. Rabbit blood coagulation factor XI: purification and properties. Thromb Res 15:475, 1979.

Wiley JS. Characteristics of the membrane defect in the hereditary stomatocytosis syndrome. Blood 46:337, 1975.

Williams DM, Lynch RE, et al. Drug induced aplastic anemia. Semin Hematol 10:195, 1973.

Winawer SJ, Streiff RR. Gastric and hematological abnormalities in a vegan with nutritional vitamin B_{12} deficiency. Gastroenterology 53:130, 1967.

Windebank KP, Tefferi A, et al. Acute megakaryocytic leukemia (M7) in children. Mayo Clin Proc 64:1339, 1989.

Winkelman JW, Morris MW, et al. Spuriously elevated band counts with an automated differential counter. J Lab Clin Automat 3:401 1983.

Winman B. Primary structure of the β-chain of human plasmin. Eur J Biochem 76:129, 1977.

Winslow RM (ed). Laboratory Methods for Detecting Hemoglobinopathies. Atlanta: Centers for Disease Control, 1984.

Wintrobe MM. The erythrocyte sedimentation test. Int Clin Ser 46:34, 1936.

Wintrobe MM. Clinical Hematology (8th ed). Philadelphia: Lea & Febiger, 1981.

Woodruff AW, Topley E, et al. The anemia of kala azar. Br J Haematol 22:319, 1972.

Woodward RH, Goldsmith PL. Cumulative Sum Techniques (ICI monograph no. 3). Edinburgh: Oliver and Boyd, 1964.

World Health Organization. Inherited Blood Clotting Disorders: Report of a WHO Scientific Group (WHO technical report series no. 504). Geneva: World Health Organization, 1972.

World Health Organization. Committee on Biological Standardization Thirty-Third Report (WHO technical report series no. 687). Geneva: World Health Organization, 1983. P 81.

Worlledge SM, Rousso C. Studies on the serology of paroxysmal cold haemoglobinuria (PCH), with special reference to its relationship with the P blood group system. Vox Sang 10:293, 1965.

Wright DJ, Jenkins DE Jr. Simplified method for estimation of serum and plasma viscosity in multiple myeloma and related disorders. Blood 36:516, 1970.

Wright J, Brosious EM. Quality Assurance in Hemoglobinopathy Testing. In RM Schmidt (ed), Hematology Procedure Manual. Atlanta: US Department of Health, Education and Welfare, 1977.

Wuepper KD, Miller DR, et al. Flaujeac trait deficiency of human plasma kininogen. J Clin Invest 56:1663, 1975.

Yam LT, Li CY, et al. Cytochemical identification of monocytes and granulocytes. Am J Clin Pathol 55:283, 1971.

Yamaguchi K, Schoefl GI. Blood vessels of the Peyer's patch in the mouse: III. High endothelium venules. Anat Rec 206:419, 1983.

Yunis JJ, Bloomfield CD, et al. All patients with acute non-lymphocytic leukaemia may have a chromosomal defect. N Engl J Med 305:135, 1981.

Zacharski LR, Kyle RA. Significance of extreme elevation of erythrocyte sedimentation rate. JAMA 202:264, 1967.

Zaizov R, Kirschmann C, et al. Alpha-globin chain synthesis in children with haemoglobin Bart's at birth. Rev Eur Etud Clin Biol 9:1457, 1973.

Zanella A, Barosi G, et al. Relative iron deficiency in hereditary spherocytosis. Am J Hematol 31:81, 1989.

Zanella A, Izzo C, et al. Acidified glycerol lysis test: a screening test for spherocytosis. Br J Haematol 45:481, 1980.

Zeineh RA, Fiorella BJ, et al. Core isoelectric focusing. Am J Med Tech 41:10, 1975.

Zimmerman TS, Ratnoff OD, et al. Immunologic differentiation of classic hemophilia (factor VIII deficiency) and von Willebrand's disease. J Clin Invest 50:244, 1971.

Zimmerman TS, Ruggeri ZM. Von Willebrand's Disease. In TH Spaet (ed), Progress in Hemostasis and Thrombosis. Vol 6. New York: Grune & Stratton, 1982. P 103.

Zimmerman TS, Ruggeri ZM. von Willebrand's disease. Clin Haematol 12:175, 1983.

Zinkham WH, Conley C. Some factors influencing the formation of LE cells. Bull Johns Hopkins Hosp 98:102, 1956.

Zucker MB. Tests of platelet adhesion aggregation and release. Thromb Diath Haemorrh 42:1, 1970.

Zucker MB. Effect of heparin on platelet function. Haemorrhage 33:63, 1975.

Zucker-Franklin D. Eosinophil function and disorders. Adv Intern Med 19:1, 1974.

Zucker-Franklin D, Petursson S. Thrombocytopoiesis: analyses by membrane tracer and freeze fracture studies on fresh human and cultured mouse megakaryocytes. J Cell Biol 99:390, 1984.

Index

WITHDRAWN
FROM STOCK
LIBRARY

WITHDRAWN
FROM STOCK
QMUL LIBRARY